Clinical Evaluation of Newborns, Infants and Children

Clinical Evaluation of Newborns, Infants and Children

Third Edition

Editor-in-Chief

S Sushamabai

MD (Pediatrics) DCH FIMSA FIAP
Former Professor and Head
Department of Pediatrics
Government Medical College
Kottayam
Former Professor and Head
Department of Pediatrics
Pushpagiri Medical College
Pushpagiri Institute of Medical Sciences and Research Centre
Thiruvalla, Kerala, India

Associate Editors

Lalitha Kailas

MD (Pediatrics) DCH
Former Professor and Head
Department of Pediatrics
Government Medical College
Thiruvananthapuram
Professor
Department of Pediatrics
Principal
Sree Gokulam Medical College
and Research Foundation
Thiruvananthapuram, Kerala, India

Darly Saramma Mammen

DCH DNB (Pediatrics)
Professor and Head
Department of Pediatrics
Government Medical College
Kottayam, Kerala, India

Suresh S Vadakedom

MD (Pediatrics) DCH DNB (Pediatrics) MPhil
(Behavioral Sciences)
Associate Professor
Department of Pediatrics
Government Medical College
Kottayam, Kerala, India

Foreword

Mohanan Kunnumal

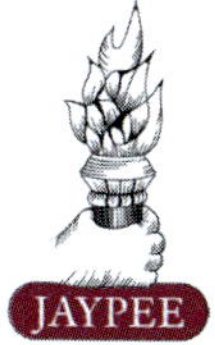

JAYPEE BROTHERS MEDICAL PUBLISHERS
The Health Sciences Publisher
New Delhi | London

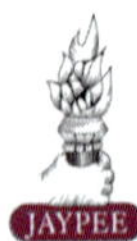

Jaypee Brothers Medical Publishers (P) Ltd

Headquarters
EMCA House
23/23-B, Ansari Road, Daryaganj
New Delhi 110 002, India
Landline: +91-11-23272143, +91-11-23272703
+91-11-23282021, +91-11-23245672
E-mail: jaypee@jaypeebrothers.com

Corporate Office
Jaypee Brothers Medical Publishers (P) Ltd.
4838/24, Ansari Road, Daryaganj
New Delhi 110 002, India
Phone: +91-11-43574357
Fax: +91-11-43574314
E-mail: jaypee@jaypeebrothers.com

Overseas Office
JP Medical Ltd.
83, Victoria Street, London
SW1H 0HW (UK)
Phone: +44-20 3170 8910
E-mail: info@jpmedpub.com

EU GPSR Authorised Representative
Logos Europe, 9 rue Nicolas Poussin
17000, La Rochelle, France
Phone: +33 (0) 6 67 93 73 78
E-mail: Contact@logoseurope.eu

Website: www.jaypeebrothers.com
Website: www.jaypeedigital.com

Inquiries for bulk sales may be solicited at: jaypee@jaypeebrothers.com

Clinical Evaluation of Newborns, Infants and Children

First Edition: 2002

Second Edition: 2009

Third Edition: **2025**

ISBN: 978-93-5696-736-6

Printed in India

Dedicated to

The medical fraternity who cares for children
and the students of Pediatrics everywhere
And
My loving husband, K Rajagopalan for the
constant support, love, and care given to me and
My son, Raj Anand for help and encouragement

Contributors

Darly Saramma Mammen DCH DNB (Pediatrics)
Professor and Head
Department of Pediatrics
Government Medical College
Kottayam, Kerala, India

Davidson Devasia
MD (Pediatrics) DM (Neurology) Fellowship in Pediatric Neurology and Epilepsy
Assistant Professor
Department of Pediatric Neurology
Amrita Institute of Medical Sciences and Research Center
Kochi, Kerala, India

Kalyani Pillai MD (Pediatrics) DCH
Professor
Department of Pediatrics
Amala Institute of Medical Sciences
Thrissur, Kerala, India

KP Vinayan
MD (Pediatrics) DNB (Pediatrics) DM (Neurology)
Professor and Head
Department of Pediatric Neurology
Amrita Institute of Medical Sciences and Research Center
Kochi, Kerala, India

KS Vijayakumar MD (Pediatrics) DCH
Former Professor
Department of Pediatrics
Government Medical College
Kozhikode
Professor and Head
Department of Pediatrics
Believers Church Medical College
Thiruvalla, Kerala, India

L Jayasree
DMRD DNB (Radiodiagnosis)
Professor
Department of Radiodiagnosis
Government Medical College
Thiruvananthapuram, Kerala, India

L Rajam
MD (Pediatrics) DCH
Former Professor
Department of Pediatrics
Government Medical College
Kottayam
Former Professor and Head
Department of Pediatrics
Amrita Institute of Medical Sciences and Research Center
Kochi, Kerala, India

Lalitha Kailas MD (Pediatrics) DCH
Former Professor and Head
Department of Pediatrics
Government Medical College
Thiruvananthapuram
Professor
Department of Pediatrics
Principal
Sree Gokulam Medical College and Research Foundation
Thiruvananthapuram, Kerala, India

M Geethadevi
MD (Community Medicine)
Additional Professor
Department of Community Medicine
Government Medical College
Kottayam, Kerala, India

M Veerendra Kumar
MD (Pediatrics) DCH
Additional Professor
Department of Pediatrics
Government Medical College
Kottayam, Kerala, India

M Vijayakumar
MD (Pediatrics) DCH DNB (Pediatrics)
FIAP FRCP PDCC
Professor and Head
Department of Pediatrics
Government Medical College
Manjeri, Kerala, India

M Zulfikar Ahamed
MD (Pediatrics) DCH DM (Cardiology)
Former Professor and Head
Department of Pediatric Cardiology
Government Medical College
Thiruvananthapuram
Clinical Professor
Department of Pediatric and Adolescent Cardiology
Child Development Center
Thiruvananthapuram
Chief
Department of Pediatric Cardiology
KIMS Hospital
Thiruvananthapuram, Kerala, India
Adjunct Professor
Department of Cardiology
Kasturba Medical College
Manipal, Karnataka, India

Manu Raj
DCH DNB (Pediatrics) MS HRM Clin Epi
Professor and Senior Consultant
Departments of Pediatrics and Health Sciences Research
Amrita Institute of Medical Sciences and Research Center
Kochi, Kerala, India

MD Fiji MD DCH
Assistant Professor
Department of Pediatrics
Government Medical College
Kozhikode, Kerala, India

P Savida
MD DCH MPhil (Behavioral Sciences and Rehabilitation)
Former Professor and Head
Department of Pediatrics
Government Medical College
Kottayam
Professor and Head
Department of Pediatrics
Mount Zion Medical College
Adoor, Kerala, India

R Bhanuvikraman Pillai
MD (Pediatrics) FAAP Board Certified in Pediatrics by American Board of Pediatrics Board Certified in Pediatric Gastroenterology by American Board of Pediatrics
Associate Professor and Head
Department of Pediatric Gastroenterology
Amrita Institute of Medical Sciences and Research Center
Kochi, Kerala, India

R Vishnu MSc Dip RP
Assistant Professor of Radiation Physics and Radiological Safety Officer
Department of Radiodiagnosis
Government Medical College
Thiruvananthapuram, Kerala, India

S Letha MD (Pediatrics) DCH
Former Professor and Head
Department of Pediatrics
Government Medical College, Kottayam
Professor
Department of Pediatrics
Pushpagiri Institute of Medical Sciences and Research Center
Thiruvalla, Kerala, India

S Radhika DNB (Pediatrics) DNB (Neonatology)
Associate Professor of Neonatology
Department of Pediatrics
Government Medical College
Thiruvananthapuram, Kerala, India

S Sushamabai MD (Pediatrics) DCH FIMSA FIAP
Former Professor and Head
Department of Pediatrics
Government Medical College
Kottayam
Former Professor and Head
Department of Pediatrics
Pushpagiri Medical College
Pushpagiri Institute of Medical Sciences and Research Centre
Thiruvalla, Kerala, India

Sheeja Sugunan DCH DNB (Pediatrics) FPIC
Associate Professor
Department of Pediatrics
Government Medical College
Thiruvananthapuram, Kerala, India

Suma Balan
MD (Pediatrics) MRCP (Pediatrics) CCST in Pediatrics and Pediatric Rheumatology
Professor and Head
Department of Rheumatology
Amrita Institute of Medical Sciences and Research Center
Kochi, Kerala, India

Suresh S Vadakedom
MD (Pediatrics) DCH DNB (Pediatrics) MPhil (Behavioral Sciences)
Associate Professor
Department of Pediatrics
Government Medical College
Kottayam, Kerala, India

Vaishakh Anand MD DM
Assistant Professor
Department of Pediatric Neurology
Amrita Institute of Medical Sciences and Research Center
Kochi, Kerala, India

VH Sankar
MD (Pediatrics) MNAMS (Pediatrics) DM (Medical Genetics)
Associate Professor
Department of Pediatrics
Consultant Geneticist, Genetic Clinic
Government Medical College
Thiruvananthapuram, Kerala, India

VK Parvathy
MD (Pediatrics) DCH
Former Professor and Head
Department of Pediatrics
Government Medical College, Thrissur
Former Professor and Head
Department of Pediatrics
Amala Institute of Medical Sciences
Thrissur, Kerala, India

VT Ajith Kumar
MD (Pediatrics) DCH DNB (Pediatrics)
Professor and Head
Department of Pediatrics
Government Medical College
Kozhikode, Kerala, India

Foreword

It is with great enthusiasm that I present the foreword for the latest edition of "Clinical Evaluation of Newborns, Infants and Children" authored by Professor S Sushamabai. As the Vice Chancellor of the Kerala University of Health Sciences, Thrissur, Kerala, India, I have had the privilege of observing the evolution of medical education in our state, particularly in the field of Pediatrics. Medical education in India has a rich history, having begun in 1835 with a curriculum heavily influenced by Western textbooks. However, it was not until the latter half of the 20th century that Indian authors began to contribute significantly to this body of knowledge. Despite this progress, the development of pediatric literature in Kerala has been relatively slow, highlighting the need for a comprehensive and locally relevant resource. Professor S Sushamabai's work stands off as a beacon of excellence in this context.

This edition of "Clinical Evaluation of Newborns, Infants and Children" is a meticulously revised manuscript that not only reflects the advancements in clinical assessment over the years but also addresses the unique challenges faced by medical students and practitioners in pediatrics. The book is structured to facilitate a deep understanding of clinical signs, with each chapter presenting clear explanations and illustrative clinical photographs that enhance the learning experience. The inclusion of practical case scenarios allows students to apply theoretical knowledge to real-world situations, fostering a more comprehensive grasp of pediatric assessments. Moreover, I am particularly impressed by the collaborative effort involved in this edition. Each chapter has been enriched by contributions from specialists in pediatrics, ensuring that the content is both authoritative and relevant. This collaborative approach not only elevates the quality of the material but also reflects the collective expertise of our esteemed faculty across various medical colleges in Kerala.

A noteworthy feature of this edition is the emphasis on research and references that are pertinent to Indian children. By incorporating studies and guidelines from Indian experts, such as the WHO-IAP growth charts, this book provides a contextually appropriate foundation for understanding pediatric growth and development. The attractive design of the book, complemented by high-quality clinical photographs, makes it an invaluable resource for students and practitioners alike. It serves as a handy reference for bedside evaluations, empowering medical students to approach pediatric patients with confidence and competence.

Professor S Sushamabai is a distinguished figure in the field of pediatrics, with extensive academic and clinical experience. Her dedication to advancing pediatric education is evident in this work, which will undoubtedly serve as an essential tool for both undergraduate and postgraduate students. I am proud to endorse "Clinical Evaluation of Newborns, Infants and Children" as a vital resource for mastering the complexities of pediatric clinical assessment. I am confident that this book will significantly contribute to the education of future pediatricians and enhance the quality of care provided to our youngest patients.

Sincerely,

Mohanan Kunnumal MD (Radiodiagnosis)
Vice Chancellor
Kerala University of Health Sciences
Thrissur, Kerala, India
Member
National Medical Commission

Preface to the Third Edition

The second edition of "Clinical Evaluation of Newborns, Infants and Children", released in 2009, was accepted widely by the undergraduates (MBBS) and postgraduates in Pediatrics and was promoted by the faculties from all medical colleges. In the same year, the Director of Medical Education (DME) of Kerala recommended it as the textbook for Clinical Pediatric study for MBBS students.

Though clinical signs remain constant, periodic updating is needed in clinical evaluation since the reference data, health indices, and disease patterns differ due to the changing socio-economic status, calamities appearing worldwide, lifestyle changes, and the cultural pattern of people. The drastic effects of the COVID-19 pandemic were reflected in the nutritional status of children with the double burden of undernutrition and obesity all over the world. Newer clinical signs and classifications came to be observed subsequent to the emergence of new infections and the reemergence of old ones with changing manifestations as well by other diseases.

Substantial effort has been made in this third edition by the learned contributors for maximum updating. In addition to the experienced senior faculty, for each system, experts specialized in that subject have also been included so that each chapter could be thoroughly revised. Clinical case scenarios are included in most chapters to substantiate the descriptions. Six more chapters are added for the assessment of the acutely ill children, for introduction to medical research, and for the basics in pediatric imaging.

Self-explanatory good clinical photographs by the chapter contributors, faculties, and residents from different medical colleges are presented in relevant areas for helping the students get a realistic impression of the diseases.

Suggestions received from many senior colleagues to improve this edition are also observed.

I was lucky again to get the helping hands of M/s Jaypee Brothers Medical Publishers (P) Ltd, New Delhi, India, the leading medical book publisher in India, to accept this third edition of "Clinical Evaluation of Newborns, Infants and Children" for publication.

I sincerely wish that this third edition will be a boon in clinical assessment for students in pediatrics.

S Sushamabai

Preface to the First Edition

Clinical evaluation of children includes history taking, physical examination and interpretation, which are the most important aspects of patient assessment ensuring quality care in medical practice. Compared to adults, mastering of clinical skills in pediatrics requires more patience, tactics, astute observation and interpretation. With the advent of innumerable diagnostic tests and expansion of various specialties in medicine there is deterioration in acquisition of clinical skills and this has ultimately resulted in loss of humane touch in patient care. Unlike the diagnostic investigations which are costly, painful and require constant updating by the doctor, clinical evaluation remains unchanging and provides confidence and self-reliance irrespective of the patient and situation wherever one works. Once mastered, clinical skills remain with the doctor forever and are not subject to errors and costly equipment are not needed.

The young medical graduates from developing countries are to work under various constraints. On one side there is the huge burden of patients with diverse spectrum of illnesses and on the other side there is scarcity of paramedical personnel for assistance, investigation facilities and essential drugs. With limited time and resources available, the diagnosis is to be made quickly, treatment has to be decided and implemented promptly and psychologic support to the family has to be extended. The physician well versed in clinical skills only will be able to rise up to this challenging situation to meet all these demands.

Children under fifteen years of age contribute to 45% of the total population in developing countries. Textbooks on clinical methods focusing the adults are many but regarding children they are scanty. Pediatric textbooks reveal elaborate description of diseases but astonishingly lack diagnostic clinical methods specially designed for children, so that the student in pediatrics has to proceed in the same tempo of adult clinical evaluation. After having acquired thirty-two years of teaching experience, to me it appears that there is a felt need for textbooks on clinical evaluation in children.

Perfection in clinical skills is to be achieved by the relentless process of constant practice, revision and improvement. One has to be aware of this continuous process of teaching and learning and hence this textbook is intended to benefit students of all ages and stages of experience who wish to practise pediatrics.

S Sushamabai

Acknowledgments

While bringing out this third edition of "Clinical Evaluation of Newborns, Infants and Children", once again I recollect the spirit of clinical assessment in patient evaluation and empathy to the sick children and their parents, obtained from my senior, Professor Dr Shanta Kurup (Late), during the period I worked as her assistant (12 years) at the beginning of my career, immediately after my postgraduation.

In bringing out this third edition, I gratefully acknowledge the timely hard work extended by all the contributors, accepting the challenges to upgrade it with maximum perfectionism. Without their dedicated and sincere effort, this mission would not have been fulfilled in time.

Further, I greatly acknowledge the excellent performance by the Associate Editors, Drs Lalitha Kailas, Darly Saramma Mammen, and Suresh S Vadakedom for their prompt editing, providing the latest growth charts, relevant clinical photographs, and all the references required for this manuscript.

My acknowledgments also go to Mr Sreeraj of Alumni Association, Government Medical College, Kottayam, Kerala, India for his expert and untiring computer work and to Mr Lekshmanan, the librarian, Government Medical College, Kottayam, Kerala, for helping me in getting the literature required for this edition and Ms Mini G Pillai, University Librarian, MG University, Kottayam, Kerala for helping me to prepare tables and data collection.

I appreciate the interest and cooperation of faculties and postgraduates of the department of Pediatrics, Government Medical College, Kottayam, Kerala for the contribution of relevant clinical photographs for the manuscript.

I am deeply indebted to the vast number of sick children I had cared for in my profession and to their parents for getting my knowledge expanded in patient examination and expertise in clinical diagnosis.

I thank God Almighty for showering blessings on me all these years from 2002 onward, from the time of release of the first edition of this book on Clinical Evaluation which was widely accepted by the undergraduates in MBBS and postgraduates in Pediatrics.

This is the third edition of my first book getting published by M/s Jaypee Brothers Medical Publishers (P) Ltd, New Delhi, India. I am extremely grateful to Shri Jitendar P Vij (Group Chairman), and Mr Ankit Vij (Managing Director) of M/s Jaypee Brothers Medical Publishers (P) Ltd, New Delhi, India for accepting the manuscript again for publication. I immensely appreciate the honest and dedicated work of Mr Naman Singh (Development Editor) of M/s Jaypee Brothers with much enthusiasm in printing the proof of the manuscript in time, clarifying the doubts as and when required.

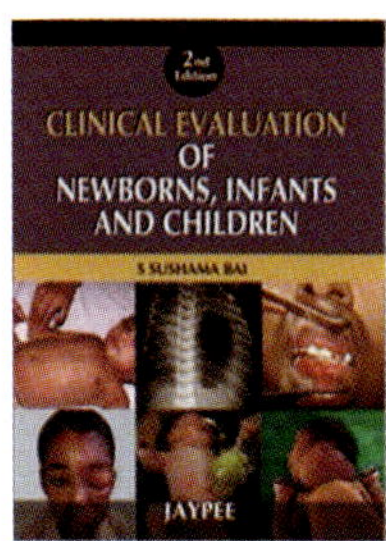

Clinical Evaluation of Newborns, Infants and Children

S Sushamabai
New Delhi: Jaypee Brothers Medical Publishers 2009
Pages 211, Price. Rs. 495.00

The strength of the book is that it asks its readers to acquire the communication skills. Elicitation of the history, which is the most important part of the patient workup, had been dealt with in good measures. It would have completed the description if prior treatment history had also been included. Dietary history lacks importance of breastfeeding and the nutritive value of breast milk has not been highlighted in the description of complementary feeding.

The description of the general physical examination and growth and development of the child have been written with a good blend of years of experience and a simple illustrative approach. The limitation is that only CDC-2000 growth tables and charts have been used. It would have been better to include WHO growth charts as well.

The examination of the newborn baby seems sufficient for an undergraduate medical and nursing student to differentiate a sick neonate. The systemic examination part is adequately written, and students will find it easy to elicit many signs and to describe abnormalities. The author has worked hard to reproduce better-quality clinical photographs liberally to help students learn the clinical situation which they may not have a chance to see as a clinical case during ward posting. Pedigree charting, reading of ECG, and skiagrams of chest are good additions. Overall, the book gives a pleasant reading and can be recommended to the undergraduate students.

MMA Faridi
Professor and Head
Department of Pediatrics
University College of Medical Sciences
New Delhi, India

Contents

SECTION

History and General Examination

1

CHAPTER

The Doctor

S Sushamabai

> Sruthe paryavadathathwam bahushodrusta Karamatha/
> Dakshyam souchamithanjeeyam vaidyaguna chathushtayam//

Nobody other than Charaka has stated the attributes of the doctor (*vaidya*) so clearly. The essential four qualities are (1) in-depth knowledge of the subject, (2) wide experience acquired from observing treatment, (3) capacity to implement and revise treatment, and (4) cleanliness of body and purity of mind.

Knowledge in medical science should be gained from constant learning, teaching, and dedicated patient care. Experience in patient care should, apart from one's own, be widely gained from observing treatment by seniors and colleagues. The capacity to implement treatment and the mentality to revise at the right time should be present. The mind should be pure and never should harm the sick, even in thought. The body should be kept clean always.

The doctor should be a good human being first and should have good listening habits so that the parent, as well as the child, should feel the receptiveness to communicate with freedom; should be gentle, kind, alert, attentive, and reveal concern for patients and parents; approach should be pleasant and attire should be modest **(Fig. 1.1)**. Such attributes add to the confidence of the patient and parent on the doctor.

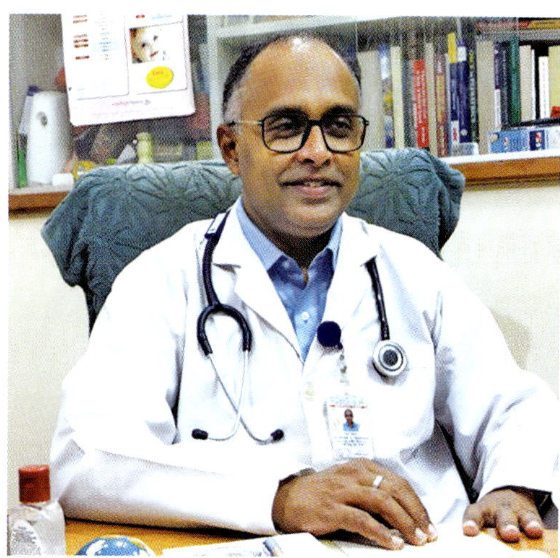

Fig. 1.1: The doctor with a pleasant face and relaxed appearance.

To have a good rapport with the child and family it is good to utilize verbal and nonverbal cues. Verbal cues are greeting the family pleasantly, calling the child by name, relaxing the situation with friendly talks not related to the illness, and praising the child for his nice shirt and squeaky shoes, attractive hairdo, or nice bangles and anklets. Nonverbal cues include pleasant smiles and a relaxed appearance as if you are ready to spend enough time with the kid.

Adequate and updated examination tools should be available with the doctor in the outpatient department, emergency area, and in all wards. Always observe hand sterilization (initially with soap and water hand wash and subsequently with alcohol-based solution) before and after examining each patient. Ours is a serving profession with the mission of relieving anxiety for which our appearance and behavior count a lot. A white overcoat has an association with cleanliness and purity, and it imparts a sense of professional authority and responsibility to the doctor and obtaining respect from parents. On the other hand, dressing in nonprofessional attire is in a way fooling the child as well as making the parents dubious. In addition, professional status also must be revealed by using the name tag.

SUGGESTED READING

1. The attributes of a pediatrician. In: Singh M (Ed). Pediatrics Clinical Methods, 1 edition. Ved Mansion, New Delhi: Sagar Publications; 2009.

The Family Interview

CHAPTER

S Sushamabai

Read Chapter 1 before you proceed

The family interview in the first instance should create confidence in the doctor from the patient and parents and is a prerequisite for history taking since the treatment begins the moment the family enters the consulting room. Being preoccupied with work, doctors never realize that the child and the parents, and the accompanying relatives are closely assessing them before the interview begins. By word and deed, the doctors should behave in such a way that every bit of patients' time is treated as valuable as our own.

Remember

The child and the parents have started assessing you well before you assess the child.

The crucial factors of success in the family interview are the doctor and the consultation room. The doctor should greet the child and parents in a pleasant and friendly manner and offer them seats. This simple act of offering seats conveys the message that the doctor is ready to spend sufficient time to evaluate the child even if the interview is brief **(Figs. 2.1A and B)**. The child should be addressed by name as far as possible. Never use the term "it" when referring to a child at any age and state the gender wrong. Important points are to be written as and when needed, maintaining eye contact in between with parents and at the same time observing the child. During subsequent visits as an outpatient or as an inpatient, before going through the charts, the doctor should greet the child by name and enquire about the progress of the illness.

Key points

Never stand and convey important messages; never keep aloof, sustain eye contact; observe the child in between.

In the overcrowded outpatient departments of less privileged hospitals in developing and underdeveloped countries,

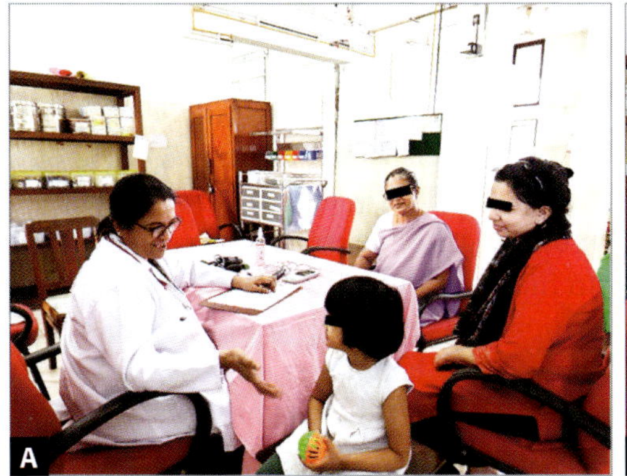

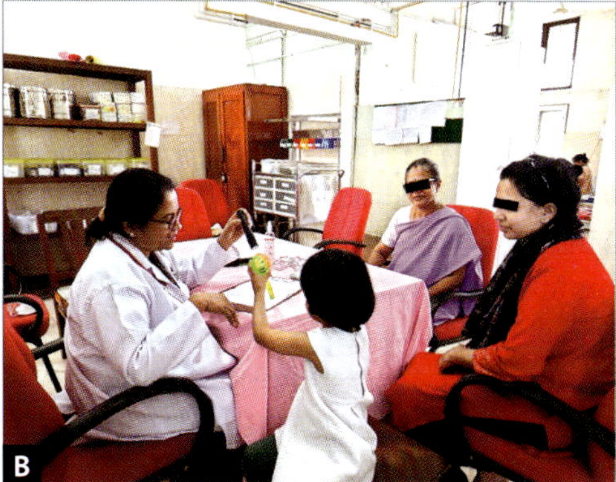

Figs. 2.1A and B: Family interview-creating confidence.

an ideal outpatient setting is difficult, but maximum comfort and privacy should be provided to the patient. These can be achieved if the doctor is committed and knows the significance of such principles in patient care. The room should be well-lit and ventilated, unfamiliar instruments (which may produce apprehension for the child) should be kept out of sight of the child. The room walls should be made attractive with a few pictures of familiar animals and birds, flowers, and natural scenery. They should at the same time provide information to the parents regarding ideal child-rearing practices on nutrition, illnesses, and immunization.

Key points

The room for the family interview should be well-lighted and ventilated. Unfamiliar instruments should be kept out of sight of the child. The wall pictures should provide information on child rearing practices.

In many parts of the world, it is common to see relatives and friends accompanying a child, especially if sick and getting involved in the interview. The interview should be restricted to the child and the parents and history should be elicited from the mother mainly. Regardless of the education and occupation of the parents, mothers (especially) of younger children yield an accurate history. Father should be allowed to express his views. The accompanying persons should be politely requested to wait outside the room. If the mother is not available, the caretaker should be considered as the responsible person. In case, the mother employed elsewhere is accompanying the child along with the caretaker, after eliciting history from the caretaker, the mother should be given a chance to express her own additional points. Age-appropriate play materials such as toys, puzzles handy picture books (of familiar animals, birds, fruits, vegetables, flowers, etc.) and coloring books of yellow, orange, and red along with wall pictures in the consulting room will aid in getting cooperation from the child. Such an environment will allay the anxiety of the child and enable the pediatrician to observe many aspects of developmental milestones. A compliment for the youngster about their appearance, dress, or hairstyle will rapidly build a friendly atmosphere and will make further encounters much easier.

A medical consultation is frequently a source of anxiety for children and their parents. Sitting at the eye level of a child is reassuring. Most children above 4 yr of age would like to get involved in the interview and they should be encouraged.

Key points

Provide privacy and comfort for the family. Consider mother as the most important person. Compliment the child to gain confidence.

Patients presenting with emergency illness or severe pain should be dealt with differently (Ref. Ch. 8). A formal family interview is not possible at the first encounter for such patients. Children coming from other states and countries (migrant laborers, businesspeople, government employees, tourists including medical tourism) are encountered by doctors very often at present. Interviewing these groups will be easier, and treatment will be better if colleagues or other hospital staff know the patient's language and are willing to be interpreters in such situations. In India, apart from the mother tongue, our national language (Hindi), English, and as many local languages as possible need to be mastered by the doctor for better patient care.

3 CHAPTER

Communication with Patients and Parents

VK Parvathy

Chapter Outline

INTRODUCTION

Please read Chapters 1, 2 and 4 for other aspects of communication.

The medical profession is the most challenging one regarding communication among all because irrespective of social, educational, and financial status, people feel helpless when they have to approach doctors and the health system for illness. Communicating with patients and parents is an art; only very few master the tactics in a short time. Most require self-effort and learning by observing their seniors and peers and from the lessons learned from their own experience, self-correction, and vast reading including fiction and nonmedical subjects. Communication skills and dialogues are essential for building, fulfilling, and enduring relationships between patients, parents, and doctors. Patients and their parents are individuals with their own characters and needs. There is no easy and uniform approach right for all, but it is mandatory that all patients and parents should be properly informed about their illness after each interview and be satisfied.

Key points

The ability to communicate effectively is a core skill required in all areas of medicine, and one should master this quality by intense effort.

CLINICAL COMMUNICATION

This is defined as any interaction between health professionals or between health professionals and patients and relatives. Effective communication by medical practitioners can increase diagnostic accuracy and adherence to treatment, minimize litigation, enhance patient satisfaction, and improve health outcomes.

To the doctor, the patient may be just one case among many; to the patient or parent, it is the only one that matters to them. When things go wrong, they will remember if the attitudes and actions of the doctor concerned were caring or defensive. Hence, all interventions must be made with the clear knowledge that the first rule of therapeutic strategy is to leave the family willing to come again for the next session **(Fig. 3.1)**.

Medical profession is the most humane of all services. The combination of medical knowledge, intuition, and judgment defines the art of medicine. Tact, sympathy, and understanding are expected of the physicians because the patient is not a mere collection of symptoms and signs, disordered functions, damaged organs, and disturbed emotions. Physicians have to approach patients not as cases or diseases (such as in the case of

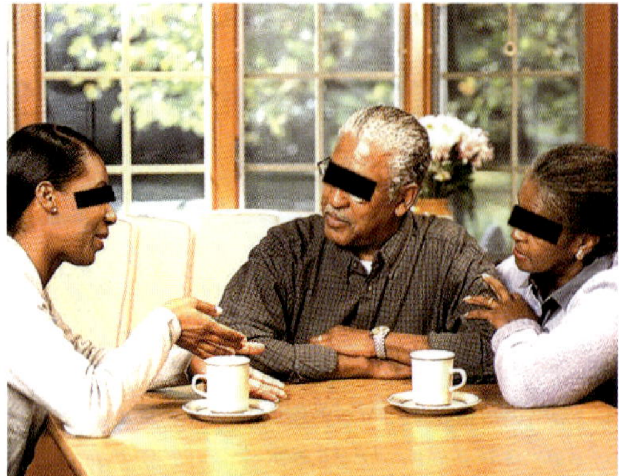

Fig. 3.1: The ability to communicate effectively is a core skill required in pediatrics.

hemolytic anemia and enteric fever) but as individuals. The beneficial effects of communication skills are applicable to both patients and doctors. Physicians are less likely to be sued for malpractice if they are able to communicate well and talk to their patients.

Most parental complaints of dissatisfaction and mismanagement originate due to lack of communication or because of the abrasive, cold, or callous attitude of the doctor or members of the health care team and not due to lack of knowledge and skills or unsatisfactory management of the patient. Hence doctors should be careful, tactful, and diplomatic in deciding not only "what to tell the parents" but also "how to tell it."

The idea is simple: Better communication skills = better understanding of patients and symptoms = better diagnosis and treatment = lower risk of negative effects.

Patients and parents must always feel that they are treated with respect and dignity. The doctor should consider his patients as clients and handle them with due confidence, humility, concern, and empathy. To communicate with the parents, we should literally come down to their level. Eye-to-eye contact should be maintained during communication. The doctor should not judge, belittle, or argue with the parents but handle them with due courtesy and consideration. The parents should be told about the condition of the child in a simple, easy-to-understand language without any medical jargon. One should be pragmatic but honest in communicating the true medical status of the child trying to keep the hope alive, which has tremendous healing capabilities. Do not allow the technology to further dehumanize medicine and try to resurrect the declining image of the medical profession. It is a must that all the medical and nursing colleges in the country should initiate regular education programs in the fields of social and behavioral sciences, the art of communication, and medical ethics for graduate and postgraduate medical and nursing students.

COMPONENTS OF COMMUNICATION

Components of communication are contents and exchange processes.

Contents (Message)

Communication becomes successful when the contents are clear, and the exchange process is not biased. These include the exact diagnosis, the particular stage of illness, diagnostic investigations, treatment options, and the expected outcome. The clarity of contents depends on good history and careful physical examination mainly (which are effective ways of communication), the minimum necessary investigations, and the doctor's ability to interpret the diagnosis and to provide the best cost-effective, and least harmful treatment. For this, the doctor must have updated knowledge on the subject, and mentality to revise the diagnosis and accept the pitfalls.

Exchange Processes

The exchange process has verbal and nonverbal aspects. Children acquire nonverbal communication before they understand the meaning of words. Nonverbal communication can be improved by *action tips* and *mechanical tips*. Some of the action tips are eye contact in between, tone of voice, rate of speech (be a good listener), facial expression, head movements, hand gestures, and body postures. Important helpful mechanical tips are:

- Offering a chair before the exchange process indicates that the doctor is willing to spend time (even though the duration is brief).
- Pulling a chair near to a bedridden patient reveals that the doctor is willing to get close to the patient's level.
- Touching, holding the hand, and patting implies empathy and consolation.
- Helping the parent (to remove the cloth, hold the baby, open the button, etc.) reveals helpfulness.

Note: Use safety precautions against contagious diseases while providing mechanical tips.

Verbal Exchange

Children as young as 3 yr of age may volunteer with verbal participation in their health care. By 13 yr of age, the youngster should be dealt with directly. Hence, in children under 3 yr of age, verbal communication is between the doctor and parent. In the 3–13 yr age group, the exchange is between parents and doctor, parents and child, between parents and between child and doctor. Some of the verbal exchange tips are:

- Always observe common courtesy—greet the patient by name and tell the purpose of the interview (e.g., for demonstrating a physical examination finding, before a procedure even if it is not painful).
- Remain patient and confident even if provoked and not be conscious of one's own dignity.
- Speak in a soft persuasive voice.
- Do not do all the talking. Should be a listener also, but ask questions related to the problem in between. Audio or videotaping of communication and review will improve one's quality of communication.
- Ask open-ended questions. Conversation should be attuned to the intellectual and social level of the child and parents.
- Encourage free communication. Spend time to clear all doubts.
- *Praise the mother for the positive aspects of baby care and encourage her to overcome the negative aspects.*
- When parents do not appear readily reassured, make it comfortable and easy for them to ask questions or express ungrateful or angry feelings.

Verbal exchange tips to be observed for children are:

- Greet by name. Compliment the child for appearance, dress, hairdo, etc.
- Talk in the manner a physician talks with any patient.
- Do not convey the feeling that their ideas are childish.
- Do not laugh at what children say.
- Do not always try to be funny to children. They know the difference between doctors and funny people.
- Never tease.
- By 4–5 yr discuss with them their symptoms, diagnosis, and treatment in terms they can understand.
- Never discuss with others the illness or treatment of hospitalized children who have acquired receptive language

functions (in their presence) unless you are discussing it with them as well.

- Noncooperation and struggling mean that children are frightened.

Problems of communication are who all, how much, what, and what not to be communicated, and the maintenance of confidentiality. A common rule is that both parents should be present at the time of communication and a relative or a close friend may also attend if the parents wish to have. If the parents are very tense, the relative or friend will be a better perceiver.

COMMUNICATION ACCORDING TO SITUATIONS

Ambulatory Care

Intercommunication is limited in the outpatient department due to the restraints in time and space. Try to maintain privacy. If a follow-up date is advised, explain the purpose. For referred patients if disposed of on ambulatory care, a provisional diagnosis should be made, appropriate treatment should be started, and a proper explanation should be given for sending back the patient by a reply note to the doctor who referred the patient. Verbal explanations to the relatives to convince them is a must. The details should be entered in the hospital record.

Emergency Room and Observation Area

Explain the treatment or procedure to be done and the reason with a duration of observation.

Routine Ward Rounds

First information should be provided observing privacy and tailored according to the educational status of the parents. On subsequent visits, enquire first about the progress of the patient, followed by physical examination and lastly review of charts. The condition of the child is to be explained after that. Listen carefully and reevaluate the child if the mother or an experienced nurse expresses concern about the child's condition. Most children above the age of 4 yr will be able to grasp serious problems from the conversation between the doctor and the parents and hence such discussion should be avoided in front of the child.

Critically Ill Children

State the probable diagnosis, treatment provided, and prognosis but do not make exact predictions about the time of death or chances of survival. It is never possible to be absolutely sure about the prognosis; the outcome may be surprising.

When a child is admitted to the pediatric intensive care unit (PICU), after establishing the treatment, family members must be given details regarding the probable diagnosis, further investigations needed, the treatment started, and also the roles played by the different healthcare providers. Ideally, the senior doctor should communicate at least once daily in the initial days or till the recovery starts. If the resident or a senior trainee is assigned with the responsibility of communicating with the family, this doctor should be specially introduced to the family and directed to act only as the spokesperson of the attending physician. He/she should be constantly in touch with the attending physician regarding the updates of the patient and the decisions thereof. The assigned resident should give full information in proper context to the family at least twice daily. This will alleviate the anxiety of the family members. It is also important to communicate that the resident may act independently in certain situations but only under the supervision of the attending physician.

Medical Accidents

If a complication or error in treatment has occurred, deal with it immediately and initiate corrective steps without delay. Tell the parents exactly what has happened. Like anyone else mistakes can occur to doctors also; parents recognize and accept this, but they will not readily forgive attempts to conceal the truth.

Noncompliance

Identify accurately the reason for noncompliance and rectify the defect. It may be due to lack of understanding, restraints with time or money, doubts not clarified properly, influence from other sources (medical/nonmedical/relatives), psychiatric or emotional upset of parents, anger toward physicians, or resistance by an angry child.

Newborns or Children with Mother Not in Sound State and Father Not Available

The doctor has to take treatment decisions for the best of the patient as far as the law permits and should be documented with reason.

Demonstration of a Physical Finding

Inform the purpose of the examination and get consent. Expose only the minimum necessary body parts.

Painful Procedures

Appropriate anesthesia must be always used. Do not lie to the child; the doctor can tell the child that there will be some pain that will wane away quickly. Praise the child as a brave one to bear the pain and remain calm. The nature of the procedure should be explained to the child and the parents. The presence of parents during the procedure will make the child more confident. In children with chronic illness (e.g., leukemia) requiring repeated painful procedures, liberal visiting by doctors and chances to act out fearful procedures in dolls are helpful.

Children with Functional Disorders

The situation should be handled with the same seriousness as an organic illness. The child is advised to wait outside, while the nonorganic nature of the disorder is informed to the parents. There will be stress factors for the child which carry equal importance as an organic disease. Tailor the explanations in such a way so that the parents are able to come up with their views regarding the situation. Sarcasm or criticism should never be expressed by the doctor.

Newborn with Congenital Anomalies or Metabolic Disorders

Repeated sessions with both parents together are needed to relieve the feelings of guilt and to accept the baby. Discuss the positive aspects of improvement with proper investigations and available treatment.

Adopted Child

Encourage the parents to speak freely and repeatedly to the child about adoption from toddler years continuing through adolescence.

Children Requiring Reference to Another Hospital

Referral should be to the apt person with a proper letter. Explain the reason for the reference to the parents. Occasionally, parents may request a reference to another hospital without a valid reason. The doctor should not get upset over this matter but should explain the prognostic issues, and the treatment available in the present institution and elsewhere. The ultimate decision is to be taken by the parents. Here also a proper referral letter should be issued detailing the treatment given and the reason for reference.

Patients Received by Referral from Another Hospital

Unnecessary comments should not be made regarding the treatment already received. The diagnostic and treatment dilemmas of referring doctors must be respected although the treatment provided may not have been up to the standards.

Children with Malignancy

For reasons already mentioned both parents should be informed together along with a relative as far as possible. Different sessions will be required to discuss various aspects and clear the doubts.

Children with Acquired Immunodeficiency Syndrome

Diagnostic investigations should be undertaken only after getting consent from parents. Always maintain confidentiality and, at the same time counsel regarding various aspects of the illness-family life, risk of transfer of infections, schooling, treatment duration, etc.

Illnesses Without a Definite Diagnosis

In the medical profession diagnosis is an efficient way to communicate. Knowing the diagnosis helps to manage the disease accordingly and counseling the parents is easier. When the definite diagnosis is not made and is on the wait up of investigation results, symptomatic treatment may be offered, but this is to be informed boldly and plainly. If a second opinion is warranted it should be arranged.

Withholding and Withdrawing Intensive Life-prolonging Treatment

The following questions are to be considered: Who should decide? What are the criteria? If treatments are withheld or withdrawn what alternative care is appropriate? Are there implications for others? What about society and law?

When the physician realizes, along with the opinion of the intensive care unit team, that further aggressive treatment is futile and harmful to a patient, the family should be compassionately informed. Decisions to curtail life-supportive measures should be based on mutual understanding about the quality of life. The law confers protection on all infants born alive at any gestational age, but it does not insist that all available treatments must be used to maintain life in all circumstances. Documentation of decision-making is important. These decisions should not be influenced by considerations of the potential use of the child's organs or tissues for transplantation or by economic reasons.

Antenatally Detected Major Congenital Anomaly

Parents have high expectations for the unknown baby and to know that something is abnormal with the baby is shocking. In such a situation one should have thorough knowledge of the condition as well as maturity and compassion for the expectant parents. Explain the pros and cons of continuing pregnancy, help them decide, and get it documented. The decision should never be of the doctors.

Asphyxiated Baby

Be gentle in explaining the outcome and be prepared to clear all doubts. Avoid saying "Nothing can be done." The dialogue should be unhurried, and parents should be encouraged to express their feelings. Talk about the positive aspects and try not to cultivate feelings of guilt in them.

Children Requiring Prolonged Replacement Therapy

Examples are congenital hypothyroidism, congenital adrenal hyperplasia, hemophilia, inborn errors of metabolism, immune deficiency disorders, etc. Spend time telling the prognosis, and the need for continued therapy and answer all the queries. Areas of concern will include growth, scholastic performance, puberty, problems regarding marriage, medical fitness, inheritance to offsprings, etc.

Chronically or Fatally Ill Children

The physician should stand for hope and relief of discomfort and be ready to help the parents and children. They should be assured that the child will not be abandoned and a skilled team will remain involved in pursuit of the revised diagnostic and therapeutic goals. In areas of uncertainty, a review of what has happened and honest and factual answers should be given.

The Dying Child

Parents need to know that everything reasonably possible has been done to save their child, by themselves and by the hospital staff. When there is no hope for survival, they need to be told clearly but compassionately. By designating one individual close to the family, to keep the parents informed on the ongoing process of resuscitation, providing them with realistic information as it evolves, and involving them in the decision-making process when the time comes to stop resuscitation, parents can be given some sense of empowerment at a time of ultimate helplessness. If the parents are willing to be in the treatment room, allowing them to witness the resuscitation may help them to come to terms with the gravity of the situation and to feel that they were with their child in the last moments. If this is to be offered a staff member must be available to stay with the parents. After resuscitation efforts have stopped, parents and family members should be provided with a private room to hold the child and say goodbye. We must remember that the goal is survival with good functional neurologic recovery.

Up to 5 yr of age, children though aware of death, do not consider it as an unpleasant event, but as a reversible incident. In this age group when questions are asked about death (Am I going to die?), truth can be told in a simplified manner that the child is going to be a star in the sky or to heaven but will not be left alone. At the age of 8–9 yr, death is personified as the one who punishes and avenges. After 9 yr only death is understood as universal and final biological. In children above 5 yr, there is no absolute rule to deal with the situation, but a sensitive and flexible approach is needed to tell the truth. Close physical contact with the parents and emotional exchange with verbal explanations are advised.

After Death

The doctor should remain with the parents till the body is properly taken care of and provide help with funeral arrangements. The spectrum of the normal response of family members may range from apparently unnatural calm to emotional decompensation and outrage. The anger of family members is often a reflection of their sense of guilt and helplessness. A visit to the family a few days after the death will be always thought of with gratitude by the family. This will provide the family with an opportunity to clear their unanswered doubts and guilt. Further, the doctor can assess their mental status and the physical as well as the mental health status of the siblings. Repeated sessions may be needed sometimes for parents to talk out their feelings. The siblings of the dead should be allowed to participate appropriately in the rituals that generally surround death and burial. They should not be interrupted from the usual social or recreational activities after death in the family, either out of respect for the death or in recognition of the grief of the remaining persons.

RATING TOOLS

Many assessment tools have been developed that provide feedback also as self-reporting scales (can be used by students themselves), external raters (or observing faculty), or by patients. The evaluation criteria for these scales are based on the Kalamazoo Consensus Statement (May 1999, Kalamazoo, Michigan, North America) which defines seven essential elements of physician-patient communication.

Kalamazoo Consensus Statement 2001

The seven elements of the Kalamazoo Essential Element Communication checklist are the following:

- *Build the doctor-patient relationship:* Greet and show the interviewee as a person; use words that show care and concern throughout the interview; use tone, pace, eye contact, and posture that shows care and concern.
- *Open the discussion:* Allow the patient to complete his/her opening statement; elicit the patient's full set of concerns; establish/maintain a personal connection.
- *Gather information:* Use open-ended and closed-ended questions appropriately; structure, clarify, and summarize information; listen actively using verbal and nonverbal techniques.
- *Understand the patient's and family's perspective:* Explore contextual factors; family, culture, gender, etc.; explore beliefs; acknowledge and respond to the patient's ideas, feelings, and values.
- *Share information:* Use language that the patient can understand, check for understanding, and encourage questions.
- *Teach agreement on problems and plans:* Encourage patients to participate in decisions, check patients' willingness and ability to follow the plan, and identify and enlist resources and support.
- *Provide closure:* Ask whether the patient has any other issues or concerns, and summarize and affirm agreement with a plan of action.

These broadly supported elements provide a useful framework for communication-oriented curricula and standards.

SUGGESTED READING

1. General Medical Council. (2009). Tomorrow's doctors: Outcomes and standards for undergraduate medical education. London: GMC. [Online] Available from http://www.gmcuk.g/Tomorrow_s_Doctors_1214.pdf_48905759. pdf [Last accessed September, 2024].
2. Howells RJ, Davies HA, Silverman JD. Teaching and learning consultation skills for paediatric practice. Arch Dis Child. 2006;91(4):367-70.

3. In: Prabhakara GN (Ed). Short Textbook of Professional Medical, 2nd edition. New Delhi: Paras Publishing; 2001.
4. JyModi JN, Anshu, Chhatwal J, Gupta P, Singh T. Teaching and Assessing Communication Skills in Medical Undergraduate Training. Indian Pediatr. 2016;53(6):497-504.
5. Keir A, Wilkinson D. Communication skills training in paediatrics J Paediatr Child Health. 2013;49(8):624-8.
6. Laidlaw A, Hart JO. Communication skills: an essential component of medical curricula. Part I: assessment of clinical communication: AMEE Guide No. 51. Med Teach. 2011;33(1):6-8.
7. Makoul G. Essential elements of communication in medical encounters: the Kalamazoo consensus statement. Acad Med. 2001;76(4):390-3.
8. McCabe ME, Servint JR. Loss, Separation and Bereavement. In: Kliegman R, StGeme JW, Blum NJ, Shah SS, Tasker RC, Wilson KM, et al. Nelson Textbook Pediatrics, 21st edition. Amsterdam: Elsevier; 2020. pp. 168-72.
9. Schirmer JM, Mauksch L, Lang F, Marvel MK, Zoppi K, Epstein RM, et al. Assessing communication competence: A review of current tools. Fam Med. 2005;37(3):184-92.
10. Shendurnikar N, Thakkar PA. Communication skills to ensure patient satisfaction. Indian J Pediatr. 2013;80(11):938-43.
11. Singh M. Communication as a Bridge to Build a Sound Doctor-Patient/Parent Relationship. Indian J Pediatr. 2016;83(1):33-7.

CHAPTER

Communication as a Student

Darly Saramma Mammen

Chapter Outline

- Introduction
- Challenges Encountered
- Difficult Problems
- Support from Professional Peers
- Bedside Clinical Examination
- Clinical Case Discussions

INTRODUCTION

Please read chapters 1, 2, and 3 for communication skills.

Medical students and residents face challenging situations in pediatrics for clinical assessment and communication. The reasons are the age difference, and the developmental status of the child compared to adult patients. The patient population in pediatrics may range from newborns to 12 yr or 18 yr of age based on the hospital infrastructure. Communication with the child is influenced by the developmental and cognitive stages of the child, interaction levels in the family, and the needs and the situation of the child and the parents. Apart from medical problems, the child may have behavioral, developmental, or psychosocial problems. Pediatrics is distinct and always requires expert communication with the parents and sometimes with family members or close friends of the parents. The quality of the relationship and communication with children and their parents affects all aspects of patient care, the diagnostic process, the treatment decision, adherence with the recommendations, and also the satisfaction of the trio—(1) child, (2) parent, and (3) physician. Difficult patient encounters (DPEs) are being experienced nowadays more often by pediatric residents. DPEs are often due to disagreement in diagnosis and/or management, strong emotions from either side, the situations in the family, and also by disease-specific factors.

CHALLENGES ENCOUNTERED

The student is put into the test of communication in pediatrics on four occasions mainly:

- Bedside clinical examination
- Clinical case discussion
- Presentation in examinations
- Presentation in conferences.

Though all these situations need good communication, the quantity and quality vary accordingly. The aspects of presentation at conferences are beyond the scope of this chapter and hence not discussed.

The key element of student training should be a progressive increase in the level of independent action in all aspects of patient care. They should be under the guidance from experienced seniors with expert supervision and direction, but motivation and effective involvement of the student is a must. The invariable qualities of a student should be the awareness of the responsibility for learning and taking a key role in patient care.

Communication skills have a prime role in achieving the goal of good training. Some communication skills are innate, but most are to be acquired by constant training. Students with good communication skills thrive better during training because of clear communication, both spoken and written, improves:

- The relationships with other pediatricians, nurses, and paramedical staff.
- Children, parents, and community as a whole.

DIFFICULT PROBLEMS

Beware of individuals with whom communication is impossible, at least for you, at that particular time. Individuals who see themselves as complex, fascinating, and informed may in fact be difficult, ignorant, and dogmatic. The benefit of the doubt should be given to each person but one's confidence should not be destroyed by individuals who complain about everything. If you find it failing to communicate, delegate the responsibility to someone else. This is important for one's own morale, for good patient care, and for medicolegal reasons.

One should expect to be challenged during training to acquire new skills and more knowledge and to provide comprehensive well-rounded care. Life involves moral and cultural standards; medicines involve risk and urgency. To avoid becoming a society of victims, we must improve our ability to share concerns, give and receive apologies, and retain an element of common sense and goodwill.

SUPPORT FROM PROFESSIONAL PEERS

Emotional support is important during training period. Hence, it is wise to identify a pediatrician to whom you can turn for emotional and intellectual support. Try to cultivate such a relationship as early as possible.

Time Management

Time management is of utmost importance in the medical profession. To avoid wasting time, keep the meetings brief and fruitful and end them on schedule. Try to complete tasks without interruption especially during ward rounds, clinical examination of patients, and order writing. The following points, if kept in mind, will be fruitful for good time management.

- Make lists and priorities for the day.
- Set deadlines, especially for reading or writing.
- Manage your free time more aggressively.
- Cultivate a full life away from the hospital to make you more efficient and committed at work.
- Recreation should be fun, stimulatory, and entirely different from the routines.
- Create a habit of doing exercises to keep in physical well-being.
- Awareness of potential problems, as well as deliberate attempts to improve your morale can ease much of the strain.
- Try to utilize the opportunities to teach others while you learn. This will improve your vocabulary, build up your presentation technique, and widen your knowledge.
- Compassion and humor will enrich your life.
- Celebrate the strength and positive attributes of your colleagues and yourself.

BEDSIDE CLINICAL EXAMINATION

- Always practice the basic qualities of a medical student, the attributes of the doctor, the points to be remembered in

diagnostic investigations, empirical antibiotics in the first hour (Golden hour), and supportive measures simultaneously.

Communication: The parents should be informed about the probable diagnoses and the need for early proper treatment and urgent CSF studies which is an invasive investigation. Proceed for permission to collect CSF and blood and to start empirical antibiotics, anticonvulsants, and supportive treatment. The parents should be informed in between about the clinical status of the child and the laboratory reports. Always see that there is no time-lapse and that documentations are proper and prompt including the communications given.

- List of investigations should be relevant and there should be adequate reason to select the particular investigation.
- Treatment offered should be according to standard protocols.
- Advances and controversies in management may be highlighted if you are aware.
- Do not do any foul play in the examination.

If you happen to get a "tip" use it wisely, otherwise you will be in trouble.

- A 9-yr-old girl presents with polyarthritis for 3 yr and grade 2 disability. She was on irregular treatment with modern and Ayurvedic medicines.

The most probable clinical diagnosis is juvenile idiopathic arthritis (JIA) but there are differential diagnoses to be ruled out.

Communication: The child requires detailed investigations to establish the diagnosis of JIA. Most of them can be done as an outpatient if there are no red flag signs, such as high fever, severe anemia, respiratory distress, and bleeding manifestations. Detailing of the illness should be done after diagnostic confirmation about the chronic nature, different modalities of treatment available and possible complications. The need for periodic follow-up should be stressed. For pain, advise paracetamol or ibuprofen. Start further treatment after diagnostic confirmation. The need for periodic follow-up should be stressed. Documentation of the clinical details, drugs, and physiotherapy given, investigations done with results and details of counseling given should be properly entered in the hospital record.

SUGGESTED READING

1. Alofisan T, Al-Alaiyan S, Siddiqui S, Hussain IB, Al-Qahtani MH. Communication skills in pediatric training program: National-based survey of residents' perspectives in Saudi Arabia. J Family Community Med. 2016;23(1):43-7.
2. Collins K, Hopkins A, Shilkofski NA, Levine RB, Hernandez RG. Difficult Patient Encounters: Assessing Pediatric Resident's Communication Skills Training Needs. Cureus. 2018;10(9):e3340.
3. Mac Nab A, Seear M. Resident/Fellow Training in The Pocket Paediatrician, Cambridge University Press 2002: 531-34.
4. Rider E A, Volkan K, Hafler JP. Pediatric residents' perceptions of communication competencies: Implications for teaching. Med Teach. 2008;30(7):e208-17.

CHAPTER

Introduction to Medical Research

Manu Raj, M Geethadevi

Chapter Outline

INTRODUCTION

Scientific research plays a significant role in maintaining health and combating disease. The word research is derived from the French word "recherche" which literally means "to go about seeking." In other words, research is a quest for knowledge through diligent search or investigation or experimentation aimed at the discovery and interpretation of new knowledge, the purpose of which varies in different branches of science.

The first clinical trial on research in modern medicine is credited to the Scottish physician James Lind (1716–1794) who developed the theory that citrus fruits cured scurvy. The clinical trial was on 12 patients affected with scurvy in the ship, who were divided into six groups. The medicines used were cider, vitriol elixir, vinegar, sea water, a mixture of nutmeg, garlic, mustard and tamarind in barley water, and citrus fruits. The group given citrus fruits got cured in a week. A systematic research work was not done further, due to the poor knowledge on research at that time.

Research starts with finding out gaps in knowledge, creates new knowledge, and develops proper tools for using existing knowledge thus providing evidence for policy making on health and development. As per revised curriculum, the National Medical Commission (NMC) has incorporated learning of Research Methodology from the undergraduate level itself so that students are motivated to do research projects and disseminate the new knowledge gained through presentation in conferences or as publication in journals.

STEPS OF RESEARCH PROCESS

Medical research basically has several steps which include (1) identifying a research theme, (2) Framing the research question, stating objectives/hypothesis (3) identifying suitable scientific methods of design, and (4) statistical analysis to get an answer to the research question.

Selection of Research Theme

The selection of a research theme is dependent on two basic things—the researcher's "interest and need" based on the existing circumstances. The topic should come from within the researcher and it should not be forced upon. If the research taken up is not interesting to the person, planning and designing will be improper; sometimes, it may stop in the middle or the end point will be an unattractive piece of work. Select the research topic based on one's own intrinsic interest, vast reading, clinical observations, discussion with colleagues, attending conferences, questions asked by others, etc.

After selection, read the topic by reviewing the available books and articles on the topic published during the last 3–5 yr, identify the gap in knowledge, i.e., what was already known and what is yet to be known. After identifying the gap in knowledge, do an in depth reading to identify the specific area of interest.

Formulate a Tentative Research Question

The entire planning, design, and analysis of research work depends on the research question. If proper care is not taken in framing the research question, the whole effort will be wasted and adds one more unscientific work to the many already existing. Evaluate the tentative question for its suitability. The *FINER* criteria is an acronym of five critical features essential for a proper research question which are *F*easible, *I*nteresting, *N*ovel, *E*thical, and *R*elevant. By asking these questions the researcher can modify the crude question to a refined and structured one before starting the research work. Never try to modify the question after starting the research work.

Define three things for structuring a research question—the population, the exposure, and outcome for an observational study. If one is dealing with an experimental study design, the items to specify include the population, the intervention, the control procedure, the outcome of interest, and the duration of intervention. A badly structured research question can never be salvaged by future modifications after the study is initiated. Deficiencies in any of the critical requirements mentioned earlier can destroy the research study and hence enough time should be spent in formulating a good research question.

Example: Can exercise reduce obesity among adolescents? This is a vague research question, which can be made more specific like—"Can 30 min of brisk walking every day for 8 w reduce body mass index by 15% among obese adolescents?"

A well developed and specific question may give certain indications:

- Suspected exposure—lack of exercise (30 min of brisk walking)
- Effect or outcome—obesity
- Magnitude of effect—15% reduction by removal of the cause.

Research Hypothesis

Research question when expressed in a statement form becomes the research hypothesis. A hypothesis is simply an approximate explanation that relates to the set of truths that can be tested by certain further investigations included in the study proper. There are basically two types of hypotheses, the null and alternative versions. A research generally starts with a research problem which has to be converted to a hypothesis to proceed further.

Example: 30 min of brisk walking every day for 8 w can reduce the body mass index by 15% among obese adolescents. The research hypothesis is a tentative guess which we wish to test and finally accept or reject in our proposed research work.

- *Null hypothesis (H0)* is the research hypothesis stated in a negative manner. 30 min of brisk walking daily does not have any effect in reducing body mass index (by 15% at least) among obese adolescents. As we proceed further (during statistical analysis) one may accept or reject the H0 and not the research hypothesis.
- *Alternative hypothesis (H1)* is the exact opposite of the H0. Conventionally, it makes a statement that points to a potential result that an investigator may expect and wish to confirm by doing the study.

Finally, write down the relevance of our research question in brief which helps to write down the introduction part of our research paper. It should include: (1) The importance of the research topic (public health and clinical practice), (2) What is already known in the area, (3) What are the gaps in knowledge that need to be filled up, (4) How the present study is able to resolve uncertainties in the area, and (5) What are the potential problems in the proposed research work and how are they proposed to be overcome.

IDENTIFYING THE APPROPRIATE RESEARCH DESIGN

Once the research question has been framed, the next step is to select the type of research design most suitable for the question. There are issues where the choice of study design did not match properly with the research question framed at the start. To avoid this mistake, while doing research, a proper understanding of various research methods are required.

Research methods are broadly classified into *observational and experimental designs.* Observational methods are again categorized as descriptive and analytical studies. Experimental (interventional) studies include randomized trials and nonrandomized studies.

Observational studies are preferred when the researcher does not assign exposure, but only observes. But in interventional studies the researcher assigns exposure to one group.

Descriptive studies simply describe a phenomenon of interest, and express it in terms of measure of health or disease (mean, median, incidence, and prevalence), a preformed hypothesis regarding cause and effect relationship is not a must and they generate hypotheses only. Descriptions are given according to time, place, and person. In descriptive design, the research question is also descriptive in type, e.g., what proportion of adolescents are doing 30 min walking every day?

Analytical Study

Here the researcher starts with a preformed hypothesis regarding cause effect relationship. The researcher investigates the cause effect relationship between a possible exposure and outcome. Analytical studies address issues related to treatment, preventive or diagnostic modalities, or regarding the role of risk factors/prognostic markers. The key word in analytical study is comparison. *The basic framework of analytical research is a 2 x 2 table as shown in* **Table 5.1***:*

For testing hypotheses, analytical studies are used. Among analytical studies cohort studies are prospective (forward looking/ exposure to outcome) in which one group with exposure and another group without exposure are followed up for a particular period of time and the outcome is compared in both groups. Strength of association is calculated by relative risk (RR).

TABLE 5.1: Basic framework of analytical research.

	Outcome		
Exposure	***Present***	***Absent***	***Total***
Present	a	b	a + b
Absent	c	d	c + d
Total	a + c	b + d	a + b + c + d

Relative risk is the ratio of incidence of outcome among the exposed and the nonexposed.

RR = a/a + b: c/c + d

Interpretation of Relative Risk

- RR 1—Incidence of outcome in exposed and unexposed is same, so the exposure is neither a risk factor nor protective factor
- RR >1—Incidence of outcome is more among exposed, so the exposure is a risk factor
- RR <1—Incidence of outcome is more among unexposed, so the exposure is a protective factor.

Case control studies are retrospective (backward looking/outcome to exposure) which include a group of cases (with the disease) and controls (without disease) and presence or absence of exposure is ascertained by history given by the participant.

Odds ratio (OR) is calculated to express the measure of risk.

- OR = Exposure odds among cases/ Exposure odds among controls,
- Exposure odds among cases = cases exposed/cases not exposed (a/c),
- Exposure odds among controls = controls exposed/controls not exposed (c/d),

OR = a/c: b/d = ad/bc

Odds ratio can be >1, 1, or <1. If it is >1 the exposure is a risk factor, <1 exposure is a protective factor, and 1 means it is neither a risk factor nor a protective factor.

In *cross-sectional analytical studies* a cross section of the population is studied. Measurement of outcome and exposure are carried out at the same point of time.

Experimental/interventional design is the most scientifically sound design where a researcher collects a group of subjects in whom neither exposure nor outcome has happened. The researcher randomly allocates these subjects into two groups (both are similar to each other). Then one group is deliberately given the exposure and the other group is not exposed.

Researchers follow up both groups for a particular period of time to see how many in each group have the defined outcome.

Basic principles of choosing the right design are shown in **Flowchart 5.1**.

Population and sample: It is not possible to study the whole population so that a subset of the accessible population (known as a sample) is selected. This accessible population *(study population)* is a representative subset of the total population (universe or reference population). The sample selected should be representative of the study population and it should be of adequate size. Ensuring representativeness and adequate number of subjects is an integral part of any research study. The required number of subjects can be calculated mathematically using data from previous studies in the same theme. If such published data is not available, a pilot study can be done and use the data for calculating sample size. Once the required sample is calculated, the same number of subjects are recruited using either random or nonrandom methods. Selection of subjects is based on inclusion and exclusion criteria that should be stated clearly in the research protocol.

Flowchart 5.1: Basic principles of study designs.

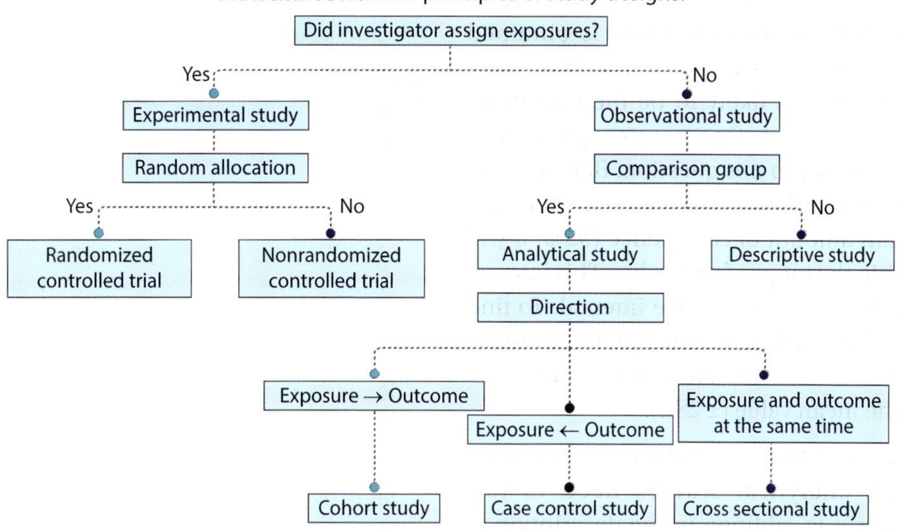

Source: Grimes DA, Schulz KF. An overview of clinical research: the lay of the land. Lancet. 2002;359(9300):57-61.

DATA ANALYSIS

Once the required number of subjects are selected, collect data needed for statistical analysis which depends on the research question, type of design, and what characteristics of the subjects are planned to investigate (variables).

Variables are any quantity or quality of subjects which can be recorded and which varies from one subject to another, and classified into quantitative and qualitative. Quantitative variables are classified into discrete and continuous types. Discrete variables are those characteristics of subjects which assume values as whole numbers (number of male/female members in a family). Continuous variables can assume any value within a specified range of minimum and maximum value [age, weight, height, serum bilirubin, body mass index (BMI)]. Qualitative variables can be nominal (gender—male/female), ordinal (cancer grading, socioeconomic status—low, middle, or high). Knowledge about the type of the variables in the study will help to decide how to represent data, to determine sample size, and also to choose the statistical test.

Probability distribution is to enumerate different values the variables can have and how frequently each value appears in the population. Common examples are binomial, Poisson, and normal distribution. Incidence of relatively common diseases follow binomial distribution and of rare diseases follow Poisson distribution. Distribution of continuous variables (height, weight, and BMI) are considered as normally distributed.

The type of analysis depends on the design of study which again depends on the research question. Thus in *descriptive studies* the unknown population values are estimated using the value calculated from the sample. One researcher has found that the mean hemoglobin value of 100 females is 12 g/dL. But it cannot be stated that the population mean is also 12 g/dL, since some uncertainty is associated with an estimate of 12 g/dL. This uncertainty can be measured by standard error (SE) which is the standard deviation of sample mean from population mean. SE can be calculated from a single study $SE = Sd/\sqrt{n}$; where Sd is the standard deviation and n is the number of samples.

Confidence interval: In descriptive studies an estimate of the parameter is obtained from the study. Next question is how close your estimate is likely to be the true value of the parameter. One cannot get a 100% certain answer to this question. But based on sampling distribution one can state that with a certain amount of confidence (95%) it will be within the range of true value. This interval is known as the confidence interval. To find out the 95% confidence interval for normally distributed variables add and subtract 2 SEs from the mean value (± 2SE).

Analytical study: In contrast to descriptive studies, analytical studies need to test hypotheses in addition to the description of population.

TESTING HYPOTHESIS

Testing hypothesis has several steps:

Identify Null Hypothesis

This is a restatement of a research hypothesis in the null form, i.e., no effect of treatment, no difference in outcome, or no difference in incidence rate.

Determine Levels of Alpha and Beta Errors Acceptable in Inference

As one conducts study in a sample it cannot always be said that the hypothesis is true or not in the population. Decision is dichotomous to accept null hypothesis (H0) or reject null hypothesis. Two types of errors are possible:

1. *Type 1 (α error)* is the probability of rejecting a true null hypothesis by which one is accepting a false alternate hypothesis stating that the treatment is effective or the difference is significant which leads to a false positive conclusion. In that sense, type 1 error should be as low as possible and fix type 1 error to a maximum of 5%.

TABLE 5.2: Type 1 and type 2 errors in testing hypothesis.

Decision based on sample results	***Truth in population***	
	H0 true	***H0 false***
Accept H0	No error	Type 2 error (β)
Reject H0	Type 1 error (α)	No error

2. *Type 2 error (β error)* happens when one accepts a false null hypothesis which leads to the rejection of a true alternate hypothesis stating that there is no effect for this treatment or that there is no significant difference leading to false negative conclusions. **Table 5.2** reveals the summary of the testing errors.

SELECTING THE BEST STATISTICAL TEST

It depends on the type of variables, the number of groups, and probability distribution of variables as revealed in **Table 5.3.**

Example 1: Considering the research question whether exercise will bring down BMI, the outcome variable is decrease in BMI, exposure variable is exercise (30 minutes brisk walking daily), the groups are one with exercise and other without exercise, outcome measured as mean reduction in BMI which is a continuous variable and there are two groups (with exercise and without exercise). As given in the **Table 5.3**, here the unpaired t-test can be used.

If another researcher wants to measure the outcome as the number (count) of adolescents whose BMI was reduced following exercise, then from the table—outcome variable expressed as count and exposure variable expressed as count, the ideal statistical test is Chi-square.

TABLE 5.3: Statistical tests based on variables and number of groups.

Variable	*Groups*	*Statistical test*
Qualitative—expressed as count/frequency	2 or more	Chi-square
Continuous expressed as mean	One (pre-post comparison)	Paired t-test
Continuous expressed as mean	2 groups	Unpaired t-test
Continuous expressed as mean	3 or more	ANOVA test
Ordinal (scores) expressed as median	1 group	Wilcoxon signed-rank test
Ordinal (scores) expressed as median	2 groups	Mann–Whitney U test
Ordinal (scores) expressed as median	3 or more	Kruskal–Wallis test

(ANOVA: analysis of variance)

Example 2: A consumer group would like to evaluate the success of three different commercial weight loss programs. Subjects are assigned to one of three programs (group A, group B, and group C). Each group follows a different diet regimen. First time and at the end of 6 w subjects are weighed and their body weight measurements are recorded.

Test to detect mean difference in body weight between groups A and B—mean weight which is a continuous variable is compared between two groups. So, the unpaired t-test is recommended for finding out statistical significance.

Is there a significant difference in body weight in group A between the first time and at the end of 6 w—here it is one group and pre- and postintervention mean weight is compared—paired t-test can be used.

Is there any significant difference in the body weight of subjects in group A, group B, and group C at the end of 6 w—here mean difference in weight is compared among three groups, the ideal test is analysis of variance (ANOVA).

CALCULATING THE VALUE OF TEST STATISTICS

Perform the test using computerized programs like Epi Info (free software), Statistical Package for the Social Sciences (SPSS), etc. This involves calculating the appropriate test statistic ($t/Z/X^2$) and comparing the computed value with the table value. If the calculated value is more than the table value, reject the null hypothesis and accept the alternative hypothesis. If the calculated value is less than the table value, accept the null hypothesis and conclude H0 is true.

p VALUE

The *p value* is the probability of rejecting a null hypothesis when it is true. So, when a true null hypothesis is rejected one may accept the alternative research hypothesis which is false. In that situation, it is said as type 1 error or α error has happened which is a grave mistake. One cannot completely eliminate this error but need to limit it. So, fix type 1 error usually as 5% (but in interventional studies it may be fixed as low as 1%) and *p* value <5% (<0.05) which means the probability of false positive conclusion is <5%. For example, a *p* value of 0.03 (α error—5%) indicates the result of the study is statistically significant and the observed results represent a real difference.

Calculate power of test: Power of a test is the probability of correctly rejecting a null hypothesis (H0) when it is false and it is complementary to type 2 error (β). In other words, a powerful test readily detects the true difference when it exists. If the null hypothesis is not rejected, statistical power (1-β) is computed. If power is acceptable, agree with the null hypothesis. Power too low, one would recommend that study be repeated with large sample size. The Minimum acceptable level of power is 80%.

HOW TO REPORT?

When a research study is conducted depending on the research question/objectives, the researcher reports one of the three measures—disease frequency, measure of association, or measure of potential impact. Descriptive studies report the measures of disease frequency in terms of prevalence and incidence. In contrast to descriptive studies, analytical studies have more than one group and there is comparison. Analytical studies also test hypotheses. The statistical test can be chosen from the type of variables in the study and number of groups as shown in **Table 5.3**. Analytical studies use measures to indicate strength of association—as relative risk and attributable risk in cohort studies and odds ratio in case control studies.

In experimental studies testing new drugs, new treatment options, new preventive measures relative risk, attributable risk reduction, and relative risk reduction are used.

RANDOM ERROR AND BIAS

Random errors are chance errors due to variability in estimation arising from unknown or uncontrollable causes. They do not follow a pattern. Random errors can be reduced by using an average measurement from a set of measurements or increasing sample size.

Bias occurs when results of a study are systematically different from truth. If a study is planned to estimate the risk of disease associated with an exposure and the result overestimates the risk then the result is biased. Bias results from faulty design and can be reduced by a proper design. Bias can be selection bias, information bias, and confounding bias. Bias can be reduced by restriction, matching, stratification during analysis and using advanced statistical methods like regression.

SUGGESTED READING

1. Bhalwar R, Patrikar SR. Basic Principles of Inferential Statistics and Statistical Estimation. In: Bhalwar R, Duneja P, Jindal A, Bhatnagar A (Eds). Texbook of Community Medicine, 4th edition, Wolters Kluwer; 2019. pp. 237-47.
2. Grimes DA, Schulz KF. An overview of clinical research: the lay of the land. Lancet. 2002;359(9300):57-61.
3. World Health Organization. Regional office for the Western Pacific. (2001). Health Research Methodology: a guide for training in research methods, 2nd edition. [online] Available from http://apps. who. int/iris/handle/10665/206929.

6

CHAPTER

History Taking

S Sushamabai

Chapter Outline

INTRODUCTION

Read chapters 1, 2, 3, and 4 before you proceed

A thorough goal-oriented history taking is the first and most important skill to be learned by the student in medicine to become an astute clinician. Successful interpretation of a patient's problems depends on careful history which will provide a strong basis for systematic physical examination. Eliciting the history is an art and is best learned through repeated practice and by observing seniors and colleagues. In 75% of patients, a possible diagnosis, system localization, and nature of illness can be streamlined by proper history taking. The method may be according to one's own style but finally should be edited in a standardized format. Such a format is shown in **Box 6.1**. On the other hand, when met with a sick child, rapid assessment and stabilization (Ref. Ch. 8) are the priority along with brief parallel history. Detailed history should be evaluated after completing resuscitation and stabilization in such a situation.

BOX 6.1: Format for history taking.

- Personal data
- Presenting complaints
- History of present illness
- History of past illness
- Antenatal history
- Natal history
- Postnatal history
- Developmental history
- Nutritional history and diet
- Immunization history
- Family history
- Socioeconomic history
- Environmental history

Children differ in their behavior in the hospital environment or in a consultation room. The student should acquire the tactics to get cooperation from the child as detailed in chapters 1, 2, 3, and 4. Contrary to adult patients, parents or caretakers are a must to provide correct history in children. Above 4 yr of age, most children will be able to communicate and contribute to their history which should be encouraged. Adolescents also need parents/caretakers to complete the history details. Most adolescents become nervous when facing a doctor and may hide their problems due to fear of illness.

Parents/caretakers differ in presenting the history; most of them will be calm and clear cut in this aspect; some will be over anxious; some may be angry and short tempered; yet another group will be elaborating vague points; some parents simply hand over the reference letter/prescriptions/lab reports and think that all details of the patient are given in these papers. Whatever be the nature of the accompanying adult, the student should master the technique of getting appropriate history within the stipulated time.

Key points

Most parents give proper history which will help to unveil the diagnosis, some may be vague but the student should acquire the tactics to get appropriate details in the stipulated time.

PERSONAL DATA

Document the child's name, sex, date of birth, and age in completed years and months, full address of the child, phone number, date and time of examination, informants name, relationship with the child, and the reliability which includes literacy of the informant and the duration of stay with the child. Address and phone number are important for follow-up in many situations. Writing should be legible for self-reference and for others to read. Age, sex, and place of residence may provide important clues for diagnosis. Maintain eye contact with the child and parent in between. The important points should be documented.

Examples include the following:

- *1 m old baby boy with increasing cough and respiratory distress from birth onward is probably having congenital lobar emphysema; it is unlikely to be hyper-reactive airway disease.*
- *Baby boy of 2 yr age with features of rickets is likely to have familial hypophosphatemia as well as nutritional rickets.*
- *Think of the possibility of Turner syndrome in a newborn girl revealing edema of both feet.*
- *A child with fever, myalgia, and conjunctival congestion, residing in an endemic area of leptospirosis, the possibility of such a disease should be thought of.*
- *A child with fever residing in an endemic area of malaria, that disease should be considered as a possibility.*

The reliability of history is to be recorded as "the informant is the aunt who is looking after the baby since the mother is working abroad and the information is reliable".

PRESENTING COMPLAINTS

Document the presenting complaints with duration in chronological sequence using the patient's words, avoiding medical terminology.

Example: Fever for 7 days, left knee pain for 2 days, and chest pain since today morning (Note: Since indicates correct time of onset).

Children with chronic diseases when brought for added acute symptoms pertaining to another system, the complaints can be modified as:

Twinkle, 7 yr old girl child, previously diagnosed to have congenital cyanotic heart disease, is now brought for abnormal body movements for 2 days and altered sensorium since 1 PM today.

Chronically-ill children without added symptoms may be brought for internal or external assessment of the students at times. The complaints on such occasions need to be modified as:

"Shyam, 1.5 yr old infant, already on treatment for liver problems, is presently brought for follow-up assessment as directed by the

doctor"(should not present to the examiner that the child is brought for examination purpose).

Long duration symptoms should be stated from the date of onset of illness.

Example: "Sona, 5 yr old girlchild is having abnormal movements involving the whole body from the 7th day of life onward and is brought for follow-up".

Review the treatment documents after entering personal data and then focus on the history. Patients or parents feel awkward if the initial treatment documents are ignored by the doctor. Read them carefully; give a nice comment even if the contents are poor. Sometimes the parent may hand over the documents and remain quiet thinking that further detailing is not necessary; they should be encouraged to speak the details so that more details can be collected.

Never be irritated with patients and parents; if they persist with unnecessary details, guide them to get relevant points.

Children who have already recovered from an illness may report for an expert opinion after getting treatment from one hospital. The complaints may then be stated as:

"Chandran, 1.5 yr old infant, was getting treatment for pneumonia for the past 10 days. He is presently asymptomatic but is brought for an expert opinion".

The reason may be that the parents would like to know whether further investigations and preventive measures are to be taken because someone else known to them would have died of a similar illness.

The doctor must be aware of the confusing complaints given by parents—nasal discharge may be stated as fever, rigors as seizures, pallor as edema or jaundice, breath holding spells as seizures, etc. With appropriate leading questions, the exact problem should be made out.

Key points

Write the chief complaints in chronological order, restricted to three or four; evaluate carefully and show respect to the treatment documents brought by the patient.

HISTORY OF PRESENT ILLNESS

The details of present illness may be elicited from the child whenever possible with age appropriate questioning. Then ask the parents to provide those details which the child is unable to give. Find out the exact date of onset of illness by asking *"When was the child last apparently well?".* Each complaint has to be elaborated and stated in medical terminology.

Example: Reema, 1 yr old baby girl, had mild fever since 4 PM with three episodes of vomiting. The fever increased in intensity at night. By 10 PM she developed one episode of abnormal movement suggestive of seizure of generalized tonic clonic type lasting for about 15 min followed by unconsciousness. She was taken to the local hospital immediately. The unconsciousness lasted for 30 min till some parenteral medicines were given in the hospital".

The evolution of problems leading up to the presenting illness, should flow clearly and sequentially. Get the precipitating factors according to the parents view, the remedial measures taken, and the response to treatment. Educated parents will be able to report the name, dose, frequency, and duration of the medicines given. These details will help the doctor plan the next step of treatment.

Elicit the negative history **(Box 6.2)** by asking relevant questions so that the involvement of other systems can be found out by simple clinical analysis.

Symptom analysis should be done in detail. Discuss the sensitive issues regarding emotional or behavioral problems of children

BOX 6.2: Eliciting the negative history.

Reema, 1 yr old infant—history of (H/O) fever, vomiting three episodes, one episode of complex febrile seizure—1 day

- Ask for—H/O irritability, fall, recent trauma, past history (P/H) of fever with seizures, family history (F/H) of afebrile seizures—to excludes CNS problems
- Any H/O food intake from the food court? Was the vomitus bilious/projectile/bloody? Any loose stools?—can rule out (R/O) food poisoning, intestinal obstruction
- Ask the amount and type of fluids given after vomiting? Plain water/oral rehydration solution (ORS)/ORS equivalent? How much?—Helps to assess the fluid and electrolyte replacement
- Ask about the urine passed passed last; What was the quantity and color of urine?—Helps to assess the renal status

in their absence only. Specific questioning is required for complaints regarding the diseases of different organs and systems (refer to respective chapters). Pain, fever, diarrhea, weight loss, and poor appetite are the very common general symptoms in children. Collect the following points at least regarding these complaints:

- *Pain*—location, intensity, character, onset, duration, frequency, associated symptoms, radiation, aggravating and relieving factors, interference with routine activities and sleep, and the details of medicines taken [some children may not report the exact details due to stranger fear (doctor, hospital staff), scared of injections or fear of getting hospitalized].

  In nonverbal children having pain parents will be able to express the intensity by the lack of interest in play activities, not getting consoled by comfort measures (cuddling, feeding) and the requirement and response for analgesics. Pain can be objectively rated in young children by asking a "little bit" "moderate amount" or "a lot" by opposing the index and thumb and by increasing the distance between the fingers.

  Faces Scales is a widely used pain rating cartoon method **(Fig. 7.20)** especially beneficial for nonverbal children.

- *Fever*—Assess the intensity, duration, diurnal variation (evening rise of temperature), rigors, associated symptoms such as chills, dysuria, abdominal/limb/throat pain, headache, ear pain, limping, body swelling, loose stools, and infected wounds.
- *Diarrhea* is the passage of watery stools (watery defined as the fecal matter which spreads over the shape of the occupying surface) at least three times in a day. Confirm the watery nature of the stool and its approximate quantity, bloody, or foul smelling, frequency of the stools, associated fever and its nature, history of food ingestion from any outside sources, etc. Whether the child is thirsty (will demand fluids and drink eagerly), associated vomiting (frequency and quantity of vomiting, whether bilious, bloody, or with fecal odor), frequency, volume and color of urine, the type and quantity of fluids and food given, and also the details of treatment taken.
- *Weight loss or poor growth*—How did the parents assess the problem, duration, how much weight loss, was it documented, what was the weight/height last measured, when and by whom? Enquire about eating habits, pica, play and activities, details of illnesses, school performance, and food faddism.
- *Poor appetite and eating*—Duration, food faddism, pica (eating inedible things such as sand, mud, soap, cotton, thread, pencil tip, raw rice), frequent snacks in between, parental attitude toward diet, supplementation of vitamins and other health boosting tonic, presence of food allergy, and details of growth assessment.

- *Evaluate the documents of the previous consultations/investigations* done and the treatment details, avoiding adverse comments.

Key points

Symptom analysis and negative history are helpful to assess the involvement of other organs/systems and to detect the cause of the illness.

HISTORY OF PAST ILLNESS

Record analysis: Verify the infant and health visitor records and baby books for disease assessment. Enquire the relevant details regarding the child's past illness, related or unrelated to the present illness and the details of treatment received. They include history of hospital admissions, common childhood illnesses such as diarrhea, respiratory infections, seizures, asthma, allergic disorders, malaria, exanthemata, pertussis, tuberculosis, urinary tract infections, etc. Document all in chronological order and according to the age of occurrence.

Key points

Treatment details should be documented. Enquire drug compliance, treatment with alternate systems of medicines for health improvement and details of drug allergy.

If the presenting illness has direct relation to the events in prenatal or perinatal period, it is ideal to start history of present illness from that period onward as revealed in the following text:

Sunitha, 3 m old baby girl, first born of a nonconsanguineous marriage with uneventful antenatal period is brought for abnormal movements from the 1st day of life onward. The delivery was full term vaginal, but had prolonged labor pains for 24 hrs. First cry was delayed and she was given bag and mask ventilation. Before giving breastfeeding, baby developed abnormal movements, was shifted to neonatal intensive care unit (NICU) and was treated there for 4 days. Could start direct breastfeeding on the 7th day of life. She was treated in the recovery room for 1 week more and was discharged on 11th day of life as she was seizure free for 24 hrs. The seizures recurred on the next day and the baby was readmitted and treated. After that there were repeated seizures and the baby is on medications; in spite of treatment the baby used to get seizures.

Menstrual history details in older girls (young girls if pubertal changes are seen) are to be analyzed; the points to be elicited are age of attaining menarche, whether the cycles are normal/irregular, menstrual flow scanty or excess, details of associated symptoms such as severe pain and vomiting, and the remedial measures taken for the problems. Abnormal uterine bleeding is considered if larger clots of 1 inch are passed, pads >5/day are required or bleeding persists >7 days. Cycles repeating before 21 days is also abnormal. Advise the need of iron therapy in the menstrual age group girls.

Key points

Baby books and health visitor records are helpful for diagnosis. In girls nearing adolescence obtain details of menstrual history.

ANTENATAL HISTORY

Document all points which include maternal age of the present pregnancy, birth order, H/O abortion/stillbirth, whether planned normal pregnancy or conceived after infertility treatment, if so what was the infertility problem and type of treatment received, the maternal medical supervision and immunization and iron folic acid supplementation received in the present pregnancy. The details of maternal nutrition and iron intake during adolescence and periconceptional folic acid intake (for all women during their reproductive years folic acid 400 μg/day is advised to prevent neural tube defects) and the day of perception of fetal movements by the mother (quickening) should be enquired. Maternal problems related to pregnancy (diabetes mellitus, toxemias, hypertension, antepartum hemorrhage, and anemia) are detrimental to the fetus. Maternal diseases of STARCH complex (syphilis, toxoplasma, AIDS, rubella, cytomegalovirus, and herpes simplex), other viral infections including corona virus disease of 2019 (COVID 19), exposure to irradiation and intake of drugs for any other illness during pregnancy, and the details of antenatal ultrasonography (USG) done and abnormalities detected should all be evaluated.

Key points

Periconceptional folic acid therapy to the mother prevents neural tube defects in the baby.

NATAL HISTORY

Enquire the details of delivery, and document the important problems, whether domiciliary, full term/preterm/postterm, spontaneous or induced, method of induction and the drug used for induction (e.g., oxytocin), normal/assisted/cesarean section (CS), the indication for CS, duration of each stage of labor and complications, interventions done, and drugs given to the mother during labor. If the delivery was conducted at home, the reason should be clarified. Ask the length of labor (prolonged or precipitous) because birth asphyxia and birth injuries can occur in these situations.

The average *length of the first stage of labor* (from the onset of true labor pains to full dilatation of the cervix characterized by bearing down pain) can be 7 hr in the nulliparous women to 4 hr in multiparous women. The *second stage of labor* (from the full dilatation of the cervix to the delivery of the baby) usually lasts for 50 min in nulliparous to 20 min in multiparous women. The *third stage of labor* (delivery of the placenta) lasts for 15 min. Prolongation of the third stage may cause postpartum bleeding in the mother as well as delay in breast-feeding initiation and inadequate baby care. Details of any postpartum problem or birth injuries encountered and the immediate care given should be enquired. Verify the details from mother and baby cards if available.

POSTNATAL HISTORY

Collect the details of baby (Ref. Ch. 14) immediately after delivery which include birth weight, maturity, Apgar score (Ref. **Table 14.1**), first cry (spontaneous, good quality, or after resuscitation?), color change (cyanosis, pallor, and jaundice), bleeding from any site, and activity (good activity of limbs and alertness or limp and drowsy baby). Meconium and urine should be passed within 24–48 hr respectively after delivery. Ask the time of first feeding and problems related to it (as frothing from the mouth, vomiting, poor sucking, and abdominal distension), abnormal movements, fever, respiratory distress, cyanosis, or bleeding from any body part. Document the time of initiation of breastfeeding, maternal fever, day of umbilical cord stump falling, and details of treatment in the first month of baby's life.

Key points

The details of problems encountered in delivery, baby details and treatment provided should be documented.

DEVELOPMENTAL HISTORY

Development is the maturation of functions or the acquisition of skills and it proceeds parallel to the age and growth of the baby. This ability is promoted by the nervous and locomotor systems and the special senses. History should be tailored according to the age of the child and the nature of the disease. In children primarily presenting with developmental delay or suspecting such problems, detailed history should be elicited (Ref. Ch. 12). In older children with good scholastic performance and physical activity, it is irrelevant to ask for the age of social smile, vocalization, standing, walking, etc.

Elicit the developmental history under six domains—gross motor (GM), fine motor-adaptive (FM-A), cognitive, language, vision, and hearing.

- *GM development* is the acquisition of skills to promote locomotion and depends on the integrity of neurologic and locomotor systems. The skills attained are head control, rolling over, crawling, sitting, standing, walking, running, and jumping.
- *FM-A behavior* facilitates the skills for purposeful manipulation of hands along with eye coordination; the skills attained are handling dolls and play materials, eating, writing, drawing, painting, and sculpting. This domain reflects the intellectual capacity of the child along with the neurologic and locomotor systems.
- *Cognitive development* denotes the interpersonal and social skills (what the family and society expects from the child) such as social smile, stranger recognition, play activities, peer and family relations, imitative behavior, interaction with other people, school performance, and bowel, bladder control.

Personal habits of the child should be enquired. They are eating, bowel habits, urine voiding and bladder control, sleeping pattern, physical activity, speech, playing, and peer group relationship. Problems in eating present as fussy and picky eating, quarreling at eating times and frequent vomiting without any organic cause. Food allergies should be excluded, if the baby has inadequate weight gain. Abnormal bowel habits are constipation and encopresis (persistent soiling of the undergarments after the age of achieving bowel control [4 yr]). Improper bladder control manifests as dribbling, involuntary passing of urine irrespective of the circumstances and enuresis after the age of attaining bladder control by 5 yrs. Children with sleep disorders present as late sleepers, reveal difficulty in getting to sleep, have frequent night terrors, somnambulism, and frequent waking up with inconsolable crying. Hyperactive children reveal constant activity as reckless running or jumping, get self-injured often, and reveal destructive habits and aggressive behavior to peer groups often injuring them. Abnormal play activities present as lone play or stereotype playing. Delay in speech development, repetition of words, regression of speech, and poor peer interactions indicate autistic features.

- *Confirm vision and hearing* in all children at the first visit itself. In a child with normal hearing and vision, deficits in cognitive and language capacity point to intellectual subnormality, developmental deviation, or defective environmental stimulation.

Key points

Elicit developmental history under six domains in all young children; screen for vision and hearing at the first visit itself.

How to suspect developmental delay? First verify whether the agewise target milestones of the child are achieved by asking simple questions to the mother as detailed in ***Table 6.1*** *along with observation. If delayed, collect detailed history in each domain and assess the developmental age of the child along with the mother's reporting. Use it as the baseline information for developmental assessment as given in Chapter 12.*

TABLE 6.1: Key developmental milestones-birth to 5 yr

Age/m	*Gross motor*	*Fine motor*	*Cognitive*	*Language*	*Vision*	*Hearing*
Birth	Moves head to side. Asymmetric tonic neck reflex (ATNR	Hands closed	Sleeps 18 hr	Cries when uneasy	Fixation of vision on examiners face	Startle reflex
1	Head lags	Visual following 90°	Sleeps 14 hr		Mother regard	Quiets to voice
2	Prone-lifts chin off mattress		Social smile		Visual following 180°	
3	Neck holding, ATNR disappears	Hands mostly open	Mother recognition	Cooing	Visual following 180° vertically	Turns to familiar voice in supine
4		Grasps rattle when placed in hands		Laughs aloud	Recognizes familiar toy	Turns head towards a sound
5	Sits with support	Bidextrous approach	Smiles at mirror image		Smiles at mirror image	Listens to conversation
6	Rolling over	Hand to hand transfer, mouthing	Smiles at mirror image	Monosyllables 'ba'' ma'	Sees and recognizes at adult distance	Turns to sounds when sitting
7	Bounces on standing	Holds objects with crude palmar grasp	Stranger anxiety		Looks at falling objects	Responds to own name
8	Sits without support		Understands 'No'	Nonspecific 'mama'		
9	Crawls, pivots	Explores objects	Mouthing of objects	Recognizes familiar words	Sees crumbs on floor	Locates sounds at greater distance
10	Stands with support	Assisted pincer grasp	Plays peak–a boo. Waves bye-bye	Specific 'dada' 'mama'		
11	Cruises around objects	Unassisted pincer grasp		Follows gesture command		
12	Stands without support. Takes first step	Turns pages of book 3 to 4 at a time. Puts objects in container	Plays simple ball games	2–3 words with meaning	Recognizes pictures of objects	Recognizes tunes
13	Walks without support. Dances to music. Sits Down from standing	Points with fingers. Spontaneous scribbling	Demands attention. Separation anxiety. Temper tantrums	3–4 words in addition to mama, dada	Visual fixation on rolling balls	-do-
14	Climbs stairs on hands and knees	Cooperates in dressing	Self play. Likes an audience. Fear of darkness	Names all family members	-do-	-do-

Contd...

Contd...

Age/m	*Gross motor*	*Fine motor*	*Cognitive*	*Language*
15	Walks alone. Gets into constant movement	Spoon feeds. Marks with pencil. Builds tower with cubes. Puts pellets in bottle. Likes push pull toys	Hugs parents. Indicates needs by pointing and when wet	• Jargon. Follows simple commands • May name a familiar object
16	Sits on a chair		Hunts for missing parents	Enjoys explanation of pictures in book
17	Stands on one foot holding on chair		• Demands personal attention • Afraid of large animals	
18	Runs stiffly, walks upstairs with one hand held. Explores drawers	Handed ness is determined Imitates scribbling	Feeds self. Seeks help when in Trouble, complains when wet or soiled. Day time bladder control	• 10 words. Uses "NO" • Names pictures
19	Kicks ball	• Builds 3–4 block tower • Flushes toilet	Enjoys swing. Pulls wagon with toys inside	10–15 words. Likes to be read to
20	Jumps	Throws ball. Puts lid on box	Possessive about toys. Puts on shoes. Imaginary play " Tea party"	• Asks "what is that?" • Shows action "pick me up"
21	Walks up steps holding railing	Folds papers	Likes bugs and other small objects	Uses pronoun "I". Uses word combinations. Echolalia
22		• Unwraps packages • Puts beads together.	Starting to cooperate.	• Listens to stories • Repeats nursery rhymes
23	Walks up and down steps alone both feet on each step. Runs all the time	Likes to fill and empty water in bottles or vessels	• "Reads" books to self • Easily frustrated	Asks for food and drinks
24	Walks backward	Matches objects. Draws horizontal lines. Circular scribbling. Turns pages of book one at a time	Does not share. Avoids bed time. Parallel paly. Bowel control. Verbalizes toilet needs	Verbalizes. Puts 3 words together (subject, verb, object)

Contd...

Contd...

Age/m	***Gross motor***	***Fine motor***	***Cognitive***	***Language***
30	Goes upstairs on alternating feet	Makes tower of 9 cubes. Draws vertical and horizontal strokes	Helps to put things away Pretends in play	Refers to self by pronoun "I" knows full name
36	Rides tricycle. Stands momentarily on one foot	Copies a circle. Imitates a cross. Makes a tower of 10 cubes. Imitates construction of bridge of 3 cubes	Parallel play with other children. Unbuttons clothing. Puts on shoes Washes. Handedness established Knows gender	Knows age and sex. Counts 3 objects correctly. Repeats 3 numbers or a sentence of six syllables
48	• Hops on one foot. • Climbs well. Throws ball over head. Uses scissors to cut out pictures.	Copies cross and square. Draws man with 2–4 parts besides hands. Names longer of 2 lines.	Group play. Role play. Goes to toilet alone. Night time bladder control	• Tells a story • Counts 4 coins accurately
60	Skips	• Copies a triangle • Names heavier of 2 weights	Enjoys jokes and riddles. Dresses and undresses. Asks questions about the meaning of words. Domestic role playing full time bladder control	• Names 4 colors. Repeats sentences of 10 syllables. Counts 10 coins correctly. Delights reciting • Gives full birthday, home address

NUTRITIONAL HISTORY AND PRESENT DIET

Let food be thy medicine and medicine be thy food"—Hippocrates (460–370 BC)

This quote from the father of modern medicine reveals the significance of nutrition in maintaining health and the healing capacity of a healthy diet. Detailed history and critical evaluation of the child's diet are a must to enable the doctor to assess (1) whether the food is adequate, balanced, appropriate, and healthy for the age of the child, (2) the cause of growth aberrations, (3) micronutrient deficiency, (4) the presence of toxic elements in the diet, and (5) to provide proper diet advice. In children the requirements, eating pattern, and the type of diet differ substantially in the age groups of <6 m, 6 m–2 yrs, and >2 yrs.

Infants of <6 m age: Exclusive breastfeeding (mother's milk or human milk feeding) is declared as the right of all babies by the World Health Organization (*WHO) in 1989*, unless there are definite contraindications (mother on cancer chemotherapy, lithium and antithyroid medicines, and baby affected with galactosemia and congenital lactose intolerance).

Human milk is designed for human babies only and is superior to bovine milk in composition **(Table 6.2)**. Clarify the following points in feeding and give correct advice to the parent/caretaker, if needed. When was the first feeding given (as early as possible—should be within 1 hr after delivery)? If delayed, what was the reason? Any prelacteal feed given? If so, what was the feed and the reason for giving such a feed? Any pacifiers used? Prelacteal feeds and pacifiers cause infections and reduce the breast milk (BM) intake and should not be given. Is the baby taking night feeds? Promote night feeds so that BM output increases and it prolongs the BM yield.

Is the baby given any other milk, and if so, what is the reason? What is the type of milk given and the method of feeding (bottle, cup and spoon, or paladai)? Find out the dilution of preparing milk feeds. Did they get the doctor's advice for giving BM substitutes? Check whether the caretaker is observing proper hygiene in preparing the feed and giving it to the baby? Advise soap and water hand washing, cleaning and boiling the vessels,

TABLE 6.2: Nutritive values of human and animal milk (per 100 mL).

Parameters	*Human milk*	*Cow's milk*	*Buffalo's milk*	*Goat's milk*
Calories (kcal)	67	70	107	72
Proteins (g)	1.1*	3.3	4.3	3.3
Fats (g)	4.2†	4.5	6.6	4.1
Lactose (g)	7	4.7	5.2	4.5
Calcium (mg)	35	120	210	134
Phosphorus (mg)	14	90	130	111
Vitamin D (IU)	0.4–10	0.3–4		
Vitamin K (μg)	15	60		
Zinc (mg)	0.53	0.38		
Ash (g)	0.25	0.75	0.7	0.7

*High quality proteins—lactalbumin and lactoglobulin, easily digestible.
†Mainly polyunsaturated fatty acids.

and proper preparation of the feeds, if not breastfed. Instruct the caretaker not to dilute cow's milk. For preparing formula feeds the caretaker should be advised to follow the manufacturer's instructions.

Assess the adequacy of BM—Is the baby contented and goes to sleep for 2–3 hr after feeding? Voids urine 6–8 times/day? Gaining weight adequately (should be monitored). If the answer is "yes" for these questions BM is adequate for the baby. If the baby is restless or reveals frequent crying, consider hunger/colic/wet diaper/illness/maternal drug intake including alternate system of medicines for postnatal care. Feeding of the baby should be observed to assess whether the method is correct if the mother complains of scanty milk, or sore nipples or the baby has inadequate weight gain.

Enquire about vitamin D and iron therapy to the baby. Vitamin D 400 IU/day and elemental iron 1 mg/kg/day are advised for all babies during the first yr of life. Higher dose may be required, if the baby is preterm or low birth weight (LBW), since BM is low in vitamin D and iron content. Most queries regarding feeding of infants <6 m of age will be clarified by these questions.

The BM yield of a healthy mother is approximately 600 mL/day; most mothers yield more amounts for the initial 6 m of postnatal period. Thereafter, BM gets reduced to 30–60 mL/feed.

Key points

Practice exclusive breast feeding (BF) up to 6 m of age; night feeding increases BM yield; advise proper hygienic instructions for formula feeding. All babies require vitamin D and iron supplementation.

More than 6 m–2 yrs of age group: BF should be continued up to the age of 2.5 yrs.

Complementary feeds should be added at 6 m of age since the activity of the infant increases, and the increased calorie and nutrient demands cannot be met with BM alone by this age. Homemade items are ideal. Chewing capacity, mouthing and swallowing, and accepting food items of different tastes and flavor—all develop during 6–10 m of age period. Also, the nutrients stored in liver (vitamins A, D, and iron) come to a nadir by 6 m of age and micronutrients (nutrients with RDA <100 mg/day) need be supplied from other food items.

Complementary foods are items added to the infant diet at >6 m of age to meet the higher energy and nutrients (calcium, iron, and micronutrients) which include vitamins and minerals demand of the body. Such foods should be locally available, nutritious, tasty, affordable to the family, and easy to prepare. Ragi, banana, rice and wheat, processed as powder or soaked and prepared as porridge adding jaggery, and coconut milk/ghee are traditional Kerala items. Cooked and mashed potato and khichdi (mixture of cooked rice and moong dal mashed) are other items. The items should be soft and tasty and fed with a clean spoon or finger. Mother should be given detailing about such complementary foods, the items to select, and the method of preparation, as her baby reaches 5 m of age.

The BM yield after 6 m of age can be approximately calculated by the number of feeds given to the baby/day and multiplied by the quantity stated by the mother as adequate or scanty. The questions to be asked to clarify the diet are—Is the baby still breast fed? If not, what is the reason for stopping BF? What else is substituted for BM? How do they prepare the item? If cow's milk is given, how much is the dilution? How is it given—using a cup and spoon/paladai/bottle? Paladai **(Fig. 6.1)** is a popular device for feeding preterm and LBW babies until they can suck breast. BM (or the substitute) is expressed into the rounded part of the device. Tip of the beaked end (should not be very sharp) is placed at

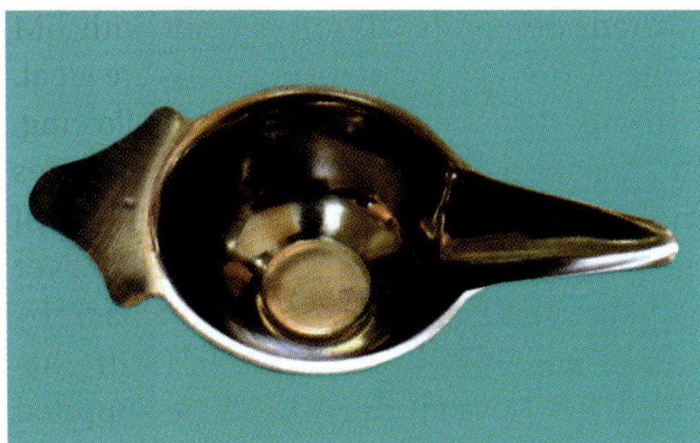

Fig. 6.1: Paladai.

the center of the baby's mouth to get the milk as drops.

Get the 24 hrs diet of the infant by recall method from the mother **(Table 6.3)**. With the help of the food value chart **(Table 6.4)**, calculate the calorie and protein content of homemade dietary items. After assessing all these together, calculate the actual intake of calories and proteins. Food items of equivalent nutritive value can be advised for acceptability of the child. Find out the deficiencies/excess in the diet and give advice regarding further feeding.

Key points

Continue BF up to 2.5 yrs of age; homemade and anganwadi complementary foods are superior to commercial products.

Enquire the changes in food given during illness: The common examples are nephrotic syndrome, diabetes mellitus, and metabolic diseases in which modifications in the diet would have been told to the parents by the doctor. Parents may restrict many food items to babies as per advice by the elders or neighbors. To increase the taste and calorie content add oil/ghee/butter to the items. Anganwadi infant foods can be given to babies as they are nutritious and free of cost.

Key points

Food restrictions made during illness with duration should be verified.

Compare the actual intake with recommended dietary allowances (RDA) for the age and sex from the Indian Council of Medical Research (ICMR) chart **(Table 6.5)** or by bedside calculation **(Box 6.3)** to find out the gap/excess in calories, proteins, vitamins, and minerals. Praise the mother if the diet is appropriate for her baby. If any deficiency is observed the statement can be: "The diet reveals a gap of —calories and —proteins as per ICMR recommendations and —calories by bedside calculation; it is inadequate in vitamin A, iron, trace elements, and proteins of high biological value". The ICMR recommendations are the ideal whereas bedside calculation is the minimum dietary requirements for a child. Explain the parents to correct the deficiencies, by increasing the quantity of food, feeding more calorie rich foods (*upma*, *pongal*, nuts, and seeds), giving small feeds in between, adding calorie dense items on food (coconut milk, oils, ghee, butter, sugar/jaggery, ice cream, and fried items). If the intake is high and the child is overweight explain the situation to the parents (and the child if old enough). Advise to reduce the quantity of food, oily and sweet items, and add more raw and cooked vegetables. Screen time should be reduced and physical activity should be increased. Also, never forget to compliment a mother revealing good child rearing practices with good eating habits.

Key points

The doctor should have reasonable knowledge of the locally available common food materials, their food values, and the preparation of the complementary diet for the baby so as to advise the mother. Deficiencies or excess in the present diet should be pointed to the family to be corrected. Physical activity should be promoted, if the child is obese.

TABLE 6.3: 24 hr diet of a baby boy of 1.5 yr prepared by recall method.

Time	*Item*	*Quantity*	*Calories (as kcals)*	*Proteins (g)*
6 AM	Breast milk (BM)*	Give after each meal 6–7 times/day (250 mL/day)	167	2.75
8 AM	• Idli • Plantain	1 1	50 50	2 0.5
	Sambar	3 tsp	20	1
10.30 AM	Banana fry	1	150	1
12.30 noon	Cooked rice	1 cup†	175	4
	Fish	½ ounce	40	3
	Cooked dal	3 tsp	20	1
	Veg curry	4 tsp	10	0.5
4 PM	Egg	1	80	6
	Biscuits	5 numbers	100	2.5
7 PM	Kanji	1 cup†	175	4
	Green gram	4 tsp	30	1.5
Total			*1,067 kcal*	*29.75 g*

Note: Calorie yield of nutrients (kcals/1 g): Proteins—4; Carbohydrates—4; Fats—9.
*Approximate amount 250 mL/day; tsp = teaspoon (5 mL). Vegetarians—replace fish and egg with curd and pulses.
†1 cup = 150 mL

TABLE 6.4: Recommended dietary allowances (RDA) for children ICMR—updated 2023.

Age	*Energy (kcal)*	*Proteins (g)*	*Fat (g/d)*	*Retinol (µg/d)*	*Calcium (mg/d)*	*Fe (mg/d)*	*Vitamin D (IU)*
0–6 m	92/kg/day	1.16 g/kg/day	–	350	500	0.46	400
7–12 m	80/kg/day	1.69 g/kg/day	19	350	500	0.5	400
1–3 yr	1,060/day	16.7 g/day	27	400	600	9	400
4–6 yr	1,350/day	20.1 g/day	25	400	600	13	400
7–9 yr	1,690/day	29.5 g/day	30	600	600	16	400
10–12 yr	*Boy:* 2,190/day *Girl:* 2,010/day	39.9 g/day 40.4 g/day	35 35	600 600	800 800	21 27	400 400
13–15 yr	*Boy:* 2,750/day *Girl:* 2,330/day	54.3 g/day 51.9 g/day	45 40	600 600	800 800	32 27	400 400
16–18 yr	*Boy:* 3,020/day *Girl:* 2,440/day	61.5 g/day 52.5 g/day	22 35	600 600	800 800	28 26	400 400

Note: Corrections on nursing mother's diet—mother with moderate activity normally requires 2,230 cals/day; to this add 600 cal and 74 g proteins/day for breast feeding (BF) for the baby up to 6 m of age; 520 cals and 68 g proteins/day for BF the babies of >6 m of age; calcium 1,200 mg/day.

TABLE 6.5: Nutritional value of local and homemade food items.

Items	*Quantity*	*Calories (kcal)*	*Protein (g)*	*Vitamins*	*Minerals*
Cow's milk	1 cup (180 mL)	120	6	A, B, K	Ca, P, K, I, Zn
Cooked rice	1 cup (150 mL)	175	4	B, A, D	Fe, Ca, P, Se
Ragi flour	6 tsp	100	2	B, A, D	Fe, Ca, P, Se
Egg	1	80	6	A, D, B	Ca, P, Fe
Fish	1 Oz	80	6	A, D, B	Ca, P, Mg, Se, I
Meat	1 Oz	80	6	B, K	Fe, P, Cu, Zn, Se, Cr, Mg, K, I
Dosai	1	70	2	B, E	Mg, Cr, Fe, Ca, P, Se
Idli	1	50	2	B, E	Mg, Cr, Fe, Ca, P, Se
Chapati	1	70	2	B, A, D	Fe, Ca, P, Se
Appam	1	70	1	B, E	Fe, Ca, P, Se
Bread	1 slice (1 Oz)	70	2	B, E	Fe, Ca, P, Se
Puri	1	35	1	B, A, D	Fe, Ca, P, Se
Vada/bonda	1	50	1	B, K, A, D	Fe, P, Cu, Zn, Se, Cr
Cooked dal	1 tsp	10	0.5	B, K	Fe, P, Cu, Zn, Se, Cr
Plantain	1	50	0.5	A, B, C	K, Cu
Upma	1 cup	250	6	B, A, D	Fe, Ca, P, Se
Sugar	1 tsp	20	0	0	0
Jaggery	1 tsp	20	0	B	Ca, Fe, Cr
Ghee/butter	1 tsp	40	0	A, D, B	Ca, K, P
Mashed potato	1 tsp	40	0	A	K, Mg
Nuts/seeds	100 g	615	19	A, D	Fe, Cu, Ca, P, I, Mg, Cr
Pappadom	1	20	0.5	B, K, A, D	Fe, Ca, P
Biscuit	1	20	0.5	B, A	Fe, Ca, P, Zn
Tapioca (tubers, roots)	100 g	157	0.7	0	K, Mg
Green vegetables	100 g	46	1–2	A, B, K, D	Fe, Ca, K, Mg, I
Other vegetables	100 g	50	0.5–2	A, B	K, Mg, I
Pongal	1 cup	415	10	B, A, D	Fe, Ca, K, Se
Grated fresh coconut	100 g	354	3.3		

Note: Measures—1 ounce (Oz = 28.4 g, 1 teaspoon = 5 mL (5 g), 1 g = 1 mL), 1 medium cup = 150 mL, 1 teacup (large) = 180 mL (180 g).

BOX 6.3: Recommended dietary allowances (RDA) for calories as per bedside calculation.

- *Up to 1 yr of age: Required calories = 100 cals/kg* (*expected weight for age)*
- *More than 1 yr of age: Required calories = 1,000 + (age in yr – 1 × 100)*

IMMUNIZATION HISTORY

Verify the vaccines received from the baby book for reliability. If it is not available, document the details with the approximate dates of immunization as reported by the parents. The reasons for missing any vaccine and complications or adverse events following immunization should be enquired. Advise the parent for completion of the schedule with prompt administration of missed doses. Verify the presence of BCG scar.

Changes in vaccination schedule occur depending on newer vaccines introduced and emergence of endemic areas for certain infectious diseases; parents may not be aware of it. **Table 6.6** gives the current National Immunization Schedule in India.

TABLE 6.6: National Immunization Schedule in India—January 1st, 2023 onward.

Age	*Vaccines advised*
Birth	BCG, OPV-0, Hepatitis B birth dose
6 w	OPV-1, Pentavalent-1*, RVV-1†, fIPV-1‡, PCV-1§
10 w	OPV-2, Pentavalent-2, RVV-2, PCV-2
14 w	OPV-3, Pentavalent-3 + fIPV-2, RVV-3, PCV-3
9–12 m	Measles and Rubella (MR)-1, Japanese Encephalitis (JE)-1‖ in endemic districts only
16–24 m	MR-2, JE-2‖, DPT-booster-1, OPV-booster
5–6 yr	DPT-booster-2
10 yr	Tetanus and adult Diphtheria (Td)
16 yr	Td
Pregnancy	Td1, 2, or Td-booster¶

*Diphtheria, tetanus, whooping cough (pertussis) (DPT) + hepatitis B (HBV) + *Haemophilus influenzae* type b (Hib)
†Rota virus vaccine
‡Fractional dose of inactivated polio vaccine
§Pneumococcal conjugate vaccine
‖In endemic areas only
¶One dose, if previously vaccinated within 3 yr

FAMILY HISTORY

Enquire the age and health details of parents, siblings, and other family members. Healthcare of children of single mothers, divorced, or step parents may not be adequate; they are more vulnerable for malnutrition, infections, infestations, and battered baby syndrome.

Enquire regarding consanguinity [*con* (with) *sanguine* (blood) *ity*], i.e., sharing the same blood between parents (which predisposes the offspring to acquire more inherited diseases). **Table 6.7** reveals the degree of consanguinity, the amount of genetic material shared, and the type of relatives. Higher the degree of consanguinity, more is the probability for inherited disorders.

History of previous abortions, stillbirths, death due to unknown diseases, birth of abnormal children, and presence of inherited diseases in the family as well as among close blood relatives are to be elicited. Details of long-standing illnesses in parents and medicines taken (whether regular or not), communicable diseases among family members, and family planning methods adopted by the parents, all should be recorded.

If the history reveals hereditary diseases in the family, get the details of a wider circle of relatives and prepare the pedigree chart, using accepted symbols as revealed in **Fig. 6.2**.

TABLE 6.7: Degree of consanguinity and percentage of shared genes between relatives.		
Degree of consanguinity	***% of shared genes***	***Relative groups***
1 degree	50%	Parents to children, between siblings
2 degree	25%	Uncle to niece, aunt to nephew, grandparent to grandchild
3 degree	12.5%	Between first cousins

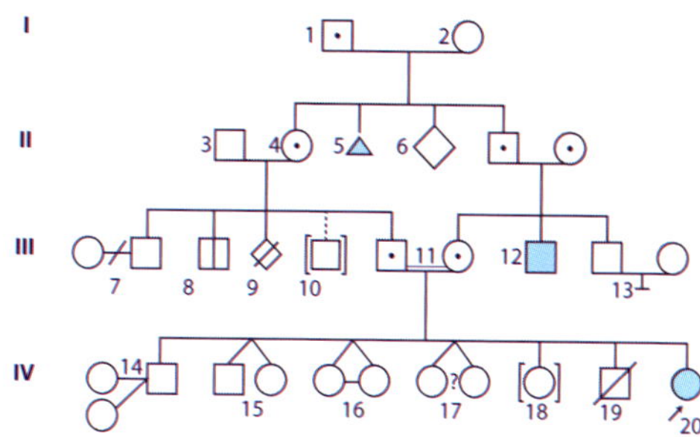

Fig. 6.2: Pedigree chart or genogram. [1: Obligate carrier male; 2: Normal female; 3: Normal male; 4: Obligate carrier female (no overt disease); 5: Miscarriage; 6; Sex unspecified; 7; Divorced; 8; Nonpenetrant carrier (may manifest disease); 9; Stillbirth; 10; Adopted into the family; 11: Consanguineous marriage; 12: Affected male; 13: No offspring; 14: Multiple unions; 15: Unidentical twins; 16: Identical twins; 17: Twins of unknown zygosity; 18: Adopted out of family; 19: Deceased male; 20: Affected female or the Index case]

A pedigree chart or genogram is a clear and informative diagram of the family history and illustrates the relationship of family members, so that within a small space maximum messages can be conveyed. A complicated family history can be better represented by such a chart as in **Fig. 6.2**. and will be an effective screening tool to detect inherited disorders.

Drawing the family pedigree should begin with parents and cover three generations if any genetic disease is suspected. Generation in the pedigree chart is identified by Roman numerals on the left end and the location of the affected persons by Arabic numerals close to the symbol. Siblings are arranged in decreasing age from left to right.

Key points

Assess whether immunization is updated; sort out the degree of consanguinity in the family circle; pedigree chart of the family quickly picks up inherited diseases and their type.

SOCIOECONOMIC HISTORY

Social background and economic status of the family play important roles in the severity and outcome of diseases. Hence, such details are highly necessary to detect the reasons of diseases and to eliminate them at grass root level. The data on occupation, education, and income of parents, and the income of all family members should be collected to assess the socioeconomic grading (SEG), which should be according to the accepted standards of the country. Kuppuswamy socioeconomic scale (KSS) periodically updated is widely accepted for classifying the SEG **(Table 6.8)** in India. The higher the total score, better will be the living conditions, child rearing, feeding, care given, environmental stimulation, and academic as well as extracurricular achievements of the children in that family.

Social customs detrimental to the baby are applying *kajal* to the baby's eyes, cow dung to the umbilical stump, instilling oil to the nostrils and then blowing it forcefully, discarding colostrum, and giving pacifiers and bottle feeding. Such practices definitely produce infections and should be abolished. Good practices are personal and environmental cleanliness, adequate

TABLE 6.8: Modified Kuppuswamy scale (MKSS) (updated 2023).

A: The scoring system used for the education and occupation of the head of the family

Parameters	***Score***
Education:	
• Professional degree	7
• Graduate	6
• Intermediate/diploma	5
• High school	4
• Middle school	3
• Primary	2
• Illiterate	1
Occupation:	
• Legislators, senior officials, and managers	10
• Professional	9
• Technician/associate professionals	8
• Clerk	7
• Skilled worker, shop and market sales workers	6
• Skilled agricultural and fishery workers	5
• Craft and related trade workers	4
• Plant and machine operators and assemblers	3
• Elementary occupation	2
• Unemployed	1

B: Total monthly income of the family

Updated monthly family income in Rupees (June 2023)	***Score***
≥146,104	12
109,580–146,103	11
73,054–109,579	10
68,455–73,053	9
63,854–68,454	8
59,252–63,853	7
54,651–59,251	6
45,589–54,650	5
36,527–45,588	4
21,914–36,526	3
7,316–21,913	2
≤7,315	1

Contd...

Contd...

C: Modified Kuppuswamy socioeconomic classes based on total score (Tables A + B + C)

Total score	***Socioeconomic class***
26–29	Upper (I)
16–25	Upper middle (II)
11–15	Lower middle (III)
5–10	Upper lower (IV)
<5	Lower (V)

physical activity, reading, selective television (TV)/screen viewing, helping nature, good relationships and communication between family members, peers, and with neighbors, healthy eating (eating the family diet at family meal time, along with family members), and sleeping habits. Children brought up in such circumstances reveal good personal relationships, helping nature, family bonding, and better achievements in life.

ENVIRONMENTAL HISTORY

The environment of the child is the house, its premises, and the school. The approachability to the house and school, transport facilities, overall awareness of medical aid and cleanliness of the area are of top priority. The house located near large markets or in large forest areas have health hazards.

Assess the internal environment contributed by the quality of the house—hut, tiled or concrete with well-finished flooring, and the number of rooms available. Overcrowding (more than two persons sharing one room) transmit airborne infections more. Poor ventilation of the rooms, unfinished or cow dung made floor, dirty carpets and upholstery, rearing pet animals inside the house (cats, dogs), domestic animals (cow, goat, buffalo) and birds (lovebirds, hen, duck) close to the house, pest infestation (cockroaches), biomass use, passive smoking, chemicals and paints storage, and carpentry work inside the house—all cause pollution leading to frequent infections and allergic diseases in children. Contact with infectious diseases, availability of safe drinking water, sanitary toilet facilities, and proper waste disposal should be asked. Details of environmental pollution are important to eliminate many health problems such as airborne infections, hyperreactive airway disease, diarrhea, parasitic infestations, skin and enteric diseases, and food and drinking water pollution. External air and water pollution can be from careless garbage disposal, poultry farms, cattle sheds, and small/large scale industries/workshops or from factories around the house and motor vehicles.

Key points

Assessing the socioeconomic and environmental factors are highly important to find out the disease etiology at the grassroot level and to eliminate the risk factors.

PRESENTING THE HISTORY

The situations faced by the student or a junior doctor in history presentation are (1) case discussion in the regular teaching sessions, (2) presentation during examinations, (3) reporting to the faculty in the outpatient department/ward rounds, or (4) reporting to a specialist to whom the patient is being referred.

The parent has to be given the option to add any further points in history at the end. Before the presentation, read the write up, recapitulate the details to make it clearer, brief, and point projected. Include only the relevant points during presentation. The narration should be in English using short and simple sentences. If the appropriate word in English is not found, use the patient's word in the same language. Try to finish the presentation in time.

Example: Sajeeda, 7 yr old girl, second child of parents with 3rd degree consanguinity has chest pain and dyspnea for 1 w (acute illness, affecting respiratory and/or cardiovascular systems).

- *3 w back, she had fever and throat pain (probably of infective or inflammatory etiology).*
- *This was followed by migrating polyarthritis which lasted for 4 days (most characteristic of acute rheumatic fever).*
- *Her father is a coolie earning INR 3,000/m and the family belongs to the low socioeconomic group—MKSS V.*
- *The 6 member family lives in a small thatched house (near a fish market) having one bedroom with a small window (where all of them sleep), kitchen, and an open veranda (overcrowded house, close to a fish market—all reveal unhealthy living environment).*
- *For the fever and joint pain, tablets from a local pharmacy (without the doctor's consultation) were given to her for 3 days (improper treatment).*

The history reveals that Sajeeda is having acute rheumatic fever with cardiac complications. The type of cardiac involvement can be diagnosed only by careful examination of the patient and diagnostic investigations.

SUGGESTED READING

1. Bennett RL, Steinhaus KA, Uhrich SB, O'Sullivan CK, Resta RG, Lochner-Doyle D, et al Recommendations for standardized pedigree nomenclature. J Genet Counsel. 1995;4(4):267-79.
2. Elizabeth KE. Nutrition and Child Development, 4th edition. Hyderabad, India: Paras Publishers; 2016. pp. 18-9.
3. ICMR. (2017). Nutritive value of human and bovine milk; Indian Food Composition Tables,

National Institute of Nutrition, ICMR, 2017. [online] Available from https://www.nin.res.in/ebooks/IFCT2017.pdf. [Last accessed September, 2024].

4. ICMR. (2017). Nutritive value of Indian foods; Indian Food Composition Tables, National Institute of Nutrition, ICMR, 2017. [online] Available from https://www.nin.res.in/ebooks/IFCT2017.pdf. [Last accessed September, 2024].
5. ICMR. (2020). RDA-National Institute of Nutrition, India. [online] Available from https://www.nin.res.in./RDA_Full_Report_2020. [Last accessed September, 2024].
6. Kliegman R, St. Geme III JW. Nelson Textbook of Pediatrics, 21st edition. Philadelphia: Elsevier Health Sciences; 2019.
7. NHM. 2018. Intensified Mission Indradhanush 5.0 Operational guidelines_240216_015005_copy.pdf, Page 75. [online] Available from https://nhm.gov.in/New_Updates_2018/NHM_Components/Immunization/Guildelines_for_immunization/Mission_Indradhanush_Guidelines.pdf. [Last accessed September, 2024].
8. Park K. Park's Textbook of Preventive and Social Medicine, 24th edition. Madhya Pradesh, India: Banarsidas Bhanot Publishers; 2015.
9. Radhakrishnan M, Nagaraja SB. Modified Kuppuswamy socioeconomic scale 2023: stratification and updates. Int J Community Med Public Health. 2023;10(11):4415-8.

7 CHAPTER

General Physical Examination

S Sushamabai

Chapter Outline

- Introduction
- Getting the Cooperation
- Preparations for Patient Assessment
- Schema of General Examination
- Clinical Case Scenarios

INTRODUCTION

Please read Ch. 1, 2, 3, 4, and 6 before you proceed; For detailed evaluation of bones and joints read Ch. 25.

Physical examination of the patient should begin with general assessment to detect serious functional impairment of organs and systems requiring immediate care (Ref. Ch. 8) which should proceed parallel to the history. Patients requiring urgent life support should be spotted out rapidly by simple clinical signs and stabilized at the "Golden hour".

Compared to adults, physical examination of children needs more patience and tactfulness, and fast completion; lengthy examinations irritate children and their parents. As the values of vital parameters for different ages vary, the doctor should have the expertise to interpret the observed values quickly.

The outpatient room should provide maximum comfort to the child patient and the family as detailed in Ch. 2; strange instruments should be kept out of sight as the child may get frightened. The doctor should be mentally well prepared for the urgent management of difficult and sick patients 'encountered' at any time; at the same time to deal with the arrogant accompanying persons without any provocation. Experienced supporting staff and well-equipped emergency care services in functioning status should be available around the clock nearby.

Undressing the child each time should be partial only and should be done with the help of the caretaker always, to maintain cooperation, prevent hypothermia, and to avoid unnecessary allegations. For a crying baby, sufficient time should be provided to get the baby consoled. The nursing staff in the outpatient department (OPD) and emergency room (ER) should be enough experienced to provide gentle and expert care to sick and irritated babies. While examining adolescent girls a chaperone should be always present.

A systematic approach should be practiced as far as possible, but prioritize the system and techniques depending on the circumstances. Uncomfortable procedures such as examination of the throat, tympanic membranes, hips, and rectum should be reserved for the last, but the schema of presentation should be according to set pattern **(Box 7.1)**. Findings to be elicited at the end of the examination should be noted down using a different color ink to be completed later.

BOX 7.1: Schema of general exam.
- Appearance
- Vital signs
- Danger signs
- Head-to-foot examination

GETTING THE COOPERATION

Small babies (<3 m of age) may be placed on the caregiver's lap or the examination table for physical examination. Infants and toddlers (6 m to 3 yr) prefer to remain on the caregiver's lap and older children (>3 yr) would like to be offered a seat. Occasionally one may come across highly irritable and noncooperative children of age group from the newborn period even up to adolescence (due to illness or fright). Breastfeeding is an effective way to pacify young infants. For the age group from 6 m to 2 yr, distraction by colorful toys is possible. In the age group 2–4 yr, colored picture books of animals, birds, fruits, vegetables, vehicles, etc., attract children and make them much more comfortable cooperative **(Fig. 7.1)**.

Older children like to hear compliments (e.g., your nail polish/hairdo is so fine, who made it for you?) which will build up friendship rapidly (Ref. Ch. 2). Alternatively, a screaming and struggling child at the sight of the doctor/nurse reveals intact vision and stranger recognition and thus gives a rough assessment of the nervous system and developmental status. Sedation of a struggling child may be needed occasionally to examine the cardiovascular system or abdominal mass evaluation.

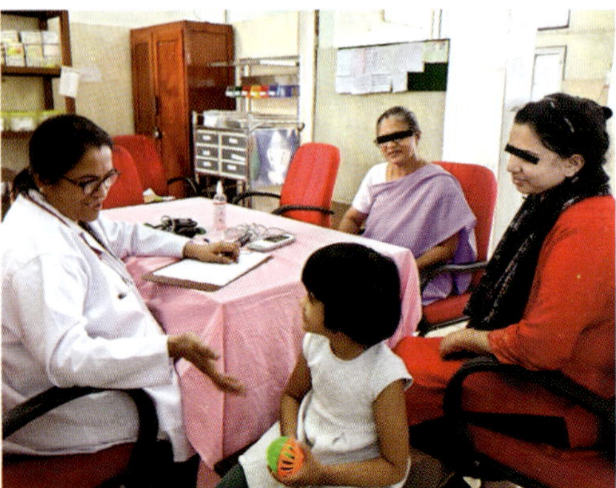

Fig. 7.1: Getting the cooperation of the youngster.

PREPARATIONS FOR PATIENT ASSESSMENT

- *The doctor* should be receptive with a welcoming smile and vigilant, searching eyes, sharp ears, and warm sensitive fingers (Ref. **Fig. 1.1**). Observe all aseptic precautions-wearing mask and sterile gown and practicing proper hand hygiene by soap and water washing or by applying hand sanitizer.
- *The tools* should include an updated pediatric stethoscope (Ref. Ch. 17), moderately bright torch light, fingertip pulse oximeter, nonstretchable tape, wooden tongue depressor, thermometers, sphygmomanometer with adequately sized cuffs (Ref. Ch. 17), pediatric knee hammer, hand lens (to assess skin lesions), and otoscope. Minimum materials for developmental screening should be at hand (a red bangle tied with a red string, a squeaky doll, few red pellets, and a small picture book of animals, birds, fruits, flowers, and vehicles). Additional tools for each system examination are specified in the concerned chapters.
- *Child and mother-friendly environment*: Warm, clean, well-aerated assessment room with white curtains and few attractive and informatory wall pictures.
- *An emergency room* near the OPD with adequate life-saving medicines and equipment, experienced, well-behaved, and adequately trained staff (doctor, nurse, and paramedical staff).

SCHEMA OF GENERAL EXAMINATION

Box 7.1 discusses how to proceed with examining the child brought to the OPD or ER.

Appearance

Is the child cheerful, alert, and cooperative, dull or inert, irritable or sick looking?

A sick child may remain with eyes closed and respond poorly to the mother's calling or may have open eyes with a *vacant aloof* look **(Fig. 7.2)**. Danger signs such as drowsiness, refusal to feed/poor breast sucking/fluid drinking, noisy breathing (stridor, wheezing, rattling, and grunting), tracheal tug (inward pulling of trachea at the suprasternal notch seen during inspiration in severe respiratory distress), apnea, cyanosis, convulsions, jaundice, severe pallor, severe malnutrition, overt bleeding, hypothermia (perceived by cold skin on holding the limb or feeling the skin warmth of the patient with the dorsum of fingers by the doctor), and severe congenital anomalies indicate serious illness. A child with any of these features should be labeled as sick.

Certain clinical parameters can be applied to assess the severity of acute illness in children. Yale Observation Scale 7 (YOS 7) with six parameters **(Table 7.1)** is found to be a valid one in many studies for the presence of bacteremia or serious disease in febrile children of age group >1–59 m.

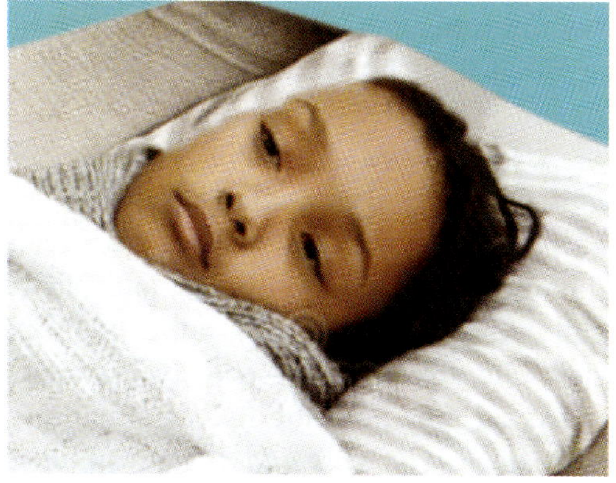

Fig. 7.2: Sick child with a vacant look.

The best possible score is 6 × 1 = 6; the worst score is 6 × 5 = 30. The probability of serious bacterial infection is 2.75% if the score is <10; 26% with a score of 11–15; and 92.3% with a score >16.

Vital Signs

Vital signs to be evaluated are pulse rate (PR), blood pressure (BP), respiratory rate (RR), body temperature, capillary refill time (CFT), hydration status, and oxygen saturation.

Pulse

Count the radial pulse for 15 sec and multiply with 4 to get the rate and rhythm; if it is irregular or poor in volume, count for 1 complete minute. The right radial pulse is the one commonly evaluated.

Counting the Radial Pulse

The patient has to extend and half pronate the forearm at the elbow and partially flex the wrist. This position can be easily procured in infants and children by offering a "shake hand". With the index and middle fingers of the other hand, approaching from the radial side of the forearm, gently press against the distal end of the radius to get the arterial pulse **(Fig. 7.3)**. Radial pulse is difficult to obtain in newborns, obese, and edematous infants and in patients with shock; if so, rapidly search for brachial (over the cubital fossa), carotid (at the carotid triangle), or femoral pulsations (press midway between the anterior superior iliac spine and the symphysis pubis below the inguinal ligament). Occasionally one's own pulse may be confused with the patient's pulse;

TABLE 7.1: Yale Observation Scale 7 (YOS 7).

Observation item	***Normal (score = 1)***	***Moderate Impairment (score = 3)***	***Severe impairment (score = 5)***
Quality of cry	Strong with normal tone *Or* Content and not crying	Whimpering *Or* Sobbing	Weak/moaning/high pitched
Reaction to parent stimulation	Cries briefly then stops *Or* Content and not crying	Cries off and on	Continual cry Or Hardly responds
State variation	If awake → Stays awake *Or* If asleep and stimulated → wakes up quickly	Eyes close briefly, awakes with prolonged stimulation	Falls to sleep *Or* Does not wake up
Color	Pink	Pale extremities *Or* Acrocyanosis	Pale *Or* Cyanotic *Or* Mottled *Or* Ashen
Hydration	Skin normal, eyes normal, and mucous membranes moist	Skin, eyes-normal, and mouth slightly dry	Skin doughy/tented and dry mucous membranes and/or sunken eyes
Response (talk and smile) to social overtures	Smiles *Or* Alerts (≤2 m)	Brief smile *Or* Alerts briefly (≤2 m)	No smile, face anxious/dull/expressionless OR No alerting (≤2 m)

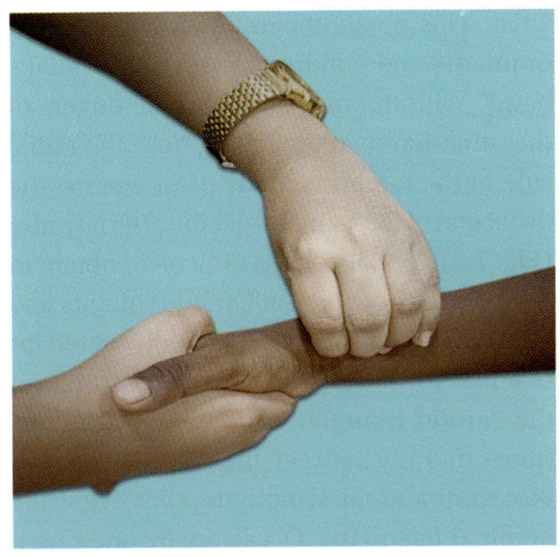

Fig. 7.3: Counting the radial pulse.

if so try to compare it with the examiner's own temporalis artery pulsations with the other hand. *Dorsalis pedis and posterior tibial* are the other peripheral pulsations to be assessed at the first visit itself; all these three should be palpated on both sides.

Assess the rate, rhythm (regularity), and force of pulsations and compare for each vessel on both sides. **Table 7.2** reveals the normal values of pulse, BP, and RRs in children in different age groups. Rapid or slow rate, irregular or feeble, or bounding pulse, all may indicate disease situations. *Physiological increase and decrease* in pulse rate during inspiration is sinus tachycardia

TABLE 7.2: Normal values of PR, RR, and BP in children.

Parameter	*Preterm baby*	*Newborn*	*Infant*	*Child*	*Adolescent*
Pulse/min	120–160	100–150	90–120	70–110	60–95
RR/min	40–60	40–60	30–40	20–30	14–18
BP (mm Hg)	As per gestational age in Ch. 15	60/40	90/60	*90 + (2 × age in yr) #70 + (2 × age in yr)	

*90 + (2 × age in yr)—systolic BP 50th percentile
#70 + (2 × age in yr)—systolic BP fifth percentile
(BP: blood pressure; PR: pulse rate; RR: respiratory rate)

and on expiration is sinus bradycardia respectively; both are normal phenomena. Benign extrasystoles are nonpathological irregularities in rhythm. *A feeble pulse* may herald shock, aortic stenosis, cardiomyopathy, or vasculitis. *Unequal radial pulses* indicate preductal coarctation. *Radiofemoral delay* is seen in postductal coarctation beyond the subclavian vessel. For more details on pulse and BP see Ch. 17.

For 95th percentile BP values refer Ch. 17.

Blood Pressure

Record the BP (Ref. Ch. 17 for details) when the child is quiet or sleeping. Values <5th and >95th percentiles indicate hypo and hypertension, respectively.

Respiratory Rate

- *Observe the RR* whether fast or slow, regular or irregular, depth of respiration, abnormalities in breathing pattern, work of breathing, and added sounds perceived by naked ears.
- *Count the RR* by inspection in children since palpation or auscultation may interfere with the RR due to the tactile stimulus. Observe the inspiratory rising of the chest for one complete minute (since the rate can be irregular) while the patient is quiet and resting. Tachypnea or fast breathing is increased RR for the age as revealed in **Table 7.3** and is the best clinical indicator of respiratory distress and hypoxia in children.

TABLE 7.3: Agewise RR for tachypnea in children.

Age	*RR/min*
<60 days	≥60
≥60 days to 1 yr	≥50
≥1–5 yr	≥40
≥5 yr	≥30

The most common cause of tachypnea is lower respiratory infection. Hyperreactive airway disease, upper airway obstruction, congenital anomalies of the respiratory system, pleural effusion/empyema, pneumothorax, foreign body impaction of the airway, congenital heart disease, cardiac failure, cardiomyopathy, pericardial effusion, renal failure, renal tubular acidosis, diabetic ketoacidosis, inborn errors of metabolism (IEM), and drug intoxication (salicylism) are the other causes (Ref. Ch. 19).

Temperature

A change in body temperature (temp) to higher or lower levels is detrimental to body functions and indicates illnesses. In children up to 10 yr of age, body temp should be recorded from the axilla or groin for safety reasons. In older cooperative children and

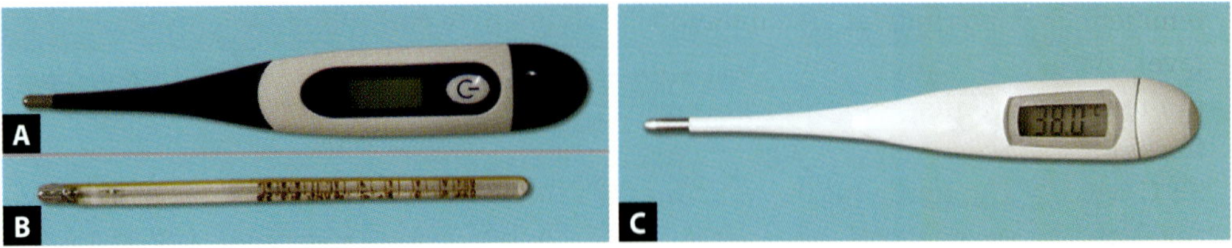

Figs. 7.4A to C: Different types of thermometers for body temperature recording. (A) Digital oral thermometer (blue); (B) Mercury rectal thermometer (yellow); (C) Digital rectal thermometer.

adults, oral recording is feasible. Hypothermia should be assessed by rectal recording. Electronic and mercury glass thermometers (oral and rectal) are equally reliable. The latter are not used at present in most places, because of the environmental poisoning hazard and danger to the patient if it breaks within the mouth or rectum. **Figures 7.4A to C** show the different types of thermometers. Rectal thermometers have shorter and more round tips compared to the oral types.

How to take body temperature?

Antiseptic (70% isopropyl alcohol) cleaning is a must before and after the use of the thermometer. Soap and water cleaning is needed for the rectal thermometer. Child should not have taken oral ice or warm water at least 30 minutes before oral temperature recording. For axillary recording, apply the thermometer tip correctly to the apex of the axilla without clothes in between; approximate the arm (which is flexed at the elbow) tightly and keep it till the beep of the electronic thermometer is heard indicating the time of reading. In the mouth, place the tip of the thermometer under the tongue, firmly close the lips, and ask the child to breathe through the nose. On hearing the beep the reading should be documented. In newborns suspecting hypothermia, sick children, and those with coma or severe protein-calorie malnutrition (PEM), rectal temperature recording is a must.

- *Rectal temperature recording:* Place the infant in lateral decubitus posture (or prone) over the parent's lap or over a table, hold the child's lower back firmly with one hand, and introduce slowly the lubricated tip of the rectal thermometer 0.5–1 inch through the anal opening. Stop the attempt if any resistance is felt. Keep the thermometer steady between the second and third fingers, cupping against the baby's bottom till the beep is heard. The oral temperature is 0.5°C higher than the axillary and the rectal temperature is 0.5°C higher than the oral. Hence, when the body temperature is reported, whether the recording is axillary, oral, or rectal should be specified (or report the temperature after adding appropriate correction).
- *Infrared thermometers* **(Fig. 7.5)** measure body temperature using infrared technology (equally reliable as electronic thermometers). Recording is easy and quick. They are costlier and accuracy may be affected by direct sunlight, lower surrounding temperature, sweaty forehead, and lack of contact with the forehead.
- *Interpretation of body temperature:* According to the American College of Emergency Physicians, fever is defined as rectal temperature >100.4°F. The three types of classical fevers are: Continuous,

remittent, and intermittent. In continuous fever, daily fluctuations are <1°C and the temperature never reaches normal. In remittent fever, daily fluctuations are >2°C without the temperature touching the baseline (e.g., typhoid fever and tuberculosis). *Hectic or septic fever* **(Fig. 7.6A)** is a type of remittent fever having >3°C fluctuation (seen in abscess, deep-seated infections, pyelonephritis, and malignancy). In *intermittent* fever fluctuations exceed 1°C which lasts for a few hours of a day, *quotidian* fever is such fluctuations occurring daily, *tertian* fever is fluctuations occurring on alternate days (typical of *Plasmodium vivax* infection); in *quartan* fever, the fluctuations occur on every third day (typical of *Plasmodium malariae* malaria). With the widespread use of antipyretics, antibiotics, and chemotherapeutics these typical patterns of fever are uncommon now. In *relapsing fevers,* the spikes are separated by few normal days in between. In biphasic fever (camelback fever) two distinct phases of fever **(Fig. 7.6B)** occur over one or more weeks for a single illness. Leptospirosis, dengue illness, yellow fever, rat bite fever, tick fever, and paralytic polio reveal such biphasic fever. Fever with relative bradycardia (<10 beats/°F reductions) occurs in typhoid, brucellosis, leptospirosis, dengue fever, viral hepatitis, and myocarditis. **Table 7.4** reveals the interpretation of body temperature.

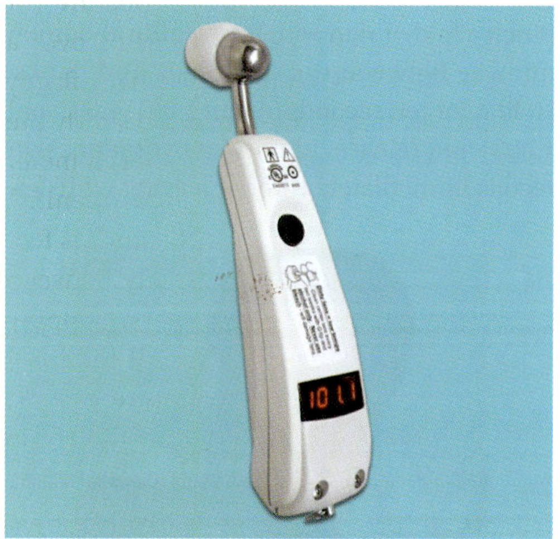

Fig. 7.5: Infrared thermometer.

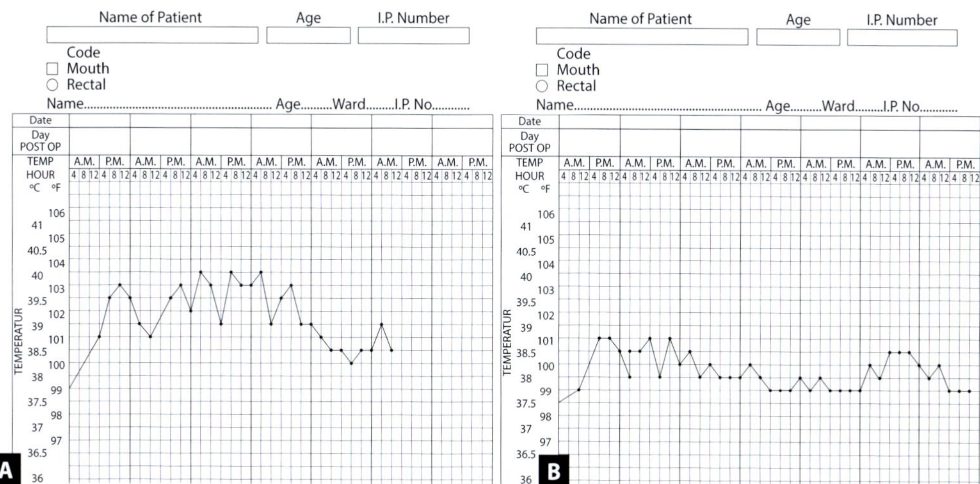

Figs. 7.6A and B: (A) Hectic fever in Acute osteomyelitis and (B) Biphasic fever in dengue illness.

Capillary Refill Time (CFT)

Capillary refill time is a bedside test to detect the peripheral perfusion of tissues. To assess CFT lift the limb 15° above the precordial level and press the pulp of the finger (sole of foot in newborns) for 5 sec (count in mind 1,001; 1,002; 1,003; 1,004; and 1,005) so as to blanch the area and release. The time for blanch to disappear or CFT is normally ≤2 sec; ≥3 sec is prolongation (Ref. **Fig. 8.2B**); ≥5 sec is inadequate systemic perfusion as in hypovolemic and cardiogenic shock. This sign may not occur in the early stage of septic shock due to capillary dilatation. Exposure to cold environments can prolong CFT in normal persons. Other sites for CFT evaluation are precordium and ear lobules (in newborns).

Hydration Status

Assess the hydration status in all sick children by asking about the fluid intake (breastfeeding in small babies) "Is the baby drinking eagerly?" and the volume and frequency of urine voiding. Symptoms of dehydration are excessive thirst, voracious drinking, and tiredness/irritability. Lethargy, sunken eyes **(Fig. 7.7)**, absent tears, dryness of tongue and buccal mucosa, loss of skin recoil, and hypotension are the signs. **Table 7.5** reveals the grading of dehydration in children.

Skin recoil is the reverting of the skin after pinching, an important sign of dehydration. Pinch a fold of skin with fat over the abdomen midway between the umbilicus and flanks. Hold it for ten seconds (count 1,001, 1,002 and 1,003) and release. In normal hydration, skin recoils immediately without leaving wrinkles.

TABLE 7.4: Interpretation of body temperature.

Body temperature	***Celsius (°C)***	***Fahrenheit (°F)***
Normal	36.6–37.2	98–99
Subnormal	<36.6 (cold stress in neonates)	<98
Hypothermia	<36	<95
Febrile	>38	>100.4
Hyperpyrexia	>41	>106

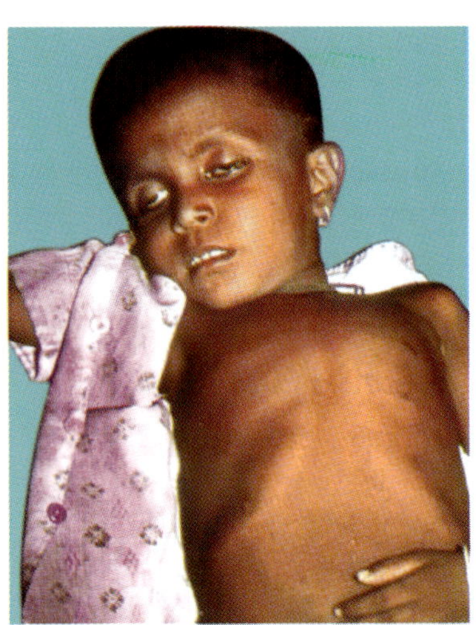

Fig. 7.7: Sunken eyes and scaphoid abdomen in severe dehydration.

TABLE 7.5: Assessment of dehydration in children.

Clinical signs	***No dehydration***	***Some dehydration***	***Severe dehydration***
Sensorium	Alert	Irritable	Altered sensorium, coma
Eyes	Normal	Sunken	Very sunken
Oral mucosa and tongue	Moist	Dry*	Dry* and parched
Skin pinch	Immediate recoil	Recoils in 2 sec	Recoils after 2 sec
Thirst	Normal drinking	Drinks eagerly	Unable to drink
Urine output	Normal	Decreased	Much decreased/absent

*Oral mucosa can be moist after fluid intake or vomiting. Can appear dry in mouth breathers.

In some dehydration recoiling occurs by two seconds. In severe dehydration, wrinkling persists >2 sec. In severely wasted children skin pinch will not recoil in normal hydration. The dryness of buccal mucosa is a reliable sign to assess dehydration in them. *To assess oral mucosal dryness,* introduce the index finger between the inner cheek and upper jaw posteriorly. Severe dehydration can lead to hypotension, anuria, renal failure, and coma.

The most common cause of dehydration in children is diarrhea. Repeated vomiting, excessive gastric aspiration, diabetic ketoacidosis, IEM, diuretic therapy, salicylism, diabetes insipidus, renal tubular acidosis (RTA), and starvation are other causes. Dehydration and anasarca may coexist in nephrotic syndrome, chronic liver failure, chronic congestive heart failure, and edematous malnutrition. In young babies presenting with unaccountable dehydration exclude congenital adrenal hyperplasia and RTA.

Oxygen Saturation

Low oxygen saturation is fatal unless corrected at the earliest. Hypoxemia can be screened by a pulse oximeter [a handy, easy to operate, reliable, cheap device, safe to home care patient also since it needs only minimal training **(Fig. 7.8)**]. The device measures the percentage saturation of hemoglobin (Hb) bound with oxygen in the blood. It is operated by applying the probe of the oximeter over a capillary-rich area of the body, ideally the pulp of the index or middle finger. Toes or ear lobules are advisable for newborns. The hand should not be cold or wet, be clean and warm, and nail polish removed. An appropriate-size probe is attached to the finger. As infrared light is passed through the fingertip, the oxygen saturation value appears along with the pulse rate. The value is noted as the reading becomes stable. Normal oxygen saturation is >95%. <90% in <5 yr children is hypoxemia and require oxygen therapy. The drawbacks are that accuracy is less in severe desaturation (<70%), hemoglobinopathies, hypotension, and carbon monoxide (CO) poisoning.

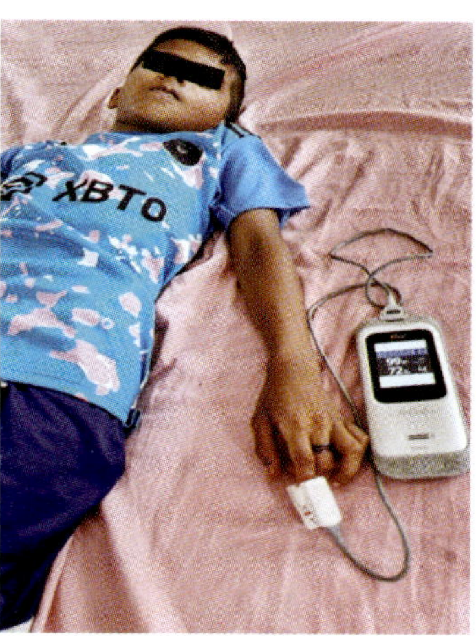

Fig. 7.8: Pulse oximeter recording.

Assessment of Danger Signs

Pallor, icterus, cyanosis, clubbing, lymphadenopathy, edema (acronym *PICCLE* signs), bleeding tendency, skin changes, subcutaneous emphysema, and bone tenderness are the danger signs.

- *Pallor* is the pale appearance of skin and mucous membranes usually due to anemia [caused by reduced number of red blood cells (RBCs)] or due to shock (subsequent to decreased perfusion). As per the WHO, anemia is Hb <11g/dL in children <4 yrs, <11.5 g/dL in 5–7 yrs, and <12 g in 8–14 yrs of age. Examine for pallor over the conjunctiva, mucosa, tongue, palms, skin, and nails. Pallor without anemia is seen in vasovagal episodes and septic shock. In severe pallor, palmar creases reveal faded appearance. Tachycardia and edema indicate the complication of congestive heart failure due to severe anemia. If there is koilonychia or spoon-shaped nails, it indicates iron deficiency. The presence of petechiae indicates platelet deficiency in number or qualitative defect and bone marrow aplasia or infiltration. Hyperpigmentation of the knuckles is pathognomonic of megaloblastic anemia seen in vegans (strict vegetarians); whereas, in congenital aplastic anemia, it is circumoral in distribution.

- *Icterus (jaundice)* is yellowish discoloration of the body due to the increase in serum bilirubin (>5 mg/dL in newborns and >2 mg/dL in older children). It is best detected in daylight by looking at the sclera **(Fig. 7.9)** and less on the undersurface of the tongue, palms, and skin (Ref. Ch. 15 for newborn jaundice). Yellowish discoloration of the body can occur in carotenemia also in which clinical manifestations and the investigations will be noncontributory. **Table 7.6** reveals the salient differentiating points between direct and indirect hyperbilirubinemias.
- *Cyanosis* is bluish color of skin and mucosa **(Fig. 7.10)** due to increased amount of reduced Hb (>5 g/dL) in superficial blood vessels. It can be *central* when both mucosa and skin are blue or **peripheral** if extremities only are blue with cold peripheries or *differential* if only upper or lower limbs are blue (Ref. Ch. 17). The causes of cyanosis are discussed in **Box 7.2**. Oxygen saturation may reach <85% in cyanosis. Hence, in severe anemia with Hb <5 g/dL, cyanosis may not be obvious clinically.
- *Digital clubbing* is selective enlargement of the distal segment of fingers or toes induced by chronic hypoxia (should be for at least 6 w) leading to increased capillary permeability

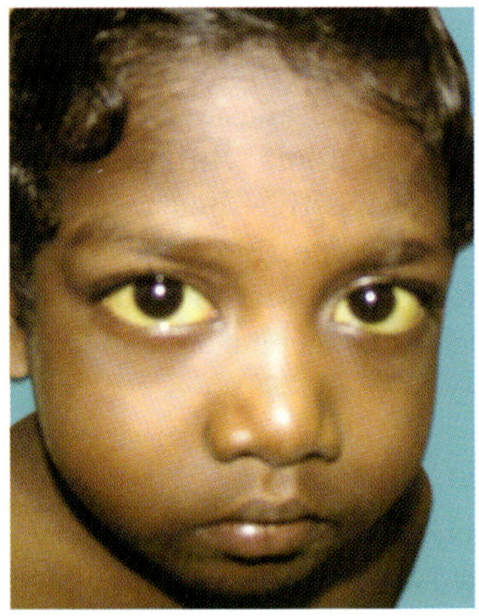

Fig. 7.9: Yellow sclera in jaundice.

TABLE 7.6: Differentiating points in two types of jaundice.

Signs	*Conjugated hyperbilirubinemia*	*Unconjugated hyper bilirubinemia*
Color of sclera	Orange yellow	Lemon yellow
Urine color	Dark yellow	Lemon yellow
Stool color	Clay color	Normal color
Body scratches	Very obvious	Absent
Liver changes	Obvious	Nil
Splenomegaly	±	Present
Urine bile salts	Present	Absent
Urine urobilinogen	+++	Absent
Bleeding tendency	Usual	Absent

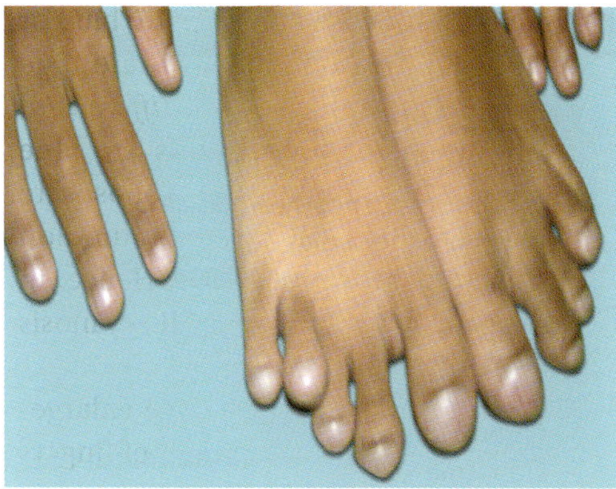

Fig. 7.10: Cyanosis, stage 3 clubbing.

TABLE 7.7: Clinical grading of clubbing.

Grade	*Clinical signs*
I	Increased fluctuation at the nail bed
II	Obliteration of the angle at the nail bed
III	Loss of longitudinal ridges of the nail, increased convexity of the nail from above downwards and from side to side "Parrot beak appearance" **(Fig. 7.10)**
IV	The terminal segment becomes bulbous like the end of a drumstick. Pain and swelling of wrist and hands

BOX 7.2: Causes of cyanosis in children.

Central cyanosis:
- Respiratory:
  - Congenital anomalies of the airways and lung
  - Foreign body impaction of airways
  - Progressive pneumonias
  - Tension pneumothorax
  - Pleural effusion
  - Suppurative lung diseases
  - Cystic fibrosis
  - Alveolar hypoventilation syndromes
  - Bronchopulmonary dysplasia
- Cardiovascular

Cyanotic congenital heart diseases (TOF, TGA with VSD, TAPVR, and pulmonary AV fistula)
- *Hemoglobin abnormalities:*
  - Methemoglobinemia
  - Sulfhemoglobinemia
  - Caboxyhemoglobinemia
- *Peripheral cyanosis:*
  - Exposure to cold
  - Shock
  - Vascular thromboembolism (arterial, venous)
  - Raynaud phenomenon

(AV: arteriovenous; TAPVR: total anomalous pulmonary venous return; TGA: transposition of the great arteries; TOF: tetralogy of Fallot; VSD: ventricular septal defect)

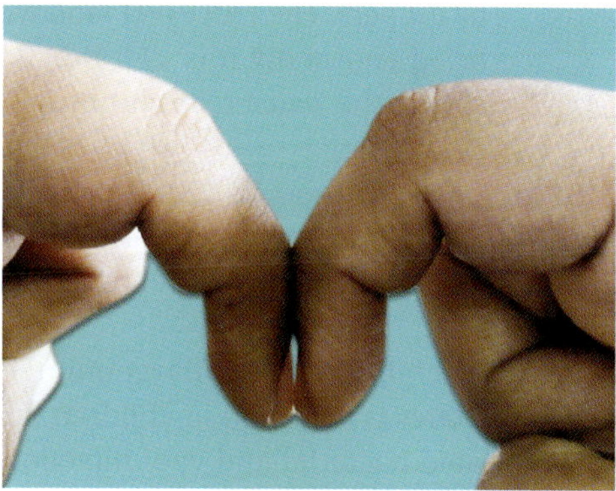

Fig. 7.11: Eliciting Schamroth sign.

and connective tissue hypertrophy by platelet-derived growth factor. Four grades of clubbing are described clinically **(Table 7.7)**. Clinical detection of advanced clubbing (grade III and IV) is easy. Grade II clubbing is best detected by:

i. *Schamroth sign* is the obliteration of the diamond-shaped space at the base of the nail bed when the dorsal surfaces of the terminal phalanges of similar fingers are placed in opposition **(Fig. 7.11)**.
ii. *Obliteration of Lovibond's angle:* The angulation between the nail plate and the skin below the nail is

normally <180°. Hold the finger in profile, horizontally at the level of the eyes to see the angle. In clubbing as the tissues at the base of the nail become thickened, this angle is lost.

iii. *Phalangeal depth ratio:* Normally the distal phalangeal depth (DPD) is smaller than the interphalangeal depth (IPD). In clubbing DPD exceeds IPD because of the basal tissue proliferation of the fingertip; look at the profile of the finger held at eye level or measure the depth by calipers. The DPD/IPD ratio will be >1 (normally it is <1). **Box 7.3** shows the causes of clubbing in children.

In *koilonychia*, seen in iron deficiency anemia, nails become soft, thin, brittle, and spoon-shaped. This sign is uncommon in children.

- *Lymphadenopathy* or enlargement of lymph nodes is common in children due to repeated bacterial and viral infections producing lymphoid proliferation.
  - *Approach:* Enlarged lymph nodes present as swellings which may be the primary complaint or they may be incidentally detected while examining the child. The first step is to exclude the nonlymphoid masses simulating lymph nodes. In the neck, there are thyroid masses (goiter, thyroglossal cyst, and thyroid abscess), branchial cleft cyst/ or infected sinus, neurofibroma, cystic hygroma, cervical rib, and sternomastoid tumor. Assess clinically and by relevant investigations. **Figure 7.12** reveals rapidly enlarging cystic hygroma with tracheal compression in an infant. Cervical, axillary, epitrochlear, inguinal, and popliteal lymph nodes can be examined clinically.

BOX 7.3: Causes of clubbing in children.

- Hereditary
- Idiopathic
- *Cardiac:*
  - Cyanotic congenital heart disease
  - Bacterial endocarditis
  - Chronic congestive heart failure
- *Respiratory:*
  - Lung abscess
  - Bronchiectasis
  - Chronic pneumonia
  - Empyema
  - Cystic fibrosis
  - Malignant neoplasms
  - Pleural mesothelioma
  - Tuberculosis (rare)
- *Gastrointestinal:*
  - Celiac disease
  - Chronic dysentery
  - Crohn's disease
  - Polyposis of intestine
  - Ulcerative colitis
- *Hepatic:*
  - Biliary cirrhosis
  - Chronic active hepatitis
- *Others:*
  - Hodgkin disease
  - Thyrotoxicosis
  - Congenital methemoglobinemia

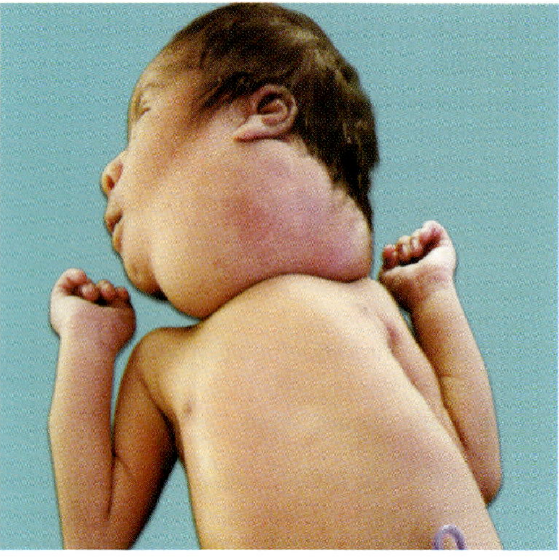

Fig. 7.12: Cystic hygroma of the neck.

- *Cervical lymph nodes:* The examiner may stand or sit facing the child; change the position as needed according to the lymph node groups and cooperation of the child. *Observe* the lymph nodes for redness, surrounding edema, ulceration, granuloma, or discharge. *Palpate* the nodes (on the left side with the right hand and vice versa) gently with the pulp of the index and middle fingers. Assess the size, location, consistency, tenderness, whether isolated or matted, presence of fluctuation, mobility/fixation to the skin or to other tissues. Palpate in order the preauricular, retro auricular, tonsillar, submandibular, submental, posterior cervical, anterior cervical, deep cervical, pretracheal, and lastly the supraclavicular groups. Examine the drainage area of the cervical lymph nodes (head and neck) for pediculosis, infections, ulcers, or swelling. **Figure 7.13** shows tuberculous lymph nodes on the posterior triangle of the neck.
- *Axillary lymph nodes:* With your left hand lift the patient's left arm to get it relaxed; palpate deeply with your right hand for the apical, medial, anterior, posterior, and lateral groups of lymph nodes; palpate the right axillary glands with your left hand in the same way. Posterior axillary lymph nodes are better palpated on standing behind the patient. Examine the drainage areas, i.e., upper limbs, breasts, chest, and upper abdomen for ulcers, infected wounds, lumps, and scratch marks.

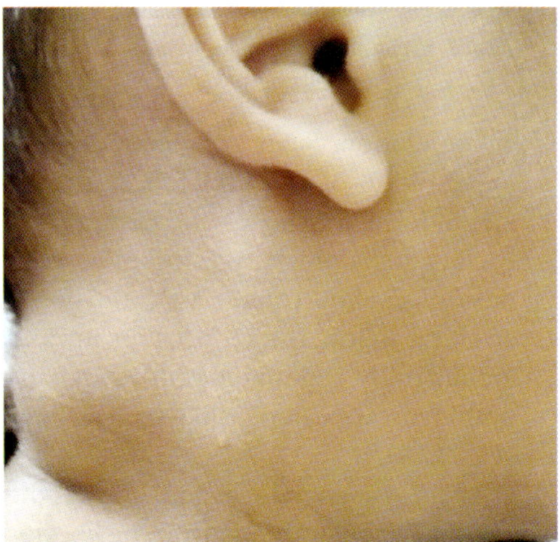

Fig. 7.13: Tuberculous lymphadenopathy neck.

- *Epitrochlear lymph nodes* are characteristic of infectious mononucleosis (IMN) and cat scratch disease (CSD). Gently hold the patient's forearm across the chest (left hand of the child with the left hand of the examiner and vice versa) and palpate with the fingers of the other hand above the epitrochlear region. Examine for scratch marks/ulcers on the forearm.
- *Inguinal lymph nodes* have superficial and deep groups; the former are visible, have vertical and horizontal groups, and are easy to see and palpate (examiner sitting and facing the child; child seated on the mother's lap/chair or standing). The vertical group is close to the long saphenous vein and drains the leg; the horizontal group is just above the inguinal ligament and drains the lower abdominal skin, anal canal, buttocks, lower vagina, and external genitalia excluding the testes.
- *Popliteal lymph nodes* are difficult to approach and need deep palpation. *Inspect the drainage area of each group of lymph nodes* for infection/scratch marks (characteristic of CSD), wounds, or insect bites to detect the etiology. Enlargement of cervical and axillary lymph nodes >1 cm and

BOX 7.4: Common causes of lymphadenopathy.

- *Generalized:*
  - Infections
    - *Viral:* IMN, CMV, rubella, HIV, measles
    - *Bacterial:* TB, syphilis, septicemia, plague, typhoid
    - *Protozoal:* Toxoplasmosis
    - *Fungal:* Coccidioidomycosis
    - *Neoplastic:* Leukemias, lymphomas, neuroblastoma
    - *Lymphoproliferative:* Histiocytosis
- *Regional:*
  - All the above causes *plus*
  - Streptococcal pharyngitis: Anterior cervical
  - *Pediculosis scalp:* Suboccipital
  - *Kawasaki disease:* Anterior cervical
  - *Oral and dental infections:* Submandibular submental
  - *Ophthalmic infections:* Preauricular
  - *Cat scratch disease:* Epitrochlear axillary
  - *Insect bites*: Regional lymph nodes
  - *Brucellosis:* Axillary
  - Leukemias, lymphoma-mediastinal
  - Lymphogranuloma venereum-inguinal
  - *Immunization reaction:* Axillary, inguinal

(CMV: *Cytomegalovirus*; HIV: human immunodeficiency virus; IMN: infectious mononudeosis; TB: tuberculosis)

inguinal lymph nodes >1.5 cm is considered significant. Smaller lymph nodes are significant if fever, pallor, bleeding tendency, and organomegaly are present or hard in consistency (shotty lymph nodes).

- *Generalized lymphadenopathy* is enlargement of more than two noncontiguous lymph node groups. **Box 7.4** reveals the common causes of lymphadenopathy in children. Failure to regress after 2 w of treatment, hard consistency, and coexisting systemic findings (anemia, bleeding tendency, presence of nodules or lumps, and hepatosplenomegaly) point to serious diseases requiring diagnostic workup.
- *Edema:* Edema is the swelling of subcutaneous tissue due to excess fluid accumulation. *Signs* are pale and shiny appearance of the affected skin with loss of normal wrinkles and doughy feel. Facial edema presents as morning puffiness of eyelids **(Fig. 7.14)** and boggy swelling below the chin when up and ambulant. In abdominal wall edema, the umbilicus appears slit-like or "smiling" **(Fig. 7.15)**.

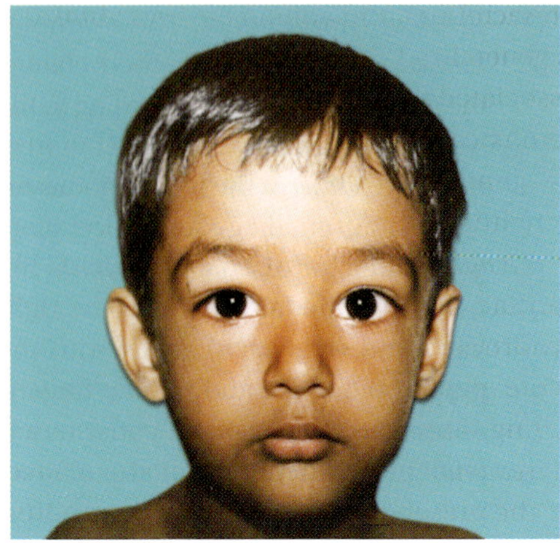

Fig. 7.14: Facial puffiness.

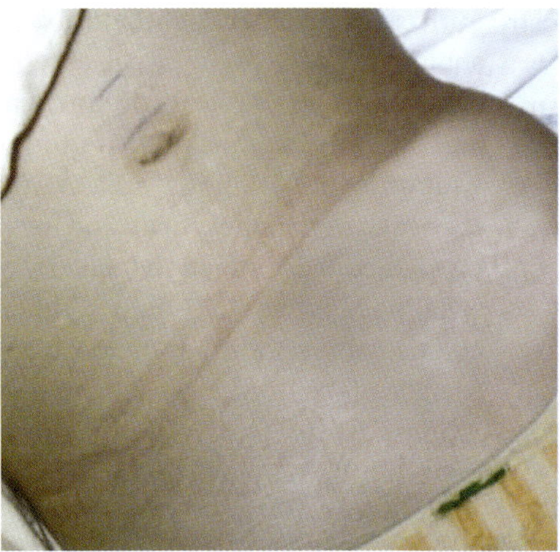

Fig. 7.15: Smiling umbilicus in abdominal wall edema.

Dependent edema is seen initially over the legs in the ambulant patient; in newborns, infants, and bedridden patients, it is over the presacral area and around the eyes. *Anasarca* is generalized massive edema and is usually associated with fluid collection in multiple serous cavities (polyserositis). Edema may be generalized or localized, pitting, or nonpitting.

Generalized pitting edema occurs in cardiac failure, liver failure, nephrotic syndrome, and severe PEM. Edema in acute nephritis and angioedema are less pitting. Examples of nonpitting edema are *myxedema* (collection of myxomatous tissue in the subcutaneous plane seen in older children with hypothyroidism) and filarial edema (localized edema due to lymphatic obstruction) in contrast to acute inflammatory edema. Pitting is elicited by applying firm pressure for at least 20 sec over bony prominences (behind the malleoli, over the shin, and presacral region). The indentation produced should persist for minimum 15 sec **(Fig. 7.16)**.

Bleeding tendency manifests as areas of reddish to bluish discoloration on mucous membranes, skin, and deeper tissues or as external oozing from intact mucous membranes, wounds, and puncture sites (Ref. Ch. 10).

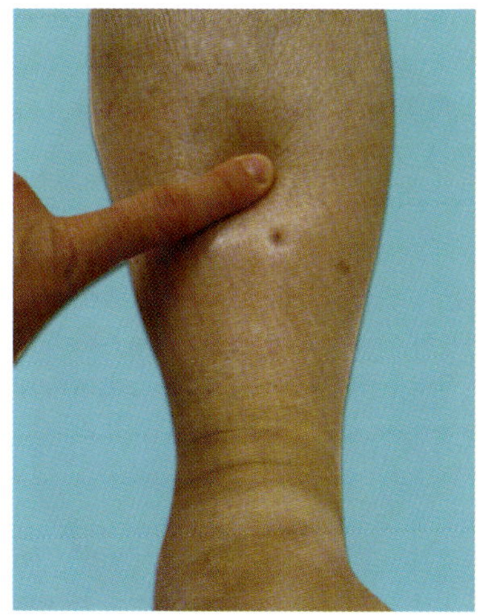

Fig. 7.16: Eliciting pitting edema over the shin.

Subcutaneous/surgical emphysema is the collection of air in the subcutaneous tissue (from the airways, lungs, paranasal sinuses, or organs near the respiratory system). Gently compress the areas around the neck, chest wall, and anterior abdominal wall up to the inguinal ligament; crackling sensation if perceived indicates surgical emphysema. Accidents causing crush injuries of the chest, rib fractures, stab and bullet injuries, and perforating lesions of the pharynx, larynx, trachea, and esophagus are the common surgical causes. Medical causes are pneumothorax, pneumomediastinum, paroxysmal cough produced by acute asthma, pertussis, foreign body impaction of the airways and rarely following thoracentesis. In orbital fracture air escaping from paranasal sinuses is collected mainly over the face.

Bone tenderness is elicited by pressing over the superficial bones (anterior border of the tibia and sternum). Fracture of the bone, vitamin D deficiency, osteomyelitis, osteogenesis imperfecta, Caffey's disease, and infiltrative disorders of the bone marrow (leukemia) are the common causes of bone pain and tenderness.

Ref. Ch. 10 for details on skin disorders.

HEAD TO FOOT EXAMINATION

- Proceed to examine the head, face, neck, chest, upper limbs, abdomen, perineum, and lower limbs.
- *Head:* Assess the size, shape, hair, fontanelle (empty areas on skull bone junctions providing space for brain growth), sutures, scalp veins, and craniotabes. Size of the head may appear small or large visually and should be confirmed by anthropometry.

- *Shape: Plagiocephaly* (asymmetrical head) is due to premature unilateral closure of coronal or lambdoid sutures. In young babies, plagiocephaly can occur by constant pressure on the skull, due to lying on one side (which can occur during the intrauterine period also) and gets corrected as the baby gradually abandons the posture. *Dolichocephaly* (scaphocephaly/elongated/"boat-shaped" head) and *brachycephaly* (broad-head, typical of Down syndrome) are due to premature closure of sagittal and coronal sutures respectively. Skull bones grow at right angles in the direction of the suture which gets closed prematurely.
- *Oxycephaly* (acrocephaly/turricephaly/"tower skull deformity") is vertical growth of the brain due to the premature closure of many cranial sutures. In *cloverleaf skull* deformity, all sutures close prematurely; and as the brain grows through anterior and temporal fontanelle, bulges appear over these regions. *Caput quadratum* is large head, seen as four quadrants (due to frontal and parietal bossing by osteoid accumulation) with a narrow base, typically seen in rickets.
- *Abnormal head shape and size* occur in rickets, achondroplasia, hydrocephalus, skeletal dysplasias, chromosomal anomalies, genetic syndromes, craniosynostosis, microcephaly, and mucopolysaccharidosis. **Figures. 7.17A and B** reveal microcephaly and hydrocephalus.

Hair

Assess the quantity, pigmentation, texture, and pluckability of hair and the number of hair whorls on the scalp. Hypotrichosis is deficient hair growth which may be partial or complete, scarring or nonscarring **(Fig. 7.18A)**. Hair becomes lusterless, sparse, hypopigmented, and easily pluckable in PEM and in deficiencies of iron, zinc, and essential fatty acids, and in chronic inflammations. "Flag sign" is alternate bands of hypo and hyperpigmentation of hair indicating repeated periods of severe undernutrition, seen very common in the past. Biotinidase deficiency is an inborn error of metabolism characterized by

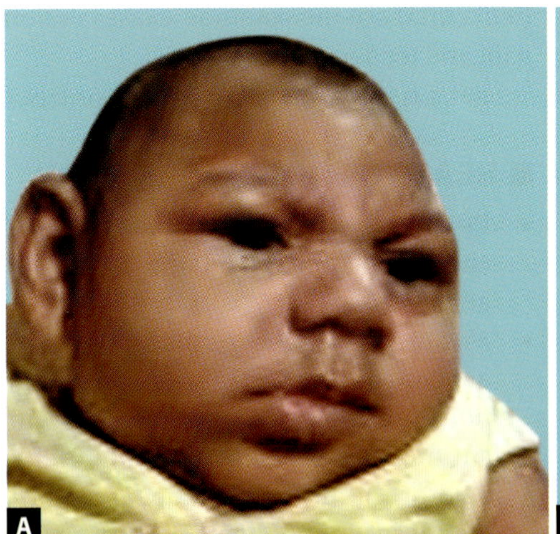

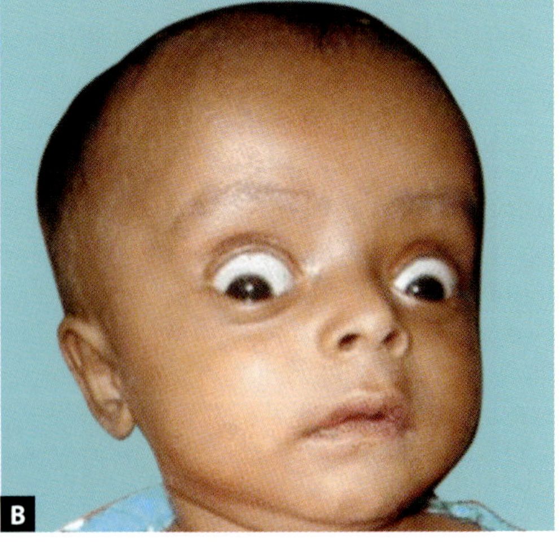

Figs. 7.17A and B: (A) Microcephaly and (B) Hydrocephalus revealing large head with setting sun sign.

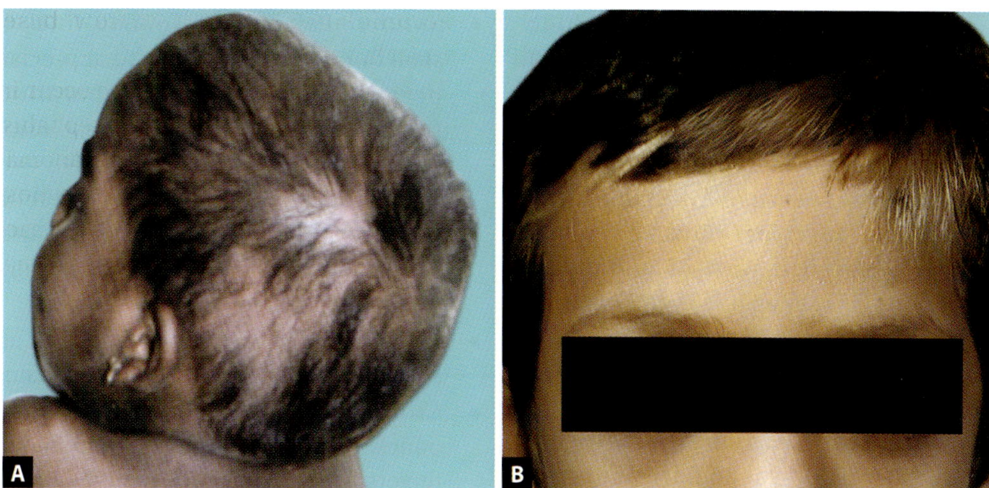

Figs. 7.18A and B: (A) Alopecia in a child with human immunodeficiency virus (HIV) disease and (B) White forelock in partial albinism.

seborrheic dermatitis, alopecia, candidiasis, hearing impairment, developmental delay, and myoclonic seizures. Hirsutism is androgen-dependent male pattern of hair growth in women. Disorders of hair are due to undernutrition, intrinsic disturbances of hair growth, underlying biochemical, endocrine, genetic, or metabolic defects, inflammatory dermatoses, and drug-induced or structural anomalies of the hair shaft. In *albinism* (congenital absence of skin pigment) hair is light colored; partial albinism can present as a white patch of hair **(Fig. 7.18B)**. Hair whorls over the scalp (deviation points of hair) more than one may indicate underlying brain anomalies.

Seborrhea (Ref. Ch. 10)

Low anterior hairline is characteristic of hypothyroidism; *low posterior hairline up to C5 vertebral level* appears in Turner syndrome **(Fig. 7.19)** and Down syndrome.

- *Fontanels:* Fontanels (fontanelle) are soft spots in the skull with defective bone formation which helps in sufficient expansion of the skull for brain growth. The palpable midline fontanelle at birth is the large anterior fontanel (AF) and the small posterior fontanel (PF) which may not be palpable. AF is a diamond-shaped area at the junction of sagittal and coronal sutures between the medial parts of the two frontal and parietal bones. Measurement is taken diagonally, i.e., from the anteromedial angle of the parietal bone to the posteromedial angle of opposite frontal bone on both sides. The normal size is 2 × 2 cm, is slightly depressed from the scalp surface,

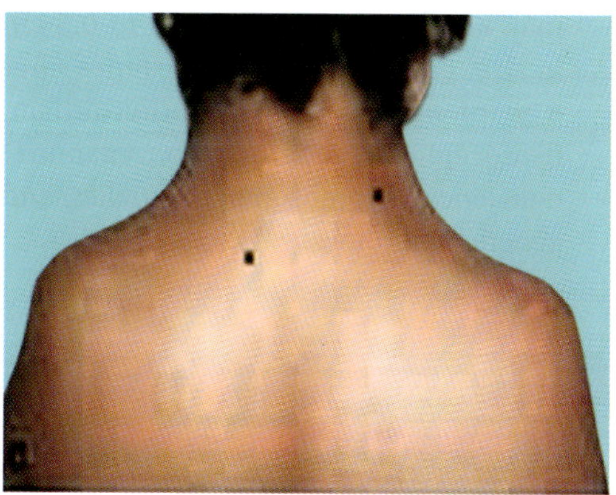

Fig. 7.19: Turner syndrome revealing low posterior hairline and webbing of the neck.

pulsatile and is best assessed when the infant is feeding, asleep or when held upright. The average age of closure is 9–18 m. Sunken AF is an important sign of dehydration in infants. Loss of pulsations followed by bulging of AF occurs in RICP and also on crying. **Box 7.5** provides the diseases with wide AF and delayed closure. Rarely it can be a normal variation. Unusually small size and early closure of fontanelle occur in microcephaly and craniosynostosis.

Trace the PF (triangular area at the junction of parietal and occipital bones in the midline) with the index finger along the sagittal suture posteriorly till it approaches the occipital bone. PF may be closed at birth or up to 0.5 cm in size. Larger size and persistence after 8 w of age suggest hypothyroidism, hydrocephalus, undernutrition, vitamin D deficiency, chromosomal anomalies, and genetic syndromes.

BOX 7.5: Causes of delayed AF closure.

- Normal variation
- Rickets
- PEM
- Hypothyroidism
- Hypophosphatasia
- Skeletal dysplasias
- Chromosomal anomalies
- Trisomy 13, 18, and 21
- Genetic syndromes

- *Sutures:* Palpate the joining lines of skull bones with fingertips to appreciate premature closure or separation. Craniosynostosis is premature closure (felt as a hard nonmovable ridge over the suture) of all sutures producing microcephaly; affection of few sutures causes abnormal skull shape only. Sutural separation is an early sign of RICP.
- *Dilated scalp veins* indicate RICP and are seen in young infants with hydrocephalus.
- *Craniotabes* is softening of the cranial bones. Press with your index and middle fingers over the occiput or parietal bone (away from the suture) to elicit the sign. The bone yields as if being pressed into a ping-pong ball and gets released. It can be normal in newborns and young infants; pathological causes are rickets, osteogenesis imperfecta, hydrocephalus, and syphilis (Ref. Ch. 21 for more details of head).

Face

Observe from the front (frontal), side (profile), above (bird's eye view), and below (worm's eye view) to see upper, middle, lateral, and lower facial abnormalities distinctly. Assess the forehead, orbits, eyes, nose, ears, mouth, cheeks, and lower jaw for abnormalities. *Grading of pain* in nonverbal children can be done by comparing their faces with the "Faces scales" **(Fig. 7.20)**; and by assessing the pain severity score from the child's facial

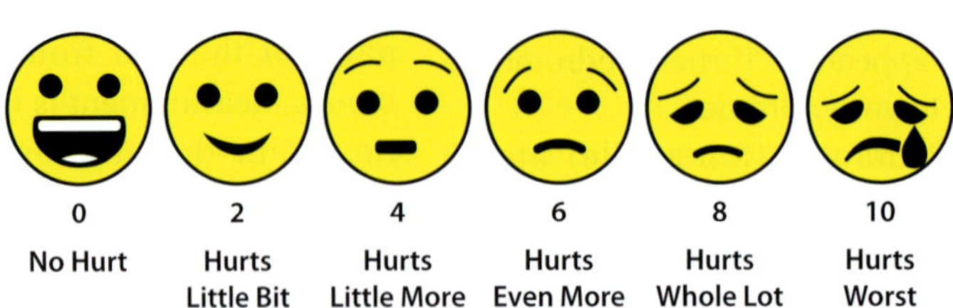

Fig. 7.20: Faces scale for pain rating.

expression; older children will be able to point to the face picture according to the severity of pain when asked. Score 1 is normal; score 10 is severe pain.

Frontal prominence is seen in rickets (due to osteoid tissue proliferation over the frontal bones), hydrocephalus, mucopolysaccharidosis, and skeletal dysplasias. A receding forehead is typical of autosomal recessive (AR) microcephaly **(Fig. 7.17A)**. Prominence of metopic suture is insignificant. *Dysmorphic facies* are seen in Down syndrome, many chromosomal anomalies, genetic syndromes, mucopolysaccharidoses, and intrauterine insults. *Hypertrichosis* is excess hair growth. It may be familial or racial if on the face. Conditions associated with hypertrichosis are Cushing's syndrome, congenital adrenal hyperplasia, genetic disorders, fetal exposure to hydantoin and alcohol, postnatal administration of hydantoin, diazoxide, cyclosporin, penicillamine, and corticosteroids. Synophrys (closely placed or continuous eyebrows in the midline) is a feature of de Lange syndrome **(Fig. 7.21)**.

- *Orbits and eyes:* Assess the size and shape of the eyes, look for squint (Ref. Ch. 21), long curly eyelashes, and palpebral fissures. Microphthalmos is abnormally small eye in all dimensions made out by microcornea; can be an isolated congenital anomaly or a manifestation of intrauterine infection. Enophthalmos is the inward placement of the eye following infection or trauma and phthisis bulbi. Colobomas are the partial absence of eyelids. In puffiness of the face orbits appear full; in proptosis the eye is pushed forward with visible sclera above and below the cornea. Bilateral proptosis is seen in craniofacial anomalies and hyperthyroidism. Exophthalmos (often used interchangeably with proptosis) is protrusion of the eyeballs due to endocrine problems. *Unilateral proptosis* often heralds serious diseases **(Fig. 7.22)**. **Box 7.6** enumerates the causes of unilateral proptosis.

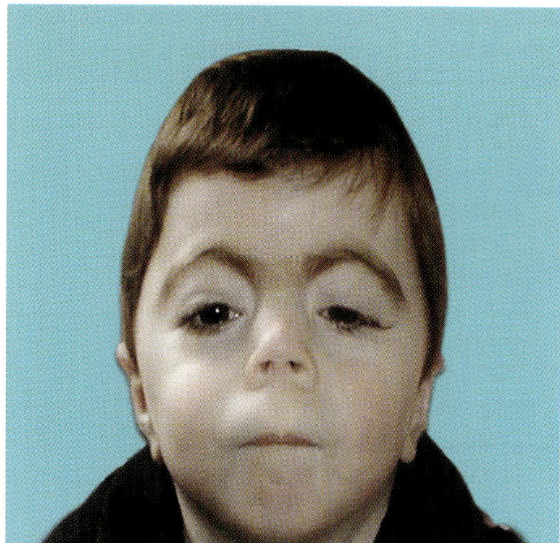

Fig. 7.21: De Lange syndrome revealing synophrys, curly eyelashes and long philtrum.

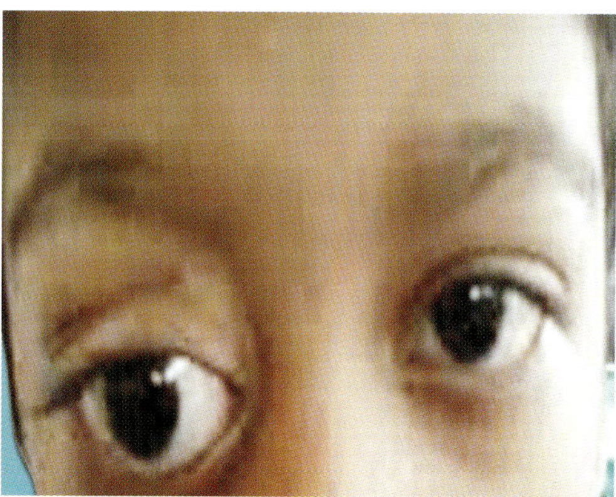

Fig. 7.22: Unilateral proptosis (R)-in a child with acute myeloid leukemia.

- *Observe the alignment of eyes:* Look for hyper or hypotelorism, i.e., increased or narrow interorbital distance respectively, by measuring the inner canthal distance **(Fig. 7.23A)**. Both these anomalies are

BOX 7.6: Causes of unilateral proptosis in children.

- *Infections:*
  - Orbital cellulitis
  - Thrombophlebitis
  - Orbital abscess
  - Osteomyelitis of orbital bones
- *Vascular problems:*
  - Aneurysms
  - Arteriovenous malformations
  - Hematoma
- *Inflammations:*
  - Myositis
  - Vasculitis
  - Sarcoidosis
- *Neoplasms:*
  - *Benign lesions:*
    - Lacrimal cysts
    - Lacrimal adenomas
    - Lipomas
    - Osteomas
    - Dermoid cysts
- *Malignant disorders:*
  - *Primary*
    - Optic gliomas
    - Retinoblastoma
    - Myeloma
    - Histiocytosis
    - Rhabdomyosarcoma
  - *Secondary malignancies:*
    - Leukemia
    - Lymphoma
    - Neuroblastoma

often morphogenetic variations. Isolated hypertelorism can be associated with frontal meningocele or encephalocele; associated visual defects or progressive primary optic atrophy can occur. Hypertelorism is a feature in Down, Zellweger, and Turner's syndromes, skeletal dysplasias, hypothyroidism, and genetic abnormalities. Isolated hypotelorism can be associated with holoprosencephaly and scaphocephaly and is found in 13 trisomy, 18p syndrome, hypopituitarism, and genetic disorders.

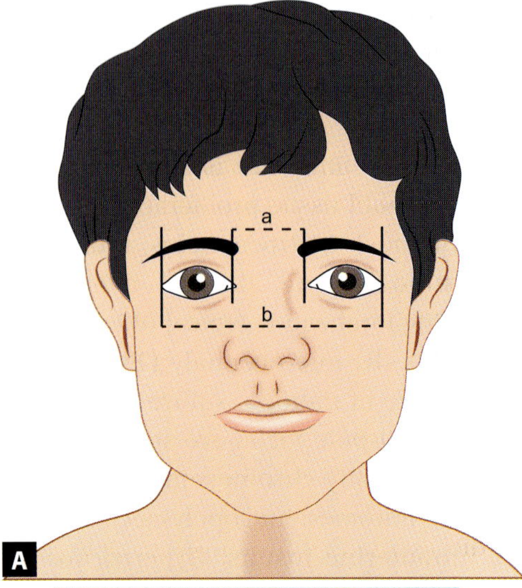

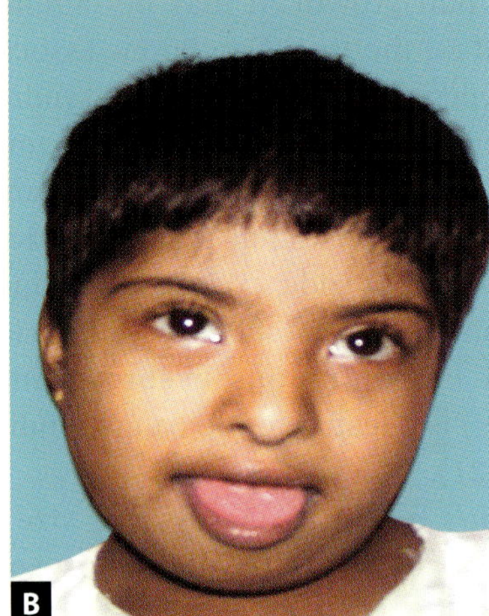

Figs. 7.23A and B: (A) Canthal distance measurement—(a) Inner canthal distance and (b) Outer canthal distance. (B) Hypertelorism in Down syndrome.

Assessment is by estimating the canthal index (100 × inner canthal distance divided by outer canthal distance). Normal values are 38 (SD: 2.4) for boys and 38.5 (SD: 2.4) for girls. The distances between inner and outer canthi should be measured with a transparent scale. Normally the distance between the two inner canthi (inner canthal distance), equals the distance between the inner and outer canthi of each eye. In hypertelorism, the inner canthal distance (a) will be wider than the distance between the inner and outer canthal distance (b).

- *Palpebral fissures:* Assess the levels of the canthi for upward or downward slant. In mongoloid slant the outer canthi are placed at a higher level than the inner canthi **(Fig. 7.23B)**. Mongoloid slant is seen in 21 trisomy, Zellweger, Prader-Willi, and 4p-syndromes. Mongoloid slant is a normal facial appearance among certain racial groups. The common diseases with antimongoloid slant (outer canthi placed at a lower level than inner canthi) are trisomy 17 and 18, Cri-du-chat (5p-), Alport, and Treacher Collin syndromes.

  Medial epicanthal folds are vertical or oblique skin folds (partial or complete) on the upper eyelids seen with increased frequency in syndromes and trisomies; their isolated presence does not carry any significance **(Fig. 7.24)**.

  Long and curly eyelashes, synophrys, and hypertrichosis are features of Cornelia de Lange syndrome **(Fig. 7.21)**.

- *Infections and infestations* of the eyelids are blepharitis (scaly, itchy, and ulcerated lid margins), hordeolum externum (stye), chalazion and pediculosis of the eyelashes (*Staphylococcus aureus* is the most common bacterial infection). Purulent discharge, sticky eyes, conjunctival congestion with hemorrhages, chemosis, and palpebral edema indicate conjunctivitis **(Figs. 7.25A and B)**.

  Examine the sclera for jaundice **(Fig. 7.9)**, pigmentation, dryness, vitamin A deficiency signs and inflammatory lesions like phlycten and episcleritis. The earliest sign of Vitamin A deficiency

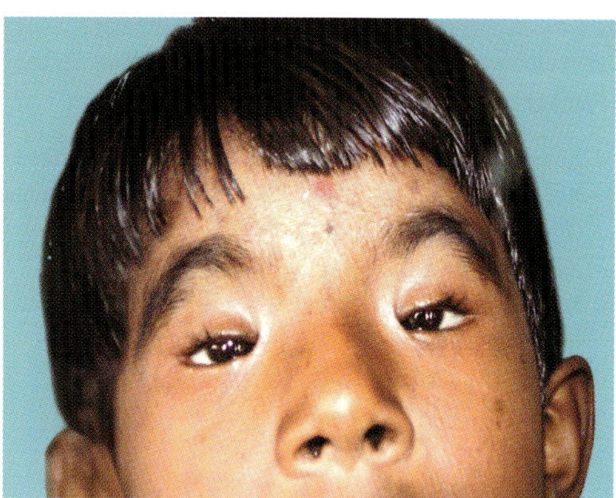

Fig. 7.24: Medial epicanthal folds in a normal girl.

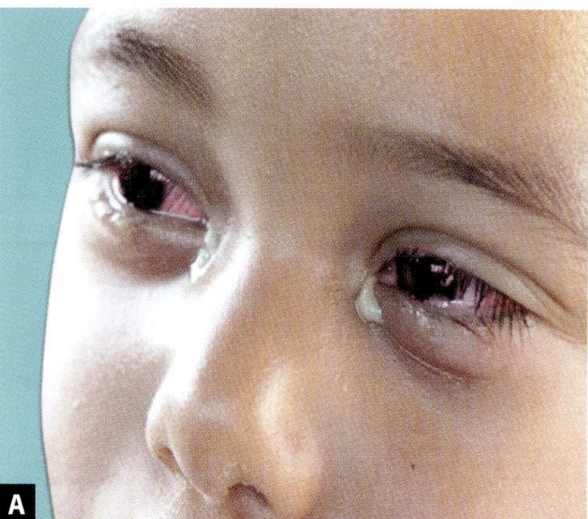

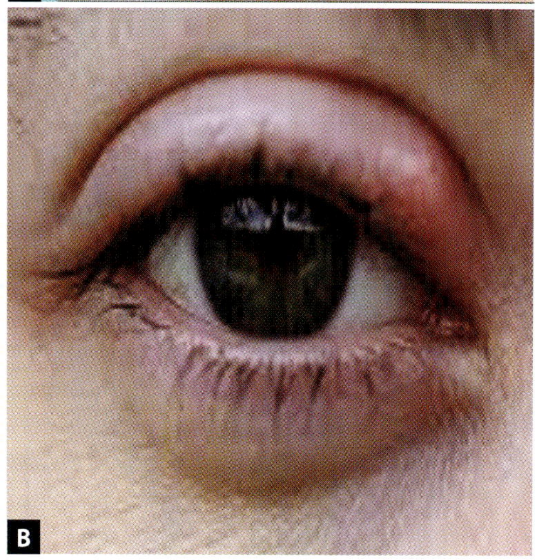

Figs. 7.25A and B: (A) Conjunctivitis and (B) Stye upper eyelid.

TABLE 7.8: WHO classification of xerophthalmia.

Primary signs	*Secondary signs*
• XIA conjunctival xerosis • XIB Bitot's spots **(Fig. 7.26)** • X2 corneal xerosis • X3A corneal ulceration (<1/3 of cornea) • X3B corneal ulceration (>1/3 of cornea)	• XN night blindness • XF fundal changes • XS corneal scarring

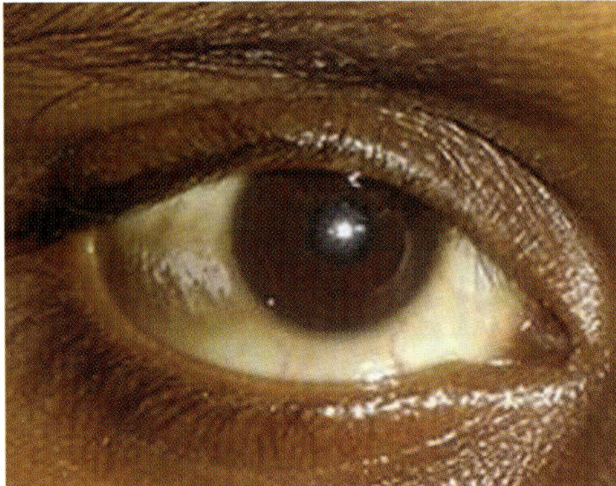

Fig. 7.26: Bitot's spot.

is xerophthalmia characterized by dryness and wrinkling of sclera. **Table 7.8** reveals the WHO classification of xerophthalmia. Bitot's spots are triangular scaly patches of keratinization with dirty white color having shiny appearance and base near the cornea.

In newborns and infants, the sclera is thin with bluish tint; by 6 m of age, the sclera acquires white color. Persistence of blue color is seen in osteogenesis imperfecta, Marfan syndrome, Ehlers-Danlos syndrome, and congenital glaucoma (Ref. **Fig. 25.9**).

- *Cornea:* Assess the size (microcornea <10 mm, megalocornea >13 mm), and look for dryness or ulceration, last is the terminal stage of vitamin A deficiency leading to blindness.

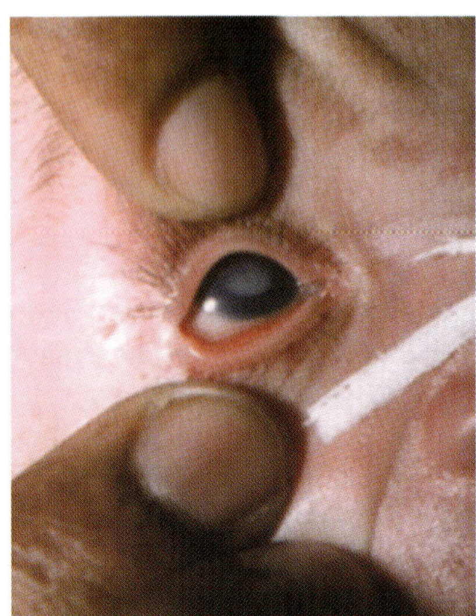

Fig. 7.27: Congenital cataract.

BOX 7.7: Causes of cataract in children.

- *Congenital:* Isolated
- *Secondary:*
  - IU infections (TORCH group)
  - Galactosemia
  - Hypoparathyroidism
  - Homocystinuria
  - Marfan syndrome
  - Radiation therapy
  - Hypoparathyroidism

- *Iris:* Aniridia is absent iris (seen in Wilms tumor). Brush field spots are salt and pepper appearance of the iris in Down syndrome.
- *Pupils (Ref. Ch. 21)* may be irregular and abnormally placed. Look for white eye reflex due to *cataract or retinoblastoma* **(Fig. 7.27)**. **Box 7.7** reveals the causes of cataracts in newborns.
  - *Ectopia lentis* is the displacement of the lens; the complaints are blurring

of vision and diplopia. Simple ectopia lentis is heritable. Disorders with ectopia lentis are Marfan syndrome, homocystinuria, and Ehlers-Danlos syndrome. In simple ectopia lentis and Marfan syndrome, the lens displacement is up and lateral; in homocystinuria, the displacement is downward and nasal. Trauma, infections, inflammations, and skeletal dysplasias are the common causes of lens displacement.

- *Epiphora* is overflowing with tears seen in babies due to nasolacrimal duct obstruction or infections. Corneal trauma, foreign body impaction, and eye infection are the common causes of epiphora in older children.
- *Vision and fundus:* Ref. Ch. 21 for details.

- *Nose* may be flat or bulbous with an upturned tip. *Depressed nasal bridge* is seen in hydrocephalus, rickets, congenital syphilis, chondrodystrophy, and Down syndrome. A small nose is typical of trisomy 21 and 13. Upper respiratory infections are common in daycare and school-going children. Persistently purulent, foul-smelling, or blood-stained discharge from the nostrils indicates foreign bodies inside the nose (small pieces of plastic or paper are the common items) and adenoid hypertrophy. In leech-infested areas, persistent and prolonged nasal bleeding can occur due to the migration of leech inside the nostrils. Very narrow nares with persistent discharge are common in Down syndrome. A horizontal crease across the lower part of the nose is seen in children with allergic rhinitis and adenoids due to repeated upward rubbing of the nose tip termed "the allergic salute" **(Fig. 7.28)**; allergic shiners are dark circles beneath the eyelids.

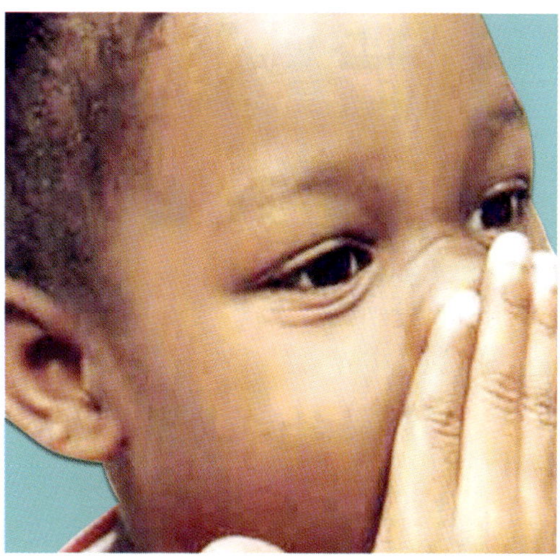

Fig. 7.28: Allergic salute with horizontal nasal crease.

Choanal atresia should be suspected in babies with severe respiratory distress during feeding but gets relieved by crying. *To detect choanal atresia* hold a wisp of cotton in front of each nostril and see its movement as the baby breaths. Lack of movement of the cotton wisp during expiration indicates choanal atresia; confirm the obstruction by passing a nasogastric tube. Look for foreign body or polyp through a nasal speculum.

Adenoid hypertrophy children present with persistent snoring, open mouth, disturbed sleep, hyponasal speech, poor attention span, and frequent URI.

Adenoid facies (long face syndrome) is revealed by dull face, pinched up nostrils, open mouth, everted upper lip, crowded upper teeth, hypoplastic maxilla, and narrow highly arched hard palate **(Fig. 7.29)**.

- *Ears:* Examine the ears for size, shape, alignment, and abnormalities. Large prominent ears (bat ears) are seen in microcephaly and chromosomal anomalies. Small rudimentary ears with intact hearing are not uncommon. Assess whether the ears

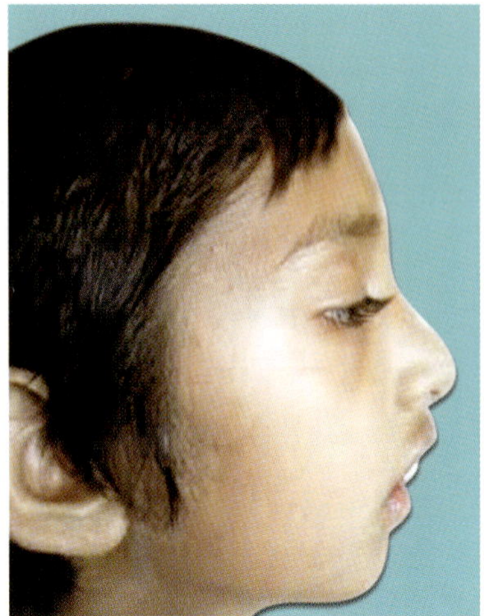

Fig. 7.29: Adenoid facies.

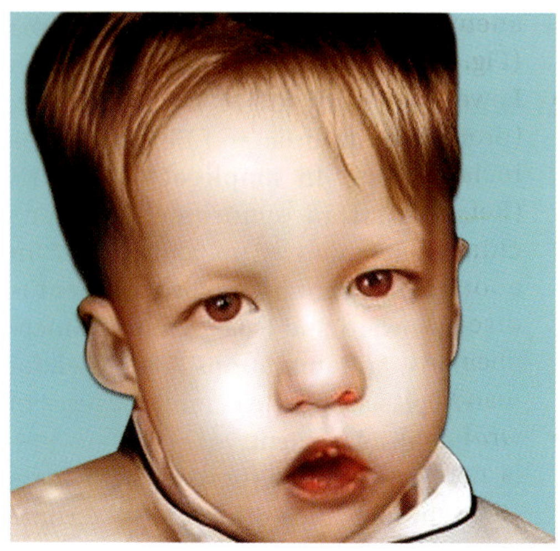

Fig. 7.30: DiGeorge syndrome—note the short philtrum.

are low set; for this examine the child from the front holding the child's head erect with eyes looking forward. A transparent paper (3 inches wide and lengthy enough to encircle the head beyond the ears) on which a horizontal central line is drawn is placed over the orbit in such a way that the line intersects both the inner canthi. Ears are considered low set if the superior attachment of the pinna is below the canthal line. Other anomalies are preauricular tag (Ref. Ch. 15) and sinuses. Ear anomalies usually indicate associated cardiac or renal anomalies, which should be looked for.

Examine the *external ear canals and tympanic membranes* (as the last item) using appropriate-sized otoscopes in all infants and children with unexplained fever, upper respiratory infection, earache, or ear discharge (Ref. Ch. 19).

- *Mouth:* Philtrum is short in Di George syndrome due to the thin and everted upper lip **(Fig. 7.30)**. Philtrum is long in fetal alcohol and fetal hydantoin syndromes and in Cornelia de Lange

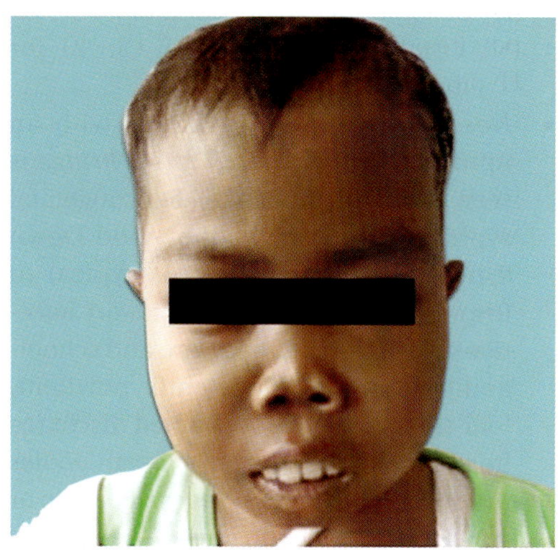

Fig. 7.31: Maxillary hyperplasia in thalassemia major.

syndrome **(Fig. 7.21)**. The most common congenital anomaly in the mouth is cleft lip which may be associated with cleft palate (Ref. Ch. 15).

Jaws: Look for abnormal shape, size, and malalignment of upper and lower jaws. Depressed nasal bridge, maxillary hyperplasia, and protrusion of the upper jaw are features of chronic hemolytic anemias, especially *thalassemia major* **(Fig. 7.31)**.

- Lower jaw anomalies such as prognathia (protruding chin beyond the maxillary incisors), retrognathia [receding chin (Ref. Ch. 15)], and micrognathia [small chin (Ref. Ch. 15)] can be isolated anomalies or associated with genetic diseases or syndromes. Difficulty in opening the mouth can occur in temporomandibular arthritis.
- *Oral cavity:* Thrush (oral candidiasis) is common in infants and resembles sticky milk curds which leave behind raw mucosa on removal **(Fig. 20.9)**. Look for abnormalities of gums, palate, uvula and tongue, bleeding tendency as revealed by gum bleeding or purpuric or ecchymotic patches inside mouth and oral hygiene. Hyperplastic gum is spongy in nature **(Fig. 7.32)**. The causes of gum hyperplasia are given in **Box 7.8**. The palate may be high-arched. A cleft palate can be isolated, or occur along with syndromes or chromosomal anomalies. Bifid uvula may indicate a submucous cleft palate which can be diagnosed by palpation of soft palate **(Fig. 19.3)**.
  - *Dentition: Primary teeth (total 20)* start erupting by 5–8 m of age and are completed before 30 m of age. The lower central incisors are the first to appear. The approximate number of primary teeth in a toddler can be roughly assessed by the formula: Number of primary teeth = Age in months-6.
  - *Permanent teeth* (differ from primary teeth by their dull white color, rough surface, and serrated biting edge) are 32 in number and erupt in the order as given in **Table 7.9**.

    Look for the number of teeth, their arrangement, color, and presence of dental caries. Delayed eruption of primary and permanent teeth (>13 m and 8 yr of age respectively) are usually familial or idiopathic. **Box 7.9** gives the causes of delayed dentition.

    Evaluate the teeth for abnormal alignment or absent teeth. Black

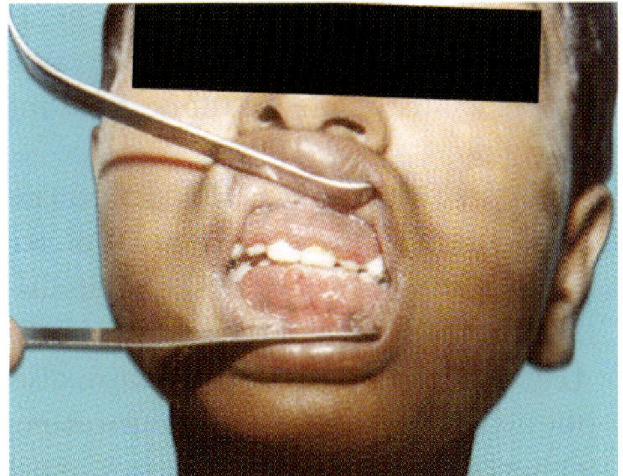

Fig. 7.32: Gum hyperplasia in acute myeloid leukemia.

BOX 7.8: Causes of gum hyperplasia.

- Gingivitis
- Drug-induced (phenytoin, amlodipine, and cyclosporine)
- Neurofibromatosis 1
- Scurvy
- Acute myeloid (monocytic) leukemia
- Xanthomatosis
- Histiocytosis X
- Hereditary gingival fibromatosis
- Granulomatous diseases
- Epulis

TABLE 7.9: Order of eruption of permanent teeth.

Category of teeth	*Age at eruption (yr)*
First molars	6
Central and lateral incisors	6–8
Canines, premolars	9–12
Second molars	12
Third molars	≥18

BOX 7.9: Causes of delayed dentition.

- Protein-energy malnutrition
- Nutritional rickets
- Hypothyroidism
- Hypopituitarism
- Hypoparathyroidism
- Genetic syndromes
- Chromosomal anomalies
- Incontinentia pigmenti
- Cleidocranial dysostosis
- Progeria

staining of teeth can occur in poor oral hygiene, oral iron therapy, fluorosis, and osteogenesis imperfecta. In hypophosphatemic rickets and dental caries, dental discoloration and decay will be present. Yellowish discoloration of teeth indicates tetracycline intake during the intrauterine period or early childhood. Dental damage can be due to caries, congenital syphilis, or ectodermal dysplasia. Natal teeth (teeth present at birth) do not have any significance **(Fig. 15.9)**. They are shed along with the primary teeth.

- *Tongue:* Examine for the size, appearance, and fibrillations. Large tongue (macroglossia)is seen in hypothyroidism, glycogen storage disease typeII (Pompe disease), Beckwith syndrome **(Fig. 20.13)**, lingual thyroid, lymphangioma, hemangioma, and mucopolysaccharidosis. In Down syndrome tongue appears large due to small jaw (relative macroglossia). The tongue is small and atrophic in hypoglossal nerve paralysis (Ref. **Fig. 21.16**). Strawberry tongue is seen in Kawasaki disease and scarlet fever (Ref. **Fig. 20.12**).
- *Neck:* Observe from front and back for shortening, webbing, torticollis (wryneck), swellings, and sinuses, and in lying posture for retraction and neck stiffness (Ref. Ch. 21). Fever with neck stiffness in children may indicate meningitis, encephalitis, brain abscess, retropharyngeal/lateral pharyngeal abscess, deep-seated neck abscess, or osteomyelitis of the cervical spine **(Fig. 7.33)**. If afebrile, consider neck trauma, battered child, tetanus, spinal caries, and Arnold–Chiari malformation. Measure the neck length if any obvious anomaly (Ref. Ch. 11) and find its ratio with the total body height. *Torticollis* (tilting of the occiput to one side and chin to the opposite side) can be congenital or traumatic injury to soft tissues or bones. **Box 7.10** enumerates the acquired causes of torticollis (acute and long-standing) in children.
- *Short neck* with webbing (best appreciated from the back by the presence of skin folds from upper neck to shoulders) is a feature of Turner and Noonan syndromes **(Fig. 7.19)**. In congenital hypothyroidism, the neck is short and thick without webbing. Other causes of the short neck are Klippel–Feil syndrome, chromosomal anomalies (trisomy 21), mucopolysaccharidoses,

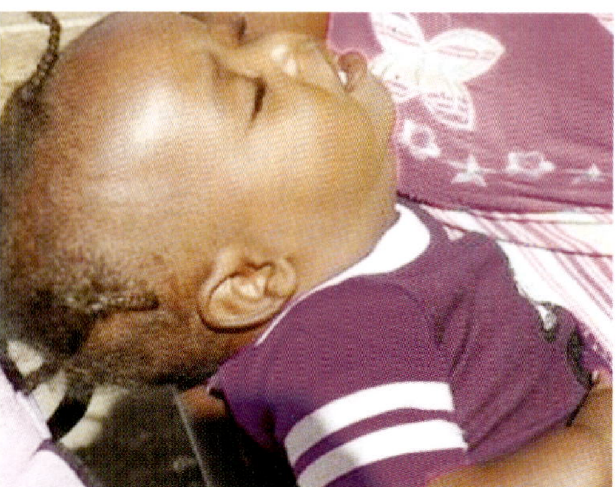

Fig. 7.33: Meningitis revealing neck stiffness.

BOX 7.10: Acquired causes of torticollis in children.

- *Neck:*
  - Traumatic injury (soft tissues, bones)
  - Infections*
  - Inflammations—JIA and myositis
  - Atlantoaxial subluxation
  - Cerebral palsy
  - Hematoma neck (coagulopathies)
- Upper lobe pneumonia
- Drug induced (phenothiazines)
- Visual defects
- Syringomyelia
- Wilson disease
- Tumors#
- GERD

*Cellulitis, abscess, and osteomyelitis.
#Posterior cranial fossa and cervical cord.
(GERD: Gastroesophageal reflux disease; JIA: juvenile idiopathic arthritis)

genetic syndromes, and cervical vertebral anomalies.

Look for pulsations of carotid arteries and jugular veins (Ref. Ch.17 for details).

Neck swellings are very common and range from congenital to neoplastic in etiology, as already discussed in the differential diagnosis of cervical lymphadenopathy in this section.

- *Chest:* Inspect and palpate for deformities and tenderness of the thoracic cage and the spine. Short sternum, pectus carinatum (pigeon breast), and pectus excavatum (funnel chest) are some of the common anomalies. Short sternum is a feature of trisomy 18.
- *Pectus carinatum* (prominence of the sternum along with cartilaginous parts of ribs, often with lateral depression of thorax) is seen in rickets, skeletal dysplasias, and long-standing heart diseases **(Fig. 7.34)**. *Pectus excavatum* (midline narrowing of the thoracic cavity due to depression of the sternum) is seen in rickets, upper airway obstruction, and Marfan syndrome; can be idiopathic also. Absent or hypoplastic ribs are usually congenital but are common in trisomy 13. Look for scoliosis (lateral convexity) and kyphosis (exaggerated posterior convexity) of the spine (Ref. Ch. 25).

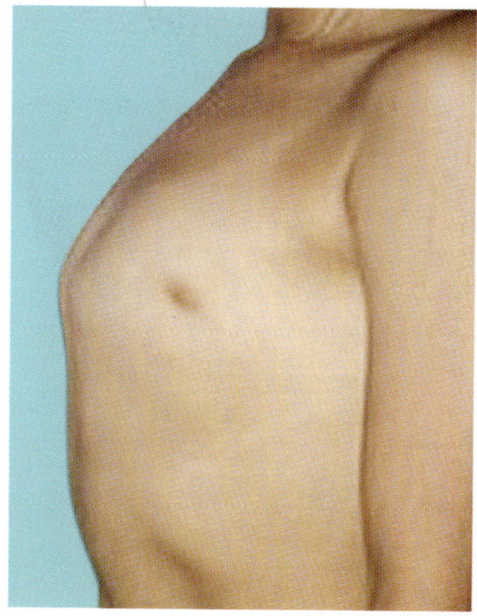

Fig. 7.34: Pectus carinatum with Harrison's groove.

BOX 7.11: Causes of Harrison's groove.

- Idiopathic
- *Acquired:*
  - Rickets
  - Chronic persistent asthma
  - Congenital laryngeal stridor
  - Chronic congestive cardiac failure (CCF)
  - Spinal muscular atrophy
  - Myopathies
  - Cystic fibrosis

- *Harrison's groove* is a horizontal depression along the lower border of the chest from the sternum to mid axillary line corresponding to the insertion of the diaphragm. The causes of Harrison's groove in children are given in **Box 7.11**.

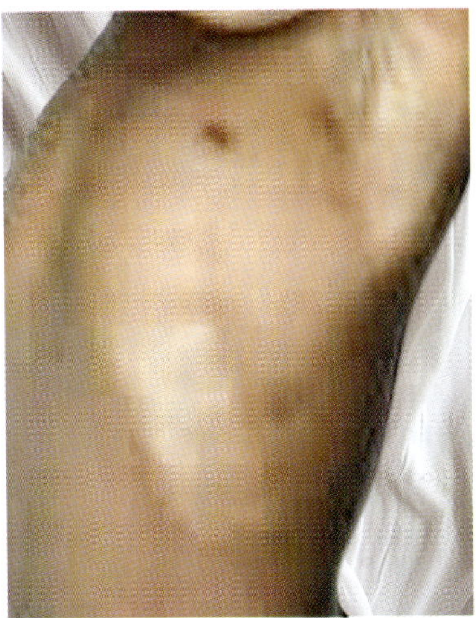

Fig. 7.35: Rickety rosary.

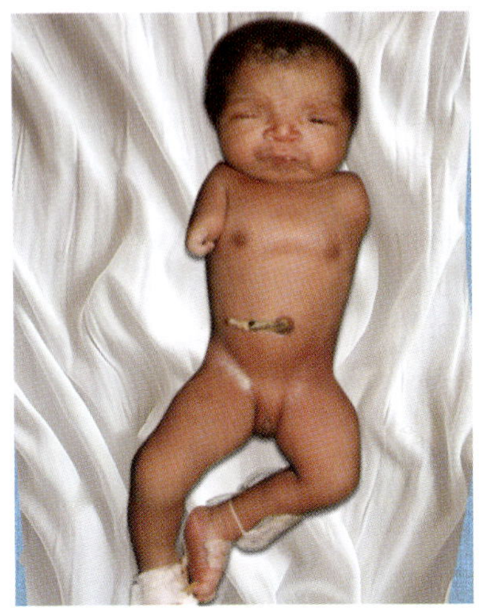

Fig. 7.36: Amelia (left) and rhizomelia (right).

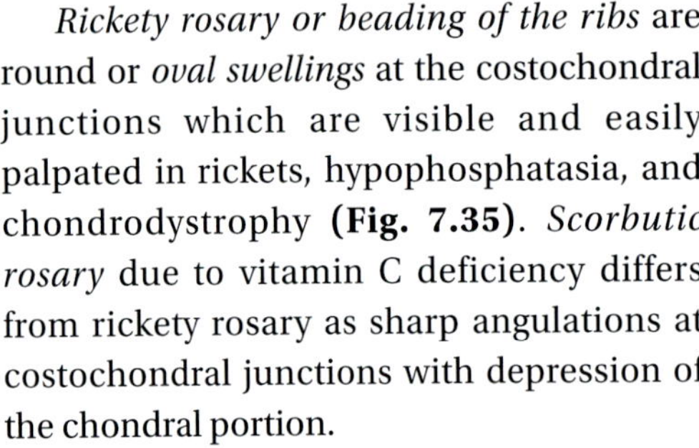

Rickety rosary or beading of the ribs are round or *oval swellings* at the costochondral junctions which are visible and easily palpated in rickets, hypophosphatasia, and chondrodystrophy **(Fig. 7.35)**. *Scorbutic rosary* due to vitamin C deficiency differs from rickety rosary as sharp angulations at costochondral junctions with depression of the chondral portion.

Nipples should be inspected for abnormal distribution and number. Measure the inter nipple distance which normally makes up 25% of chest circumference. A ratio >30% indicates *widely spaced nipples*, characteristic of Turner syndrome in which they are hypoplastic also. The presence of accessory nipples indicates possible association with congenital heart disease. Examine for deformities, pain, tenderness, or lump, which can be solid (soft or firm) or cystic. The skin over the swelling may be adherent or ulcerated in various diseases. Assess the pubertal stage of the child (Ref. Ch. 11 for SMR). *Axillae* should be inspected for *hair growth (pubarche)*, a normal phenomenon in puberty. Isolated pubarche indicates adrenal cortical stimulation in young children which should be investigated.

- *Upper limbs:* Standing on the back of the patient observe the upper limb length in relation to the body stature. Ask the child to keep the arms by the side of the body; normally the fingertips fall between the iliac crest and the upper one-third of the thighs. If the fingertips remain above the iliac crests, it is clinical disproportion indicating short limb. *Sprengel* deformity is scapula located at an abnormally high position due to the failure to descend to its normal location. Evaluate the limbs. *Amelia* is absent limb. Relative shortening is *rhizomelia*, *mesomelia*, and *acromelia* (proximal, middle, and distal segments, respectively **(Fig. 7.36)**. Fingers may show brachydactyly (generalized shortening of fingers), clinodactyly (incurving of fingers), syndactyly (fusion or webbing of fingers), arachnodactyly (long thin fingers resembling spider legs), camptodactyly (restricted extension) and hyperextensibility. Polydactyly (excess number of fingers) may be on the thumb side (preaxial) or on the little finger side [postaxial **(Figs. 7.37A and B)**]. Finger anomalies are usually associated with congenital heart diseases.

Assess the *length of the little finger*. Normally it should be up to the distal flexion crease of the fourth finger. Single flexion creases and clinodactyly of fingers indicate hypoplasia of the middle phalanx, a common feature in chromosomal anomalies.

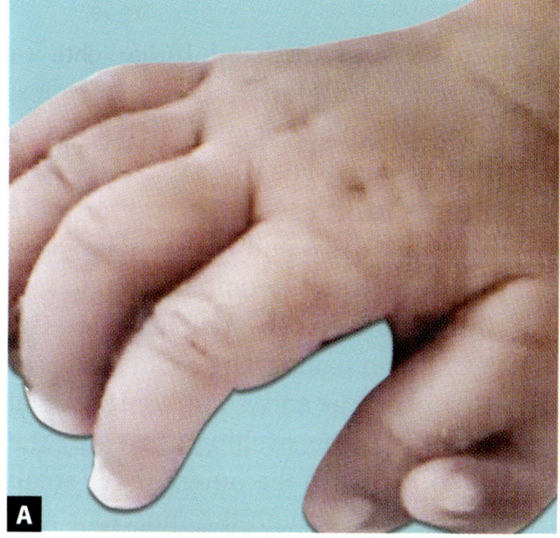

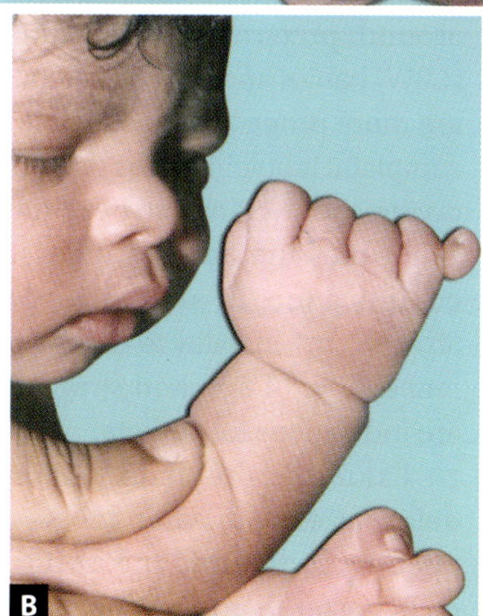

Figs. 7.37A and B: (A) Preaxial polydactyly and (B) Postaxial polydactyly.

- *Thumb:* Examine for hyperplasia, tri phalanx, proximal or distal alignment. Thumb anomalies are found in various genetic syndromes and chromosomal disorders.

The long thumb in arachnodactyly (seen in Marfan syndrome and homocystinuria) is detected by the *thumb sign* (protrusion of the thumb beyond the palm when the hand is fisted with thumb adducted on palm) and *wrist sign* (thumb overlapping the fifth finger when encircling the opposite wrist). *Cortical thumb* (Ref. Ch. 21) is a thumb constantly held adducted on the palm. It is a sign of cerebral cortical damage from birth asphyxia if it persists beyond 2 m of age. The presence of a web of skin tethering the thumb is prenatal adduction deformity.

The fists: If the metacarpals are short, the relevant knuckles will be absent and get replaced by dimples—this "Archibald's metacarpal sign" **(Fig. 7.38)**, seen in Turner syndrome and pseudohypoparathyroidism,

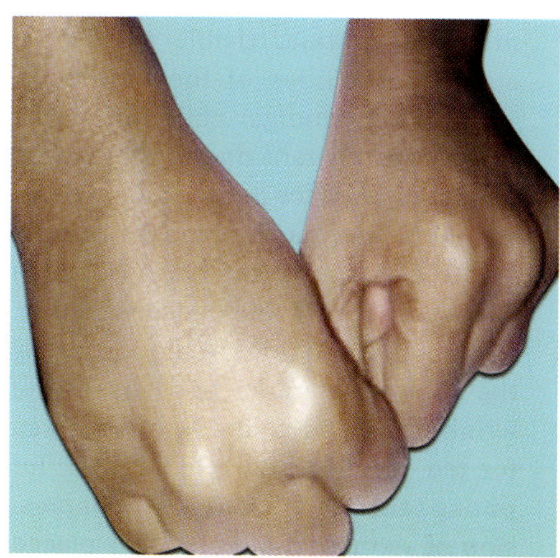

Fig. 7.38: The metacarpal sign.

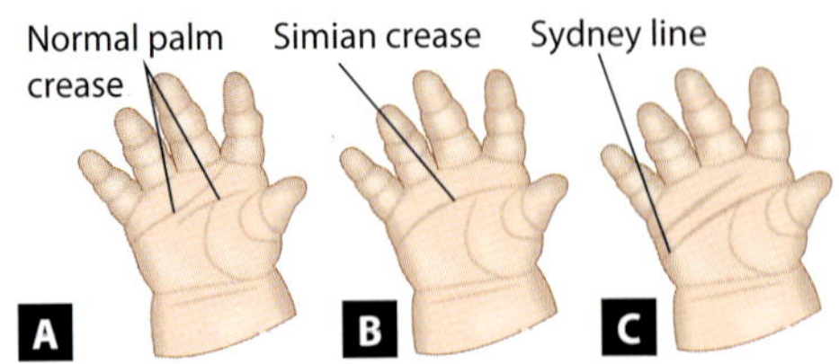

Figs. 7.39A to C: Palmar flexion creases. (A) Normal; (B) Simian crease; and (C) Sydney crease.

is due to the hypoplasia of fourth and fifth metacarpals.

Evaluate the palmar flexion creases: A transverse crease, widely known as the "simian crease" (terminology now abandoned) is single distal crease or bridging of two creases and reflects a short palm **(Figs. 7.39A to C)**. Bilateral single palmar crease is found in 50% of children with Down syndrome and also in 10% of normal children. Unilateral single palmar crease is seen in 4% of normal children. *Sydney crease* is the proximal palmar crease transversely placed over the entire palm; they occur in higher frequency in chromosomal disorders and genetic syndromes but are not considered as diagnostic criteria.

- *Abdomen:* Observe the size, shape, pigmentation, striae, visible peristalsis, and abnormalities of the umbilicus. Abdomen in younger children will be slightly protuberant due to the normal lumbar lordosis for the age and appears scaphoid in diaphragmatic hernia, severe marasmus, intrauterine growth restriction (IUGR), and duodenal atresia. Look for abdominal wall edema by the shiny appearance and absence of wrinkles; pinch a fold of skin and keep for ten seconds and release; look for pitting (alternately, look at the impression of stethoscope diaphragm placed for abdominal auscultation). "Phantom hernia" is a localized bulge due to paralysis of abdominal wall muscles, pathognomonic of paralytic poliomyelitis (rarely seen nowadays).

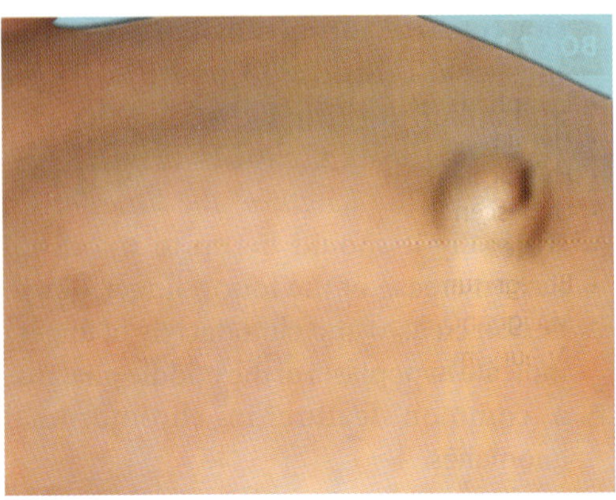

Fig. 7.40: Umbilical hernia with divarication of recti.

- *Umbilicus (Ref. Ch. 15, 20 for more details):* Pain and foul-smelling discharge from the umbilicus indicates infection due to poor hygiene. The common pathogens are *Streptococcus* hemolyticus and *S. aureus*. Umbilical hernia is the swelling caused by the protrusion of the omentum or small intestine through the muscular ring around; preterm or low birth weight (LBW) babies and the black population are more prone **(Fig. 7.40)**. The usual complaint is bulging of the umbilicus on crying; the swelling can be reduced by gentle pressure. Strangulation is a rare complication in umbilical hernia. Size (>5 cm), inability to reduce, persistence >6 yr of age, and strangulation are indications for surgery.

Examine the back for spinal deformities and *pilonidal sinus* (an opening in the midline of the natal cleft posterior to the anal opening) which may be concealed by a tuft of hair.

BOX 7.12: Causes of groin swelling.

- Lymphadenopathy
- Hernia
- Hydrocele
- Undescended testis
- Abscess
- Benign tumors—lipoma and cyst
- Malignancies—lymphoma and neuroblastoma
- Aneurysms

Inguinal region or groin is the area between the lowest part of the abdomen and the beginning of the thigh. Examine carefully for any groin swelling. See **Box 7.12** for the causes of groin swellings. Assess the size, and consistency (soft/firm/hard) and look for the signs of inflammation, (tenderness/painful restriction of movements, warmth, redness), adherence to the skin/other tissues, presence of draining sinuses, ulcers over the surface, transillumination, and reducibility. Examine the drainage areas (lower half of the abdomen to upper half of thighs) for infected lesions. Lymphadenopathy due to viral/bacterial/filarial infections is the most common cause for groin swellings. TB lymph nodes are firm, usually multiple, matted, nontender, adherent to the overlying skin, may have draining sinuses/superficial ulcers; can present with cold abscess. Hernia and hydrocele present as inguinoscrotal swelling, soft in consistency and nontender (unless the hernia is strangulated). In hernias, the upper border of the swelling cannot be reached, can get impulse on crying/coughing and the size gets reduced on lying down. Lipomas are soft in consistency. Malignant tumors are hard in consistency, will be fixed to the deeper tissues, and are immobile.

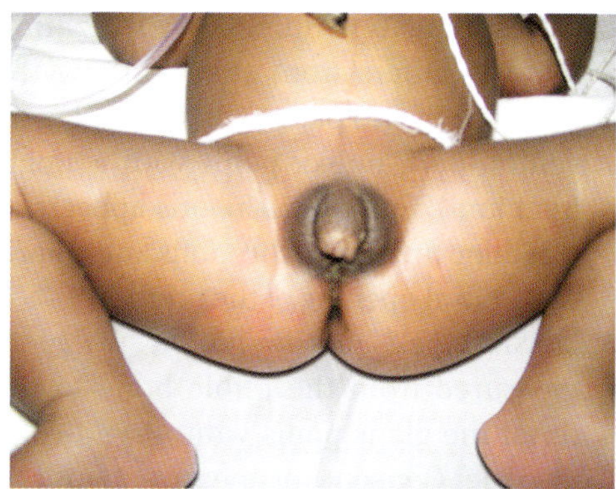

Fig. 7.41: Ambiguous genitalia revealing enlarged phallus and absent testes.

- *External genitalia:* Supine frog-leg position is preferred for examination. Infants should be placed on mother's lap. In older children, gently explain the situation and get the child's consent. Assess for cleanliness, redness, pink color with secretion (in girls), injuries, warts, and parasitic infestations (scabies and pubic lice). Assess the configuration of the genitalia for normality. In girls look for purulent vaginal discharge, bleeding, ulcers, adherent labia, hymenal configuration, hematocolpos (in adolescents), ambiguity, virilization, stage of pubertal development, evidence of sexual abuse, presence of any foreign body, and neoplasm (sarcoma botryoides resembling grape-like fleshy mass coming out from the vaginal orifice, seen in young girls). The scrotum is darkly pigmented in newborns and infants with virilizing adrenal hyperplasia. Genitalia is considered ambiguous if two or more abnormalities are found **(Fig. 7.41)**. Describe the ambiguity. Look for *epispadias* (dorsally deficient urethra), *hypospadias* (urethral opening at the ventral surface of the penile shaft), *chordee* (ventral penile curvature), *micropenis, cryptorchidism* [undescended testis (UDT)], *clitoromegaly, adherent labia*, and *absent vaginal opening.*

Clitoromegaly indicates virilization (clitoris differs from the penis by the presence of two paramedian frenulae on ventral part, unlike penis with a single frenulum). Epispadias in girls appears as a midline division of the mons and clitoris with dorsal opening of the urethra.

Stretched penile length (SPL) is measured from the pubic bone to the tip of the glans penis with a rigid ruler or scale. Consent for measurement is a must in older children. Child in supine position, press the ruler firmly against the pubic symphysis depressing the suprapubic fat pad to the maximum. The phallus is gently grasped by its lateral margin and stretched. SPL is measured on the dorsum of the penis from the pubic symphysis to the tip of the glans penis, excluding the foreskin. Penile length is approximately 3.5 cm in a term baby. Increment of 0.5 cm/yr occurs up to the age of 6 yrs and, thereafter penile growth increases according to the pubertal stage (Ref. Ch. 24).

- *Micropenis* is small penis, 2.5 SDs below the mean in length, but anatomically correct in terms of urethral development. *Inconspicuous penis* is the type that appears to be small but of normal size (seen in obesity and when buried within the scrotum by skinfold or fat). The causes of micropenis are given in **Box 7.13** (Details in Ch. 24).

Phimosis is inability to retract the prepuce which may be primary or secondary. The former is caused by physiological adhesions and spontaneously separates over the first 10 yrs of life. Secondary phimosis is due to scarring following inflammation or surgery. Examine the urethral meatus for purulent discharge or ulceration.

BOX 7.13: Causes of micropenis.

- Isolated
- *Secondary:*
  - Hypopituitarism
  - Hypogonadotropic hypogonadism
  - Hypergonadotropic hypogonadism
  - Partial androgen insensitivity
  - Chromosomal disorders
  - Genetic syndromes

Surgical consultation is advised if the child gets repeated urinary infections, or prepuce is not retractable by 10 yrs of age.

Priapism (persistent abnormal and painful erection of the penis) may occur due to local irritation, urethral or bladder calculi, leukemia, sickle cell anemia, spinal cord lesions, urethritis, scorpion envenomation, thrombosis of the corpora cavernosa or Fabry's disease.

Examine the scrotum for inflammation, trauma, hyperpigmentation, and anomalies of the scrotal contents. Grasp the testicle between the thumb and the first two digits to palpate. The epididymis is palpated on the posterior and superior aspect of the testicle. Normally both testes are approximately equal in size, up to 2.5 cm in length before puberty; if the length is <1 cm in the prepubertal period, karyotyping is a must.

Testicular volume must be measured by the Prader orchidometer **(Fig. 7.42)** devised by *Dr Andrea Prader, Swiss Endocrinologist, 1966* or by ultrasonography (normal 0.8 ± 0.1 mL at 2 yr, 3.5 ± 0. 2 mL at 11 yr) (Ref. Ch. 24 for more details). If the testis is nonpalpable consider UDT, ectopic testis, or absent (vanishing) testis, usually characterized by an atrophic remnant in the scrotum or inguinal canal. Small testis is seen in hypopituitarism or Klinefelter syndrome. Large testis

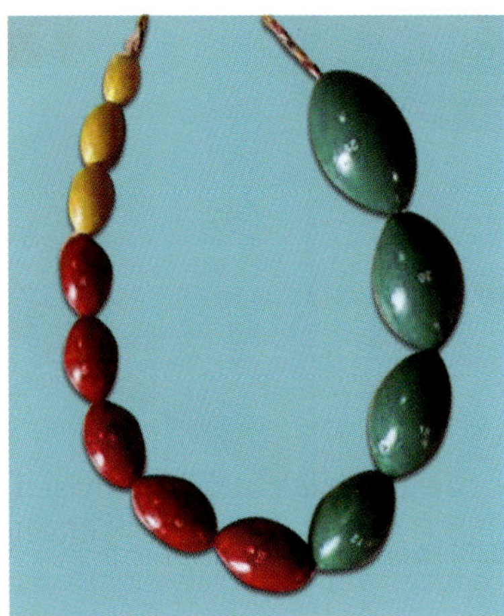

Fig. 7.42: Prader orchidometer.

BOX 7.14: Causes of scrotal masses in children.

- *Painful:*
  - Traumatic damage
  - Cellulitis
  - Abscess
  - Epididymitis
  - Hematoma
  - Incarcerated inguinal hernia
  - Orchitis (mumps and other viral)
  - Ruptured testis
  - Torsion testis/appendix
- *Painless:*
  - Hydrocele
  - Inguinal hernia
  - Idiopathic scrotal edema
  - Spermatocele
  - Varicocele
  - Henoch–Schonlein purpura
- *Neoplasms:*
  - Primary malignancy
  - Secondary leukemic infiltrates

(macroorchidism) is a feature of Fragile X syndrome. **Box 7.14** reveals the causes of scrotal mass in children.

Blunt injuries and hematoma indicate trauma; consider sexual assault in penetrating injuries. Recurrent ulcerations of genitalia (in boys and girls) indicate Behcet's disease.

- *Anus:* Evaluate in the left lateral position (alternate is knee-chest position) after explaining to the child. Gently separate the gluteal folds. Encopresis is fecal soiling (after attaining bowel control) which usually indicates emotional problems. Anterior placing of anal orifice is seen in chromosomal anomalies. Look for abscesses, fistula, fungal infections, traumatic lesions, and ulcers. Eversion of the anal orifice indicates forceful penetration, often due to sexual assault. Rectal prolapse occurs in malnutrition, amoebiasis, giardiasis, whipworm infestation, and cystic fibrosis. Primary and secondary syphilitic ulcers (condyloma lata) are painless nodular ulcers seen around the vulval orifice or anal opening (Ref. Ch. 20 for more details).

  Perineum is the area bounded by pubic symphysis, ischial tuberosities, and coccyx. Evaluate for cleanliness, ulcers, abscesses, congenital fistula, candidal infections, and diaper dermatitis. Frequent watery stools and lactose intolerance can cause redness and excoriation.
- *Lower limbs:* Examine for inequality in size, congenital dislocation of hip (Ref. Ch. 15), bony deformities, swelling and tenderness over bones and joints, and for toe anomalies (number, shape, and alignment). Wide space between first and second toes [sandal gap **(Fig. 7.43A)**] and prominent plantar longitudinal crease [Kennedy crease **(Fig. 7.43B)**] over the corresponding area are characteristic features of Down syndrome. (Ref. Ch. 25 for more details).

CLINICAL CASE SCENARIOS

Clinical Case Scenario 1

Sara, 5 yrs old girl child, was brought to the casualty at 5 AM with six episodes of

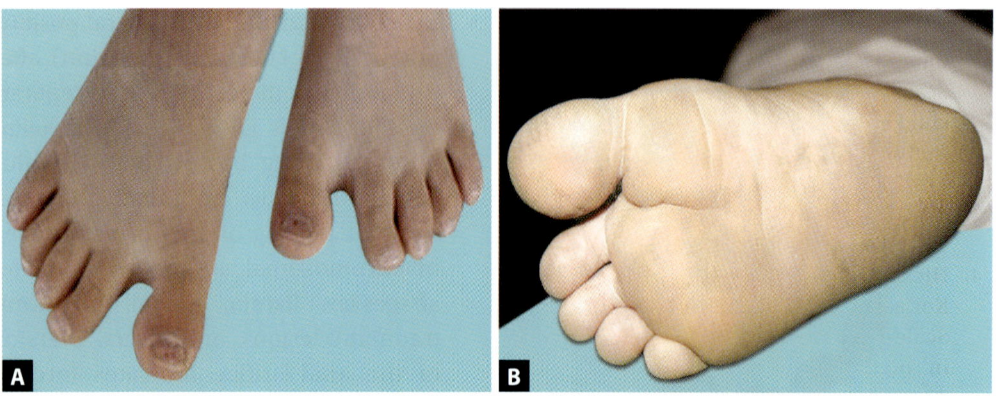

Figs. 7.43A and B: (A) Sandal gap and (B) Kennedy crease.

vomiting and profuse watery stools four times since 1 AM onward. The last vomitus was coffee ground. The girl had chicken sandwiches and ice cream from a festival food court by 7 PM. She took only 150 mL of boiled plain water after 1 AM. Parents are not aware of the time of urine she had voided last.

On examination, she is drowsy, and not responding to calls. Pulse feeble, 140/min, regular. BP 60 mm Hg (systolic). RR 22/min. Temperature 101°F by axilla. Eyes sunken, mouth dry, skin pinch not recoiling after 10 sec. CFT >6 sec. Extremities cold up to the knees and elbows.

Questions:

1. What is the complete diagnosis and probable etiology?
2. What is the cause of coffee ground vomiting?
3. Enumerate all the complications you anticipate in this child.
4. Discuss the immediate treatment you give to this child.

Clinical Case Scenario 2

Aswin, 6 yrs old boy, is brought to the OP with complaints of passing bloody urine for 2 days. No history of fever, dysuria, abdominal pain, pyoderma, wound infection, fall, or blunt trauma over the abdomen. On examination, Arjun is active, no edema, BP 90/60 mm Hg; appears normal on general and systemic examination. His investigation reports (repeated twice in the laboratory) are (1) urine-albumin trace, plenty of RBCs, and two to three pus cells/high-power field on microscopy, culture sterile; (2) abdominal ultrasonography reveals normal findings; (3) blood urea—20 mg/dL, serum creatinine 0.5 mg, serum cholesterol 126 mg/dL, serum proteins—normal. On repeat physical examination a recently healed scar of 1 cm is seen on his right leg. On repeated questioning Aswin admits of getting injured 2 w back while playing which was not disclosed to the parents as he was scared.

Questions:

1. What is the possible clinical diagnosis?
2. What are all the complications you anticipate in this child?

Remember

Reviewing the history and physical examination will help to achieve the diagnosis when the clinical diagnosis and the lab reports are not tallying.

SUGGESTED READING

1. Bang A, Chathurvedi P. Yale Observation Scale for prediction of Bacteremia in Febrile children. Indian J Pediatr. 2009;76(6):599-604.
2. Butt W. Septic shock. In Pediatr Clin North Am. 2001;48:601-25.
3. Hall BD. Approach to skeletal dysplasia. Pediatr Clin North Am. 1992;39(2):279-305.
4. Hicks CL, von Bayer CL, Spafford P, van Korlaar I, Goodenough B. The Faces Pain Scale-Revised: Toward a common metric in pediatric pain measurement. Pain. 2001;93(2):173-83.
5. In: Green M (Ed). Pediatric Advanced Life Support Study Guide, 2nd edition. United States: Mosby; 2005. pp. 97-103.
6. Isaacman DJ, Shutts J, Grows TK, Harper M. Predictors of bacteremia in febrile children 3 to 36 months of age. Pediatrics. 2000;106(5):977-82.
7. Jones KL. Smith's Recognizable Patterns of Human Malformations, 5th edition. Philadelphia: WB Saunders; 1997. p. 759.
8. Mangala S, Jain H. Yale Observation Scale for bacterial infection in febrile children. Int J Contemp. Pediatrics. 2020;7(2): 424-27.
9. McCarthy PL, Sharpe MR, Spiesel SZ, Dolan TF, Forsyth BW, DeWitt TG, et al. Observation scales to identify serious illness in febrile children. Pediatrics. 1982;70(5): 802-9.
10. Ministry of Health and Family Welfare. Government of India. Control of acute respiratory infections. [Online] Available from https://ncdc.mohfw.gov.in/wp-content/uploads/2024/07/National-Guidelines-for-IPC-in-HCF-final1.pdf [Last accessed September, 2024].
11. Smyth A. Physical examination signs. In: Silverman M, Ocollabhan CL (Eds). Practical Pediatric Respiratory Medicine, 1st edition. New Delhi: Viva Books Pvt. Ltd.
12. The genitalia. In: Green M (Ed). Pediatric Diagnosis, 5th edition. Philadelphia: WB Saunders.

8

CHAPTER

Assessment of a Sick Child

Sheeja Sugunan, S Sushamabai

Chapter Outline

INTRODUCTION

Read chapters 1, 2, 3, 4, 6 and 7 before you proceed

Systematic assessment of a sick child is of utmost importance to identify life-threatening conditions and provide timely and appropriate intervention to prevent death and disability. Evaluation, identification, and intervention is a cyclical process that must be repeated throughout the examination of the sick child. That is, once a life-threatening problem is identified immediate intervention must be provided followed by a continuation of assessment in a systematic manner.

- *Child encountered in a place outside the hospital:* Quickly survey the scene around to detect imminent dangers (fire, high voltage electricity, blasts, etc.) and extricate the child to a safe place, protecting the cervical spine (the first priority).
- *Child when encountered in the hospital proceed with systematic evaluation as per the following steps:*
    1. Initial impression
    2. Primary assessment
    3. Secondary assessment
    4. Diagnostic tests
    5. Tertiary assessment

INITIAL IMPRESSION

Initial impression/doorway or hands-off assessment begins as soon as the child is brought to the emergency room (ER) or the outpatient department (OPD); should be a few seconds only to form an impression and to identify whether the child is having a life-threatening illness or not. The three parameters that help to decide the urgency of intervention are the *appearance* of the child, *breathing,* and *color* as revealed in the pediatric assessment triangle **(Fig. 8.1)**.

Appearance

Appearance or consciousness of a child can be assessed by looking at the *tone* or general posture (can be hypo/hypertonia), interaction [depends on varying degrees

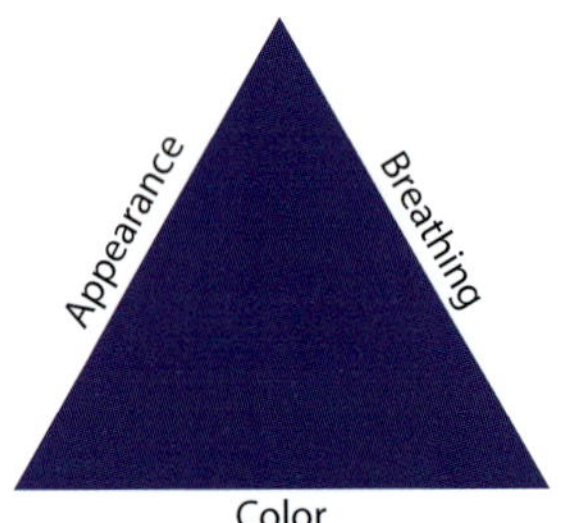

Fig. 8.1: Pediatric assessment triangle.

of sensorium (Ref. **Fig. 9.1**)], *consolability* [excessive crying, irritability, refusal to breastfeed-all reveal inconsolability), *look/gaze,* and *speech* (TICLS)]. Ref. **Fig. 7.2** for poor alertness.

Breathing

Quickly perceived by the chest and abdominal movements. Look for:

- *Respiratory rate (RR):* **Table 8.1** discusses the normal values; *assess* whether increased (tachypnea), decreased (bradypnea), or absent (apnea).
- *Work of breathing (Ref. Ch. 7, 19):* Look for the presence of *tracheal tug, chest retractions,* and *flaring of alae nasi,* all indicate increased work of breathing.
- *Abnormal pattern of breathing (Ref. Ch. 19).*
- *Listen for abnormal respiratory sounds (can be heard with naked ears)*—snoring, grunting, stridor, rattling, and wheezing *(Ref. Ch. 19 for more details).*

Tachypnea is a better sign compared to bradypnea, apnea, and abnormal breathing patterns; the latter signs indicate very serious illness.

- *Color:* Look at the skin and mucous membrane for the color
- Pallor denotes anemia, shock, or blood loss
- *Skin mottling and cyanosis* indicate shock or blood loss.

Based on the initial impression determine if the child's problem is:

- Life-threatening
- Not life-threatening

If any of the above parameters is abnormal, proceed to emergency supportive care.

PRIMARY ASSESSMENT

Proceed next to the *primary assessment* which should be quick and systematic. Screen the *blood glucose* status by estimating the capillary blood glucose. Most sick children will be *hypoglycemic*; *hyperglycemia* (occasionally encountered) heralds the serious disease-diabetic ketoacidosis. Provide appropriate intervention immediately to the life-threatening abnormalities before proceeding to the next step.

Assess-identify-intervene is the cycle to be repeated as and when needed **(Fig. 8.2A)**.

Primary assessment has five parameters: ABCDE [Assessment pentagon **(Fig. 8.3)**]

Airway

Airway is the passage that connects the lungs to the atmosphere. Observe whether the airway is obstructed with secretions, vomitus,

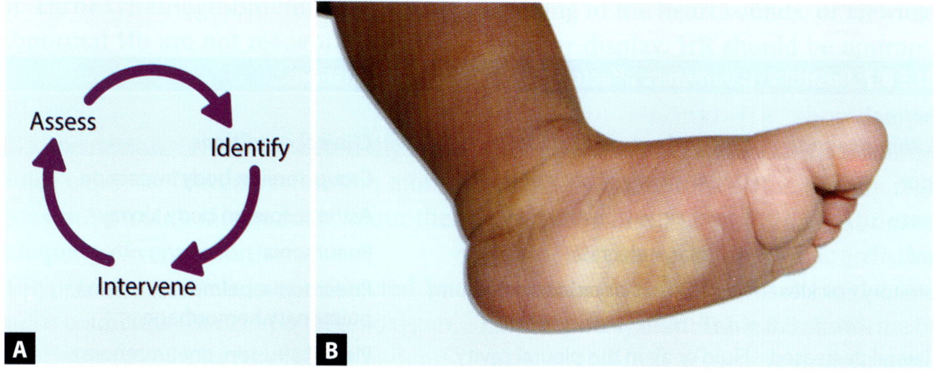

Figs. 8.2A and B: (A) Assess-identify-intervene cycle; (B) Prolonged capillary refill time (CRT).

TABLE 8.3: HR in children as per age and sleep-wake status.

Age	*Mean HR/min*	*Sleeping HR/min*	*Awake HR/min*
0–3 m	140	80–160	85–205
>3 m to 2 yr	130	75–160	100–190
>2–10 yr	80	60–90	60–140
>10 yr	75	50–90	60–100

TABLE 8.4: Central and peripheral pulses.

Central pulses	*Peripheral pulses*
Carotid (older children/ adults)	Radial
Brachial (in infants)	Dorsalis pedis
Femoral	Posterior tibial
Axillary	

TABLE 8.5: Age-wise systolic blood pressure (BP) to diagnose hypotension.

Age group	*Hypotension (systolic BP)*
<1 m (term neonate)	<60 mm Hg
1–12 m	<70 mm Hg
1–10 yrs	70+ (age in yrs × 2) mm Hg
>10 yrs	<90 mm Hg

Central and Peripheral Pulses

Palpate both central and peripheral pulses in all children. Central pulses are normally stronger than peripheral pulses as they are located closer to the heart. Exaggeration of difference in quality between central and peripheral pulses due to peripheral vasoconstriction is seen in shock. Weak central pulses are an ominous sign which requires immediate intervention to prevent cardiac arrest. **Table 8.4** reveals the central and peripheral pulses to be approached.

Blood Pressure (Ref. Ch. 7, 15)

Hypotension is defined as BP < fifth centile. **Table 8.5** reveals the BP values for hypotension.

At the end of circulatory assessment based on severity, circulatory insufficiency (shock) can be classified as *compensated or hypotensive*. Compensated shock is characterized by tachycardia with poor perfusion with maintained BP. Tachycardia is the body's compensatory mechanism to increase cardiac output, while poor peripheral perfusion is due to vasoconstriction of blood vessels in the skin so that shunting of blood can be done to more critical organs, such as the brain and heart. Based on the underlying etiology, shock can be further classified as *hypovolemic, distributive, cardiogenic, and obstructive*. Methodical history and physical examination are enough to make the differentiation between the four groups.

Disability

It is a quick assessment of brain function (Ref. Ch. 9) to be done in two steps—cortical and brainstem:

1. *Cortical dysfunction:* Assess by Glasgow Coma Scale (GCS) or AVPU (alert, voice, pain, and unresponsive); the latter is the easiest scale (Ch 9). GCS score ≤8 needs aggressive management. **Box 8.1** reveals the common causes of decreased consciousness in children.
2. *Brainstem dysfunction:* Evaluate by observing the pupillary responses **(Fig. 8.4)** and oculocephalic eye movements. Examine the pupils for size, asymmetry, and

reaction to light. Trauma, drugs, hypoxia, and poisoning can cause abnormalities in pupillary size. Unequal pupils indicate brain stem herniation due to RICP, the larger one will be abnormal.

Full Outline of Unresponsiveness (FOUR) Score

Includes parameters for cortical and brain-stem assessment (pupil, corneal, and cough reflex along with respiratory pattern) and hence useful as a single test for a full evaluation of the brain.

> **BOX 8.1:** Causes of decreased consciousness in children.
>
> - Traumatic brain injury [accidental, intentional (battered child)]
> - CNS infections-meningitis, encephalitis, brain abscess
> - Sepsis
> - *Metabolic:* Hypoglycemia and hyponatremia
> - Hypoxia and hypercarbia
> - Poor cerebral perfusion
> - Drug intoxication (accidental and intentional)

Exposure

This is the last component of primary assessment. Undress the child completely, (taking care to avoid cold injury), and examine for bite marks, hypothermia, bleeds, bruises, burns, rashes, swelling, wounds, and deformities. Examine for tenderness of extremities.

Primary assessment aims to identify the physiological status of the child at the end of which one would be able to identify the severity and type of involvement of cardiovascular, respiratory, and neurological systems. See **Table 8.6** for impressions after primary assessment.

SECONDARY ASSESSMENT

After completion of the primary assessment and stabilization of the child, perform the secondary assessment. In most situations,

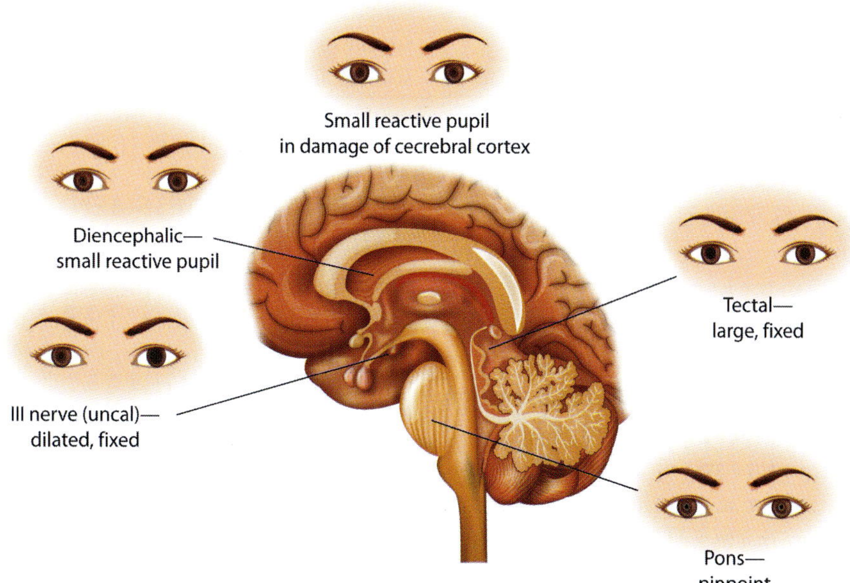

Fig. 8.4: Pupillary responses and affected brain areas.

TABLE 8.6: Impressions after primary assessment.

Cardiovascular		***Respiratory***		***Neurological***
Severity	***Types***	***Severity***	***Types***	
Compensated shock	Hypovolemic shock	Respiratory distress	Upper airway obstruction	Cortical dysfunction
Hypotensive shock	Cardiogenic shock	Respiratory failure	Lower airway obstruction	Brainstem dysfunction
	Distributive Shock		Lung parenchymal disease	
	Obstructive Shock		Disordered control of breathing	

a working clinical diagnosis can be established by the end of this assessment.

Assess by two components: Focused history and focused physical examination. History may not be relevant always if the child is brought from an accident area by a lay person, from the place of disaster, a lone unconscious child, a battered baby, or the victim of child abuse.

Focused History

It has 6 components, known by the mnemonic **SAMPLE**.

1. *S:* Signs and symptoms
2. *A:* Allergies
3. *M:* Medication received (if on long-term medications)
4. *P:* Past medical history
5. *L:* Last meal taken (for planning procedures and sedation)
6. *E:* Events leading to the child being brought to the hospital

After eliciting a focused history, proceed to systematic physical examination from head to toe followed by focused examination of the primary area of concern which can be the respiratory system in case of respiratory distress or a complete neurological examination in case of altered sensorium. Pay special attention to areas that have not been covered in the primary assessment which include the nose, throat, meningeal signs, murmurs, and organomegaly.

DIAGNOSTIC TESTS

Investigations selected should be relevant to detect and identify the presence and severity of respiratory/circulatory/neurological problems and confirm the diagnosis. If the hospital settings are adequate, do complete blood count, blood chemistry, liver and renal function tests, coagulation profile, blood gas analysis, chest radiography, echocardiography, and other radiological/imaging studies according to the clinical situation. If the facilities are inadequate, after stabilization transfer the child to a higher center after explaining the situation to the parents and informing the higher center.

TERTIARY ASSESSMENT

Based on the secondary assessment and investigation reports, proceed to tertiary assessment, the duration of which may vary depending on the type and severity of the illness.

CASE SCENARIOS

Case Scenario 1

Shalini, 9 m old, baby girl brought by her parents to the ED at 9 PM, is found in decorticate posture, cyanosed, and has irregular noisy breathing. Discuss the stepwise assessment and management.

Initial Impression (Doorway Assessment)

- *Appearance:* Unconscious child, breathing irregularly, and noisy.
- *Color:* Cyanosed
- *Impression:* Life-threatening event requiring immediate attention. Start oxygen with a nonrebreathing mask.

Primary assessment:

- *Airway:* Partially obstructed revealed by noisy breathing. Intervention—suction, chin lift, head tilt maneuver, and if needed apply oropharyngeal airway.
- *Breathing:* Irregular, support breathing with bag and mask ventilation as it is a disordered control of breathing. If breathing remains irregular or the oxygen saturation does not improve above 94%, proceed to mechanical ventilation.
- *Circulation:* Extremities cold, systolic BP 60 mm Hg, HR 168 beats/min, peripheral pulses feeble.
  Impression: Hypotensive shock. *Intervention*: 20 mL/kg saline intravenous (IV) bolus over 20 minutes. Reassess the child after the bolus fluid to decide further fluid therapy and intervention.
- *Disability:* AVPU—pain responsive with decorticate posturing. Pupils equal and reacting, Doll's eye movement present. *Impression*: Primary cortical dysfunction.
- *Exposure:* Child febrile. Temperature 102°F. No rashes, bite marks, or ecchymosis. General random blood sugar (GRBS) 120 mg/dL.
  Intervention: Paracetamol suppository to decrease fever.

Primary assessment impression: Hypotensive shock, respiratory failure—disordered control of breathing, primary cortical dysfunction.

Secondary Assessment

Focused History

- *Signs and symptoms:* Had fever for 2 days, poor feeding, and poor activity of 1 day duration.
- *Allergies:* No previous history of any allergy.
- *Medication history:* Child was on paracetamol for fever for the last 2 days. Not on any long-term medicines.
- *Past medical history:* Previously normal child.
- *Last meal:* Same morning the baby had expressed breast milk with a spoon as she was not feeding at the breast.

Events leading to medical consultation: This morning the baby had fever. She developed uprolling of her eyes with tonic posturing and was taken to a local hospital from where she was referred.

Focused Examination

Anterior fontanelle-tense and bulging, eyes, ear, and throat normal, chest and abdomen normal, skull and spine normal, GCS-E1V1M3 (no eye-opening, no verbal response, decorticate posturing), pupils equal and reacting, Doll's eye movement present, deep tendon reflexes exaggerated bilateral (B/L), plantar upgoing B/L.

Diagnostic Tests

A 9 m old critically ill child with fever, neurological symptoms, and bulging anterior fontanelle points to a CNS infection. The baseline investigations would include CBC, urine routine and culture, blood culture, renal and liver function tests, and lumbar puncture for CSF study (cytology, sugar and protein analysis, microscopy with Gram stain, and culture and sensitivity). Brain imaging [computed tomography (CT) or magnetic resonance imaging (MRI)] is also indicated.

Final Diagnosis

Acute pyogenic meningitis with hypotensive septic shock and respiratory failure.

Case Scenario 2

Amal, 4 yrs old boy, was brought by his parents at 5 PM to the emergency department (ED), for unresponsiveness and profuse sweating. Apparently a healthy child, was found sleeping at 1 PM when he was called for lunch. As he did not wake up even after 4 PM and was unresponsive he was brought to the hospital.

Initial Impression (Doorway Assessment)

- *Appearance:* Unconscious child, shallow breathing, and sweating.
- *Impression:* Life-threatening event—immediate attention needed. Start oxygen with nonrebreathing mask.

Primary Assessment

- *Airway:* Clear
- *Breathing:* Regular, RR 20 breaths/min, shallow breathing, chest movements symmetrical, bilateral air entry equal, no added sounds.
- *Circulation:* Extremities cold, CRT 5 sec, HR 158 beats/min, irregular feeble peripheral pulses, BP 64 mm Hg (systolic).

  Impression: Hypotensive shock.
- *Intervention:* Secure IV line and start IV Ringer's lactate (RL) 30 mL/kg in 30 minutes.
- *Disability:* AVPU—pain responsive. Pupils are equal and reacting. Doll's eye movement is present.

  Impression: Secondary cortical dysfunction.
- *Exposure:* Child afebrile. Temperature 98°F. No rashes, bite marks, or ecchymosis. GRBS 20 mg/dL.

  Intervention: IV 25% dextrose 10 mL/kg as rapid push followed by continuous IV infusion of 10% dextrose and GRBS monitoring.
- *Primary assessment impression:* Hypotensive shock, hypoglycemia, secondary cortical dysfunction.

Secondary Assessment

Focused history:

- *Signs and symptoms:* Apparently healthy child (weight: 16 kg). Did not go to the nursery as it was the post-anniversary day. Grandmother found him asleep at lunchtime which was unusual. His parents had gone to the office and the child was with the grandparents.
- *Allergies:* No previous history of any allergy.
- *Medication history:* Not on any medicines.
- *Past medical history:* Previously normal child.
- *Last meal:* Same-day breakfast along with his parents by 8.30 AM.
- Events leading to: apparently nil.

Focused examination: Eyes dry, pupils normal, reacting, doll's eye movements present, no tears, oral mucosa dry, sweating, skin turgor prolonged >6 sec, CRT >5 sec, pulse feeble irregular, tachycardia, and hypotension. No cardiomegaly or hepatomegaly, external genitalia normal.

Impression: Severe dehydration, hypotension, unconsciousness, tachycardia with irregular pulse, hypoglycemia.

Intervention—Start RL 30 mL/kg over 30 minutes followed by 70 mL/kg in 2.5 hours. Reassess the child after fluid resuscitation and decide on further fluid administration. Continue 10% dextrose IV infusion for 24 hours with blood glucose monitoring to see whether glycemic status is steady.

Diagnostic Tests

A previously healthy child with unresponsiveness, hypotension, dehydration, tachycardia, cardiac irregularity, and hypoglycemia.

History in detail: Grandfather is a known diabetic for the past fifteen years and is on oral hypoglycemic agents (metformin + vildagliptin). Amal used to help his grandfather with medicine ingestion when at home.

Routine blood examination, serum electrolytes (serum Sodium and serum Potassium), blood gas analysis to assess acidosis, blood urea, serum creatinine, and 12-hour fasting blood glucose are needed.

Final diagnosis: Hypotension, coma, dehydration, and cardiac irregularity following accidental ingestion of oral hypoglycemic agents.

SUGGESTED READING

1. American Heart Association. Pediatric advanced life support provider manual. https://ebooks.heart.org/product/pediatric-advanced-life-support-provider-manual-ebook50160971 [Last accessed September, 2024].
2. In: Kliegman RM (Ed). Nelson Textbook of Pediatrics, 21st edition. Amsterdam: Elsevier Health; 2019.
3. Jayashree M, Kulgod V, Sharma AK. IAP ALS Handbook. New Delhi: IAP National Publication. New Delhi: Indian Academy of Pediatrics; 2018.
4. Maconochie IK, Aickin R, Hazinski MF, Atkins DL, Bingham R, Couto TB, et al. on behalf of the Pediatric Life Support Collaborators. Pediatric life support: 2020 International Consensus on Cardiopulmonary Resuscitation and Emergency Cardiovascular Care Science With Treatment Recommendations. Circulation. 2020;142(Suppl 1):S140-84.
5. Sugunan S, Bindusha S, Geetha S, Niyas HR, Kumar AS. Clinical profile and short term outcome of children with SARS-CoV-2 Related Multisystem Inflammatory Syndrome (MIS-C) Treated with pulse Methyl prednisolone.Indian Pediatr 2021;58:718-22. (https://doi.org/10.1007/s13312-021-2277-4.

9

CHAPTER

Evaluation of the Unconscious Child

S Sushamabai, Sheeja Sugunan

Chapter Outline

- Introduction
- Scoring Systems
- Patient Evaluation
- Causes of Unconsciousness according to Clinical Presentation
- Features of Brain Herniation
- Brain Death
- Clinical Case Scenario

INTRODUCTION

Read chapters 1, 2, 3, 4, 6, and 7 before you proceed.

Unconsciousness is global unawareness of one's self and the environment as the child shown in **Figure 9.1**.

Pediatricians often encounter children with unconsciousness; early diagnosis and timely intervention are crucial for rapid recovery from coma, to have better prognosis and survival with minimum disability.

Confusion, drowsiness, disorientation, stupor, delirium, and coma are terminologies that specify varying degrees of altered sensorium with associated symptoms. Rather than using such terminologies, it is more logical to quantify unconsciousness by applying scoring systems.

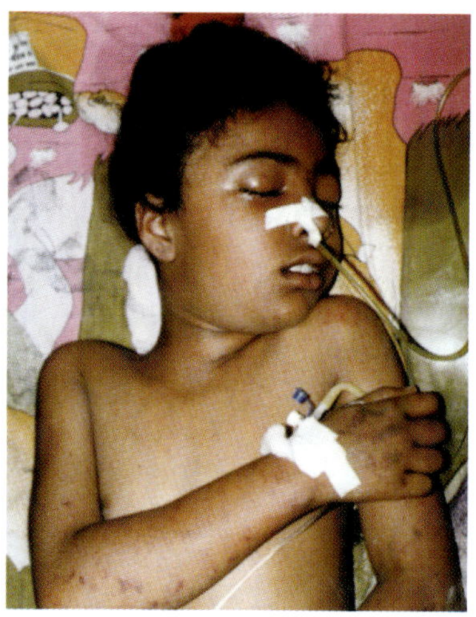

Fig. 9.1: Coma due to meningococcemia.

SCORING SYSTEMS

- *AVPU* score is a rapid assessment of sensorium (*A*—response awake, *V*—response to verbal command, *P*—response to pain, *U*—unresponsive). Stages *P* and *U* carry bad prognosis and can be akin to GCS values <8 to *U* and 9–12 to *P* in AVPU.
- *Pediatric Glasgow Coma Scale (pGCS)* gives a more precise assessment of the status of sensorium by quantifying eye opening, motor response, and verbal response. The best score is 15 and the worst is 3 **(Table 9.1)**. Periodic evaluation of the GCS helps to prognosticate the coma stage and plan further intervention.

GCS score ≤8 indicates the need for aggressive intervention **(Table 9.2)**.

TABLE 9.1: Glasgow Coma Scale (GCS).

Parameter	*Adult/child*	*Score*	*Infant*
Eye opening	• Spontaneous • To verbal command • To pain • No response	4 3 2 1	• Spontaneous • To verbal • To pain • No response
Verbal response	• Oriented • Disoriented • Inappropriate words • Incomprehensible sounds • No response	5 4 3 2 1	• Coos, babbles • Irritable cry • Cries only to pain • Moans to pain • No response
Best motor response	• Obeys commands • Localizes pain • Withdraws from pain • Abnormal flexion (decorticate) • Abnormal extension (decerebrate) • No response	6 5 4 3 2 1	• Moves spontaneously • Withdraws from touch • Withdraws from pain • Abnormal flexion (decorticate) • Abnormal extension (decerebrate) • No response
	Total = E + V + M	3–15	Total = E + V + M

TABLE 9.2: Interpretation of GCS Score.

*Score**	*Impairment*	*Intervention*
15	• Nil	• Nil
13–14	• Mild	• Observation, Investigation
9–12	• Moderate	• Investigation, Intervention
≤8	• Severe	• Investigation, Intervention
3	• Brain dead	• Re-evaluation, Intervention

*Fall of 3 scores from the previous value also indicates bad prognosis.

TABLE 9.3: Assessment of pupil reaction.

Pupil unreactive to light	*Pupil reaction score*
• Both pupils	2
• One pupil	1
• Neither pupil	0

- *Full Outline of UnResponsiveness (FOUR) score* assesses eye response, motor response, brainstem reflexes, and respiration (EMBR), and thus incorporates the brainstem parameters also compared to GCS. Each parameter has the best score of "4" and the worst is "0" (total best score = 16; worst score = "0"). Though the parameters appear better in FOUR score, large scale comparative studies in unconscious adult patients (of differing etiology) have not revealed any statistical significance in predicting prognosis that FOUR score is superior to GCS. Clinical assessment of GCS is easier than FOUR score.
- *GCS-pupil reaction score (PRS)* is the score obtained after deducting the PRS from the total GCS score as given in **Table 9.3**.

Common causes of unconsciousness in children are given in **Table 9.4**.

PATIENT EVALUATION

The approach should be assessment, identification, intervention, and reassessment cycle (Ref. **Fig. 8.2**). Assess the airway, breathing, and circulation, simultaneously eliciting a parallel brief history.

TABLE 9.4: Common causes of unconsciousness in children.

Infections	Metabolic	Noninfectious CNS causes	Miscellaneous
• Septicemia • Meningitis • Encephalitis • Cerebral malaria • Brain abscess • Cortical-thrombophlebitis	• Hypoglycemia • Hyponatremia • Diabetic ketoacidosis • Salicylism • Renal/hepatic failure • Inborn errors of metabolism	• Head trauma-accidental • Battered child • Status epilepticus • Tumors • Cerebrovascular accidents	• Drug overdose • Poisons • Snake envenomation • Hypotension • Hypertension • Raised ICP • Psychogenic

(ICP: intracranial pressure)

Stabilization and Evaluation

Airway and Breathing

Stabilization of the airway is of paramount importance; the protective airway reflexes may be absent leading to aspiration; blocking of the airway can occur by falling back of the tongue or by secretions. Assess the *breathing status* of the patient by counting the RR, inspecting the tidal volume adequacy by the *chest rise*, auscultating the chest to hear the *air movement* and objectively by *pulse oximetry*. Normal oxygen saturation by pulse oximetry does not rule out respiratory failure especially if the child is on supplemental oxygen. Neurological causes can lead to *type 2 respiratory failure* by hypoventilation causing carbon dioxide retention. Hence, in a child getting supplemental oxygen, late development of hypoxia should be anticipated.

After stabilizing the *airway proceed to evaluation of the child* **(Box 9.1)**.

Children with GCS ≤8 will require stabilization of the airway by intubation, history, resuscitation, and evaluation in a logical order. Assess for hyperventilation which in a comatose child may be due to many causes given in **Box 9.2**.

BOX 9.1: Evaluation of the unconscious child.

- Brief history
- Acute illness observation scale (Ref. Ch. 7)
- Vitals (Ref. Ch. 7)
- Establish ABC
- Blood sugar
- Pediatric GCS or GCS-PRS
- Evidence of head injury
- Neck—injury, stiffness
- Pupils—size, reaction
- Eye movements—doll's eye
- Limbs—posture, tone, movements
- Reflexes, plantar response
- Fundus
- Focal neurological signs
- Other systems

(ABC: airway, breathing, and circulation; GCS-PRS: Glasgow coma scale-pupil reaction score)

BOX 9.2: Causes of hyperventilation in comatose children.

- Metabolic acidosis
- Diabetic ketoacidosis
- Salicylism
- Brainstem lesions
- Raised intracranial pressure (RICP)
- Hepatic failure
- Renal failure
- Pneumonia

Vitals

Temperature, pulse, respiration, blood pressure, and pulse oximetry (Ref. Ch. 7, 8) reveal the gravity of RICP and metabolic problems and the possibility of infectious causes. Shock should be corrected by fluid resuscitation with normal saline and vasopressors.

- *Look for features of RICP* by assessing the asymmetry of pupils, tonic posturing, or papilledema. *Cushing triad* (bradycardia, irregular respiration, and hypertension) indicates *medullary compression*, a late sign of RICP. Measures to reduce RICP should be rapidly instituted IV mannitol or 3% saline as rapid infusion].
- Estimate the *blood sugar* initially in all patients with altered sensorium. If the child is hypoglycemic (blood glucose <40 mg/dL), rapidly push in IV 10% dextrose in 2–4 mL/kg dose.

Head to Foot Examination

Head injury: Look for *Battle* sign [known after Dr William Henry Battle who described the sign in 1800s **(Fig. 9.2)**]. It is an oval-shaped *bruising* over the mastoid bone, *behind* the ear, which indicates *basal skull fracture* usually the petrous temporal bone due to severe head injury, often blunt trauma, is seen along with *bleeding* or cerebrospinal fluid (CSF) (leakage from external auditory meatus or nostrils in comatose patients). The common situations producing head injury with Battle sign are motor vehicle accidents, blunt trauma, sports injuries, falls, assault and child abuse.

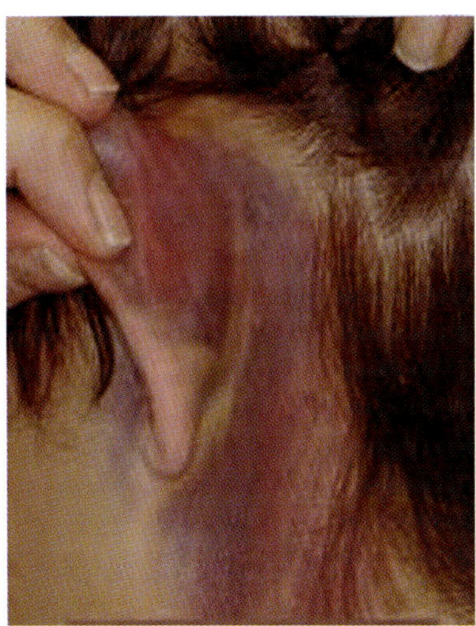

Fig. 9.2: Battle sign.

Cervical spine injury should be excluded by CT scan of the spine in children with trauma and altered sensorium and in lone children found unconscious. Such patients should be nursed in the neutral position with immobilization of the cervical spine till the possibility of cervical spine injury is ruled out.

Skin: Look for skin bleeds (bleeding disorders), rashes (infective causes such as dengue illness, encephalitis, meningococcemia, scrub typhus, and other hemorrhagic fevers), and bite marks (neurotoxic snake bite envenomation).

Abnormal smell: Consider the possibilities of poisoning, diabetic ketoacidosis, or fetor hepaticus.

Pupils: Examine the size and reaction; along with that respiratory pattern and body posture are helpful to assess the extent of brainstem herniation which proceeds from higher to lower brain centers **(Table 9.3; Fig. 8.4)**.

Eye movements: Assess by "doll's head" maneuver (Ref. Ch. 21). Normally, the patient's eyes tend to deviate in the opposite direction of head movement and remain in the straight ahead position. Loss of doll's eye phenomenon indicates extensive structural damage of the brainstem.

Reflexes: Asymmetry of reflexes and extensor plantar response indicate focal neurologic deficit and physiologic impairment.

Focal neurological signs can be made out from the presence of cranial nerve palsy, abnormal flaccidity of limbs, and absence of spontaneous movements. Limb movements can be induced by lightly touching the skin and mucous membrane around the nasal orifices with a cotton wisp. Common causes of coma with focal neurological signs are seizure episodes, meningitis, encephalitis, cerebrovascular accidents, brain abscess, brain tumors, and cortical vein thrombosis.

Other Systems: Rapidly search to detect contributory factors to coma or any evidence of multiorgan failure. If intracranial infection is suspected, administer the first dose of antibiotics within 1 hr of admission *(golden hour)* preferably after collecting CSF for study. Delay in doing lumbar puncture should not affect the administration of antibiotics.

CAUSES OF UNCONSCIOUSNESS ACCORDING TO CLINICAL PRESENTATION

Table 9.5 reveals causes of unconsciousness according to clinical presentation.

FEATURES OF BRAIN HERNIATION

Table 9.6 reveals the features of brain herniation.

BRAIN DEATH

In clinical practice, at times brain death has to be ruled out in an unconscious child to declare the patient as expired. If an unconscious patient is on ventilator support, without evidence of spontaneous breathing or brainstem reflexes (*pupillary, corneal, vestibulocochlear, cough, and gag reflexes*), brain death should be certified by at least two physicians after doing apnea test (Ref. Ch. 23). The law states that two observations with apnea test should be made by two different physicians at intervals depending on the age of the patient (≥37 w–30 days: 24 hr apart, 1 m–18 yr: 12 hr apart).

The format for stating the final diagnosis should be in the order of functional impairment followed by physiologic and topographic involvement, etiology, and pathologic lesions (level and nature) as shown in the following text:

Unconsciousness (GCS-6), upper motor neuron (UMN) facial palsy, hemiplegia on the right side, and seizures. Etiology—pyogenic meningitis. Level of lesion—diffuse cortical and left subcortical. Type of lesion—vascular occlusion, inflammation, and brain edema.

TABLE 9.5: Causes of unconsciousness according to clinical presentation.

Coma with focal signs	*Coma without focal signs and signs of meningeal irritation*	*Coma with signs of meningeal irritation*
Intracranial hemorrhage	Drugs and poisons	
Stroke	*Metabolic:* Hypoglycemia, hepatic encephalopathy, inborn errors of metabolism, uremia, Reye's syndrome, hyponatremia, hypernatremia	Meningitis
Tumors	*Infections:* Cerebral malaria, Shigella encephalopathy, enteric encephalopathy	Encephalitis
Brain abscess	ADEM, hypertensive encephalopathy	
ADEM	Nonconvulsive status, postseizure state, snake envenomation	Subarachnoid hemorrhage

(ADEM: acute disseminated encephalomyelitis)

TABLE 9.6: Features of brain herniation.

Area affected	***Pupils (Fig. 8.4)***		***Posture (Fig. 9.3)***	***Respiration***
	Size	***Reaction***		
Cerebral hemisphere	Small	Present	Decorticate	Cheyne–Stokes
Midbrain	Mid-size	Nil	Decorticate	Deep regular
Lower pons	Pinpoint	Nil	Decorticate	Rapid shallow
Medulla	Dilated	Nil	Flaccid	Irregular gasping
Unilateral uncal	Ipsilateral dilatation	Nil	Variable	Variable

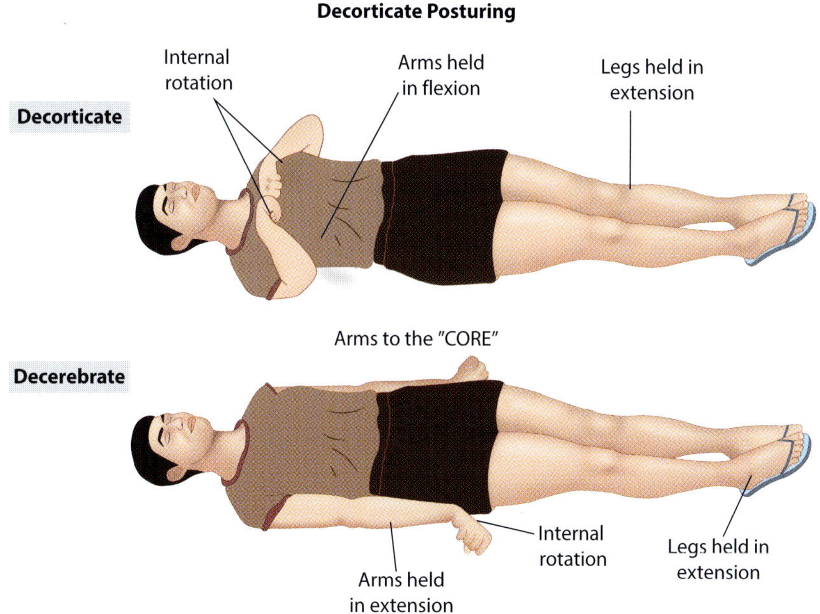

Fig. 9.3: Decorticate and decerebrate postures.

■ CLINICAL CASE SCENARIO

Sagar, an 18-month-old infant boy is brought unconscious by 4 PM in the ER; he had three episodes of seizures in the past 6 hours; was having high fever, irritability, vomiting, and several episodes of frequent, loose, and blood-stained stools for the past 2 days. History of ingesting ice cream from a parlor one day prior to the onset of the symptoms. Child was on paracetamol, Kanji water with salt added, and oral rehydration solution (ORS) as advised by the local Anganwadi teacher. Had scanty urine output in the past 2 days.

On examination, temperature 103°F, pulse 138/min, feeble, systolic blood pressure 62 mm Hg, RR 42/min, deep, regular, oxygen saturation (SpO_2) 90% in room air, extremities cold up to the knees and elbows, skin pinch >4 sec; GCS-8 (E2 + V2 + M4), pupils normal and reacting well, no focal neurological deficit, and no neck stiffness.

Final diagnosis: Unconsciousness—GCS-8, seizures, dysentery, severe dehydration, and metabolic acidosis; Etiology—Shigella encephalopathy; Level of lesion—diffuse cortical involvement; Pathology—hypernatremia, Shigella toxicity.

SUGGESTED READING

1. Foo CC, Loan JJM, Brennan PM. The relationship of the four score to patient outcome. a systematic review. J neurotrauma. 2019;17:2469-83.
2. GCS. What is the Glasgow Coma Scale Pupils Score? [online] Available from https://www.glasgow comascale.org>what-is-gcs-p. [Last accessed September 2024].
3. Kliegman RM, Samenow S. Nelson Textbook of Pediatrics, 19th edition. Gurugram: Elsevier; 2019.
4. Sushamabai S. Comatose Child. In Handbook of Pediatric and Neonatal Emergencies 1/e 2019.Ed Sushamabai S, Jaypee Brothers Medical Publishers (P) Ltd, New Delhi 110002, India.

CHAPTER 10

An Approach to Skin Lesions

Lalitha Kailas, Kalyani Pillai

Chapter Outline

- Introduction
- Dermatological History
- Examination of the Skin Lesions
- Location and Distribution
- Dermatological Terminologies
- Differential Diagnosis of Common Skin Lesions
- Transient Vascular Phenomena
- Hair Disorders in Children
- Nail Disorders

INTRODUCTION

Read chapters 1, 2, 3, 4, 6, and 7 before you proceed.

Skin and the appendages, hair and nails, form the largest and most accessible organ of the body and serve as a window for the evaluation of internal health and diseases. Studies reveal that over 20% of children have medically significant dermatology problems as primary disorders or along with systemic diseases. Recognition of the morphological patterns helps to diagnose the common skin lesions and give first clues to the underlying serious systemic and genetic diseases. Understanding the terminologies in dermatology is very important, since it will enable one to convey a clear picture of the lesions. An organized approach to the skin lesions is immensely useful, since many skin lesions are superficial reflectors of systemic diseases.

DERMATOLOGICAL HISTORY

Proper history is essential to establish the etiology and prognosis as usual, though most skin diseases can be diagnosed by inspection.

Sandwich format history, i.e., a preliminary history and physical examination, followed by leading questions based on clinical findings, is more rewarding in dermatology. Enquire the site of onset and duration of skin lesions, progression, distribution, treatment undertaken, and the response to treatment.

Associated symptoms such as itching, paresthesia, fever, joint pain, abdominal pain, vomiting, etc., should be clarified.

Details of drug intake from any system of medicine used as topical, nasal, oral, or as injections should be clarified.

Contact history of cosmetics application, environmental plants and insects, and pet animals and birds (all these become often forgotten by patients/parents) should be obtained.

Provocative/aggravating factors: Enquire exposure to sun, heat, cold environment, drugs, exercise, and season. History of similar symptoms among household contacts is helpful to diagnose highly contagious infections like scabies. Fever and associated respiratory infections may indicate viral infections. Consider child abuse, sexual abuse, and sexual activity in adolescent age group, when confronted with unexplainable skin lesions.

Past history: Ask for previous illnesses with similar manifestations, allergy, food intolerance, transfusion of blood or blood products, and recent travel to any areas.

Family history of simulating skin lesions can be obtained in inherited diseases such as tuberous sclerosis, neurofibromatosis, psoriasis, atopic dermatitis, and in infections such as leprosy and scabies.

Personal habits and living conditions should be specifically enquired. Overcrowding and poor personal hygiene predispose to rapid spread of contagious diseases such as scabies and leprosy.

EXAMINATION OF THE SKIN LESIONS

Prerequisites

- The room should be warm with good daylight and walls having light paint
- Provide privacy to the child with closed doors and curtains
- Parents should be with their children during examination. Adolescents may be examined alone, if they prefer
- A chaperone should be present while examining a girl child
- Handheld magnifying lens and pocket flashlight to examine small lesions or aberrations are needed at times
- Sterile glass slides to assess blanching of the lesion on pressure and to detect scaling
- Wear appropriately-sized sterile disposable gloves while examining wet/oozing lesions/orogenital mucosa and the babies cared for in the nursery
- Remove the child's clothes partly only during examination to avoid cooling and to get the child's cooperation; parent can assist.

Examine the skin covering the entire body surface, mucous membranes (conjunctiva, oropharynx, nasal mucosa, and anogenital mucosa), hair, and nails. Inspect, palpate, and then classify the lesions on the basis of morphology, size, numbers (single or multiple), color, texture, firmness, configuration, edges (sharp and well-defined or vague and ill-defined), location, and distribution. Assess whether the features are those of the *primary* lesion itself or the clinical pattern has been altered by a *secondary* factor such as infection, trauma, or therapy.

Specific Signs Elicited in Certain Skin Lesions

- *Darier's sign:* Scratch any area of the patient's skin with the fingernail or a sharp object (can be a pencil tip). An erythematous linear streak (*tache cerebrale*) appears within 30–60 sec in patients with acute CNS inflammatory diseases (meningitis, encephalitis).
- *Diascopy* is pressure applied with a glass slide over a red macule. Blanching of the lesion due to vasodilatation is characteristic of viral exanthems and hemangiomas. In capillary blood leaking lesions such as purpura and ecchymosis the lesions will not blanch.
- *Koebner phenomenon* is the appearance of similar skin lesions along the line of injury or scratch. Seen in molluscum contagiosum, psoriasis, lichen planus, vitiligo, and pityriasis rubra pilaris.
- *Nikolsky's sign* is elicited in children with blistering disorders, e.g., pemphigus, toxic epidermal necrolysis, and staphylococcal scalded skin syndrome. Apply lateral pressure with your thumb on normal skin of the patient over a bony prominence. The force breaks off the upper layer of

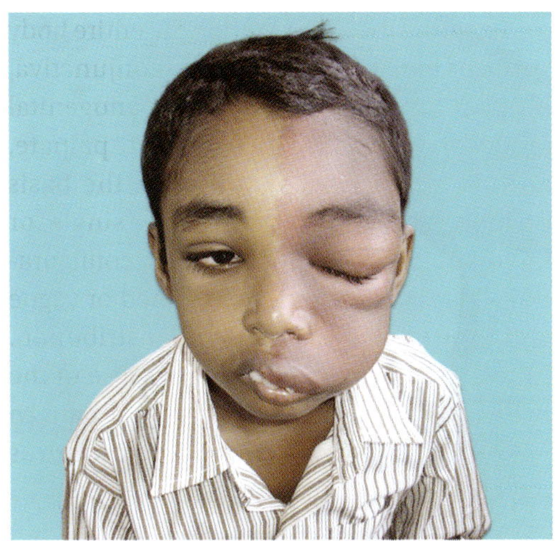

Fig. 10.1: Sturge–Weber syndrome with hemangioma on (L) side.

epidermis in diseases with intraepidermal cleavage leading to peeling of the skin.

- *Auspitz sign* is elicited in psoriasis. The thick white scales of psoriasis, if gently scraped from the surface of a plaque, reveal tiny bleeding points.

Examination of other systems and organs, especially the nervous system, liver, and gastrointestinal tract, on the basis of the skin lesions is a must. One example is the neurocutaneous marker hemangioma **(Fig. 10.1)** in Sturge–Weber syndrome.

LOCATION AND DISTRIBUTION

Symmetrical lesions imply systemic causes; *asymmetry* usually denotes external causes. A centrifugal distribution is characteristic of chickenpox and pityriasis rosea. Erythema multiforme has centripetal predilection. Atopic dermatitis affects flexural areas (antecubital and popliteal fossae); psoriasis has extensor surface distribution (elbows and knees). Papular urticaria (papules and blisters inflicted by insects) appears on exposed areas of the body. Lesions are predominantly seen in *sun-exposed* areas in systemic lupus erythematosus (SLE), dermatomyositis, polymorphous light eruption, and porphyria. Herpes zoster generally has a characteristic dermatomal distribution and is usually unilateral.

Morphology

Assess by inspection and palpation. Gently palpate the lesion and assess blanching on pressure by diascopy. Scaly nature of lesions can be noticed by rubbing with the edge of the glass slide. Observe whether the lesions are primary only or altered by secondary factors such as infection, trauma, or therapy.

DERMATOLOGICAL TERMINOLOGIES

The terms used to describe dermatologic lesions are unique, specific, and highly important for accurate diagnosis and communication. Assess whether they are primary or secondary.

Primary skin lesions are the direct result of a pathologic process **(Box 10.1)**.

Secondary skin lesions are the result of alteration or evolution of a primary lesion,

BOX 10.1: Primary skin lesions.

- Macule—nonpalpable lesion of altered color of <1 cm, e.g., freckle
- Patch—larger area of altered color
- Papule—palpable elevated area <5 mm, e.g., wart
- Plaque—palpable flat topped lesion >2 cm
- Pustule—raised lesion containing pus
- Nodule—palpable are of >5 mm–5 cm, e.g., enlarged cervical lymph node
- Tumor—elevated area of >5 cm
- Wheal—elevated flat lesion of various sizes with red margin **(Fig. 10.2)**
- Vesicle—fluid-filled lesion <5 mm
- Bullae—fluid-filled lesion >5 mm **(Fig. 10.3)**
- Cyst—circumscribed thick-walled fluid-filled lesion located deep in the skin

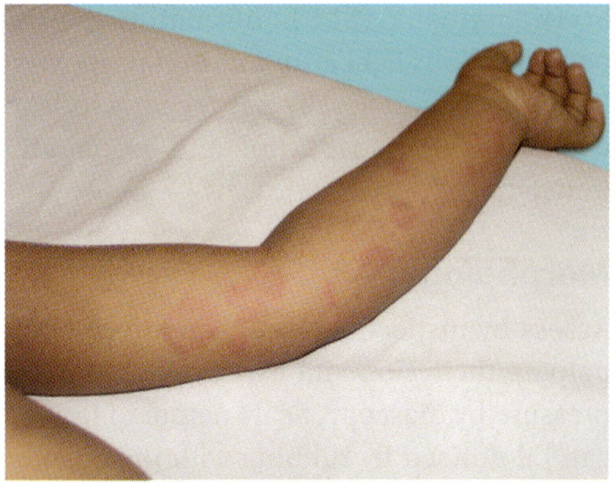
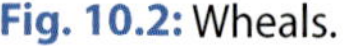

Fig. 10.2: Wheals.

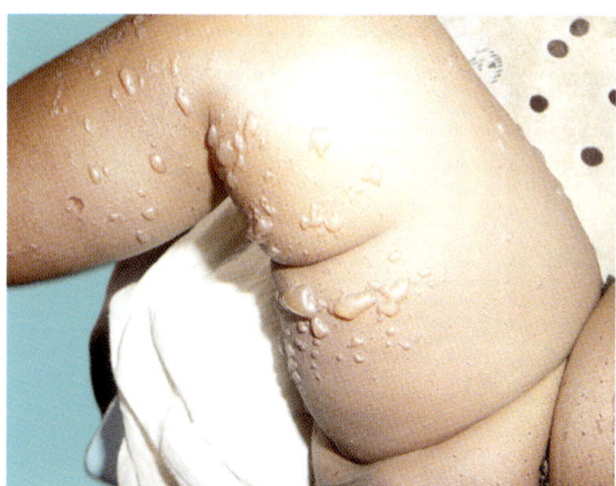

Fig. 10.3: Bullae.

BOX 10.2: Secondary skin lesions.

- Scale—loose excess horny layer, e.g., dandruff
- Excoriation—scratch
- Lichenification—thickening of epidermis with exaggerated skin margin
- Erosion—partial loss of epidermis which heals without scarring
- Ulcer—full thickness loss of epidermis which heals with scarring
- Scar—healing with fibrous tissue replacement.
- Keloid—excessive scar
- Atrophy—thinning of the skin due to shrinkage of epidermis, dermis, or subcutaneous tissue
- Striae—atrophic pink or white linear lesion due to change in connective tissue
- Fissure—slit in the skin
- Sinus—a channel that allows the escape of fluid

e.g., rubbing, scratching, or infection **(Box 10.2)**.

The leading skin lesions in children are maculopapular and vesicular types; **Box 10.3 and 10.4** reveal the common causes for these lesions. In most diseases history, asking for the details of evolution and observing the distribution of lesions, nature of lesions on examination, and associated symptoms will help in arriving at the diagnosis.

BOX 10.3: Common causes of maculopapular lesions.

- *Infections*
  - *Viral:* Measles, rubella, erythema infectiosum, exanthem subitum, infectious mononucleosis, dengue fever
  - *Bacterial:* Scarlet fever **(Fig. 10.4)**
  - *Rickettsial:* Scrub typhus
  - *Fungal:* Cutaneous candidiasis
- *Inflammatory diseases:* Kawasaki disease, systemic lupus erythematosus
- *Drug induced:* Ampicillin, amoxicillin
- *Malignancies:* Histiocytosis **(Figs. 10.5A and B)**, leukemias.

BOX 10.4: Common causes of vesiculobullous lesions.

- *Inherited:* Acrodermatitis enteropathica **(Fig. 10.7)**, epidermolysis bullosa **(Fig. 10.6)**, Incontinentia pigmenti **(Fig. 10.8)**
- *Infections*: *Viral*—Herpetiformis dermatitis, hand foot mouth disease **(Figs. 10.9A and B)**, Varicella, molluscum contagiosum **(Fig. 10.10)**, *Bacterial*—bullous impetigo, staphylococcal scalded skin syndrome **(Fig. 10.11)**, *Fungal*—Candidiasis, dermatophytosis, *Parasitic*—scabies **(Fig. 10.12)**, Cutaneous larva migrans **(Fig. 10.13)**
- *Hypersensitivity reactions*—Erythema multiforme, Steven-Johnson syndrome, toxic epidermal necrolysis **(Fig. 10.14)**

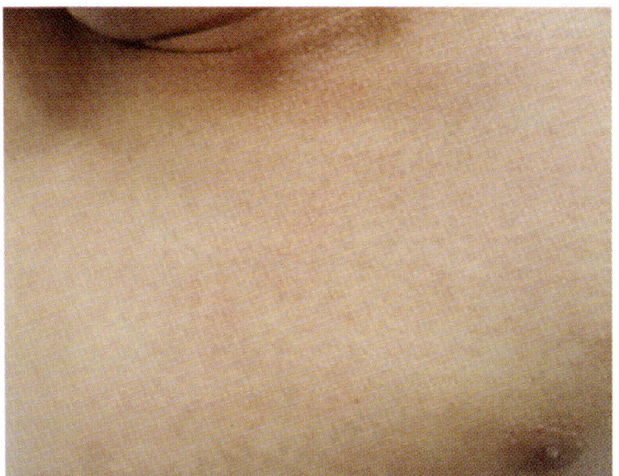

Fig. 10.4: Scarlet fever rashes.

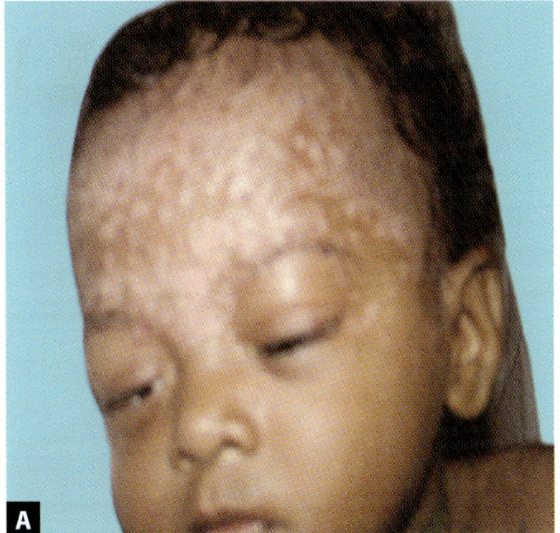

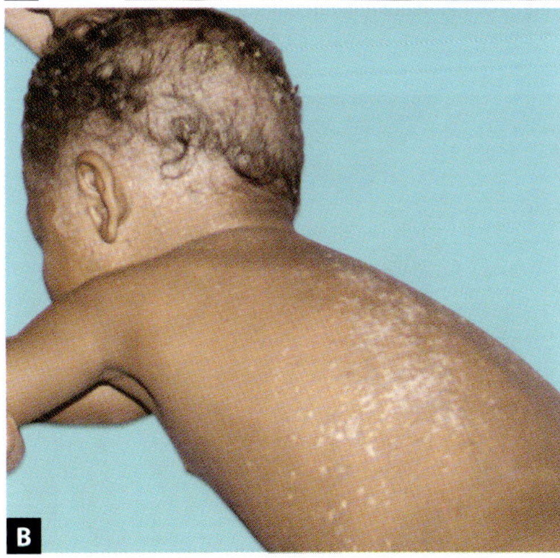

Figs. 10.5A and B: Maculopapular rashes in histiocytosis.

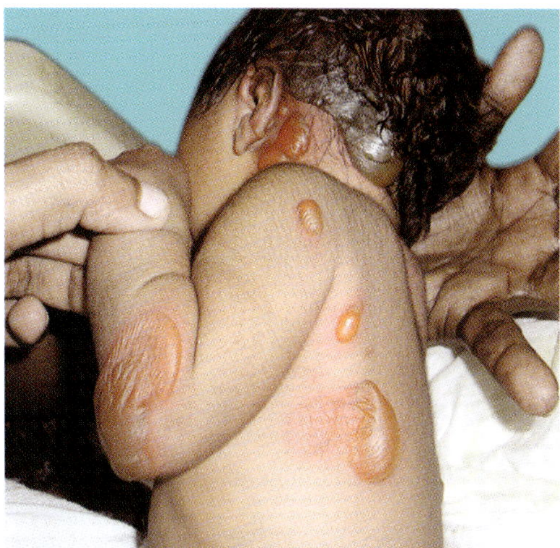

Fig. 10.6: Epidermolysis bullosa

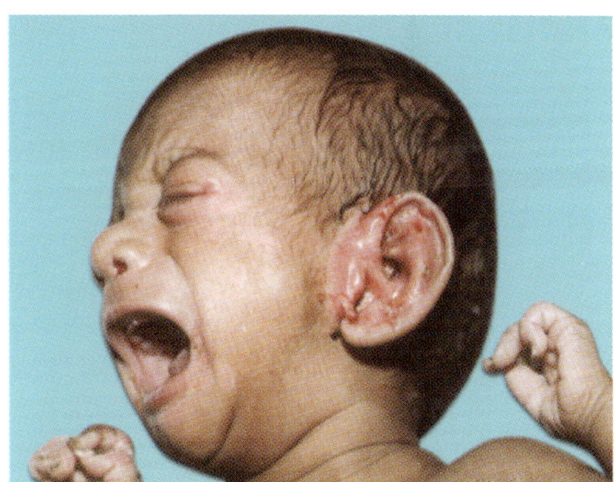

Fig. 10.7: Acrodermatitis enteropathica.

Acrodermatits enteropathica is a disorder of defective dietary zinc absorption of autosomal recessive inheritance, characterized by vesiculobullous/eczematous skin lesions with peeling affecting the limbs, cheeks, and perineum from infancy onward. Stomatitis, alopecia, and reddish tint of hair color, and chronic diarrhea are common associations.

Epidermolysis bullosa includes a group of disorders of autosomal dominant or recessive inheritance characterized by bullous lesions from birth onward.

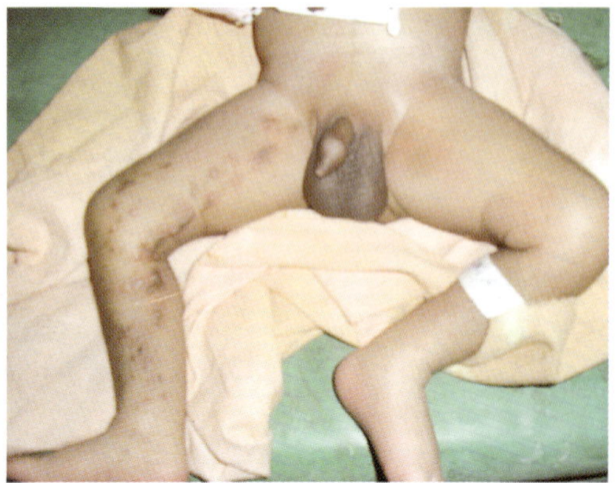

Fig. 10.8: Incontinentia pigmenti.

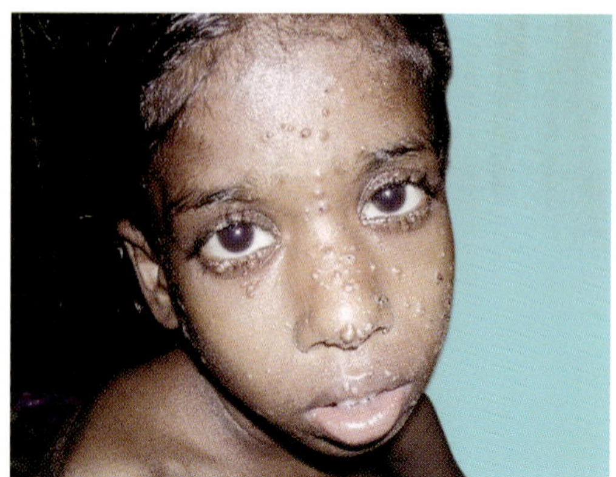

Fig. 10.10: Molluscum contagiosum.

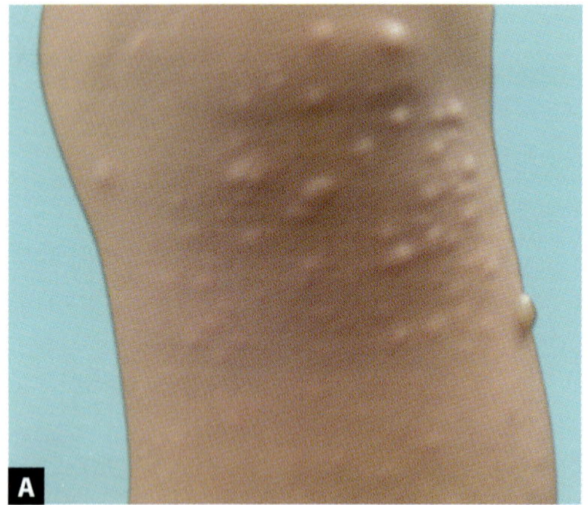

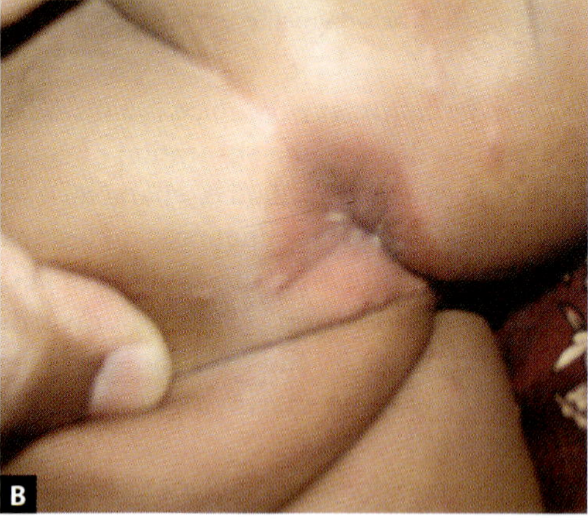

Figs. 10.9A and B: (A) Hand, foot, mouth disease; (B) Hand, foot, mouth disease revealing—perianal vesicles.

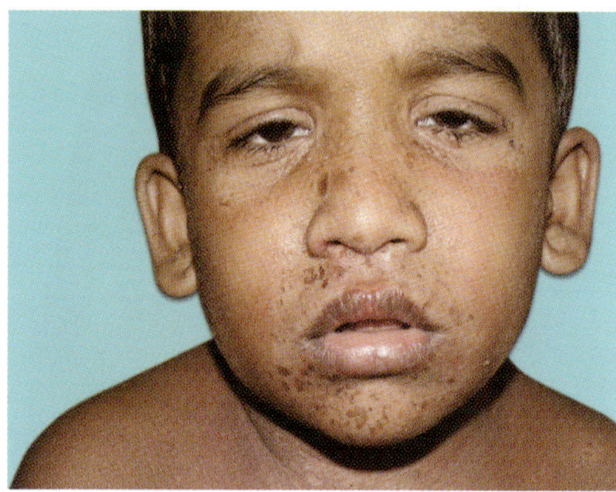

Fig. 10.11: Staphylococcal scalded skin syndrome.

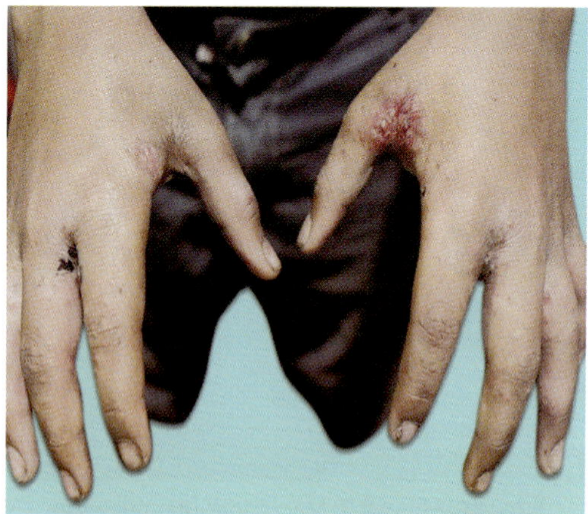

Fig. 10.12: Scabies affecting finger webs.

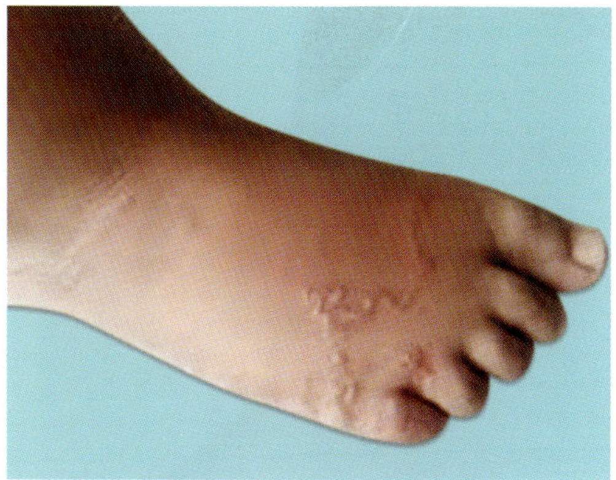

Fig. 10.13: Cutaneous larva migrans.

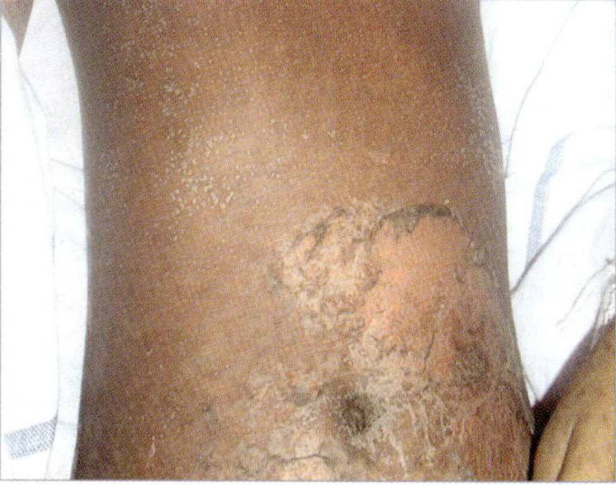

Fig. 10.14: Toxic epidermal necrolysis.

Incontinentia pigmenti is an inherited multisystem disorder with vesiculobullous lesions appearing from newborn period onward.

Hand, foot, mouth disease is infection by coxsackievirus presenting with fever and vesicles in the mouth, perianal region, hands, elbows, knees, and feet.

DIFFERENTIAL DIAGNOSIS OF COMMON SKIN LESIONS

Pruritic lesions: The common ones are scabies, atopic dermatitis, urticaria, insect bites, and papular urticaria. *Scabies* caused by *Sarcoptes scabiei* or hominis presents as small, symmetrical, pruritic lesions, and erythematous papules. Itching is typically intense at night and disturbs sleep. Hands (especially the web spaces of the fingers **(Fig. 10.12)**, flexural aspects of wrists, elbows anterior axillary folds, nipples, buttocks, and genitalia (widely known as *"circle of Hebra"* based on an imaginary circle drawn through these points) are the most affected areas. In infants face, scalp, toes, and soles are mostly affected. Family members are often affected which is a strong supportive point in the diagnosis.

Cutaneous larva migrans (creeping eruption) is caused by the larvae of dogs and cats (other animals also). They penetrate into the skin and migrate. An intensely pruritic raised erythematous serpiginous track with occasional bullae is formed on the migrating body part, most often the legs **(Fig. 10.13)**.

Toxic epidermal necrolysis is a potentially fatal blister forming hypersensitivity reaction **(Fig. 10.14)** (to drugs such as sulfonamides, amoxicillin, phenobarbitone, hydantoin, and allopurinol) manifesting as widespread blisters, erythema, and tenderness of skin with rapid progression.

Atopic dermatitis or infantile eczema is an inherited chronic inflammatory reaction of skin, often associated with family history of asthma. The lesions have a characteristic age-dependent distribution over face, scalp, and extensor areas in infants and young children, and predilection to flexural areas in the older age group **(Fig. 10.15)**. Pruritus and xerosis are common features. Acute lesions are pruritic papules with erythema, excoriations, and serous exudates; in the chronic stage change to fibrotic nodules and lichenification. Family history of skin atopy, asthma, or hay fever are common.

Urticaria are transient wheals with pruritus, excoriation, and secondary dermatographism **(Fig. 10.16)**.

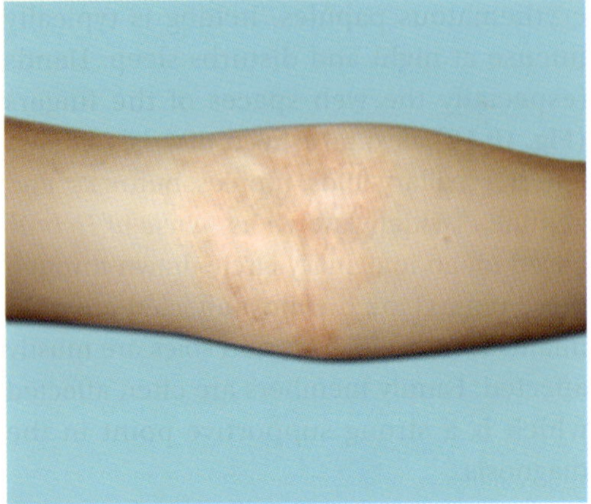

Fig. 10.15: Flexural eczema.

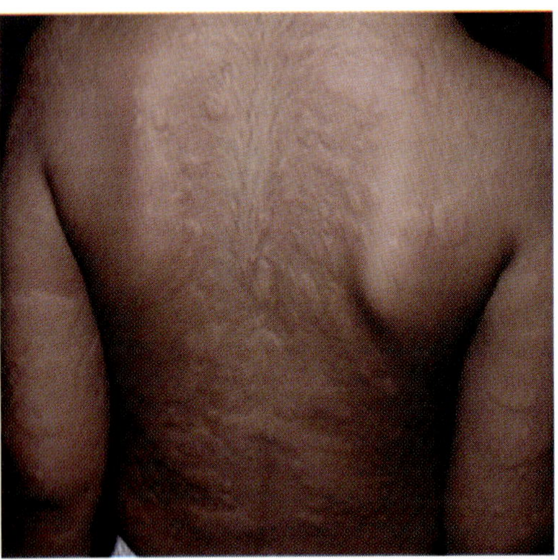

Fig. 10.16: Urticaria.

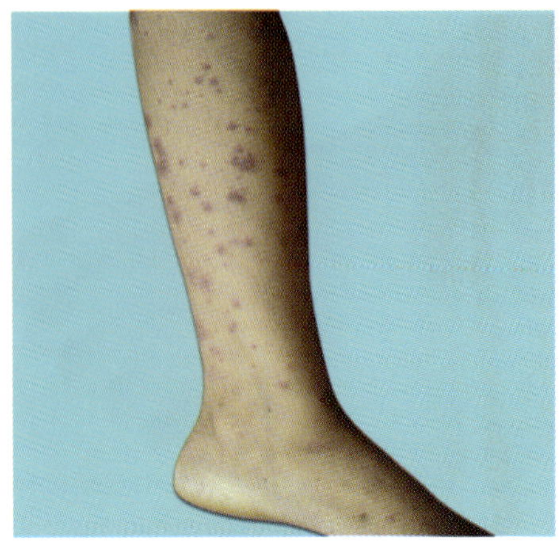

Fig. 10.17: Purpura.

BOX 10.5: Causes of skin, mucosal, and deep bleeds.

- Platelet disorders
  - Qualitative
  - Quantitative
- Coagulation factor defects
  - Congenital (Hemophilias)
  - Acquired (DIC)
- Blood vessel wall integrity disruption
  - Trauma
  - Infection
  - Vasculitis
    - Henoch–Schönlein vasculitis
    - Vitamin C deficiency
  - Collagen vascular diseases: SLE
  - Cutis hyperelastica (Ehlers–Danlos syndrome)

Hemorrhagic Skin Lesions

Purpura is bleeding under the skin or into mucosa **(Fig. 10.17)**. Lesions may be petechiae (pinpoint bleeds) and ecchymoses (larger confluent lesions). They do not blanch on pressure on diascopy as other erythematous rashes or vascular skin lesions.

Skin bleeds occur due to the disorders of platelets, coagulation factors, or blood vessel integrity. **Box 10.5** briefly reveals the causes of skin, mucosal, and deeper bleeds. Superficial skin bleeds indicate platelet disorders and larger deep seated bleeds such as hematoma and hemarthrosis are characteristic of coagulation factor defects. Mucosal bleeds and intracranial hemorrhage occur in both disorders. Hemophilia A and B, von Willebrand disease, vitamin k deficiency, and liver failure are the important causes of superficial bleeds. Purpura can also occur due to the disruption in blood vessel integrity as in trauma, infections, vasculitis

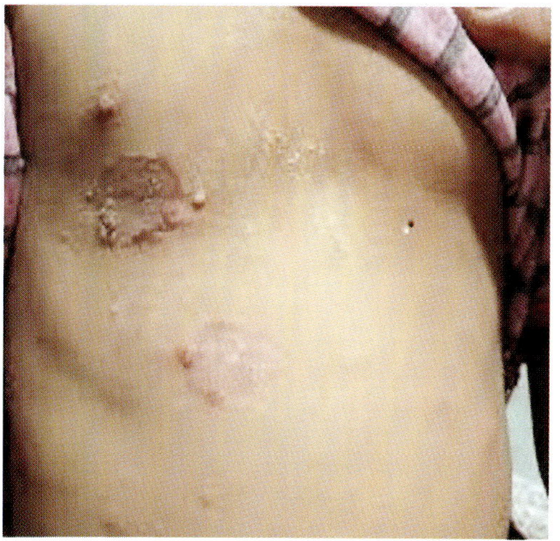
Fig. 10.18: Impetigo.

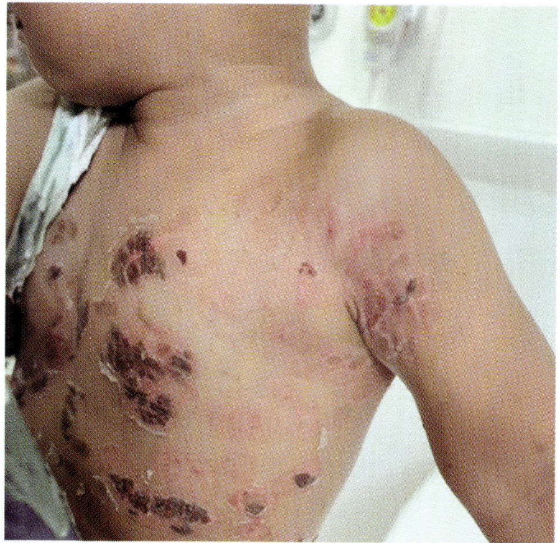
Fig. 10.19: Bullous impetigo.

[Henoch-Schönlein purpura (HSP)], scurvy, and collagen vascular diseases.

Infections

Pyoderma is bacterial infections of the skin very commonly seen in infants and young children; can predispose to sepsis, pneumonia, meningitis, and glomerulonephritis.

Impetigo **(Fig. 10.18)** is the most common superficial skin infection, seen often over the exposed parts of the body (face, hands, neck, and extremities). *Impetigo contagiosa* is the crusted variety seen in older age groups caused by streptococci and staphylococci. *Bullous impetigo* is the blister forming variety often caused by staphylococci **(Fig. 10.19)**. Ecthyma is a deeper chronic infection of skin covered by an adherent crust that contributes to the persistence of infection by certain bacteria. *Ecthyma gangrenosum* **(Fig. 10.20)** is a necrotic ulcer covered with a gray black scar characteristic of *Pseudomonas* sepsis.

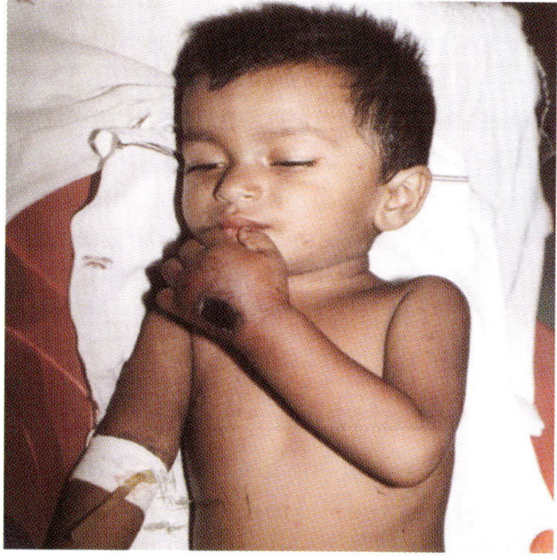
Fig. 10.20: Ecthyma gangrenosum.

Cellulitis is the infection of skin and subcutaneous tissue.

Erythema nodosum are tender red nodules (involve the dermis and subcutaneous tissue) distributed over the shin and are due to hypersensitivity reactions to infection **(Fig. 10.21)**. Organisms involved are *Streptococcus*, tuberculosis, *Mycoplasma*, *Yersinia*, and fungi, but can be the first sign of inflammatory bowel disease and connective tissue disorders. The lesions should be differentiated from perifolliculitis, insect bites, and fungal infections by the characteristic distribution of lesions.

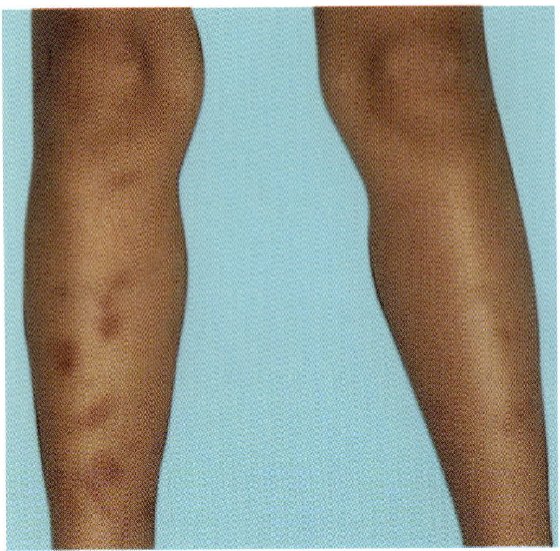

Fig. 10.21: Erythema nodosum.

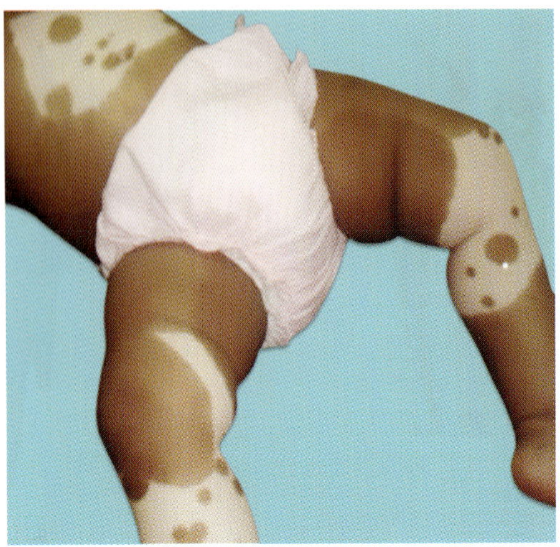

Fig. 10.22: Vitiligo.

Acne are papular or pustular lesions of sebaceous follicles, typically seen over face, upper chest, back, and deltoid area in adolescents; may cause temporary postinflammatory pigmentation. Acne in prepubertal children indicate endocrine disorders or drug intake (steroids, isoniazid, anticonvulsants, lithium carbonate, and vitamin B_{12}). Neonatal acne is due to maternal androgens and is self-regressing.

Disorders of Pigmentation

Hypopigmented lesions: The common hypopigmented lesions in children are pityriasis alba, pityriasis (Tinea) versicolor, vitiligo, postinflammatory hypopigmentation, and nevus depigmentosus. Pityriasis alba presents as scaly hypopigmented patches with ill-defined borders often on the face of children with an atopic diathesis. Pityriasis versicolor has well-defined borders, often described as pencil lines and scaly. *Vitiligo* is an acquired, localized depigmentation; may rarely affect whole skin and become a progressive disorder **(Fig. 10.22)**.

Postinflammatory hypopigmentation can follow any form of infection, dermatitis or drug exposure, and is evident by history. Nevus depigmentosus is characterized by nonprogressive, well-circumscribed, macules or patches of hypopigmentation, usually apparent from birth. In Hansen's disease (indeterminate leprosy) patches are hypopigmented, but not scaly, have ill-defined margins and loss of sensation.

Congenital Disorders of Hypopigmentation

Albinism is characterized by varying degrees of hypopigmentation of skin, hair, and eyes with generalized absence of melanin. Albinism can occur in inborn errors of tyrosine metabolism and in Prader–Willi, Angelman, and Hermansky–Pudlak syndromes.

Piebaldism is congenital localized albinism associated with white forelock. Albinism is localized in Waardenburg syndrome and partial in Chediak–Higashi syndrome.

Hypomelanosis of Ito is bizarre hypopigmented macules arranged in a marbled pattern usually present at birth or may appear by 2 yr of age.

Ash leaf macules are hypopigmented lesions of *tuberous sclerosis* usually present at

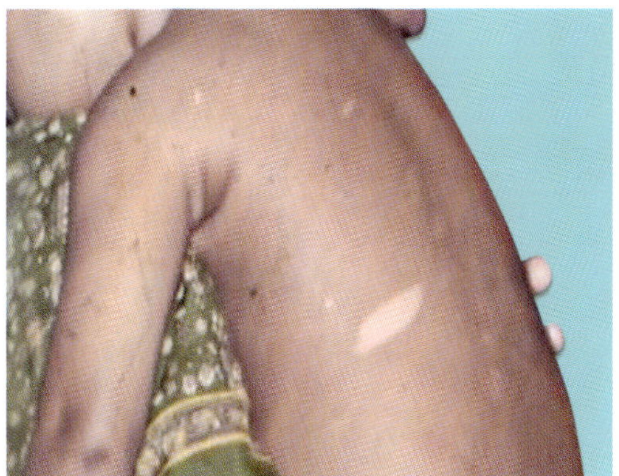

Fig. 10.23: Ash leaf macule.

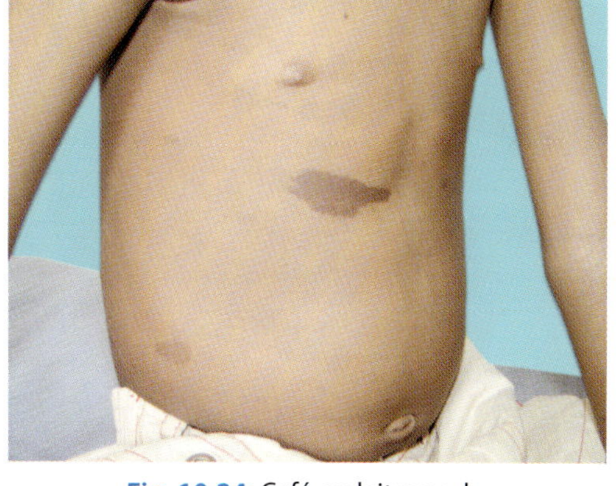

Fig. 10.24: Café-au lait macule.

birth or develop during the first 2 yr of life. They can be better made out by wood lamp ultraviolet and have the appearance of an ash leaf, often associated with other features of tuberous sclerosis **(Fig. 10.23)**.

Hyperpigmented Lesions

Café au lait macules are well-circumscribed brown macules, oval to round in shape and of various sizes appearing at birth or early childhood **(Fig. 10.24)**. Café au lait macules of smaller size and fewer in number are a common occurrence. Multiple and larger ones are associated with syndromes such as tuberous sclerosis, neurofibromatosis, Fanconi anemia, Gaucher disease, and McCune-Albright syndrome. Six or more spots >5 mm in greatest diameter in the prepubertal and >15 mm in greatest diameter in the postpubertal children are the hallmark of neurofibromatosis.

Acanthosis nigricans is characterized by distinctive velvety, warty hyperpigmentation in intertriginous areas such as neck, axilla, and groin and is usually associated with obesity, insulin resistance, and the risk for type 2 diabetes mellitus **(Fig. 24.9)**.

Freckles are small light brown macules seen on light exposed areas. They are seen in genetically predisposed children with sun exposure causing an increase in the melanin production temporarily, e.g., neurofibromatosis.

Lentigines are small macules not limited to sun-exposed areas. If multiple lentigines are present they may be a part of multiorgan syndromes (Leopard, Peutz-Jeghers).

Incontinentia pigmenti is an ectodermal disorder with hyperpigmentation mainly on the trunk in the form of whorls, reticulated patches, and linear streaks.

Melanocytic nevi are considered *congenital* if present at birth or within 2 yr of age. They can be *small* (<1.5 cm diameter), *large* (1.5–20 cm), or *giant* (>20 cm) and are deeply pigmented, slightly elevated with surface textural changes, and hypertrichosis. The giant bathing trunk nevus is commonly seen in lower back and thigh area **(Fig. 10.25)**; *satellite nevi* are small lesions in large numbers in other areas. Acquired melanocytic nevi are seen in older children and adolescents.

Acquired generalized hyperpigmentation is seen in *Addison disease* and *Fanconi anemia*. In the former, hyperpigmentation is seen mainly over the face, mucosa, hands, axilla, nipples, umbilicus, genitalia, and around joints. Generalized hyperpigmentation with

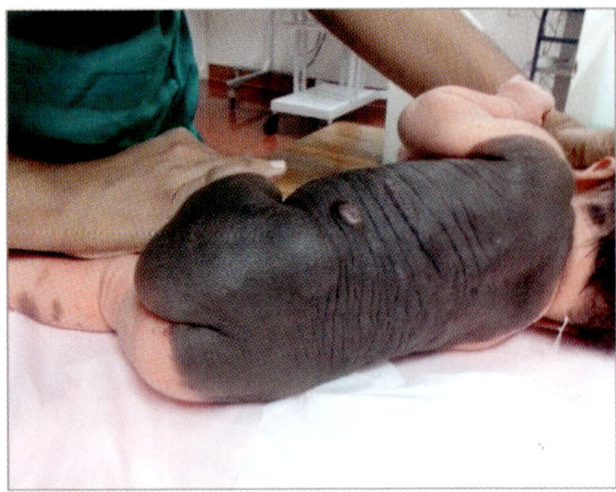

Fig. 10.25: Giant bathing trunk nevus.

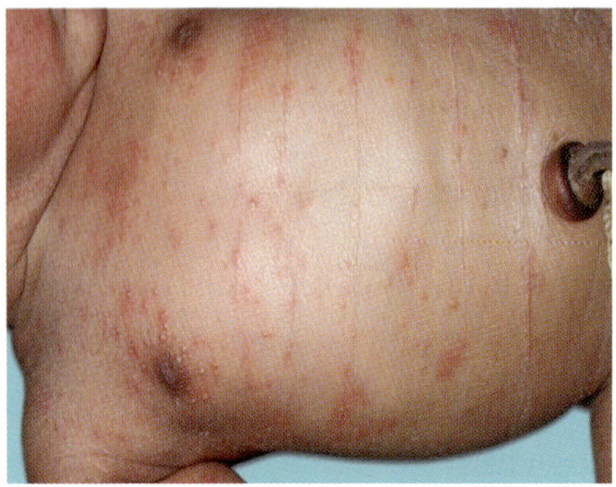

Fig. 10.26: Erythema toxicum neonatorum.

circumoral predominance is characteristic of Fanconi anemia. The common conditions producing acquired *localized* hyperpigmentation are contact dermatitis, post-inflammatory lesions, papular urticaria, and fixed drug rashes.

Postinflammatory hyperpigmentation occurs as a sequelae of skin disorders such as infection, allergic reactions, injuries, drug reactions, inflammatory diseases (SLE), etc.

Neonatal Skin Lesions (See Ch. 15 for more details)

Skin lesions are common in newborns and are a significant source of parental concern though most of them are self-limited.

TRANSIENT VASCULAR PHENOMENA

Acrocyanosis is bluish discoloration of hands and feet due to exposure to cold environments. It fades away with warming of the extremities or when the newborn stops crying. Clinical examination differentiates it from central cyanosis by the absence of cyanosis of the mucous membrane due to cardiovascular and respiratory diseases.

Cutis marmorata (a physiological response of skin to temperature change as acrocyanosis) is reticulated mottling of the skin that symmetrically involves the trunk and extremities during the first 2–4 w of life. The condition resolves when the skin is warmed. The mottling persists with trisomy 18, Down syndrome, hypothyroidism, and Cornelia de Lange Syndrome.

Harlequin color change is transient erythema covering half of the body of the newborn with simultaneous blanching of the contralateral side with a pronounced demarcation that develops suddenly and persists for 30 sec–20 min. It is more common in preterm babies and is of benign nature.

Erythema toxicum neonatorum are erythematous 2–3 mm macules and papules evolving into pustules **(Fig. 10.26)**. Each pustule is surrounded by a blotchy area of erythema, leading to a classically "flea-bitten" appearance. Lesions usually occur on the face, trunk, and proximal extremities.

Transient neonatal pustular melanosis are vesiculopustular rashes that lack surrounding erythema, rupture easily, leaving a collarette of scale and a pigmented macule (unique to this condition) that fades over 3–4 w.

Milia, a common neonatal disorder (seen in up to 30–50% of newborns) are 1–2 mm pearly white or yellow papules on the nose, cheeks, forehead, chin, and rarely on the trunk and extremities. They are epidermal cysts caused by retention of keratin within the dermis and disappear spontaneously usually within the first month of life. The lesions on the palate are called Epstein's pearls.

Miliaria affects up to 40% of infants and results from sweat retention caused by partial closure of eccrine structures. Subtypes are miliaria crystallina and miliaria rubra.

Mongolian spots are blue gray or blue green patches seen usually over the sacral gluteal area due to interrupted melanocyte migration from the neural crest through the epidermis crest **(Fig. 15.12)**. Lesions expand in the first year of life and fade in 3–5 yrs. *Acne neonatorum* occurs in 20% of newborns and consists of closed comedones on the forehead, nose, and cheeks.

Cradle cap is generalized scaling of the scalp caused by seborrheic dermatitis; canal-so affect the face, ears and neck. Erythema is more in the flexural folds and intertriginous areas (especially diaper area), whereas scaling predominates on the scalp. *Sucking blisters* are caused by vigorous sucking by the baby in the womb. Intact blisters or erosions may be found on the forearm, wrist, hands, or fingers and resolve within a few days. *Suckling blisters* are firm swellings on the upper lip and are hyperplastic responses to suckling.

Hemangiomas **(Fig. 10.27)** are benign vascular neoplasms, with an initial proliferation and spontaneous involution by 5 yr of age. Head and trunk are commonly involved, the lesions are firm, red, rubbery, and tense.

Systemic disorders with cutaneous manifestations: Several systemic disorders of childhood are characterized by cutaneous stigmata, and these skin signs can serve as important diagnostic clues **(Table 10.1)**.

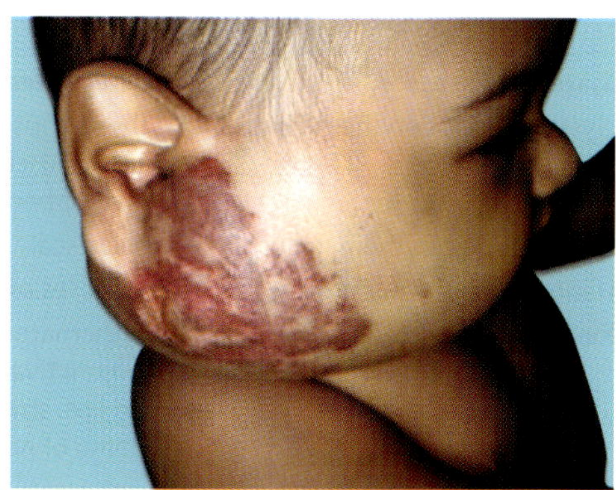

Fig. 10.27: Hemangioma face.

HAIR DISORDERS IN CHILDREN

Excessive and abnormal hair growth if generalized, it is *hypertrichosis,* and *hirsutism* if androgen dependent male pattern of hair growth in women.

Hair loss in children and adolescents can be due to acquired or congenital causes and range in severity. They are tinea capitis (TC), telogen effluvium (TE), traction alopecia (TA), trichotillomania, alopecia areata (AA), and congenital alopecia. Very common causes are malnutrition, chronic infections **(Fig. 7.18A)**, iron deficiency anemia, hypothyroidism, SLE, diabetes mellitus, and structural abnormalities of the hair shaft.

Tinea capitis is a common dermatophyte infection that primarily affects children; the presence of black dot hairs [broken hairs within the lesion **(Fig. 10.31)**], significant erythema and scaling, and posterior cervical lymphadenopathy are diagnostic points.

Alopecia areata is a common form of autoimmune hair loss with a family history of other autoimmune disorders such as vitiligo or thyroid disease. Nonscarring, well-demarcated areas of complete hair loss with exclamation mark hairs are seen at the lesion peripheries.

Trichotillomania is a compulsive disorder characterized by repetitive, compulsive, and self-induced hair pulling from the scalp, eyebrows, and/or other parts of

TABLE 10.1: Skin lesions in common systemic diseases.

Systemic disease	*Cutaneous lesions*
Systemic lupus erythematosus	Erythematous patches and plaques—malar distribution **(Fig. 10.28)**; palpable purpura, livedo reticularis **(Fig. 10.29B)**, Raynaud phenomenon **(Fig. 10.29A)**
Discoid lupus erythematosus	Annular, scaly plaques; atrophy—photodistribution
Henoch–Schönlein purpura	Purpuric lesions of buttocks; lower extremities
Kawasaki disease	• Erythematous maculopapular rash • Conjunctival congestion • Red lips, strawberry tongue • Edema of hands and feet, periungual desquamation **(Fig. 10.30)**
Juvenile dermatomyositis	• Erythematous to violaceous scaly macules over upper eyelids—heliotrope rash • Discrete papules overlying joints—Gottron papules

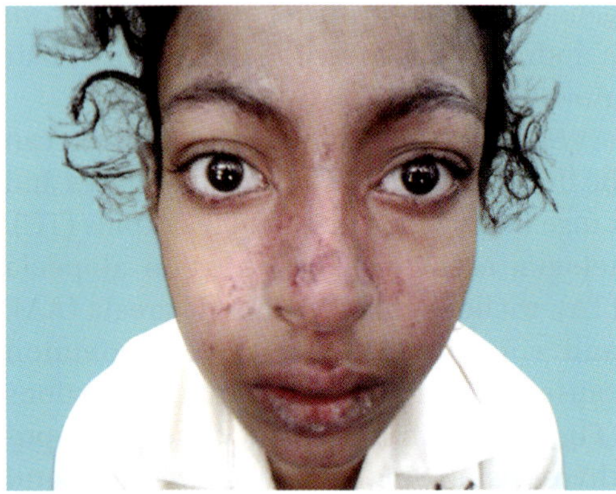

Fig. 10.28: Malar rashes in systemic lupus erythematosus (SLE).

the body. The peak incidence is in the age group 9–13 yr and is more in girls. Clinical presentation includes multiple nonscarring and focal patches of hair loss with irregular borders.

Traction alopecia is caused by prolonged traction of scalp hair by tight braids, pony tails, etc., though reversible, but if it persists chronic permanent alopecia may occur.

Color changes of hair (refer to Ch. 7) are hypopigmentation, characteristic of PEM, part of vitiligo, and premature graying of hair (if the scalp hair is gray). After the age of 20 yr graying is physiologically accepted.

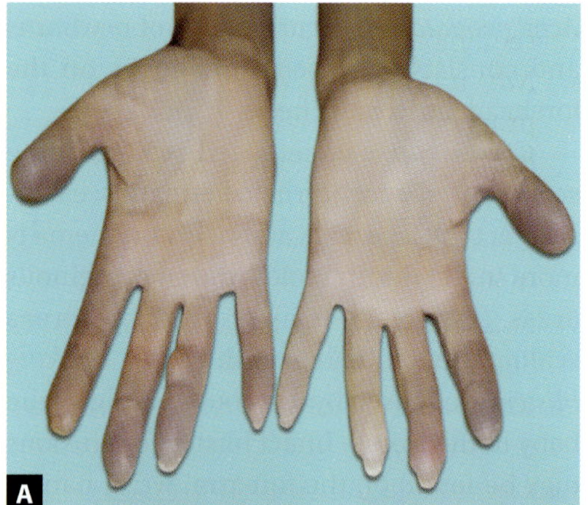

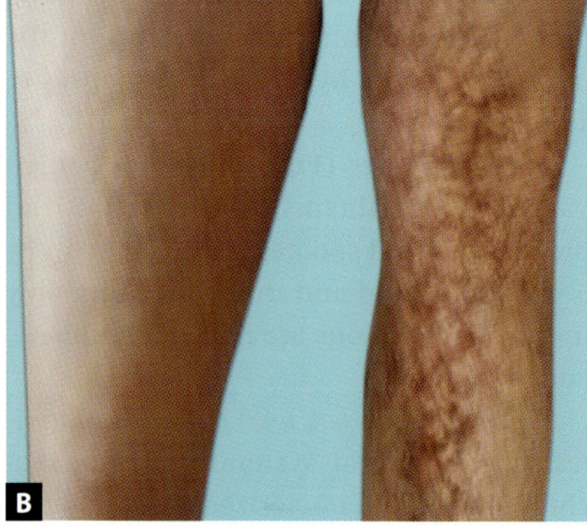

Figs. 10.29A and B: (A) Raynaud's phenomenon; (B) Livedo reticularis.

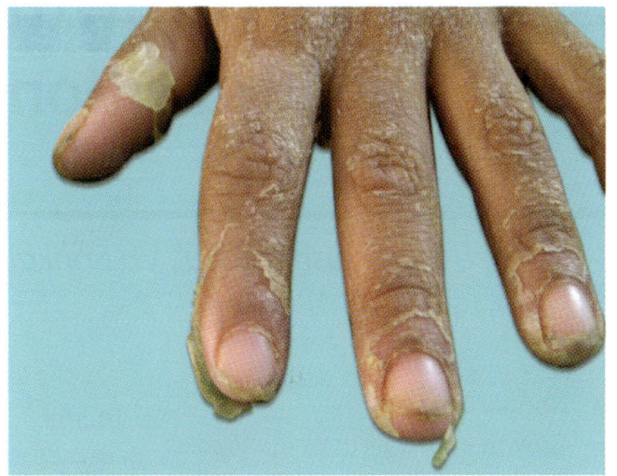

Fig. 10.30: Periungual desquamation in Kawasaki disease.

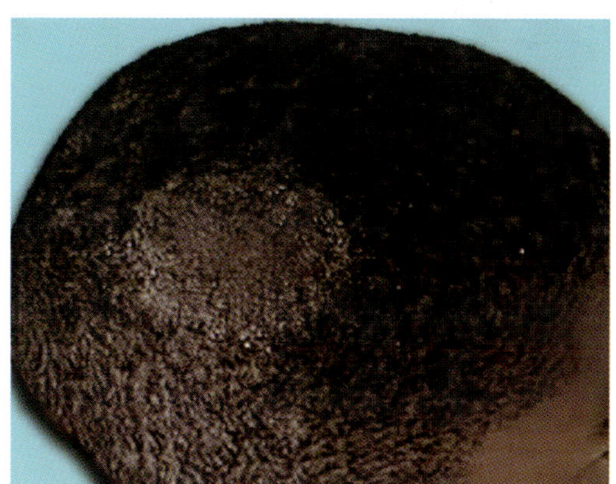

Fig. 10.31: Tinea capitis—see broken hairs and scaling within the lesion.

NAIL DISORDERS

Few commonly seen nail disorders are:

- *Nail pitting* is a common problem and presents as small-to-large punctate depressions seen in psoriasis and atopic dermatitis.
- *Beau's line* is a transverse groove or furrow that develops as a reaction to stress that temporarily interrupts the nail growth. Seen after trauma and illnesses as in Kawasaki disease and Hand, foot, and mouth disease.
- *Koilonychia is* thin depressed, concave nails seen in iron deficiency anemia (rare in children) and Lichen planus.
- *Platonychia is* flat nails seen in cirrhosis.
- *Leukonychia* is white, opaque nails seen in cirrhosis and renal failure.

SUGGESTED READING

1. Baxter S, McSheffrey G. Chapter 5. Dermatology. In: Baxter S, McSheffrey G (Eds). Toronto Notes, 2010, 26th edition. Toronto: Toronto Notes for Medical Students, Inc.; 2010.
2. Bezzant JL. (2000). Dermatology Image Bank. [online] Available from http://library.med.utah.edu/kw/derm/ [Last accessed September, 2024].
3. Buxton P. ABC Atlas of Dermatology, 4th edition. London: BMJ Publishing; 2003.
4. Elecbullet. (2009). Blackheads. [online] Available from http://en.wikipedia.org/wiki/file:Blackheads.JPG [Last accessed September, 2024].
5. Fruitsmaak S. (2010). Inflamed epidermal inclusion cyst. [online] Available from http://en.wikipedia.org/wiki/File:Inflamed_epidermal_inclusion_cyst.jpg. [Last accessed September, 2024].
6. NHS. (2022). Scarlet fever. Home. Health A to Z. [online] Available from https://www.nhs.uk/conditions/scarlet-fever/. [Last accessed September, 2024].
7. Paller AS, Mancini J. Hurwitz Clinical Pediatric Dermatology, 4th edition. Amsterdam: Elsevier (Saunders); 2011.
8. Pande V, Maroo M, Agarkhader SR, Deshpande NS. Cutaneous Larva Migrans: A case report. Int J Applied Research. 2018; 4(11):218-9.
9. Silver442n. (2007). Milia. [online] Available from http://en.wikipedia.org/wiki/file:Milia_big.png. [Last accessed September, 2024].
10. Williams G, Katcher M. (2003). Primary care dermatology module nomenclature of skin lesions. [online] Available from http://www.pediatrics.wisc.edu/education/derm/index.html [Last accessed September, 2024].
11. Wolff K, Johnson A. Fitzpatrick's Color Atlas and Synopsis of Clinical Dermatology, 6th edition. New York: Mcgraw-Hill; 2009.

11

CHAPTER

Assessment of Growth and Nutrition

S Sushamabai, VH Sankar

Chapter Outline

INTRODUCTION

Growth is the net increase in the size of the individual (due to increase in number and size of cells producing increased tissue mass) which distinguishes the child from an adult. Appropriate growth is the best index of one's health. Assessment of growth is to detect the following:

- To detect whether the child is having normal growth.
- To implement early correction if abnormal.
- To know the growth pattern of children of a country which is an index of public health and economic wellbeing.

The *gold standard* of nutritional assessment is *anthropometry*, the science which deals with the measurement of the size, weight, and proportions of the human body. Other methods of nutritional assessment are radiological and dental age estimation, which can provide added advantages; biochemical estimation and histological methods though contributory, are restricted to research purposes.

Anthropometry is simple, cheap, easy to learn and adapt, noninvasive and reliable if performed correctly. The disadvantages are the need for training the methods, difficulty of accurately measuring small changes in nutritional status, and limitations in children with body deformities. Ideally the doctor should do the measurement, but a trained staff nurse or paramedic can be entrusted in small hospitals or clinics where a single doctor has to carry out all duties.

EQUIPMENT

Equipment should be available in the outpatient department (OPD), immunization clinic, inpatient wards, and teaching rooms.

- Weighing machines **(Figs. 11.1A and B)**
- Infantometer for length measurement **(Figs. 11.2A and B)**.
- Anthropometer or stadiometer for height measurement **(Figs. 11.3A to D)**.
- Nonstretchable but flexible plastic tape.
- Harpenden skinfold caliper **(Fig. 11.7)**.
- Growth charts and reference data **[Appendix 1-Growth Charts-Fig. 11.5 (Charts 1 to 19)]**.

The parameters routinely measured are weight, length/height, lower segment (LS), head circumference (HC), mid upper arm circumference (MUAC), and chest circumference (CC). Arm span, segmental length, skinfold thickness, abdominal girth,

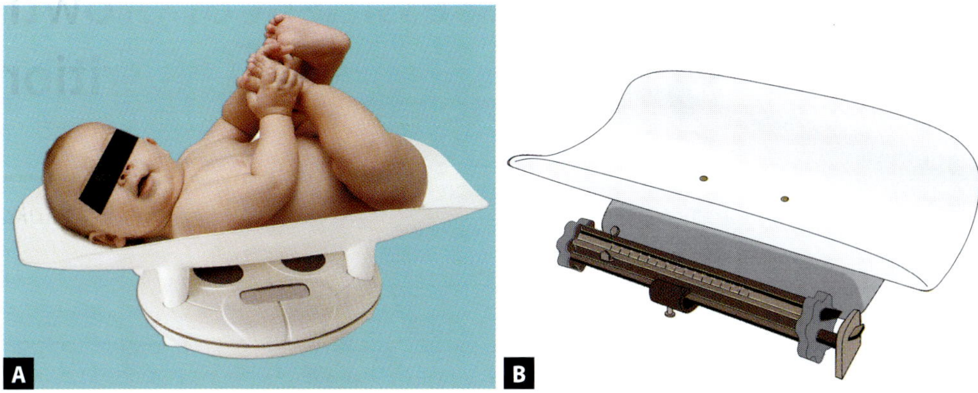

Figs. 11.1A and B: (A) Baby on electronic weighing scale; (B) Beam type weighing scale.

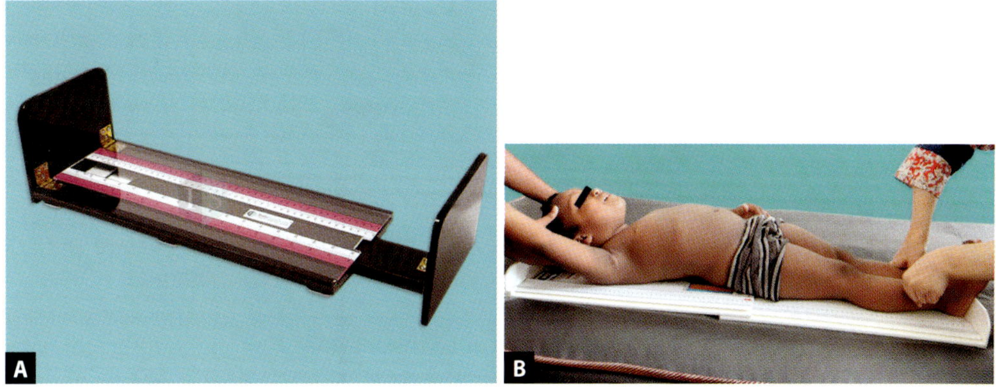

Figs. 11.2A and B: (A) Infantometer; (B) Measuring the length by infantometer.

midthigh and midcalf circumferences are some other parameters measured in relevant situations. Waist and hip circumferences are parameters to detect obesity in school age children as simple easy screening methods.

TECHNIQUE OF MEASUREMENT

Weight is the best measurement of growth and nutrition and can be easily measured. Before recording, correct the Zero error on the weighing scale. Place the scale on a flat horizontal surface. Remove the child's shoes, change the soiled napkin; clothing should be the minimum as the custom permits caring to avoid hypothermia. Child should not be in contact with any other object. Value is read directly in the electronic type. In the beam type, value is read when the beam is steady at its balance point or as the pointer becomes stable **(Figs. 11.1A and B)**.

Double weighing can be done for older children if they are unable to stand or very ill or highly uncooperative, though the accuracy is less. The parent is weighed alone first, then the combined weight of the parent and child is recorded and the difference is noted.

Length/height: Length is the linear body measurement in lying posture and stature is the standing position measurement. This measurement is comparatively difficult to

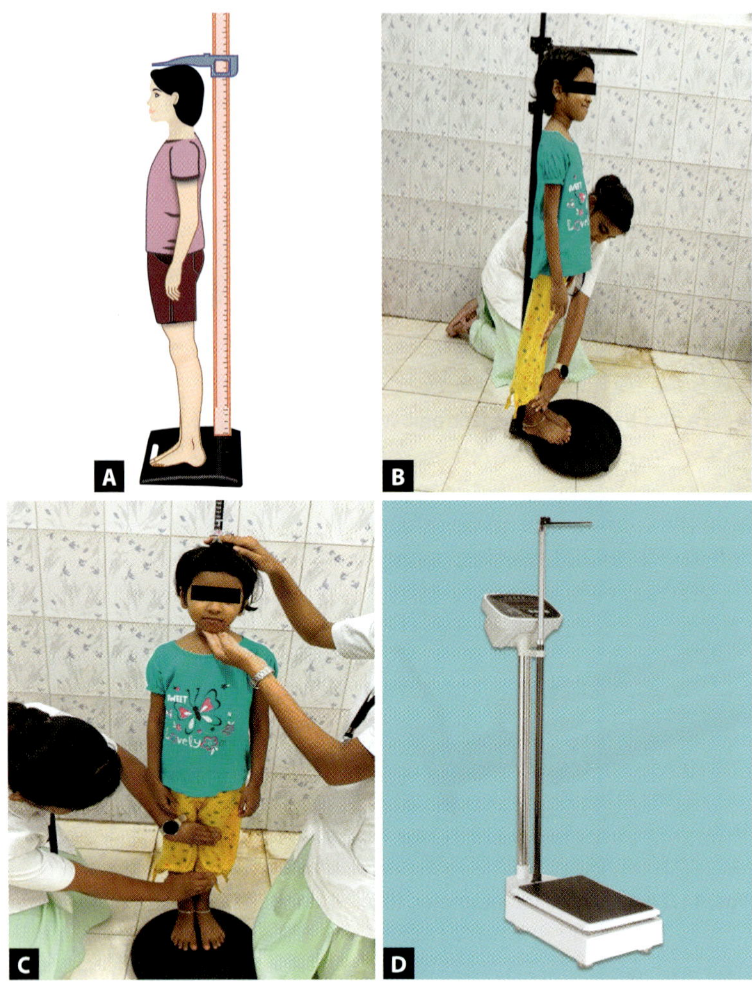

Figs. 11.3A to D: (A to C) Height measurement using the stadiometer; (D) Electronic weight cum height measuring equipment.

record but is the best indicator of nutritional deprivation of longer duration (at least 3 m) and is not affected by an acute illness or food deprivation for few days.

Length (recumbent or lying measurement) is recorded in children under 2 yr of age, since the infants cannot stand and it is difficult to make toddlers stand for the measurement in proper position. Length is 1 cm more than the height above the age of 2 yr, since the lumbar lordosis (develops by 2 yr of age) gets corrected in lying posture. Measurement is done by an infantometer with the help of a health staff or parent **(Fig. 11.2B)**. The tool has a calibrated horizontal board with two vertical boards attached at head (fixed head piece) and foot (movable foot piece) ends. Length of the baby (up to100 cm) can be read directly from the horizontal board.

How to measure the length: Remove the hair braids, ornaments, clothes to the maximum allowed, and change the napkin to get the most accurate measurement. Infant is placed on the resting board of the infantometer and the assistant is instructed to hold the head firmly in position against the fixed head-board so that the *Frankfurt line* (an imaginary line joining the external auditory canal and the lower margin of the orbit) of the child is perpendicular to the lying board. The examiner straightens the legs by pressing the knees and keeps the feet at right angles to legs with toes pointing upward. The mobile foot board is brought into firm contact with the child's heels and the reading is noted down **(Fig. 11.2B)**. Accuracy must be nearest to 0.1 cm and should be confirmed by rechecking.

Height is ideally measured with a stadiometer in older children who are able to stand. A vertical rod attached to the lever type machine or graded wall (ensure that the zero measurement is at the angle formed by the wall and the ground) may also be used, if a stadiometer is not available. Remove the shoes, head braids, and other hairdos of the child, who is made to stand on the platform of the stadiometer with the back against the graded scale (or on the floor in front of the graded wall) with heels together, feet slightly apart, legs straight, and shoulders relaxed. The heels, calves, buttocks, shoulders, and occiput of the child should touch the background **(Fig. 11.3A)**.

The head is positioned in such a way that the child looks straight ahead with the Frankfurt line horizontal to the ground. Exert gentle upward pressure on the mastoid process to position the head. Ask the child to take a breath, relax the shoulders, and stretch up to be tall to the maximum, taking care that the heels remain on the ground. A gentle push on the tummy will help the child to stand to full height. The headpiece of the apparatus (or a plastic scale kept firmly over the vertex if the graded wall is used) is brought down to compress the hair **(Figs. 11.3B and C)**. The maximum measurement is then recorded to the last completed millimeter. In children with unequal leg length, measure the length of the longest limb (this fact should be recorded). Modern electronic weight cum height-measuring equipment are available **(Fig. 11.3D)** in which weight and height values can be read simultaneously.

Lower segment: LS of the body extends from symphysis pubis to the soles, and the upper segment (US) is from vertex to symphysis pubis representing the growth of long and membranous bones, respectively. LS measurement is necessary to assess the ratio between the two segments upper/lower (U/L), which is altered in various growth disorders. To measure the LS, palpate the upper border of pubic ramus and mark it on the overlying skin carefully. In older children, LS is measured from this point to the lower medial margin of the right heel, up to the floor in the standing position using a nonstretchable tape. In infants, LS reading is noted from the infantometer by placing a scale horizontally over this point. US is the difference between total body length and LS.

Head circumference value indicates the brain growth and status of the ventricles. Children <2 yr of age can be placed on mother's lap; older children should be informed gently about the procedure and allowed to sit on a chair or stand, if they prefer so. The braids and other ornaments over the hair should be removed. The measurement should record the greatest volume of the cranium. The examiner sits or stands facing the child and holds the proximal end of the tape over the patient's supraorbital ridge by the thumb of the nondominant hand supported by the fingers placed on the patients scalp. The tape is then extended circumferentially to include the most prominent portion of the occiput, and the occipitofrontal circumference (OFC) is measured by bringing the tape to the proximal end to the nearest 0.1 mm as shown in **Figure 11.4**. Press the hair well to get the maximum correct value.

Head circumference of parents and siblings should be measured if the patient's head is abnormal in size or shape. *Errors in measurements* can occur due to scalp swellings, extravasation of intravenous fluids administered through scalp veins, and in newborns due to overriding of skull bone sutures and cephalohematoma. Average value of OFC at birth is 35 cm. Head grows very fast during the earlier months of life **(Table 11.1)**. Increments are to be ideally compared with the values in standard growth charts. Compare with the *WHO* growth charts on HC in **Appendix 1-Growth Charts-Fig. 11.5 (Charts 1 to 19)**.

Mid upper arm circumference (MUAC) is measured on the relaxed left arm. The examiner sits facing the child and marks the tips of acromion and olecranon processes over the arm and measures the upper arm length. Midpoint of the upper arm is marked and the arm circumference accurate to the nearest 0.1 cm is measured. The tape should not be tightly applied **(Fig. 11.6)**.

Chest circumference is measured at the level of nipples in recumbent posture.

Arm span: Arm span is the distance between the tips of the middle fingers when the upper limbs are outstretched at right angles to the side of the body. The measurement

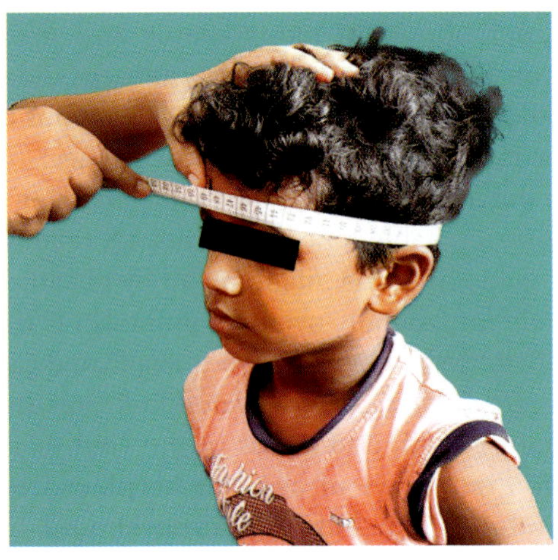

Fig. 11.4: Measuring the occipitofrontal circumference.

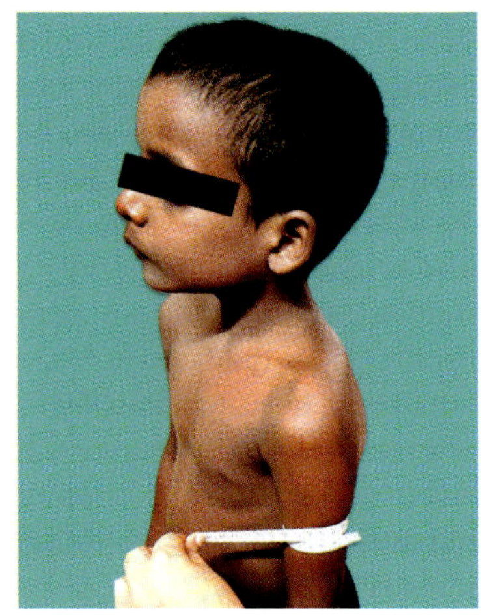

Fig. 11.6: Measuring the mid upper arm circumference.

TABLE 11.1: Approximate increments of weight, length and head circumference in infancy.

Age (m)	*Weight gain (g)/day*	*length increments (cm)/m*	*OFC increase (cm)/m*
1–3	30	3.5	2.0
4–6	20	2.0	1.0
7–9	15	1.5	0.5
10–12	12	1.2	0.5

(g: gram; m: month/months; OFC: occipitofrontal circumference) is ideally done while the child is standing in front of a wall as for measuring height. The tips of middle fingers are marked on the wall and the distance between the two points are measured. If the child is unable to stand, arm span can be measured in recumbent posture with outstretched upper limbs. The tips of middle fingers are marked on the lying surface and the arm span is measured.

Skin fold thickness (SFT) is the best measurement to assess subcutaneous fat to detect the degree of adiposity especially in community surveys to assess overweight/obesity. Sites of measuring of skinfold are the triceps, subscapular, and over the anterior superior iliac spine regions. Normal standards for the former two sites are available (Tanners and Whitehouse). The skin fold calipers [most popular is Harpenden and Best type **(Fig. 11.7)**], should be standardized before taking the measurement. The examiner should sit or stand, facing the back of the child. Triceps SFT is measured at the *midpoint of the relaxed right upper arm*. A fold of skin with the subcutaneous tissue is grasped between the left index finger and thumb by the examiner and with the right hand calipers is applied over this fold. Value nearest to 0.1 cm is noted when the pointer becomes stable (approximately 30 sec).

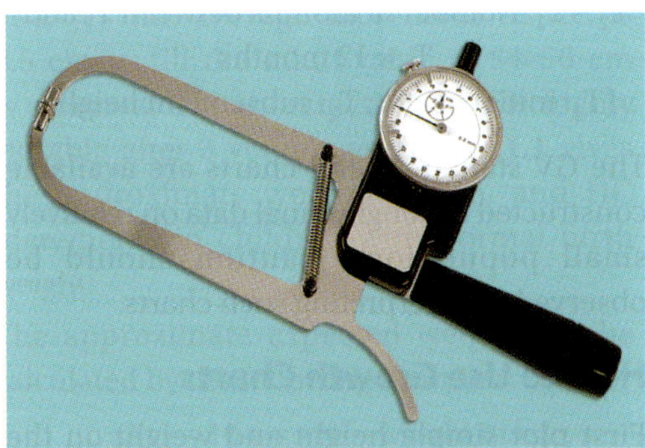

Fig. 11.7: Harpenden calipers.

GROWTH CHARTS AND REFERENCE DATA

Growth charts are the reference standards for assessing each child after completing the measurements. These charts are the graphic representations of the data presented in tables and typically depict 3rd, 10th, 25th, 50th, 75th, and 97th percentiles. The child's measurements are compared to these references or standards using the reference tables or ideally by plotting the values on a growth chart. Growth charts are available separately for both genders, which include weight-for-age, height-for-age, weight-for-height, head circumference-for-age, and body mass index (BMI)-for-age. Growth charts help to keep a longitudinal record of an individual child.

Common growth reference data being used in clinical practice include:

- World Health Organization charts 2006
- Centre for Disease Control and Prevention charts (CDC) 2000
- Indian Academy of Pediatrics (IAP) charts 2006 and 2015; and
- Combined charts—e.g., WHO-IAP.

WHO (2006) chart is currently accepted for growth monitoring in children <5 yr age. The Government of India and the IAP also endorsed this chart for growth monitoring in under-five children. For growth monitoring of children above 5 yr, nationally representative references should be used. The IAP 2015 growth charts can be used for children above 5 yr. Refer Appendix 1, **Fig. 11.5**: Growth Charts in Indian Children (WHO 2006 and IAP 2015) 1 to 10.

Interpretation of growth parameters can be done in following three ways:

1. *Percentile:* Percentile (p) means the location of a child among the peer group and is obtained by dividing an ordered set of data into 100 equal-sized groups. An observed measurement at 50th p indicates the

TABLE 11.2: IAP classification of malnutrition—weight for age.

Grade of PEM	Percentage of observed weight against expected
Normal	>80
Grade 1	71–80
Grade 2	61–70
Grade 3	51–60
Grade 4	<50

Postfix "K" to the grade if the patient has nutritional edema.

(IAP: Indian Academy of Pediatrics; PEM: protein energy malnutrition)

TABLE 11.3: Wellcome trust classification of malnutrition.

Weight for age (% of expected)	Edema	Type of PEM
60–80	Absent	Undernutrition
60–80	Present	Kwashiorkor
<60	Absent	Marasmus
<60	Present	Marasmic Kwashiorkor

(PEM: protein energy malnutrition)

age and presence of edema for the classification of PEM **(Table 11.3)**. Other widely accepted classifications of PEM according to weight for age are put forward by Gomez and Jelliffe.

Percentile tracing in growth charts: By plotting the observed measurements in standard growth charts, percentile of growth is assessed. Values below 3rd and above 97th percentiles need evaluation to exclude pathological conditions.

Standard deviation scores (SD or Z) of observed value: SD indicates the degree of dispersion or deviation of observed measurement away from the mean which is the 50th percentile of a normal distribution curve **(Fig. 11.8)**. Values beyond 2 SD (above and below) from the mean are abnormal. One SD is 12.5% for

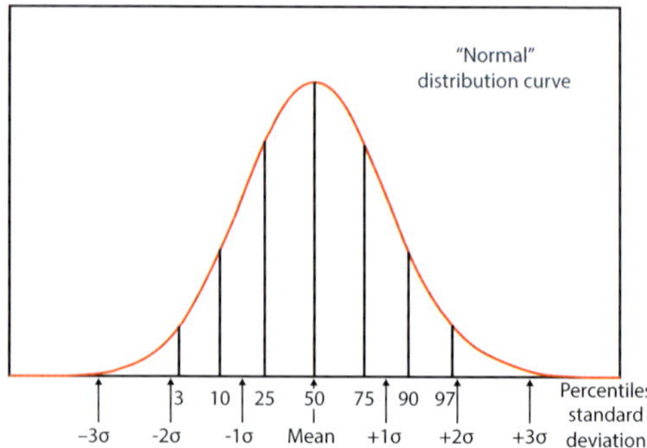

Fig. 11.8: The normal distribution curve.

weight, 4% for height/length, and 2.5% for OFC of the expected normal values (CDC 2000 mean).

While the first two approaches are most widely used in clinical nutritional assessment, the third approach—calculation of SD scores is considered more appropriate.

Weight age: From the standard growth charts find the age at which the 50th percentile weight equals the child's present weight, e.g., a 4 yr old child with 10 kg weight has the median weight of a 1 yr old child, and thus the weight age of the index case is 1 yr.

Length/height for age: The measurement is important to look for growth retardation. Malnutrition for prolonged periods (>3 m) only can cause stunting. In all patients with significant growth retardation, pathological SS must be evaluated. Waterlow's classification for stunting is the widely accepted one for stunting in relation to malnutrition **(Table 11.4)**.

If the child needs evaluation for growth retardation, the length/height should be plotted in the appropriate growth charts for analysis. Height/length <3rd percentile or <2 SD below the median value are considered as SS. If values exceed >97th percentile or >2 SD above median, patient is considered as TS.

Weight for length/height: Weight for length/height is a measure of weight compared to the weight of children of the same gender and length/height from a reference population. It is an indicator of acute malnutrition irrespective of age. The WHO and the CDC weight for length/height standards are available for children. A child with weight for length/height <2 SD is considered as wasted and <3 SD is considered to have severe wasting. Waterlow's classification for wasting is the widely accepted one in clinical practice for wasting **(Table 11.5)**.

TABLE 11.4: Waterlow's classification of stunting (height for age).

Grade of stunting	*Height for age (% of expected)*
Nil	>95
I	90–95
II	85–89
III	<85

TABLE 11.5: Waterlow's classification of wasting (weight for height).

Degree of wasting	*Weight for length/height in %*
No wasting	>90%
I degree	81–90
II degree	71–80
III degree	≤70

WHO classification of undernutrition: The WHO has recommended classification of undernutrition using terms wasting and stunting. *Wasting* is acute deficit in tissue and fat mass. *Stunting* indicates retardation of linear growth for yrs. Including edema along with wasting and stunting, in clinical settings undernutrition is categorised as in **Table 11.6** as per WHO categorization.

To assess the magnitude of undernutrition among under-five children in large screening programs the percentage of W/H and H/A are used as revealed in **Table 11.7**.

Head circumference (OFC): Interpretation should be done by percentile tracing in standard growth charts or tables, standard deviation values, and by OFC length ratio. The approximate rate of increment of OFC for different age groups is shown in **Table 11.8**. The increment is highly variable after 3 yr of age.

In growth charts, OFC values below 3rd percentile indicate microcephaly and above 97th percentiles denote macrocephaly, respectively. Values >3 SD below and above the mean indicate micro- and macrocephaly, respectively. Mean value is the 50th percentile in CDC 2000 table available up to 36 m, to which 0.5 cm/yr increment can be added up to 56 cm to get the maximum

TABLE 11.6: WHO classification of undernutrition.

Parameter	*Moderate undernutrition*	*Severe undernutrition*
Symmetrical edema	No	Yes*
W/H	– 2 SD to – 3 SD score (70–79% of expected)	<– 3 SD score (<70% of expected)
	Wasting	*Severe wasting*
H/A	– 2 to – 3 SD score (85–89% of expected)	<– 3 SD score (<85% of expected)
	Stunting	*Severe stunting*

*Edematous malnutrition: Kwashiorkor, Marasmic Kwashiorkor

(H/A: height for age; SD: standard deviation; W/H: weight for height; WHO: World Health Organization)

TABLE 11.7: WHO screening of undernutrition in <5 yr in large screening programs.

W/H	*H/A*	*Nutritional status*
≥80%	≥90%	Normal
≥80%	<90%	Stunted
<80%	≥90%	Wasted
<80%	<90%	Wasted and stunted

Note: Reference value is 50th percentile of CDC 2000. (H/A: height for age; W/H: weight for height)

TABLE 11.8: Rate of increments in OFC.

Age	*Rate of increment per month*
Birth to 3 m	2 cm/m
4–6 m	1 cm/m
7–12 m	0.5 cm/m
Second yr	2 cm/yr
>2 yr age	0.5 cm/yr till the adult value of 54–56 cm is attained

BOX 11.1: Causes of microcephaly.

- *Primary (genetic)*
  - Autosomal recessive*
  - Autosomal dominant
  - Syndromes (chromosomal, genetic)
- *Secondary*
  - Prenatal
    - Craniosynostosis
    - Drug induced (fetal alcohol, hydantoin)
    - Hyperthermia
    - Infections (TORCH)
    - Metabolic
      - Maternal diabetes
      - Maternal hyperalaninemia
    - Radiation
  - Natal, postnatal
    - Hypoxic insult
    - CNS infections
    - Malnutrition
    - Metabolic encephalopathies
    - Head trauma

Characterized by receding forehead, prominent ears, severe mental retardation, seizures* *(Fig. 7.17A)***.

adult value. **Boxes 11.1** and **11.2** reveal the causes of microcephaly and macrocephaly, respectively.

Mid upper arm circumference (MUAC) is an age-independent measurement in children between 6 m and 5 yr of age, since during this period fat of early infancy is gradually replaced by muscle mass, with the MUAC value remaining the same. See **Table 11.9** for the interpretation of MUAC values.

Body disproportion: Upper segment (US)/lower segment (LS) (U/L) is approximately 1.7 at birth and becomes 1.6 at 6 m and 1 at 7 yr due to the rapid growth of long bones (of the lower limbs) being more than the flat [membranous bones (skull, spine)] bones. In the age group above 6 m–7 yr the ratio may be found out by the following formula:

$$US/LS = 1.6 - (\text{age in yr} \times 0.1).$$

The U/L ratio is important to classify SS, to proportionate SS (with normal U/L), or disproportionate SS (altered U/L).

Altered body proportion (U/L) may be due to short trunk or short extremities. A ratio more than expected in a child with SS is suggestive of SS due to short extremities like achondroplasia (Ref. **Fig. 11.13**). A ratio less than expected for the age is suggestive of short trunk which may be due to a skeletal dysplasia involving spine (spondyloepiphyseal dysplasia), vertebral abnormalities (Klippel-Feil syndrome) or significant scoliosis.

Arm span is 2 cm less than height in children up to 5 yr age. Between 5 and 10 yr of age the difference is <1 cm. Span equals height at 10 yr and in adults it is 2 cm more than the height. The value is disproportionately more than height/length in

BOX 11.2: Causes of macrocephaly.

A. Increased cranial fluid content
- Hydranencephaly
- Hydrocephalus
- Porencephaly
- Subdural fluid

B. Increased brain matter
- Familial
- Gigantism
- Lipidoses
- Metachromatic
- Leukodystrophy
- Brain tumors

C. Thick skull bones
- Achondroplasia
- Leontiasis ossea
- Osteopetrosis
- Pycnodysostosis
- Rickets

TABLE 11.9: Interpretation of MUAC values.

MUAC value (cm)	*Nutritional status*
13.5–17	Normal
12.5–13.5	Borderline undernutrition
<12.5	Severe undernutrition
<11.5	Severe acute malnutrition (SAM)
<9 (Newborns)	IUGR

conditions with short trunk SS, arachnodactyly, coarctation of aorta, eunuchoidism, homocystinuria, Klinefelter and Marfan Syndromes.

Limb length discrepancy: Asymmetry in the limb length occurs in congenital hemiplegia, hemihypertrophy/hyperplasia syndrome, Russell-Silver syndrome, hip deformities and isolated limb malformations.

Segmental length measurement is applied to assess the approximate body length in children with deformities which prevent proper positioning (e.g., cerebral palsy, contractures, and skeletal deformities). Length of body segments is measured separately from superficial bony points and finally added to make the total body length approximately.

Body mass index is used to assess the nutritional status of children >*5 yr* of age and is calculated by the following formula:

$$\text{BMI} = \text{weight in kg}/(\text{height in m}^2)$$

The normal value of BMI in adults ranges from 18.5 to 24.99 kg/m^2. Adults are referred to as undernourished and overweight below or above this value, respectively. Since this is based on cardio metabolic risk, Asian adults have a lower cut-off value (>23 as overweight and >27 as obese). For children, there is no specific cut-off value since BMI changes with age. Age and gender specific BMI percentile curves are available for reference in all data sets. The IAP 2015 BMI charts have percentile values for 3rd, 5th, 25th, 50th, adult equivalent of 23 (overweight cut-off) and adult equivalent of 27 (obesity cut-off). Refer Appendix 1, Fig. 11.5: Growth charts No 18 and 19 for BMI in children of age group 5 to 18 yrs for adult equivalent (AE) values of overweight and obesity.

Chest Circumference: At birth, OFC is 3 cm more than the CC. The difference is >3 cm in preterm and small for date babies. CC equals OFC by 9–12 m of age and thereafter chest grows faster. In microcephaly CC exceeds OFC earlier than 9 m and in hydrocephalus the head continues to remain larger than the chest even after 1 yr of age. Growth of the chest is adversely affected in PEM, thoracic cage abnormalities (congenital and acquired), progressive neurologic disorders such as spinal muscular atrophy and congenital lung anomalies (agenesis, sequestration, diaphragmatic hernia, and congenital lobar emphysema),

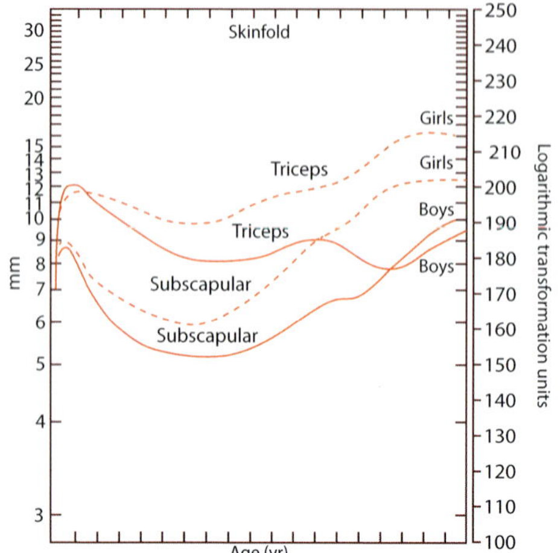

Fig. 11.9: Skin fold thickness values. (yr: year)

and in such conditions CC may not exceed OFC as the age advances.

Skin fold thickness: The normal value of *triceps SFT* is 10 mm or more in healthy children **(Fig. 11.9)**. Values <6 mm and >20 mm indicate undernutrition and obesity, respectively.

Waist Circumference (Ref. Ch. 24)

Derived anthropometric indices are the parameters made by applying the body measurements (weight, height, OFC, and MUAC) which are helpful to detect aberrations in nutritional status. Most of them are age independent and are based on the principle that rapid changes in nutrition produce alterations in labile body tissues (fat and muscle) compared to the skeleton which is a static tissue. The ratio between labile and static tissue measurements are made and compared with the normal. They are the following:

- *Weight for height:* Waterlow's classification to assess wasting **(Table 11.5)**.
- Body mass index (detailed earlier).
- Kanawati index helps to detect and grade PEM in the age group 4 m–4 yr. It is obtained by dividing MUAC (in cm) by OFC (in cm). See **Table 11.10** for the grading.
- *Ponderal index (PI)* is applied to differentiate between hypoplastic (symmetric) and malnourished (asymmetric) newborns as detailed below:

TABLE 11.10: Kanawati index.*

Grade of PEM	***Kanawati index***
Normal	>0.32
Mild	>0.28–0.32
Moderate	0.25–0.28
Severe	<0.25

*The index is not applicable if head is abnormal.

$$PI = \frac{\text{Weight in g} \times 100}{(\text{Height in cm}^3)}$$

Normal value is above 2.5. In malnourished newborns, it is <2 and in hypoplastic newborns it is between 2 and 2.5.

Bone Age (Ref. Ch. 24, Table 24.4 for Details)

Skeletal maturity of the child can be assessed by epiphyseal maturation of various bones and time of fusion of the epiphysis with the respective long bones. In familial short stature (FSS) bone age (BA) is equivalent to chronological age (CA) whereas in constitutional delay BA is less than CA but equal to height age (HA). In endocrine and other major pathological causes of SS, BA is less than HA and CA. In precocious puberty, BA is more than CA. BA is to be followed closely during therapy for any form of growth retardation.

GROWTH IN LOW BIRTH WEIGHT BABIES

Low birth weight (LBW) is defined as birth weight <2.5 kg irrespective of gestational age.

They are of two groups—preterm appropriate for gestational age (AGA) and term or preterm small for gestational age (SGA). SGA babies may be malnourished, hypoplastic, or of mixed groups and can be differentiated by PI. Preterm AGA and malnourished SGA babies usually acquire good catch up growth by 2 yr of age and this may extend up to adult age.

Growth parameters of LBW babies should be plotted on *intrauterine growth charts* up to 42 w of gestation **(Appendix 1, Fig. 11.5: Growth charts of preterm babies No 11 to 16)**. Thereafter, the WHO growth charts must be used in which parameters of preterm babies should be plotted with corrected or adjusted age based on expected date of confinement (EDC), thus deducting the period of prematurity as shown below:

Corrected age of the baby =
Chronological age – (EDC – date of birth)

ADOLESCENT GROWTH

Adolescence is the period of life during which secondary sex characters develop along with somatic growth spurt and its termination extending from 10 to 20 yr of age. The average duration of growth spurt is 2.5–3 yr which starts at the age of 10 yr in girls and 12 yr in boys. The mean height and weight increments during this period is 27 cm and 29 kg in boys and 25 cm and 24 kg in girls. Sexual maturity is completed by the attainment of menarche in girls and spermarche in boys *approximately* 2–2.5 yr after the onset of the first sign of puberty. Correlating the body growth and sexual maturity rating (SMR), adolescence is divided into three phases as in **Table 11.11**.

Nutritional status of the adolescent is best detected by plotting the height and weight in Eliz health path (EHPA) and finding the BMI **(Fig. 11.10)**.

TABLE 11.11: Phases of adolescent growth.

Parameter	*Early*	*Middle*	*Late*
Age (yr)	9–13	14–16	17–20
Weight gain/yr	2 kg	3.5 kg	1 kg
Height gain/yr	6–8 cm	8–10 cm	2–3 cm
SMR stages	1, 2	3, 4	5

(SMR: sexual maturity rating)

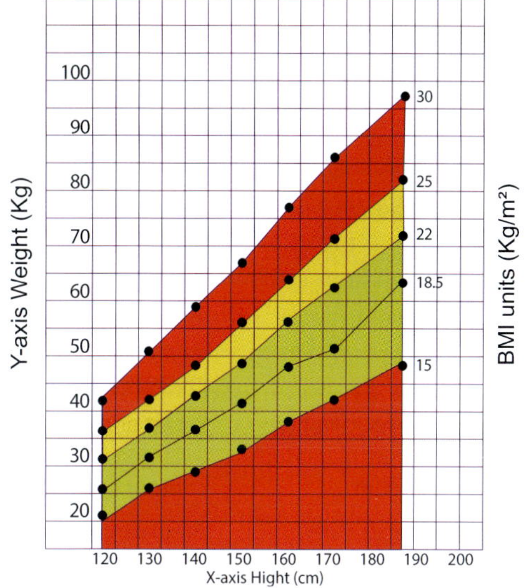

Fig. 11.10: Eliz health path for adolescents. (BMI: body mass index)

Sexual maturity rating: The stage of puberty must be defined precisely as part of growth assessment by evaluating the secondary sexual characters. SMR by Tanner is the presently accepted system worldwide. **Tables 11.12 and 11.13** reveal the SMR stages in girls and boys, respectively.

The normal age of puberty is between 8 and 13 yr in girls and 9–14 yr in boys. Puberty should be considered abnormal if age of onset is early *(precocious)* or late *(delayed)*, or altered sequence of pubertal changes or associated abnormal signs or symptoms occur.

ABERRATIONS IN GROWTH AND PUBERTY

These are under and overnutrition and precocious and delayed puberty. Undernutrition presents as varying degrees of PEM, wasting, failure to thrive (FTT), and SS. Obesity and TS represent overnutrition.

TABLE 11.12: Sexual maturity rating (SMR) stages in girls.

SMR stage	*Pubic stage*	*Breasts*
1	Preadolescent	Preadolescent
2	Sparse, lightly pigmented, straight, medial border of labia	Breast and papilla elevated as small mound; areola diameter increased
3	Darker, beginning to curl, increased amount	Breast and areola enlarged, no contour separation
4	Coarse, curly, abundant but amount less than in adult	Areola and papilla form secondary mound
5	Adult feminine triangle, spread to medial surface of thighs	Mature, nipple projects, areola part of the general contour

Protein Energy Malnutrition

The term indicates a wide spectrum of disorders due to deficient nutrient supply of mainly calories and proteins and to varying extent of vitamins and minerals. Though used in the perspective of undernutrition, literally it includes overnutrition also. The main etiology of undernutrition is *primary* or defective supply of nutrients due to poverty and ignorance. *Secondary* PEM is precipitated by various systemic diseases resulting in defective food intake, assimilation, and utilization, excess catabolism or body loss. The differentiation between the two groups can be easily made out by careful history and physical examination. Severe acute malnutrition *(SAM)* is defined as weight for length/height <3 Z score, MUAC <11.5 cm, visible wasting and/or nutritional edema. See **Figs. 11.11A to D** for different grades of undernutrition.

Wasting or thinness is decreased body weight due to loss of body fat and reduction in muscle mass. The diagnostic features are wasted appearance **(Figs. 11.11A and B)**, reduced weight for height (≤90% Waterlow, <80% WHO), reduced SFT and BMI for the age. See **Box 11.3** for the causes of wasting in children. The most common cause of wasting

TABLE 11.13: Sexual maturity rating (SMR) stages in boys.

SMR stage	*Pubic hair*	*Penis*	*Testes*
1	None	Preadolescent	Preadolescent
2	Scanty, long, slightly pigmented	Minimal change/enlargement	Enlarged scrotum, pink, texture altered
3	Darker, starts to curl, small amount	Lengthens	Larger
4	Resembles adult type, but less quantity, coarse, curly	Larger, glans and breadth increase in size	Larger, scrotum dark
5	Adult distribution, spreads to medial surface of thighs	Adult size	Adult size

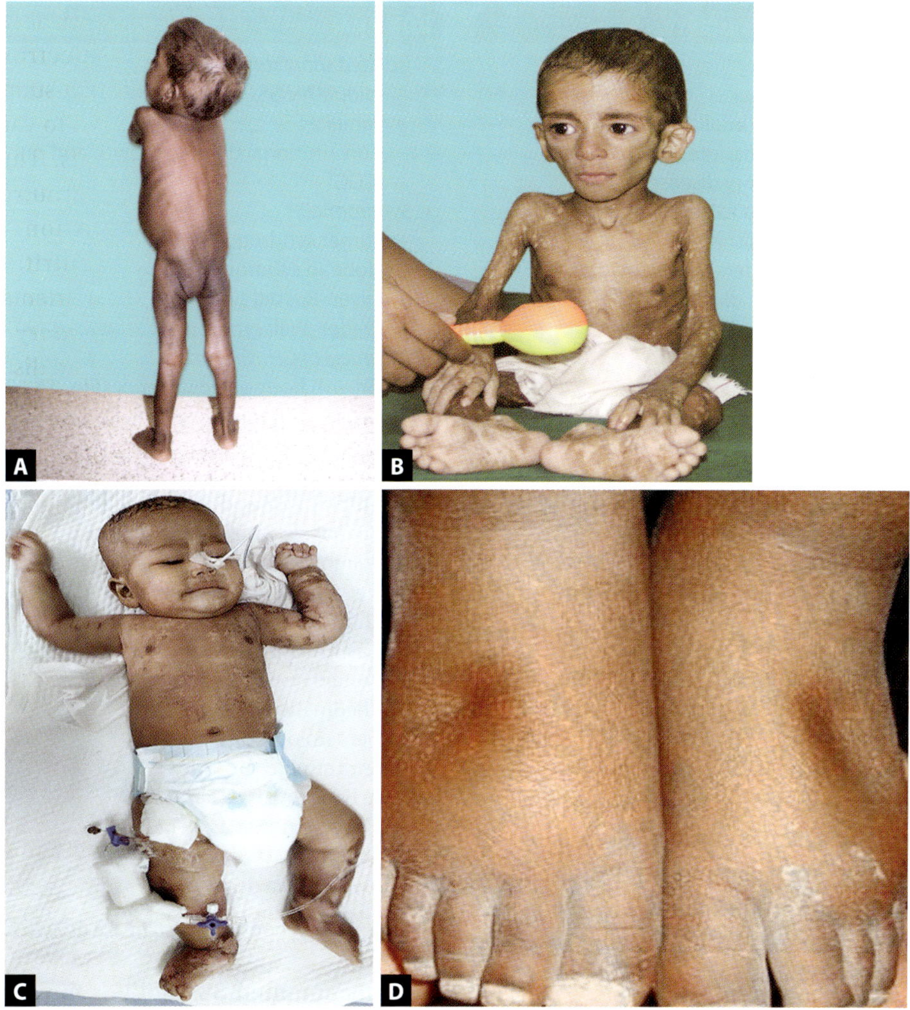

Fig 11.11A to D: (A) Early wasting-child with human immunodeficiency virus (HIV) disease; (B) Severe marasmus with loss of buccal pad of fat; (C) Kwashiorkor with flaky paint dermatosis; (D) Pitting pedal edema in kwashiorkor. Courtesy (C): Dr. Jiji Mary Antony, Associate Professor Pediatrics, Government-Medical College, Kottayam, Kerala, India.

is deficient calorie intake, but underlying diseases must be excluded in all patients with wasting. Kwashiorkor is the form of SAM characterized by growth retardation, psychomotor changes, and edema **(Figs. 11.11C and D)**. Different types of skin lesions can develop (due to zinc deficiency) in these children indicating poor prognosis.

Failure to thrive is inability to maintain the expected rate of growth over a period without any apparent etiology in children below 5 yr of age. Terminology is so vague that it is more specific to use undernutrition. The diagnosis of FTT can be made if growth parameters are persistently below 5th percentile with weight being more affected than height/length and HC, failure for

BOX 11.3: Causes of wasting in children.

- *Constitutional*
- *Secondary*
  - Deficient calorie intake
  - Chronic infections, infestations
  - Chronic respiratory diseases
  - Cardiac disorders (congenital, acquired)
  - Malabsorption disorders
  - Endocrine disorders (hyperthyroidism, Addison disease, diabetes mellitus, and diabetes insipidus)
  - Chromosomal disorders
  - Malignancies
  - Marfan syndrome
  - Anorexia nervosa
  - Progeria

appropriate weight gain over a period of 2 m or if weight drops two or more major percentiles without a decline in length percentile over 6 m. Hence, unless the child's growth parameters are clearly stated by the parent or growth cards are presented, the diagnosis of FTT is not possible with a single observation; the minimum interval for subsequent evaluation is 2 m. Causes of FTT are nonorganic (psychosocial deprivation and child abuse) or organic, i.e., secondary to a large number of underlying systemic diseases as for wasting.

Growth retardation (SS): SS is considered as length or height <2 SD of the mean for age and sex or height <2 SD of the target health or <3rd percentile of national standards (combined WHO-IAP growth chart for Indian children). *If the child is excessively short for the calculated MPH also, he/she is considered short even if the height is within the normal population percentile.* A significant decrease in height SDS is defined as a deflection of at least 0.3 SDS/yr. **Box 11.4** reveals the causes of SS in children.

Most children with SS do not have pathological growth retardation. In children

BOX 11.4: Causes of short stature in children.

- *Isolated short stature (SS)*
  - Idiopathic SS
  - Familial SS
  - Constitutional delay in growth and puberty (CDGP)
- *Syndromic*
  - Turner syndrome
  - Noonan syndrome
  - Silver–Russell syndrome
  - Prader–Willi syndrome
- *Disorders of GH-IGF-I axis*
  - Growth hormone deficiency **(Fig. 11.12)**
  - Growth hormone Insensitivity
  - *Chronic systemic illnesses*
  - Celiac disease
  - Chronic kidney diseases
  - Cardiac diseases (Congenital, acquired)
  - Pulmonary diseases
  - Neuromuscular disorders
  - Endocrine diseases
  - Gastrointestinal disorders
  - Protein energy malnutrition
  - Rheumatic diseases
  - Hematologic disorders
- *Skeletal disorders*
  - Achondroplasia **(Fig. 11.13)**
  - Hypochondroplasia
  - *Small for gestational age*
  - *Psychosocial deprivation*

(GH-IGH: growth hormone–insulin-like growth factor)

with documented SS, look for the *red flag signs* of pathological SS such as height ≤3 SD, growth velocity <25th percentile, abnormal body proportion, dysmorphic facial features, skeletal anomalies, abnormal neurological or eye findings, goiter, and chronic systemic diseases.

Tall stature and overgrowth syndromes: Length or height >97th percentile or >2 SD above the mean indicate TS, which can be physiological or pathological. **Box 11.5** reveals the causes of TS.

Marfan syndrome is characterized by TS with arm span more than height, arachnodactyly, hyperextensible joints,

BOX 11.5: Causes of tall stature and overgrowth syndromes.

- *Physiological*
  - Constitutional
  - Overeating
- *Pathological*
  - Arachnodactyly
  - Marfan syndrome
  - Klinefelter syndrome
  - Precocious puberty
  - Pituitary gigantism
  - Cerebral gigantism (Sotos syndrome)
  - Homocystinuria

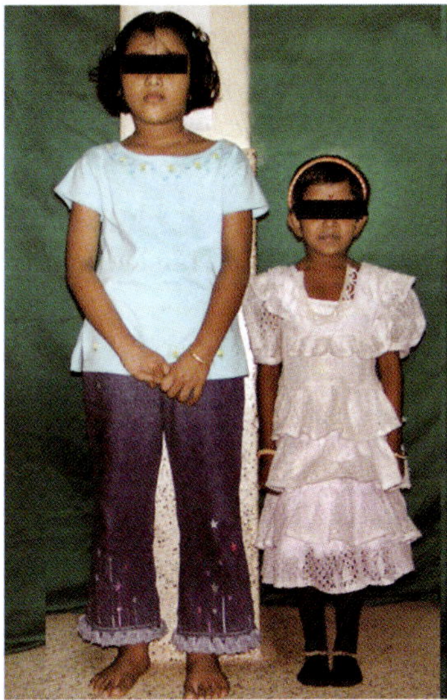

Fig. 11.12: Pituitary short stature (SS) girl—8 yr old with her younger sister of 6 yr.

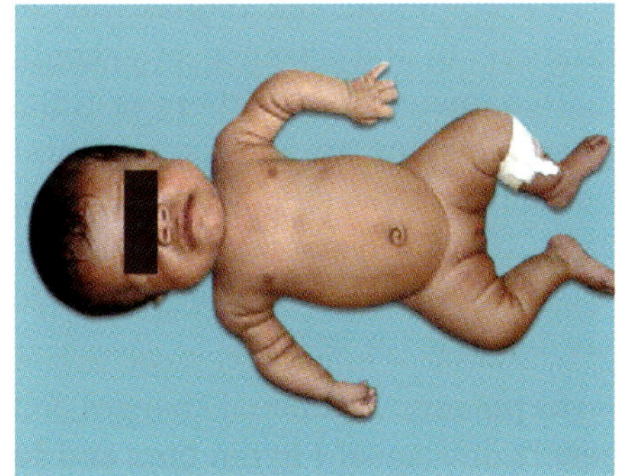

Fig. 11.13: Infant with achondroplasia and short limb-short stature.

scoliosis, dislocation of lens, aortic root dilatation, and mitral valve prolapse (MVP). *Homocystinuria* is a metabolic disease with defect in the degradation of homocysteine with phenotypic features of Marfan syndrome along with the subluxation of lens and mental retardation. *Klinefelter* syndrome is a chromosomal abnormality (47, XXY) with TS, arachnodactyly, gynecomastia, infertility, and poor scholastic performance. Examples of overgrowth syndromes are *Sotos syndrome* and *Beckwith Wiedemann syndrome*. Excessive production of growth hormone causes gigantism characterized by TS and other features of acromegaly. Children with *precocious puberty* are taller than their peers due to the effect of gonadal steroids at the initial stage of pubertal growth.

Obesity is increased body weight due to generalized excessive accumulation of fat. The diagnostic features are *obese appearance, weight for height >2 SD, weight >120% of ideal body weight for height (IBWH), BMI >95th* percentile and *SFT >90th* percentile for age. **Box 11.6** reveals the causes of

BOX 11.6: Causes of obesity in children.

- *Exogenous (simple)*
  - Constitutional
  - Sedentary life **(Fig. 11.14)**
  - Overeating
- *Endogenous (pathologic)*
  - Chromosomal disorders
  - Endocrine disorders (hypothalamic, pituitary thyroid, parathyroid, pancreas, adrenals, ovaries)
  - Genetic syndromes—monogenic obesity
- *Iatrogenic (drug-induced)*
  - Corticosteroids **(Fig. 11.15)**
  - Cyproheptadine
  - Diazepam
  - Haloperidol
  - Lithium
  - Meclizine
  - Tricyclic antidepressants

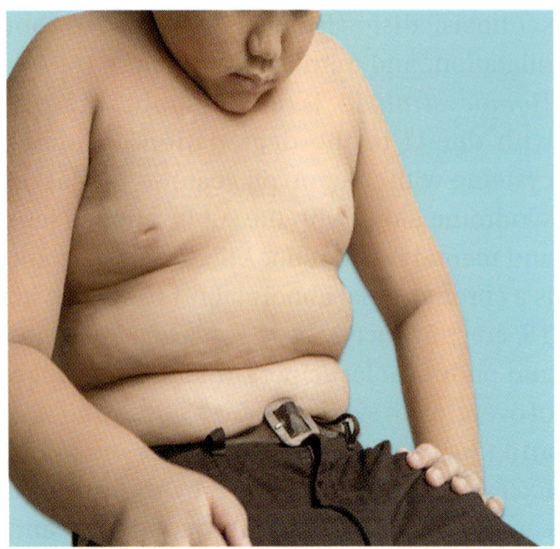
Fig. 11.14: Exogenous obesity revealing central adiposity.

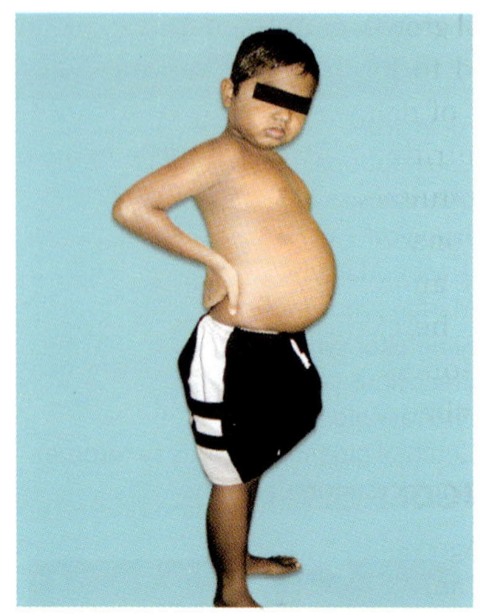
Fig. 11.15: Boy 6 yr, on prolonged steroid therapy.

obesity in children. From detailed history (especially regarding the diet and lifestyle) and physical examination, the cause of obesity can be diagnosed in most children. In exogenous obesity, patient's height will be above the MPH, but in endocrine disorders and genetic syndromes height will be below the mean for age. The obese child should be examined for features of endocrine diseases, dysmorphism/malformations (Prader-Willi syndrome, Bardet-Biedl syndrome), mental retardation (genetic syndromic cause), and other system abnormalities.

In the BMI chart for children, value >85th percentile is overweight and >95th percentile is obesity. In the age group >5 yr to 18 yr, overweight and obesity are defined as adult equivalent of 23 and 27 respectively [Ref. Appendix 1, **Fig. 11.5**: Growth Charts No 18, 19 for adult equivalent (AE) values of overweight and obesity in children] Morbid or severe obesity is BMI >99th percentile for age and gender. Increase in the muscle mass (especially in boys) can also cause increase in BMI during early puberty. Waist circumference is a better indicator of visceral obesity (Ref. Appendix 1, **Fig. 24.5**: Growth Charts No 20, 21 for waist circumference values in Indian children).

Precocious puberty is the appearance of any secondary sex characteristics before the age of 8 yr in girls and 9 yr in boys, or onset of menarche before the age of 10 yr in girls. It can be central (true or gonadotropin dependent), peripheral (pseudo or gonadotropin independent), or combined. Conditions producing precocious puberty are many (Ref. Ch 24 for details) Sexual precocity can be isosexual or heterosexual, complete or partial. Premature menarche is a rare condition and requires detailed evaluation. In the absence of secondary sexual characteristics, if there is isolated vaginal bleeding, trauma, sexual abuse, vulvovaginitis, foreign body vagina, urethral prolapse, bleeding diathesis, and malignancies (sarcoma botryoides) are to be excluded (More details in Ch. 24).

Delayed puberty: If pubertal changes do not appear by the age of 14 yr in boys and 13 yr in girls, or if >5 yr have elapsed between the first signs of puberty and completion of genital growth or onset of menarche, puberty is said to be delayed. The most common cause of delayed puberty is constitutional. Malnutrition, chronic illness, drug intake, hypopituitarism, conditions with hyper or hypogonadotropic hypogonadism, chromosomal anomalies and genetic syndromes are to be excluded before diagnosing the situation as constitutional delay in growth and puberty (Ref. Ch 24 for more details)

SUGGESTED READING

1. Agarwal R, Sankhyan N, Jain V. Growth. In: Paul VK, Bagga A (Eds). Ghai, Essential Pediatrics, 9th edition. New Delhi: CBS Publishers and Distributors Pvt Ltd; 2019. pp. 7-37.
2. Forfar JO, Arneil GC. History taking and physical examination. Standard deviation values. In: Campbells AG, Mcintosh N (Eds). Forfar and Arnails Textbook of Pediatrics, 5th edition. New York: Churchill Livingstone; 1998. pp. 14-20.
3. GrahamS, Holmes RA. Stepwise approach to the evaluation of undernutrition and failure to thrive. Pediatr Clin North Am. 1998;45(1):169-97.
4. IAP, Standard Guidelines. Approach to short Stature. [online] Available from https://iapindia.org/pdf/Ch-017-Approach-to-Short-Stature.pdf. [Last accessed September, 2024].
5. Intergrowth-21st. Standards and tools. [online] Available from https://intergrowth21.tghn.org/standards-tools/ [Last accessed September, 2024].
6. Kliegman R, W. St. Geme III J. Assessment of Growth In: Bamba V, Kelly A (Eds). Nelson Textbook of Pediatrics, 21st edition. International edition, India: Elsevier; 2020. pp. 151-7.
7. Nair MKC. The Eliz Health Path for Adolescents and Adults (EHPA). In: Nair MKC (Ed). Teens Journal of Teenage care and premarital counseling. Thiruvananthapuram, Kerala: Child development Centre, Medical College; 2001.
8. Parekh BJ, Khadilkar V. Paediatrician friendly iap growth charts 0-18 years. [online] Available from https://iapindia.org/pdf/4422_Pediatrician-friendly-growth-charts-for-0-18-year-old-Indian-children-Dr-Bakul-Parekh-and-Dr-Vaman-khadilkar.pdf. [Last accessed September, 2024].
9. Vaughan VC III. Growth and development-the normal distribution curve. In: Vaughan VC, Mckay RJ, Nelson WE (Eds). Nelson Textbook of Pediatrics, 10th edition. Philadelphia: WB Saunders and Company; 1975. p. 15.
10. Waterlow JC. Classification and definition of protein calorie malnutrition. BMJ. 1972; 3(5826):566.
11. Waterlow JC. Evolution of kwashiorkor and marasmus. Lancet. 1974;2(7882):712.

12 CHAPTER

Assessment of Development

S Sushamabai, Suresh S Vadakedom

Chapter Outline

- Introduction
- Prerequisites
- Medical and Developmental History
- Physical Examination
- Functional Developmental Estimation
- Target Milestones
- Early Markers of Cerebral Palsy
- Developmental Screening Tools
- Clinical Case Scenario

INTRODUCTION

Please read chapters 1, 2, 3, 4, 6, 7, and 15 before you proceed.

Development is the maturational process in structure and function from fetal viability to full growth. Developmental assessment is necessary for the early detection of physical and mental disability so as to provide early treatment and to prevent future handicapping. It is mandatory for suitability of adoption of babies and to assess the outcome of medicolegal aspects of fetal therapy as well as obstetric procedures.

Timely identification of developmental delay in infants is a challenge to all pediatricians. It is difficult to differentiate between infants who have delayed acquisition of skills ultimately reaching normal and those who are truly deviating from expected patterns.

All babies require periodic developmental assessment. Normal babies should be evaluated at birth (Ref. Ch. 15) and every 3 m for the first yr and every 6 m till school entry. High-risk babies require more frequent evaluation—every m for the first 1 yr and thereafter once in 3 m (or more frequently) as long as they are under the pediatrician's care for developmental backwardness.

PREREQUISITES

The assessment room should be well-ventilated with good light and least disturbance, equipped with age-appropriate test materials—cheap, attractive, and culturally acceptable. Ideally *both parents* should be present during evaluation, information, and counseling. In young babies (below 1 yr) assessment is to be done *1 hr after feeding*. Babies should be *comfortable with warm surroundings* and should not be in a sick state. Infants may be on the mother's lap. The older child can have a suitable chair and table or cot to sit.

The age group of children brought for developmental evaluation may range from neonate-to-late childhood. *Getting the cooperation* of the child and parents is very important (Ref. Ch. 1, 2). The *test materials* (should be culturally acceptable) needed are a squeaky doll, rattle, red ball, few pellets of orange, red or yellow color, moderately bright pen torch, pencil, picture book of thick pages, paper, mirror, cup and spoon, and a temple bell **(Fig. 12.1)**.

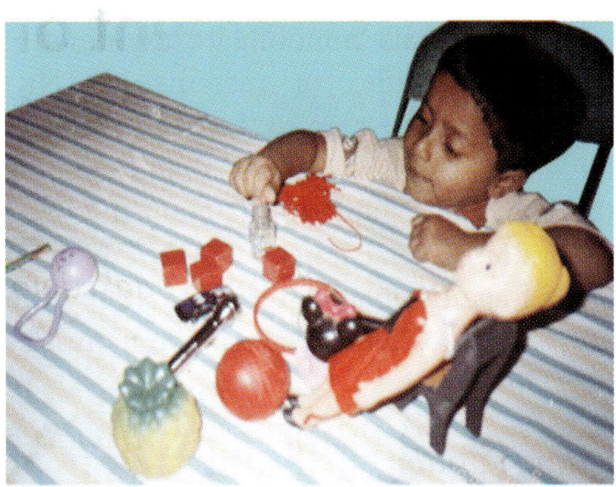

Fig. 12.1: Test materials for development assessment.

Assessment process should have three parts: (1) Medical and developmental history (Ref. Ch. 6), (2) Physical and neurological examination (Ref. Ch. 7, 15, 21), and (3) Functional developmental estimation.

MEDICAL AND DEVELOPMENTAL HISTORY

The pattern of development is remarkably constant, within fairly broad limits, but the rate at which goals are achieved varies from child-to-child. Skills are acquired sequentially, with one milestone acquired after another. Later milestones often depend on the achievement of earlier ones within the same field—for example, children must learn to sit independently, before they can stand and then walk.

Descriptions of normal development, linked to the ability to perform a particular task at a particular age, relate to the performance of the average child. The acquisition of a *key performance skill*, such as walking, is referred to as a milestone. For each skill, the normal age range for attainment of the milestone varies widely. A *median age* is the age at which *half a population of children acquire* a skill. A *limit age* is the age at which a skill should have been achieved and is two standard deviations above the mean.

Start by asking for *parental concerns* regarding their child's development. Often the *mother is right* and apprehensive about the issue. The problem may be either a *delayed normal* pattern, *pathological* delay or a *deviant* pattern. All these must be elicited through appropriate history and confirmed by examination.

Details of prenatal, perinatal, and postnatal events, including maternal health during pregnancy should be enquired. Ask about the child's acquisition of developmental milestones. The birth records and follow-up cards of the child (if available) must be reviewed at this point; if not available, the parents should be directed to bring the documents at the next visit. A sensitive but thorough environmental, social, and family history is essential, especially regarding consanguinity and developmental problems, or learning difficulties, which may point to metabolic problems or recessively inherited disorders.

Most parents in this advanced era are very clever and make *video recordings* of their child's activities which will be invaluable for assessing the developmental profile of the patient. Ask and observe specifically vision and hearing always as *the priority areas* even if the parents have not felt any impairment.

Begin with the history *all the time observing the child's* behavior and interaction with the parents (Ref. Ch. 2, 3). This period of talking to the parents enables the child to get used to the environment and to become *confident that the parents accept the stranger*. The medical and social history provides information regarding biological and environmental risks for developmental disability (such as adverse prenatal and perinatal events, maternal illness, maternal substance abuse, genetic disorders, sociocultural factors, etc.). The presence of multiple risk factors increases the chance of developmental disability. *Parental assessment* of a child's function is an important historical information. *Observe the child* entering and moving around the clinic and playing with toys (such as blocks, toy cars, pull-along toys, paper, and crayons). This will provide much information regarding the selection of toys and age-appropriate handling. Observation of the child at home or nursery can also prove invaluable, as can the reports from other caregivers at daycare, nursery school, or in the school.

A baseline knowledge regarding the developmental progression and the developmental age of the child can be obtained from developmental history **(Table 6.1)**. **Table 12.1** shows the physical examination clues to certain conditions associated with developmental disability.

PHYSICAL EXAMINATION

See **Table 12.1**.

FUNCTIONAL DEVELOPMENTAL ESTIMATION

Functional level of development should be estimated under four domains along with extended neurological examination as revealed in **Box 12.1**. First assess the age-wise developmental parameters of the child. If any delay is observed, proceed to systematic assessment of each domain.

Gross Motor Development

Gross motor (GM) development involves acquisition of skills for locomotion. Assess the GM development in supine, prone, ventral suspension, sitting, and standing positions.

Supine

Place the baby in supine position and observe the posture.

Baby reveals nonobligate asymmetric tonic neck reflex or response (ATNR) which will persist up to 3 m **(Fig. 15.25)**. By 4 m of age, ATNR is abandoned by the baby and is able to maintain the head in midline. Persistence of ATNR beyond 6 m of age or obligate response at any age are abnormal which can prevent further development.

Sitting Position

Pull the baby gently to the sitting position by holding at both wrists, noticing the movement of the head and curvature of the spine. In a newborn infant, the head lags completely behind and the back remains rounded **(Fig. 12.8A)**. Baby attains head control gradually by 12–20 w **(Fig. 12.8B)**, the spinal curvature becomes less prominent; by 8 m of age the spine becomes completely straight.

In *hypotonic babies,* head control and straightening of spinal curvature are delayed. *In spastic babies,* advanced development may be wrongly diagnosed, since they straightly go to standing posture without sitting ("*the log sign*" revealed as spastic trunk and limbs moving like a single wood piece).

Prone Position

Place the baby in prone position and observe the response.

- Full term baby—protects from suffocation by turning face to one side
- 1 m—lifts up the chin momentarily
- 3 m—lifts up head and upper chest
- 6 m—lifts up head and chest supporting weight on extended arms. Rolls in bed—first from prone to supine and then from supine to prone.
- 8 m—crawls in bed.
- 10 m—creeps keeping abdomen off the ground.

TABLE 12.1: Physical examination clues.

Growth parameters	Small for gestational age, obesity, macrosomia, marasmus, short stature, tall stature, microcephaly **(Fig. 7.17A)**, macrocephaly **(Fig. 7.17B)**
Head	Flat or prominent occiput, delayed or early closure of fontanelle and sutures
Hair anomalies	Double whorls, fine, friable, kinky, sparse, or absent hair, premature graying or white forelocks **(Fig. 7.18B)**, hirsutism, and low hairlines (anterior and posterior)
Eyes and orbit	Hyper- or hypotelorism, synophrys, microphthalmia, proptosis, squint, mongoloid **(Fig. 12.2)** or antimongoloid slant, bilateral lid ptosis, epicanthic folds, coloboma of iris or retina, brush field spots, corneal clouding, eccentrically placed pupils, nystagmus, cataract, ectopia lentis, retinal pigmentation changes, cherry red spot, lipemia retinalis, optic atrophy
Ears	Low set, small, posterior rotation, bats ear, large or malformed pinna, simple or abnormal helix, preauricular tags **(Fig. 15.5)** or pits, atretic ear canal
Nose	Small or prominent, flattened or broad bridge, upturned nares
Face	Triangular, flat or round shape, midface hypoplasia, coarse features, long philtrum (Ref. **Fig. 7.21**), hypoplasia of maxilla or mandible, prominent nose and chin
Mouth	Inverted V shape of upper lip, cleft lip and palate, macroglossia, high-arched palate
Teeth	Anodontia, notched incisors, late dental eruption, wide spaced teeth, abnormal enamilogenesis
Tongue	Macroglossia (Ref. **Fig. 20.13**), protruded tongue, glossoptosis
Neck	Webbing (Ref. **Fig .7.19**), retraction or flexion, short or long, torticollis, sinuses
Chest	Shield chest, scoliosis, malformed ribs, pectus carinatum (Ref. **Fig. 7.34**) or excavatum, absent pectoralis major, absent clavicles **(Fig. 25.8)**
Abdomen	Umbilical hernia **(Fig. 12.3)** hepatosplenomegaly, surgical scars **(Fig. 12.4)**
Genitalia	Ambiguous genitalia, macro-orchidism with inguinal hernia **(Fig. 12.4)**, undescended testis
Extremities	Short, long, or unequal limbs, phocomelia, joint dislocation or laxity, arachnodactyly, brachydactyly, polydactyly, syndactyly, clinodactyly, broad thumb, triphalanx **(Fig. 12.5)**, cortical thumb, abnormal dermatoglyphics, transverse palmar crease, overriding of toes or fingers, deep crease leading from the angle of 1st and 2nd toes, valgus or varus deformities **(Fig. 12.6)**, absent plantar arch
Spine	Sacral dimple, hairy patch, spina bifida, myelomeningocele **(Fig. 15.16)**
Skin and nails	Hypo- or hyperpigmented patches, Café au lait spots **(Fig. 10.24)**, neurofibromatosis, linear depigmented nevi, shagreen patches **(Fig. 12.7)**, facial port-wine nevus, adenoma sebaceum, hypoplastic or absent nails
Systemic diseases	Congenital heart disease, organomegaly, renal anomalies, major anomalies clustered together as a syndrome

Ventral Suspension

Hold the baby in prone position providing support with your hands under the upper abdomen. The head is held in line with the trunk by the full-term newborn.

- 4–12 w—baby lifts head up to the horizontal plane and gradually above the plane with limbs kept at partial flexion of joints.

In *hypotonic babies,* head and limbs flop down and spine curves with convexity upward

BOX 12.1: Functional developmental estimation.

- *Main domain:*
  - Gross motor
  - Fine motor adaptive
  - Personal, social, and cognitive
  - Language
- *Extended neurologic examination:*
  - Vision
  - Hearing
  - Muscle tone
  - Primitive reflexes

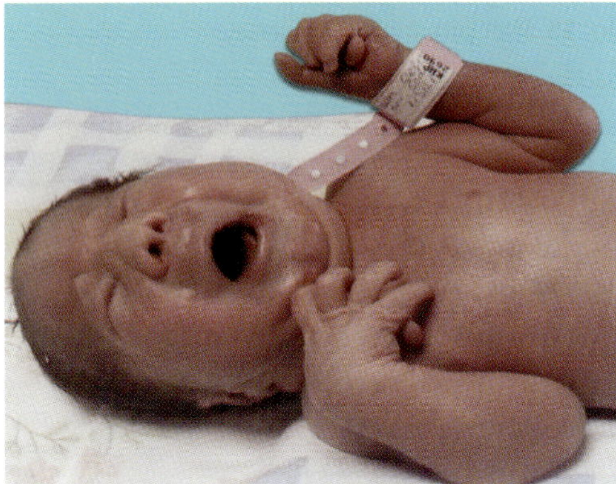

Fig. 12.2: Baby with facial dysmorphism, microcephaly, postaxial polydactyly—Trisomy 13.

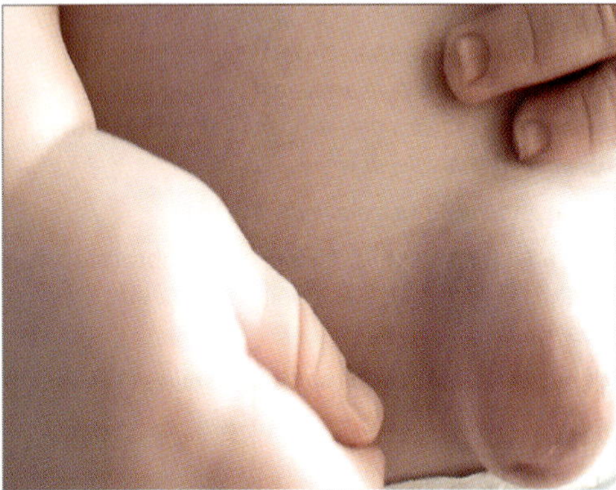

Fig. 12.3: Infant with large umbilical hernia.

(*"inverted U shape" or umbrella shape* as in spinal muscular atrophy) **(Fig. 12.9)**.

Hypertonic babies show early head lift and extension with straightening of limbs.

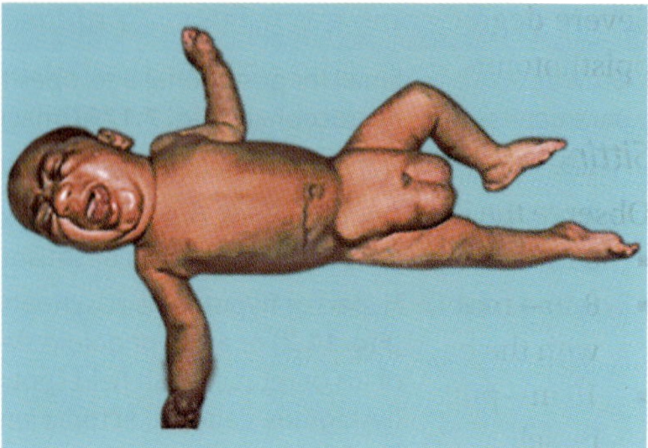

Fig. 12.4: Baby with dysmorphic face, hernia, abdominal scar and macroorchidism.

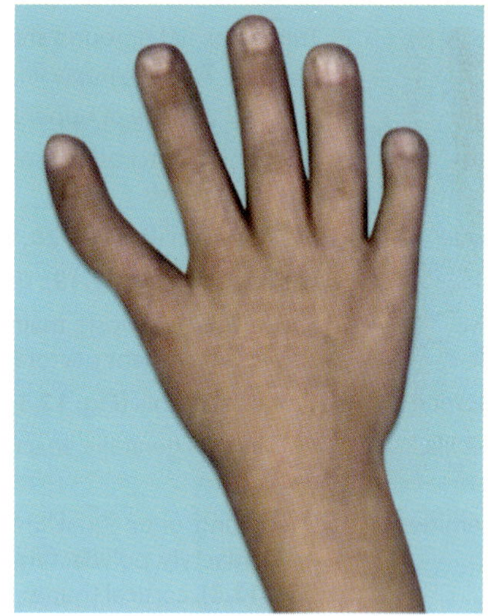

Fig. 12.5: Triphalanx.

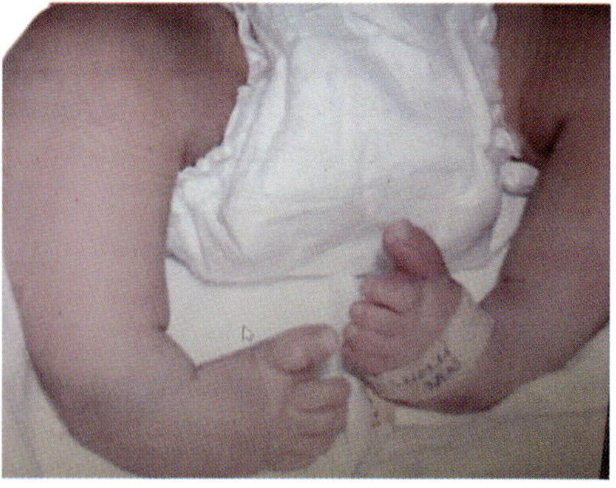

Fig. 12.6: Bilateral congenital talipes equinovarus.

Severe degree spine extension can produce opisthotonus, e.g., spastic cerebral palsy.

Sitting

Observe the baby in the sitting posture.

- 5 m—sits with support **(Fig. 12.10)**
- 8 m—maintains a steady sitting position with the back straight
- 10 m—pulls from prone to sitting position by self
- 18 m—climbs up on a chair, stands, turns, and sits down.

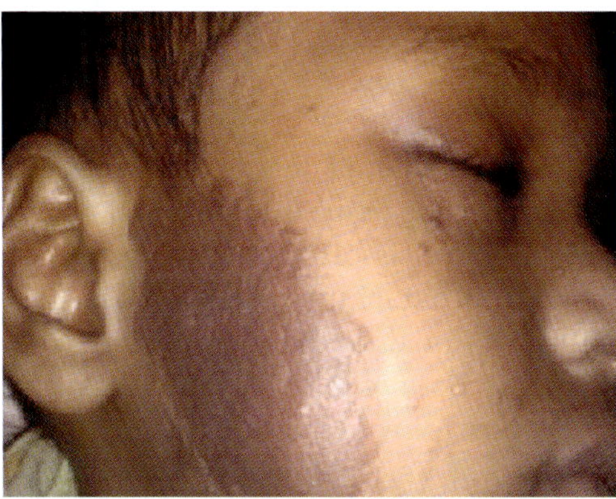

Fig. 12.7: Shagreen patch (R) side of cheek.

In *hypotonia* sitting and straightening of spinal curvature is delayed.

In *hypertonia,* infants, prefer *"W" sitting* (because of the hamstrings spasm) with the knees folded backward **(Fig. 12.11)**.

Standing

Hold the baby at axilla with both hands and observe the posture, movements, and weight bearing by lower limbs.

- 4 m—some bearing of body weight with straight legs.
- 6 m—partial weight bearing, downward parachute response—feet meet ground plantigrade when rapidly lowered; bottom shufflers reveal sitting posture.
- 7 m—full weight bearing, bounces.
- 9 m—early stepping movements when feet are placed on the table surface; pulls to standing with support.
- 10 m—cruising around the furniture.
- 1 yr—stands without support with a wide base **(Fig. 12.12)**.
- 18 m—squat and rise.

Isolated GM delay can be a normal variation. Pathologically, it indicates

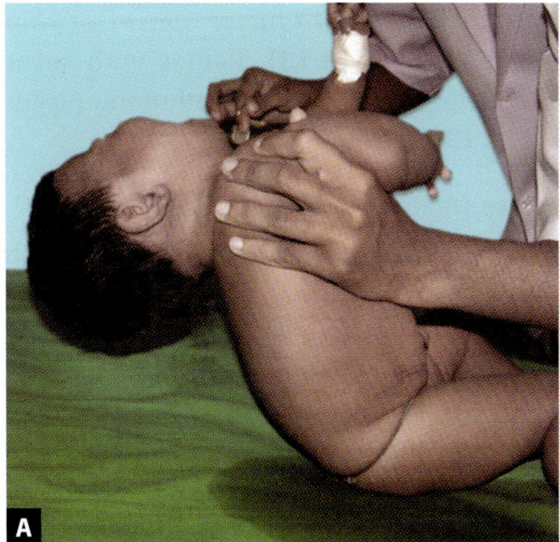

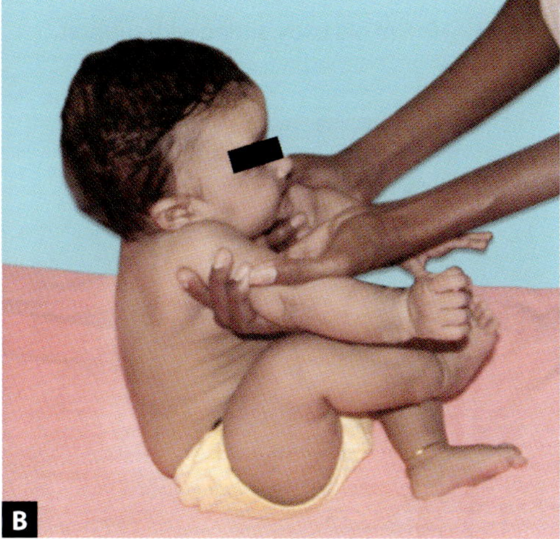

Figs. 12.8A and B: (A) Infant 2 w age—complete head lag; (B) 10 w age—partial head control.

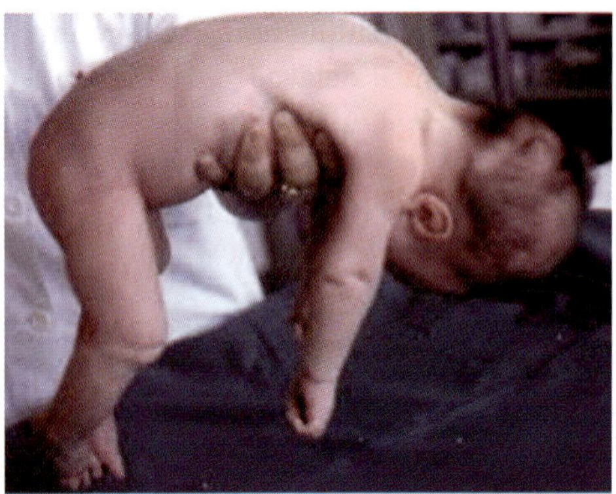

Fig. 12.9: 5 m old hypotonic baby—inverted "U" shaped posture on ventral suspension.

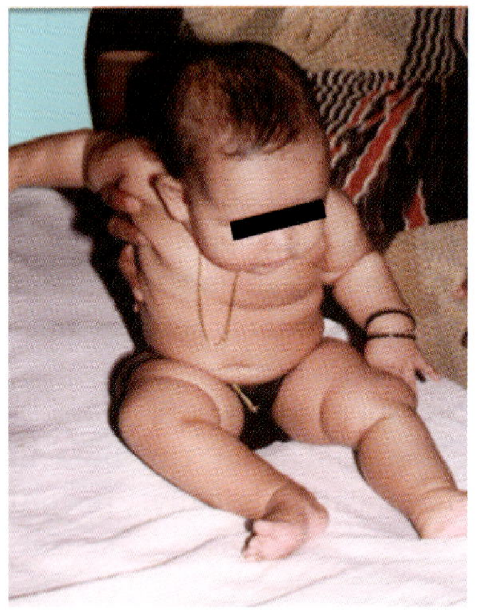

Fig. 12.10: 5 m old baby, sitting with support.

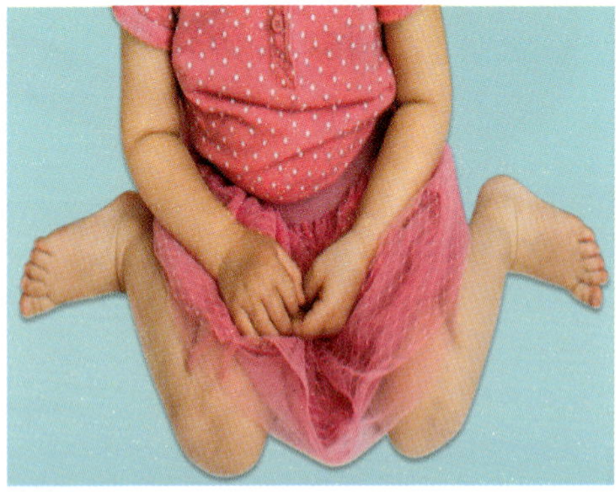

Fig. 12.11: "W" sitting due to hamstring spasm.

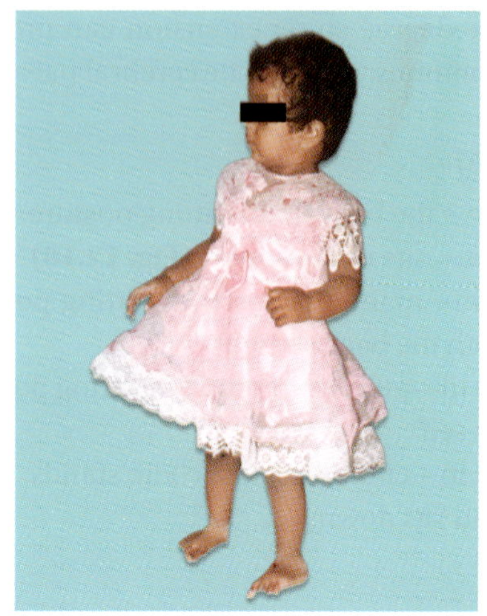

Fig. 12.12: Stands without support with a wide base at 1 yr age.

hyper- or hypotonia due to neuromuscular and connective tissue disorders and mental retardation. Scissoring, sitting posture on downward parachute, and toe stance are indicators of underlying neuromuscular disorders. *Bottom shuffling* indicates pelvic girdle muscle hypotonia and can be a manifestation of Vit D deficiency; toe walking denotes calf muscle spasm; both may occur due to genetic predisposition. In severe spasticity, lower limbs reveal *scissoring posture due to adductor spasm of thigh muscles* **(Fig. 12.13)**. Babies with severe kernicterus can develop opisthotonic posture **(Fig. 12.14)**.

Fine Motor Adaptive Skills

Fine motor adaptive skills enable the baby to *acquire skilled movements of fingers* for manipulation and coordinated activities (such as eating, writing, drawing, painting, i.e., all skilled activities needed for a successful life), along with hands and eyes. The parameters to be evaluated include eye coordination, hand eye coordination, hand mouth coordination, and hand skills.

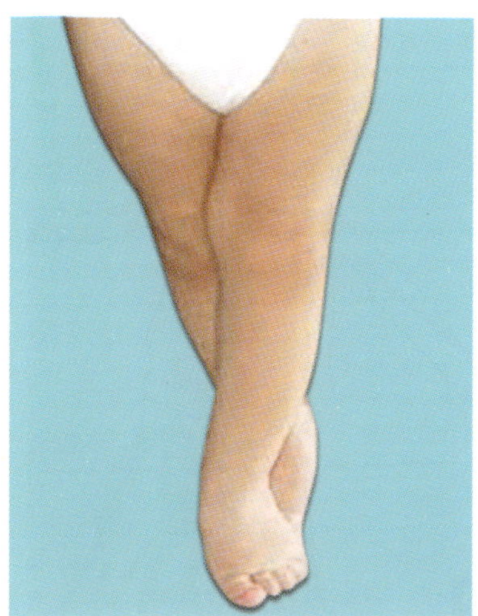

Fig. 12.13: Scissoring of legs due to adductor spasm in spastic cerebral palsy.

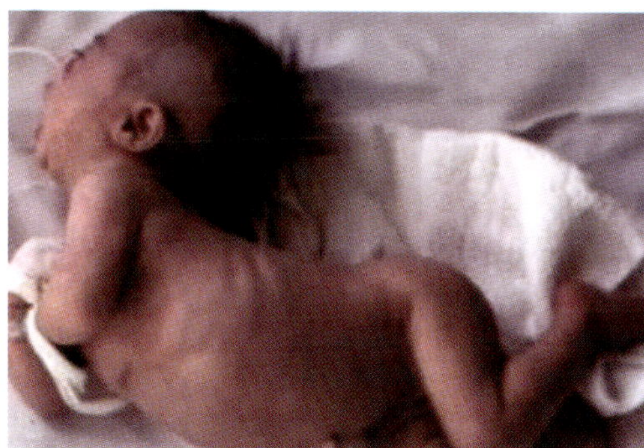

Fig. 12.14: Baby revealing opisthotonic posture—head tilted to back and arching of spine.

Eye Coordination

Bring a moderately lighted torch in front of the infant's eyes (at a distance of 20 cm) and move from side to side. Observe visual fixation and following (Ref. **Table 6.1** for target milestones).

Hand Eye Coordination

Test objects (doll, rattle, pellets, book, pen, etc.) are offered to the baby; observe the hand approach and movements (Ref. **Table 6.1**).

Hand Mouth Coordination

Observe *feeding behavior* with cup and spoon.

- 12 m—tries to self-feed with a cup and spoon but spills the contents;
- 15 m—feeds self with a spoon; no spilling of contents;
- 18 m—feeds self from a cup with only slight spilling.

Hand Skills (Ref. Table 6.1): Offer test objects; observe spontaneous activity; demonstrate and ask to copy

- 12 m—spontaneous scribbling **(Fig. 12.15A)**
- 13 m—turns 2–3 pages of a book at a time
- 24 m—turns pages of a book one at a time; draws horizontal and vertical lines (=, ||)
- 3 yr—draws a circle and plus sign (O, +); dresses and undresses
- 4 yr—draws a rectangle (▭), draws a man with 2–4 parts besides head **(Fig. 12.15B)**
- 5 yr—draws a triangle and tilted cross (Δ, X).

Personal-social-cognitive skills (Ref. **Table 6.1**) This domain relates to interpersonal, social, and cognitive (aspects of intelligence, conscious thoughts, and problem-solving ability) skills.

Language (Ref. Table 6.1)

Note: Except for GM, for other milestones information obtained from history should also be considered which are to be collected from **Table 6.1**.

Vision: Eye Coordination (Ref. Table 6.1)

- Birth—visual fixation and following in a range up to 45°. Bright light produces blinking along with constriction of pupils.
- 4 w—follows up to 90°; reveals mother regard.

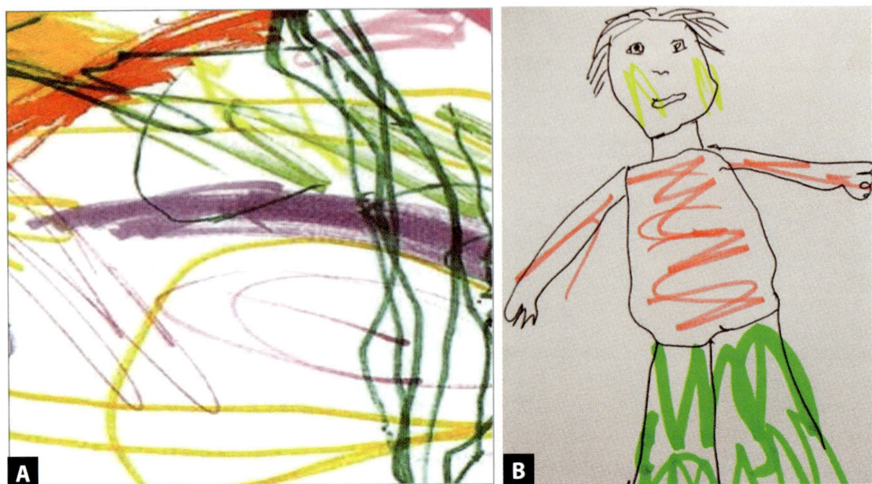

Figs. 12.15A and B: (A) Spontaneous scribbling at 1 yr; (B) Draw a person's picture at 4 yr.

- 2 m—social smile (is smiling on seeing a human face, can be the picture also. Indicates intact vision and recognition of human face).
- 3 m—follows up to 180°; fixates all near objects, doll's eye response disappears.
- 4 m—binocular vision is established.
- 6 m—adjusts position to see objects.
- 1 yr—follows rapidly moving objects; recognizes pictures of objects.

Hearing

Clinical testing to assess hearing of the very young child is more accurate than audiometry. The room should be quiet, and the baby should be alert, seated on mother's lap. Up to 6 m of age, the test sounds (rattle, squeaky doll, bell, cup and spoon, soft paper, and whispered voice) are to be produced on a level with the ear approximately 18 inches away, the examiner standing behind the baby, so as to be outside the field of vision of the baby. Above the age of 6 m, the examiner stands facing the infant but should cover the mouth to avoid facial expression if voice is delivered for testing. Above 2.5 yr of mental age, children can be tested by asking to point to body parts, toys, or pictures (examiner with covered mouth to avoid lip reading). Above 5 yr age, audiometric screening is recommended in school. The sequence of development of sound localization are:

- <3 m—quietens to familiar voices. Responds to loud noise by startle reaction, facial grimace, blink, cry if quiet, increase in heartbeat, slowing of respiration, etc.
    - *Acoustic blink*—clap the hands about 30 cm from the infant's head taking care to avoid air stream across the face. A sudden blink indicates hearing capacity.
- 3 m—turns head to the side from where sound is heard.
- 4 m—turns head toward sound and eyes look in the same direction.
- 5-6 m—turns head to one side and then downward if the sound is made below the ear.
- 6 m—turns head to one side and then upward when the sound is made above the level of the ear, imitates sounds.
- 6-7 m—turns head in a curving arc toward the sound source; responds to own name.

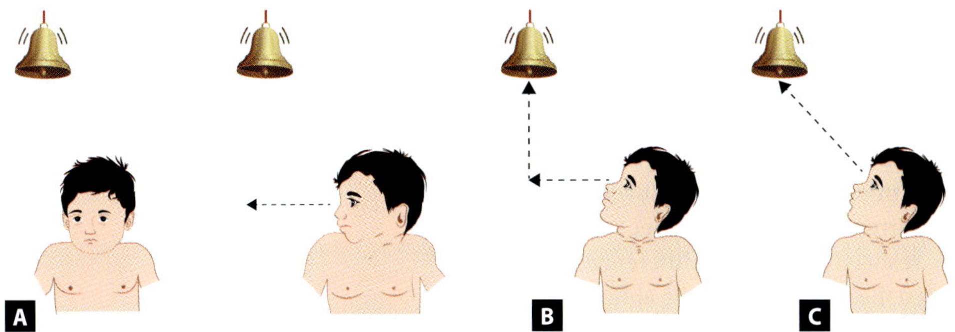

Figs. 12.16A to C: Orienting to sound of bell: (A) 4 m; (B) 6 m; (C) 10 m.

- 8-10 m—head is turned directly and diagonally toward the sound **(Figs. 12.16A to C)**.
- 9-12 m—knows the meaning of several words, including the name of members in the family.
- 1 yr—able to localize a sound source.

Defective vision at 4/12 and hearing at 6/12 if perceived by clinical testing, the infant should be referred for detailed evaluation. The common *risk factors for these defects* are family history, maternal TORCH infections, severe preeclampsia, birth trauma, prematurity, hypoxic ischemic encephalopathy, craniofacial anomalies, microcephaly, hydrocephalus, bacterial meningitis, and osteopetrosis. Additional risk factors for hearing defect are maternal exposure to ototoxic drugs, neonatal hyperbilirubinemia and mechanical ventilation, and congenital anomalies of ear and pinna.

Muscle Tone (Ch. 15)

Healthy newborns have physiological hypertonia and there is gradual reduction of muscle tone during the first yr of life.

Evaluation of Muscle Tone

Begin with neck muscles by pulling to sit posture followed by ventral suspension 180° examination and scarf sign (Ref. Ch. 15).

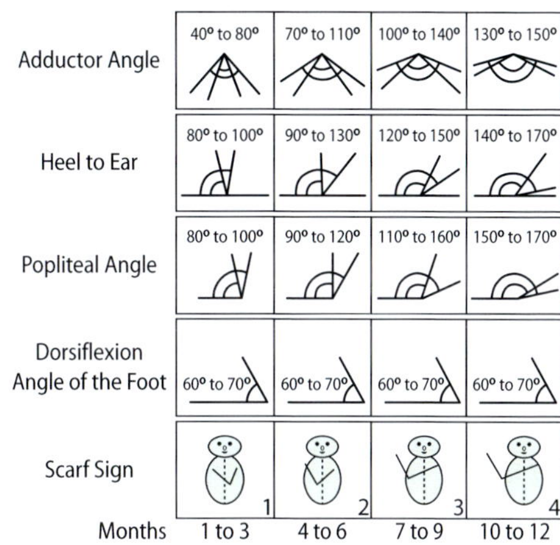

Fig. 12.17: Normal pattern of muscle tone during infancy.

Age-inappropriate head lag or neck stiffness indicate hypo- or hypertonia, respectively. The responses observed in scarf sign are three, as seen in **Fig. 12.17**: (1) Elbow does not reach the midline (up to 3 m), (2) Elbow crosses the midline (4-6 m), and (3) Arm encircles the neck (>6 m).

The range of movements at major joints during infancy is tested by *Ameil Tison* method which includes adductor angle, popliteal angle, dorsiflexion angle of foot and heel to ear maneuver (Ref. Ch. 15). **Fig. 12.17** shows the normal pattern of muscle tone during infancy. The adductor angle if bisected, the two halves should be equal. Unequal angles indicate developmental dysplasia of the hip. The difference of 20° between two sides of popliteal angles indicates significant asymmetry. Dorsiflexion angle is usually 60–70° and persists throughout infancy. Slow and rapid angle formation indicate hyper and hypotonia, respectively; also, a difference of >10° between the two sides indicate abnormality.

Indirect assessment of muscle tone is by deep tendon jerks.

Transitory tone abnormalities especially hypotonia may be noted during the first 6 m of life which normalizes by 1 yr.

Abnormalities in tone are hyper and hypotonia. Hypertonia is seen in various forms of static and progressive encephalopathies, cerebral dysgenesis, microcephaly, hydrocephalus, and 18 trisomy. In congenital (developmental) dislocation of hip, limitation of abduction of affected hip occurs which can be detected on early days itself from the *reduced adductor angle* value.

Floppy infant is the terminology to indicate persistent hypotonia in infants. It is most commonly pathological and requires detailed evaluation (Ref. **Box 12.2**).

BOX 12.2: Important causes of floppy infant.

- *Central nervous system (CNS) disorders:*
  - Atonic cerebral palsy
  - Congenital cerebellar ataxia
  - Chromosomal disorders
  - Genetic defects
  - Cerebral lipidoses
- *Spinal cord affection:*
  - Spinal muscular atrophy
  - Birth injuries
  - Congenital poliomyelitis
- *Peripheral nerves-polyneuritis:*
  - Guillain-Barré syndrome
  - Degenerative disorders
  - Metabolic diseases
  - Heavy metal poisoning
- *Neuromuscular junction diseases:*
  - Drug induced
  - Myasthenia gravis
  - Infantile botulism
- *Muscle diseases:*
  - Congenital myopathies
  - Congenital muscular dystrophies
  - Endocrine myopathies—hypothyroidism
  - Metabolic myopathies—Pompe disease
  - Polymyositis
- *Protein energy malnutrition*
- *Benign central hypotonia*

Primitive reflexes (Ref. Ch. 15 for eliciting Moro reflex, palmar, and plantar grasp).

Landau reflex: When the infant is held in ventral suspension, the head, spine, and legs extend. When the head is depressed the hips, knees, and elbows flex. The reaction is normally present from the age of 3 m and disappears by 1 yr.

Parachute reaction is elicited by holding the infant in ventral suspension around the waist and suddenly lowering toward the couch. Infant's arms extend with spreading of the fingers *as if to protect from falling.* The reflex appears at 6–9 m age and persists throughout life.

For assessing the development of preterm babies, corrected age should be followed (Ref. Ch. 11).

TARGET MILESTONES

The developmental milestones are achieved by healthy normal children within a narrow range of several weeks. *Target milestones* **(Table 12.2)** are those milestones, *which if not acquired in the specific age,* indicate future mental and/or physical retardation.

If target milestones are not achieved detailed assessment by experienced developmental specialist is needed. Isolated delay in one domain except hearing and vision may not be significant. Global developmental delay indicates defects in more than one domain.

TABLE 12.2: Target milestones.

Milestone	*Age of attainment (months)*
Social smile	2
Head control	4
Visual perception	4
Hearing	6
Independent sitting	8
Creeping	9
Standing without support	12
Mature pincer grasp	12
Walking without support	18
Scribbling	18
1–2 words with meaning	12

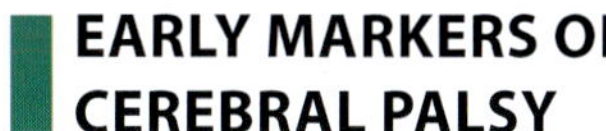

EARLY MARKERS OF CEREBRAL PALSY

Certain clinical signs and symptoms are diagnostic of cerebral palsy at the earliest which include: (1) episodes of inconsolable crying, chewing movements, and lip smacking, (2) excessive sensitivity to light and noise, (3) spontaneous Moro reflex, (4) persistence of neonatal reflexes (Moro, grasp, and ATNR) beyond 5 m of age, (5) persistent fisting with cortical thumbs beyond 8 w **(Fig. 12.18)**, (6) abnormalities in tone assessed by various angles, (7) persistent asymmetry of posture, tone, movements, and reflexes, (8) microcephaly. Early diagnosis facilitates early implementation of therapy which will ameliorate the future disability in these children due to the plasticity of the immature brain.

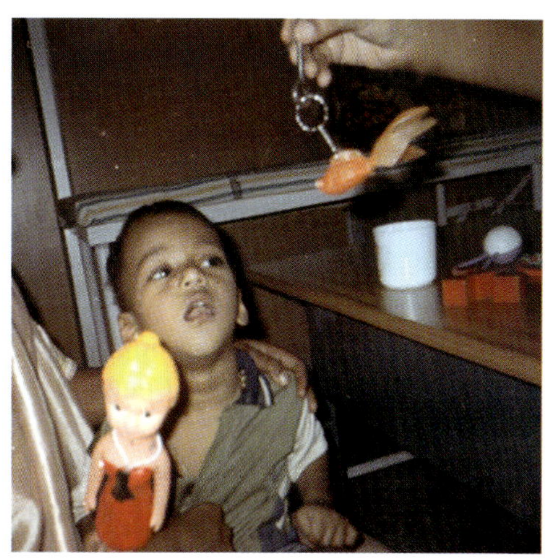

Fig. 12.18: Infant, 1.5 yr with spastic cerebral palsy (CP)—has poor head control, constant fisting, and cortical thumb.

DEVELOPMENTAL SCREENING TOOLS

Numerous developmental tools are available for screening infants and children. The pediatrician should select the most accurate, easy, and culturally acceptable method for screening purposes. The aim of developmental screening is to identify children who need a comprehensive evaluation. The salient features of few well-known tools are given in the following text:

Gessel's scale provides four major areas of development (motor, adaptive, language, and personal social) in the age group 0–5 yr. On the basis of performance, a child may be diagnosed as normal, retarded, or accelerated in development, with respect to chronological age. The scale provides an estimate of developmental quotient (DQ) for each area separately and also for overall DQ which is assessed as:

$$\text{DQ} = \frac{\text{Maturity age}}{\text{Chronological age}} \times 100$$

A child having DQ between *65 and 75 is at risk* for developmental delay.

Denver Developmental Screening Test-II

Denver developmental screening test-II (DDST-II) has 125 test items and is used for the age range from birth to 6 yr. The test meets most of the required criteria for an ideal screening and is widely used for population screening; the time required for the test is 20–30 minutes.

Trivandrum Developmental Screening Charts

Suitable screening tests are devised for children of different age groups by the faculty of Child Development Center (CDC) Thiruvananthapuram. **Fig. 12.19** reveals the simplified screening parameters for developmental assessment in the age group 0–3 yr. The test items are based on the Bayley scale of infant development. Age is plotted in months along the *"X"* axis; the lines inside the chart represent the milestones of development. The left and right edges of each line of the chart represent the 3rd and 97th percentiles of the particular developmental milestones for that age.

To administer the test, keep a plastic ruler or pencil vertically at the level of the chronological age of the child who is being tested. If the child fails to achieve any parameter on the left side of the age marker, developmental delay is suspected and is to be referred for detailed evaluation. Assessment time is 5–7 minutes. The method is simple to master so that paramedical staff can be trained to conduct the test. Since developmental delay should be detected early for effective therapy, this test can be considered as a unique one to screen infants

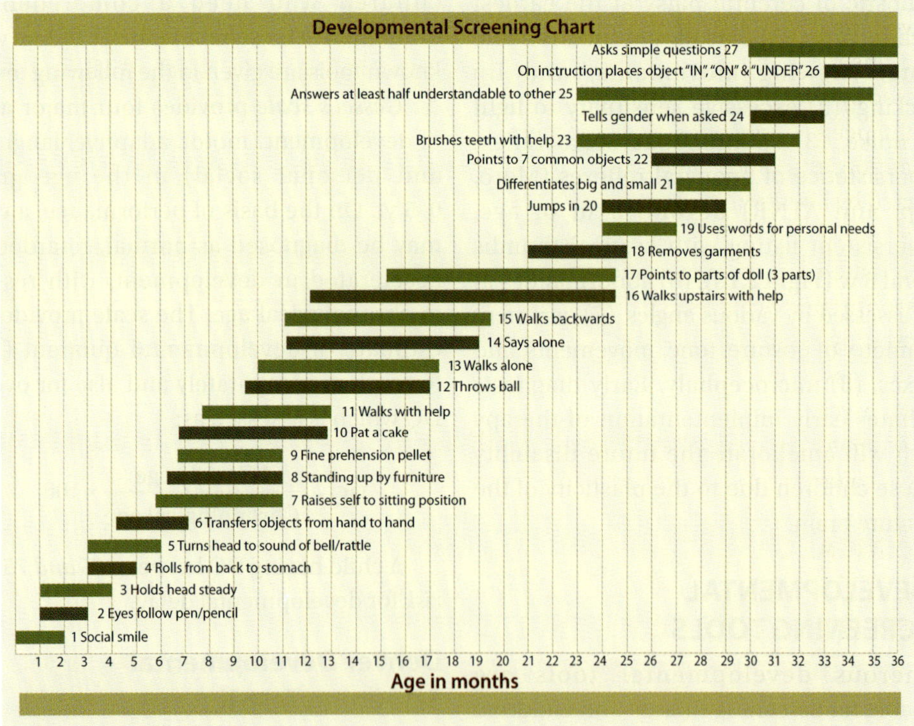

Fig. 12.19: Trivandrum developmental screening chart (TDSC) 0–3 yr.
Source: CDC, Medical College, Thiruvananthapuram. Trivandrum developmental screening chart (TDSC) 0–3 years. Indian J Pediatr. 2013.

in community by field staff. Trivandrum developmental screening charts (TDSC) for 3–6 yr and Language evaluation scale Trivandrum (LEST) for 0–3 yr are also devised and are available.

Development During Early School Years (6–12 yr) and Adolescence (10–20 yr)

Though maximal motor development is achieved by 6 yr of age, muscular strength, coordination and stamina increase progressively. This imparts ability for complex movements such as dancing, shooting, basketball playing, piano handling, etc. Personal social aspects include dealing with the peers, cooperation, eagerness to please adults, competitiveness, willingness to work for a delayed reward, belief in one's abilities, and volunteering to risk trying when success is not ensured. These parameters are to be assessed by interviewing the child, the parents and the peers. Cognitive capacity (aspects of perception, thinking, and remembering) is reflected by attention in classrooms, capacity for receptive and expressive language, age-appropriate mathematical skills, and overall classroom performance. This is usually assessed by reports from teachers. A more detailed assessment should be done by a clinical psychologist.

Common developmental problems encountered in children are given in **Box 12.3**.

BOX 12.3: Common developmental problems in children.

- Cerebral palsy (Prenatal, perinatal and, postnatal insults)
- Global developmental delay (Genetic and chromosomal abnormalities)
- Hypothyroidism
- Hearing impairment
- Autism spectrum disorders
- Intellectual disability
- Specific learning disability
- Attention deficit hyperactivity disorder
- Chronic systemic diseases

CLINICAL CASE SCENARIO

Case 1

Seethal, 15 m old baby girl, is brought for cough, noisy breathing, and increasing respiratory distress for 3 days, and feeding difficulty with vomiting for 1 day. She is the first child of the parents—father 30 yr old, mother 28 yr old. Pregnancy was uneventful with full term normal delivery. Birth wt of the baby was 3.2 kg. Attained social smile at 3 m, turned over at 6 m, but no independent sitting, crawling, or standing till now for which medical checkup was not done. No legible speech till now.

On examination, her wt is 8 kg (–2 SD), length 68 cm (<–3 SD), occipitofrontal circumference 42 cm (–3 SD), anterial fontanel 2.5 × 2.5 cm, has brachycephaly, small low set ears, hypertelorism, nonparalytic medial squint on right eye, narrow nasal passages with thick discharge, protruded tongue, small umbilical hernia, and bilateral single palmar crease.

Developmental assessment—no weight bearing, sits with support, has hypotonia, adductor angle 160°, and deep tendon reflexes sluggish. No pincer grasp, no crude palmar grasp, has occasional hand-to-hand transfer. Social smile present, no stranger recognition, no mouthing. No meaningful words, says nonspecific *ba-ma*. Vision and hearing present. Parachute reflex not elicited.

Growth parameters reveal moderate undernutrition, severe stunting, and microcephaly.

System examination shows upper respiratory infection (URI) with wheeze and normal cardiovascular system.

Final impression: 15 m old baby girl with global developmental delay (GM 5 m, fine motor 4 m, personal-social 7 m, and language 8 m), microcephaly, dysmorphic features, squint and hypotonia, undernutrition, and short stature.

Diagnosis: URI with wheeze, global developmental delay (DQ 26–53), microcephaly, hypotonia and dysmorphism with undernutrition and short stature.

Etiology for growth retardation and developmental delay—Down syndrome.

Case 2

Master Jebin, 2 yr old child, is brought for limping and abnormal walk. Child was delivered normally and had normal development up to 1 yr. There was delay in attaining self-walking. Independent walking was attained at 2 yr which was found abnormal. On examination, all the parameters are normal except for the shortening of the left lower limb and reduced adductor angle on the left side.

Diagnosis: Developmental dysplasia of left hip.

SUGGESTED READING

1. Agarwal R, Sankhyan N. Development. In: Paul VK, Bagga A (Eds). Ghai Essential Pediatrics, 10th edition. New Delhi: CBS Publishers & Distributors Pvt Ltd; 2023.
2. Bear LM. Early identification of infants at risk for developmental disabilities. Pediatr Clin N Am. 2004;51(3):685-701.
3. Day RE, Baired G, Salt A. Developmental Pediatrics. In: N McIntosh, PJ Helms, RL Smyth (Eds). Forfar and Arneil's Book of Pediatrics, 6th edition. Philadelphia, USA: Elsevier Ltd.; 2003.
4. First LR, Palfrey JS. The infant or young child with developmental delay. New Engl J Med. 1994;330:478-83.
5. Levy SE, Hyman SL. Pediatric assessment of the child with developmental delay. Pediatr Clin North Am. 1993;40(3):465-77.
6. Menkes JH. Neurologic examination of child and infant. In: Menkes JH, Sarnat HB, Moser FG (Eds). Textbook of Neurology, 5th edition. Baltimore: Williams and Wilkins; 1995. pp. 1-28.
7. Nair MKC, George B, Harikumaran Nair GS, Suma N, Neethu C, Leena ML, et al.; CDC NRHM and Childhood disability Project Team. Trivandrum Development Screening Chart 0–3 years. Indian J Pediatr. 2013.
8. Growth, Development, and Behaviour; In Nelson Textbook of Pediatrics 22/e, 2024: Kliegman R, Geme lll J, Blum, Tasker, Wilson, Schuh, Mack, International Edition, pp. 136-201.

SECTION

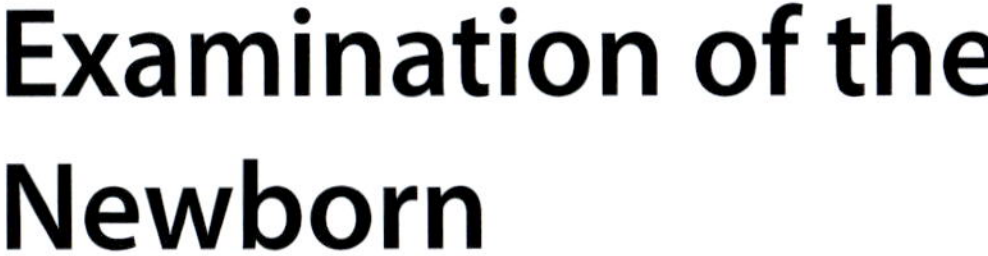

Examination of the Newborn

13

Before You Proceed

CHAPTER

L Rajam, S Radhika

Chapter Outline

- Introduction
- Timing for Examination
- Points to be Observed

INTRODUCTION

The newborn is entirely different from an older child in appearance, functions, and needs of the body and response to the environment. Since the body functions are not mature, the baby may respond in an identical manner to different external noxious factors. The pediatrician caring for the baby should have sound knowledge of the physiology of the newborn and the clinical picture of different disease states in the baby for proper assessment of the situation and management.

Examination of the newborn during the first few days of life is described as though looking through a kaleidoscope. The appearance and the findings will be changing day by day. The pediatrician should be familiar with all the factors concerned with the well-being of the baby during the antenatal period and the physiological changes during the first few days of life. The skill of examining the newborn should be developed by careful systematic and repeated attempts.

It is difficult to do a complete examination of the newborn in a definite order. Most of the examinations can be done by close observation of the baby such as the activity, color, and general state of the body. Examination of the systems should ideally be done in detail when the baby is quiet and relaxed.

An experienced pediatrician should examine the newborn and find time and patience to talk to the mother and listen to her. The junior doctors must train themselves to do the work in a satisfactory way.

TIMING FOR EXAMINATION

All newborns require immediate evaluation after delivery. If the baby is otherwise well, a detailed examination should be done before discharge from the hospital on the second or third day after birth. Babies having neonatal problems require more frequent evaluations as decided by the pediatrician.

POINTS TO BE OBSERVED

- The room must be warm and comfortable.
- The baby must be preferably under a radiant warmer.
- A good source of light should be available.
- The examiner's hands must be properly washed and warm **(Fig. 13.1)**.
- The baby must be placed on a flat surface at a height convenient to the physician.

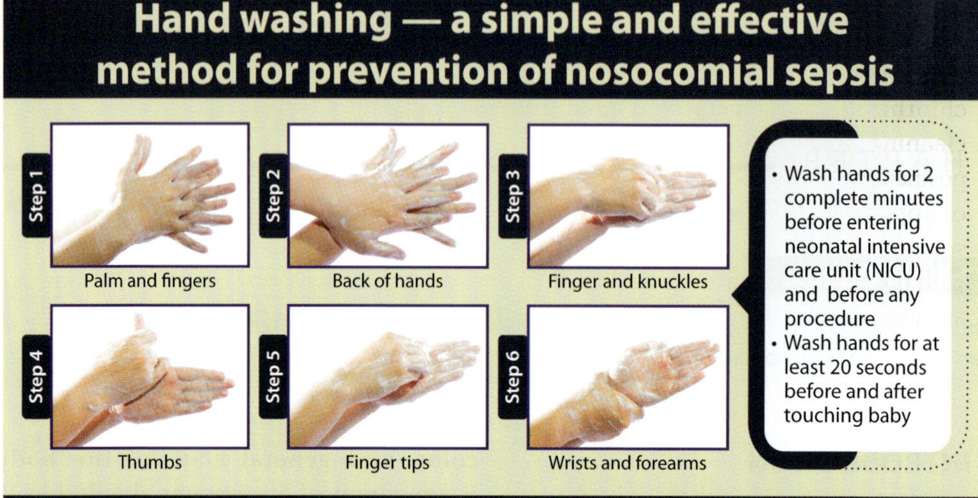

Fig. 13.1: Six steps in hand washing.

Courtesy: Division of Neonatology, Department of Pediatrics, AIIMS, New Delhi.

- The baby should be completely undressed.
- All aseptic precautions should be practiced to prevent the transmission of infections.

Hand washing is the cheapest and most effective method of sepsis prevention:

- Use an elbow-operated tap so that the tap is not touched after washing.
- Washing the hands thoroughly for 2 min in six steps should be insisted as a standard practice in all neonatal units. 20 sec should be devoted to each step.
- Both hands should be washed before and after touching each baby.
- The sleeves are to be rolled above the elbows; keep the forearms, wrists, and fingers completely free by removing watches, bangles, and rings.
- Open the tap with your hand or elbow. Clean and plain water without any added chemicals is advised.
- First wet the hands up to the forearm and then apply a nonmedicated soap; wash both hands as described in **Figure 13.1**.
- Keep elbows always dependent.
- Do not close the tap with your hands; close it with your elbow only.
- Dry your hands with a single-use sterile napkin or sterilized paper.
- Discard the napkin or the paper in the bin kept for the purpose.
- After washing your hands, do not touch pens, door handles, telephones, etc., till the required job is over.

- Rinsing the hand with alcohol is not a substitute for the initial handwashing.
- Alcohol (isopropyl alcohol, ethanol, and chlorhexidine diacetate) containing cleaning agents can be considered in postnatal wards for the routine ward rounds of apparently normal babies. Use 5 mL solution, apply on both hands, and proceed with the same sequence of hand washing and allow it to dry before touching the baby.

SUGGESTED READING

1. Abraham J, Bai SS. Handwashing and Sepsis Prevention. In: Handbook of Pediatric & Neonatal Emergencies, 1st edition. New Delhi: Jaypee Brothers Medical Publishers Pvt. Ltd. pp. 469-70.
2. Division of Neonatology. (2015). [Online] Available from http://www.newbornwhocc.org/pdf/module8_infection_prevention_WD.pdf [Last accessed September, 2024].

CHAPTER

Initial Examination of the Newborn

L Rajam, S Radhika

Chapter Outline

INTRODUCTION

Initial examination of the newborn should be *performed as early as possible* after delivery to detect any functional or structural anomalies that require immediate treatment and to establish a baseline for subsequent examinations. Conduct the examination in the delivery room itself, where the resuscitation corner should always be kept ready.

APGAR SCORE

Apgar score, devised by Dr Virginia Apgar, a Professor of Anesthesiology of Columbia University College in 1952, is a non invasive practical method of systematically assessing the newborn immediately after delivery to identify any functional impairment and to provide immediate resuscitation **(Table 14.1)**. It is done 60 seconds after the complete birth of the baby (disregarding the cord and placenta). Infant with a score of 0–3 requires immediate resuscitation. Repeat the Apgar scoring at 5 minutes and if <7 repeat at 10, 15, and 20 minutes. A score ≤3 at 20 minutes predicts high mortality and morbidity.

FIVE ORIFICES

Examine the five orifices (mouth, ears, nares, urethra, and anus), and check their patency and anomalies around them. These include cleft palate, ear anomalies, choanal atresia, absent or abnormal opening (hypospadias/epispadias) of the urethra, common anogenital opening, ambiguous genitalia, and ectopic or closed anus. Frothing at mouth and drooling of saliva if observed, pass a stiff rubber catheter or orogastric tube

TABLE 14.1: The APGAR score.

Sign	*0*	*1*	*2*
Appearance (color)	Blue/Pale	Body pink, extremities blue	Completely pink
Pulse	Absent	<100/min	>100/min
Grimace	Nil	Grimace	Cough or sneeze
Activity (muscle tone)	Flaccid	Some flexion of extremities	Active motion
Respiration	Nil	Slow and irregular	Good and crying

BOX 14.1: Common causes of hydrops fetalis.

- *Anemia:*
  - Hemolytic disease of the newborn
  - Donor in twin-to-twin transfusion
  - Fetomaternal hemorrhage
  - Alpha thalassemia
- *Cardiac failure:*
  - Supraventricular tachycardia
  - Congenital heart block
- *Intrauterine infections:*
  - Parvovirus, syphilis, Cytomegalovirus (CMV), rubella
  - Toxoplasma
- *Chromosomal anomalies:*
  - Turner syndrome
  - Trisomies
- Congenital nephrosis
- Osteogenesis Imperfecta
- Storage diseases
- Cystic adenomatoid malformation of lung

into the stomach to check the patency of the esophagus. Difficulty in insertion or coiling of the tube suggests tracheoesophageal fistula/ esophageal atresia.

Decide whether the baby is fit to be handed over to the mother in the postnatal ward or to be *transferred to the special care nursery for further management.* Indications for transfer to the special care nursery are weight <2 kg, gestational age <34 w, sick appearance, respiratory distress, postresuscitation care, edema, major congenital malformations, birth injuries, and those born to diabetic mothers.

Hydrops fetalis is excessive abnormal fluid in two or more fetal compartments (skin, pleura, pericardium, placenta, peritoneum, and amniotic cavity). **Box 14.1** reveals the common causes of hydrops fetalis.

EXAMINE THE PLACENTA

Examine the placenta for all deliveries. Normal weight is 400–500 g and is 12–15% of baby's weight. The placenta is small in babies with intrauterine growth restriction (IUGR), trisomy 18, and intrauterine infections, such as rubella. It is large in polyhydramnios, erythroblastosis, maternal diabetes mellitus, congenital nephrosis, syphilis, toxoplasmosis, and cytomegalic inclusion disease. Note the surface and color. In intrauterine infections, the appearance is dull and milky white on the fetal side and liquor is foul-smelling. *Gray yellow color of the placenta and liquor* is seen in meconium staining and erythroblastosis. In placental dysfunction, central infarction and calcification on the maternal side will be seen. Granular brown nodules (amnion nodosum) indicate oligohydramnios. Retroplacental hemorrhage may be due to fetal blood loss. Evaluate whether monochorionic or dichorionic in twin delivery. Histopathologic examination should be done when there is amnionitis or placentitis.

EXAMINE THE UMBILICAL CORD

Grayish yellow color indicates meconium staining. Examine the cut end for blood vessels—two umbilical arteries, placed lower and are smaller, rounded, and thick-walled and one umbilical vein seen above, larger, thin-walled, and slit-like. Single umbilical artery is associated with internal congenital anomalies, the common being esophageal atresia, imperforate anus, and genitourinary problems.

SUGGESTED READING

1. Bernstein S,Heimler,Sasidharn P. Approaching the management of the neonatal intensive care unitgraduate through history and physical assessment. Pediatr Clin North Am. 1998;45:79-105.

pelvic examinations done, *chorioamnionitis* (indicated by maternal fever and foul smelling amniotic fluid), other details of amniotic fluid (volume, meconium staining), cephalopelvic disproportion, cord accidents and type of anesthesia, and name and time of analgesics given to the mother.

DETAILS OF THE BABY

Enquire about the first cry whether delayed, Apgar score (at 1 min and 5 min), resuscitation required, whether the baby was kept with the mother or in a separate nursery, general activity, feeding habits, and time of passage of urine and meconium (should be within 48 and 24 hr, respectively, after delivery).

Present illness of the baby: Usual complaints in the neonate are respiratory distress (apnea, irregular, rapid or labored breathing, chest indrawing, stridor, cyanosis, pallor, edema, lethargy, poor sucking, choking, frothing, jaundice, vomiting, convulsions, delay in passing urine and meconium, irritability, incessant crying, hyperactivity, fever, diarrhea, failure to move an extremity, bleeding, umbilical discharge, abdominal distension, and congenital malformations; all are *danger signs.*

Most symptoms are common to several diseases that may originate in utero, during birth or in the immediate postnatal period. The causes may be acquired diseases and injuries, inborn errors of metabolism, genetic mutations, or chromosomal aberrations so that each complaint should be analyzed in this perspective after physical examination. Newborns can present with minor developmental peculiarities and physiologic problems which should be differentiated from serious problems requiring immediate care.

PHYSICAL EXAMINATION OF THE BABY

Ideally do 1 hr after feeding, systematically under the following headlines:

- Vital signs
- General assessment
- Measurements
- Head to foot examination
- Assessment of gestational age
- System examination

Vital signs (Ch. 7): Assess the HR, RR and BP, and temperature. Brachial pulsations are easier to palpate in newborns. Assess femoral pulsations on both sides, which if absent or weak, may suggest left-sided cardiac obstructive lesions or coarctation of the aorta. Normal values for HR and RR are double and BP 50% of that of adult values **(Table 7.2)**. Assessment of skin temperature (normal 36.5°C) by touch method (using the dorsum of examiner's fingers) is reliable. The body and the extremities should be warm and the limbs should be pink. Cold and pale extremities indicate hypothermia; mottling of the skin may herald bacterial sepsis. The difference between central and peripheral skin temperature should be <1.5°C. Evaluate capillary refill time (*CRT*) by gentle pressure over the sternum for 5 sec. The blanching should disappear in <3 sec (assess by counting 1,001, 1,002, and 1,003 in mind).

Pulse oximetry screening should be done *after 24 hr* of life to detect *critical congenital heart disease (CHD).* The saturation is measured on the *right upper limb (preductal)* and both *lower limbs (postductal).* Normal oxygen saturation (SpO_2) is >95%. The difference between pre- and postductal is <3%. If the screen fails, consider pediatric cardiology consultation, so as to have detailed evaluation.

General assessment (Ref. Ch. 7): Evaluate the color of the baby, pattern of respiration, limb movements, posture, activity, and nature of cry. Frequent face and limb movements and respiratory sounds are produced by the normal baby during sleep. Incessant or excessive crying indicates cerebral irritation; high pitched cry is due to raised intracranial tension.

Measurements (Ref. Ch. 11): Weight—use a sensitive type weighing scale with accuracy up to ±10 g. Prevent cross infection between newborns by using a sterile disposable paper on the weighing scale before placing the baby. Normal birth weight is 2.5–4 kg. Weight loss of 5–7% is normal in the first days of life but should not exceed 10% of the birth weight.

Appropriate for gestational age (*AGA*)/ small for gestational age (*SGA*)/large for gestational age (*LGA*)*:* Weight <10th percentile for gestation is SGA, >90th percentile is LGA, and in between 10th and 90th percentile is AGA.

Ponderal index (PI) is assessed to detect asymmetrical IUGR as calculated by:

$$\text{PI} = \frac{\text{Weight in g} \times 100}{(\text{Length in cm}^3)}$$

Value <2 indicates asymmetric IUGR

Crown-heel length is recorded using an infantometer (Ref. Ch. 11). Normal range is 45–54 cm.

Head circumference (Ch. 11) is measured ideally 24 hr after birth when caput succedaneum and overriding of sutures have subsided (normal range 32–38 cm). In a term baby, head circumference is around 34–35 cm with a crown-heel length of 48–50 cm.

Chest circumference (Ref. Ch. 11) is measured at the level of nipples. The difference between head and chest circumferences in normal babies is <3 cm and is >3 cm in IUGR babies.

Mid upper arm circumference (Ref. Ch. 11) in newborns is between 9 and 11 cm. Value <9 cm denotes IUGR.

Head to Foot Examination

In the supine position the newborn usually lies with the head turned to one side, with partial flexion of the extremities **(Fig. 15.3)**. *Caput succedaneum* is the edema of the presenting part.

Cephalohematoma is a fluctuant swelling of subperiosteal blood collection usually seen over the parietal bone due to injury during labor. The swelling will not cross the suture lines or midline, can be bilateral and may take weeks or months to resolve. Large cephalohematomas **(Fig. 15.4)** present with jaundice and anemia and the parents may not be pointing the scalp swelling. Subgaleal hemorrhage is the collection of blood below the aponeurosis and manifests as extensive swelling on the posterior aspect of the scalp from ear-to-ear; usually follows forceps or vacuum extraction.

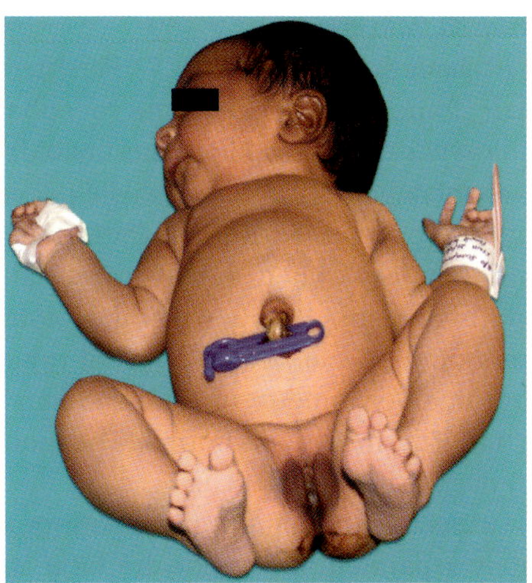

Fig. 15.3: Normal newborn-head turned to one side, limbs in partial flexion.

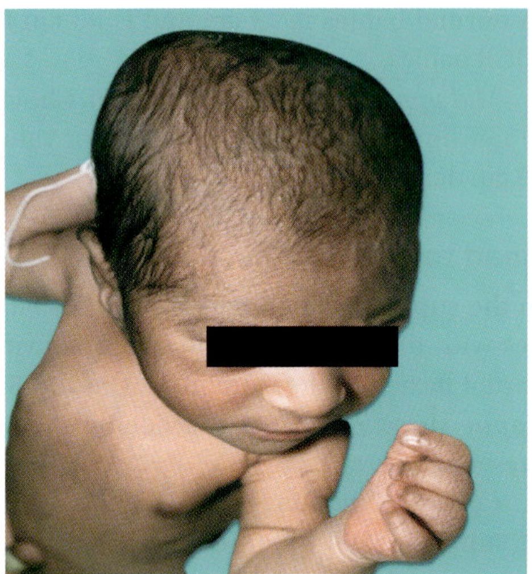

Fig. 15.4: Cephalohematoma (R) parietal region.

May indicate coagulopathies which should be investigated.

Forceps marks are seen usually on the sides of frontal and temporal or parietal bones. *Encephalocele* (meningeal sac containing portions of brain matter) and *meningocele* [cerebrospinal fluid filled meningeal sac and is transilluminant] are swellings seen along the midline sutures. They differ from other scalp swellings by *the positive impulse perceived from crying.*

Evaluate the *fontanelle* (Ch. 7). Persistently small fontanelle suggest microcephaly, craniosynostosis, congenital hyperthyroidism or wormian bones. Large fontanelle (>2 cm) may be normal variation. Pathological conditions associated are hydrocephalus, hypothyroidism, IUGR, trisomies, osteogenesis imperfecta, and congenital rubella syndrome. Asymmetry of the head can be normal, if the head size is normal. The sutures may overlap in the first 48 hr.

Suspect *hydrocephalus* if the sutures are widely separated, fontanelle are large and the head circumference is increased. Sagittal suture can be separated up to 0.5–0.75 cm in the first few weeks due to rapid growth of the brain. The squamo-parietal suture is usually closed. It may be open in premature or IUGR babies and in hydrocephalus. Metopic suture may remain open or be closed with a ridge. Suspect craniosynostosis when all the sutures are closed with ridging. Soft areas in the occipital region suggest irregular calcification and wormian bones and are seen in osteogenesis imperfecta, lacunar skull, cleidocranial dysostosis, hypothyroidism and Down syndrome.

Craniotabes is softening of the skull which can be indented like a ping-pong ball and elicited away from the suture line normally seen in preterm babies. Cradle cap is seborrheic crusting over the scalp and is usually self-regressing.

Face

Examine the hairline and face for dysmorphism. Assess the skin color. Pallor indicates blood loss or sickness. Babies born to diabetic mothers or having polycythemia appear unusually pink. Facial palsy usually follows forceps delivery; rarely, it may represent Moebius syndrome. Hypoplasia of the depressor anguli oris muscle (DAOM) may simulate facial palsy and is diagnosed by the asymmetry of the face when the baby cries with retaining of wrinkling of the forehead and closure of the eyes. Cardiovascular lesions and congenital dislocation of hips may coexist with hypoplasia of DAOM. Babies with Down's syndrome have a flat facial profile, flat occiput, upslanting palpebral fissures, epicanthal folds, dysplastic ears, protuberant tongue, and loose skin folds in the back of the neck.

Ears

Look for size, shape, position, and abnormalities such as preauricular sinus, skin tags,

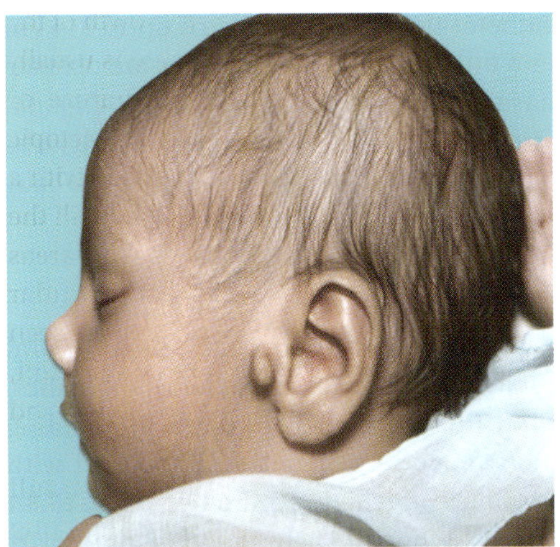

Fig. 15.5: Baby with preauricular skin tag.

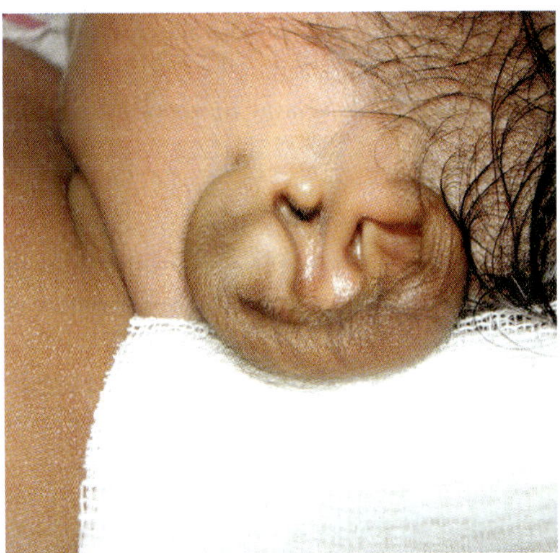

Fig. 15.6: Infant of diabetic mother with hairy pinna.

etc., **(Fig. 15.5)**. Ear abnormalities are often associated with anomalies of the kidneys. Hairy pinna is seen in infants of diabetic mothers **(Fig. 15.6)**. Low set ears (Ref. Ch. 7) may be seen in renal agenesis, trisomy 13, 18, Turner's, Down's and in Treacher Collins syndromes.

Eyes

Observe the position, distance between the two eyes, their alignment, and any inequality in size and presence of conjunctivitis. Examine the eyelids for defects and infection. Assess the cornea for size (normal 9–10 mm) and transparency. Corneal size >1 cm and raised ocular pressure indicate glaucoma. Examine the iris for color difference or defects and the lens for *cataracts* or opacity of lens **(Fig. 7.27)**. See **Box 15.1** for common causes of cataract in newborns.

BOX 15.1: Common causes of cataract in newborns.

- Inherited (dominant, recessive, and X-linked)
- Prematurity
- Intrauterine infections
- Chromosomal anomalies (Trisomy 13, 18, 21, Turner)
- Galactosemia
- Hypoparathyroidism
- Multisystem genetic disorders
- Ocular anomalies

Look for the normal *red reflex* in the eye. An ophthalmoscope is focused on the pupil of the baby about 18 inches away from the eyes. Normally, the red reflex should be symmetrical. Absence of red reflex or white pupillary reflex (leukocoria) suggests cataracts, chorioretinitis, persistent hyperplastic primary vitreous, retinopathy of prematurity or tumors, and warrants immediate ophthalmologic evaluation.

Examination of the eyes by forcing the lids apart is difficult in newborns. The eyes open spontaneously or with minimal force applied to lids, if the infant is held up and tipped gently forward and backward, a response of labyrinthine and neck reflexes. Brushfield spots (gray to white spots around the periphery of the iris) may be seen in Down syndrome. *Transient setting sun appearance* (the eyes are rolled down so that the upper sclera becomes visible) is normal especially in preterm and SGA babies but persistence indicates pathology as hydrocephalus **(Fig. 7.17B)** or kernicterus.

Retinal or subconjunctival hemorrhages unless associated with bleeding from other sites are usually benign **(Fig. 15.7)**. Epiphora (lacrimation) usually indicates an obstructed nasolacrimal duct which can be uni or bilateral. Purulent discharge indicates secondary infection.

Nose

Examine the nose for size and shape. Choanal atresia causes severe nasal obstruction, feeding difficulty, and cyanosis, and can be diagnosed by the inability to pass a firm nasal catheter through each nostril up to 3–4 cm into the nasopharynx. Neonates are obligate nasal breathers; bilateral severe choanal atresia can cause severe respiratory distress and cyanosis which is relieved when the baby cries or an oral airway is inserted.

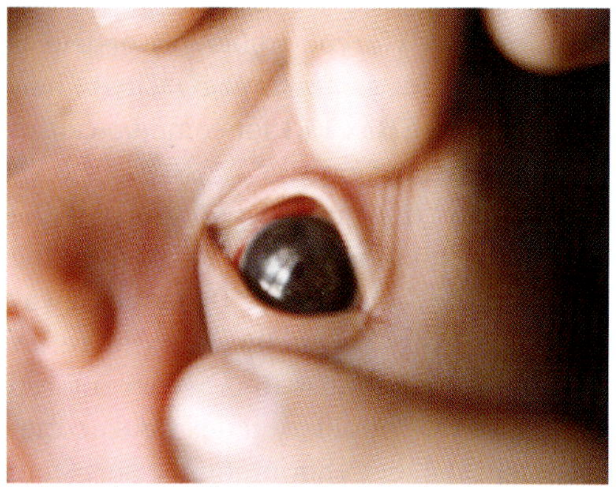

Fig. 15.7: Subconjunctival hemorrhage.

Mouth

Assess the overall size and shape of oral cavity and chin for congenital anomalies. Cleft lip and cleft palate are the leading ones; may be isolated or associated with trisomies or genetic syndromes **(Figs. 15.8A and B)**. When the baby cries, the oral cavity should be inspected for palatal anomalies, lingual thyroid (at *foramen*), Epstein pearls (white spots on the hard palate which are the epithelial inclusion cysts) and congenital teeth **(Fig. 15.9)**. Natal teeth need not be removed unless they interfere with feeding or are highly mobile. Tongue tie is a thin membrane on the under surface of the tongue from the tip of tongue to the floor of the mouth. Short, thick, and fibrous tongue tie causes notching at the tip and may interfere with the movement of the tongue. Ranula are bluish mucous retention cysts seen on

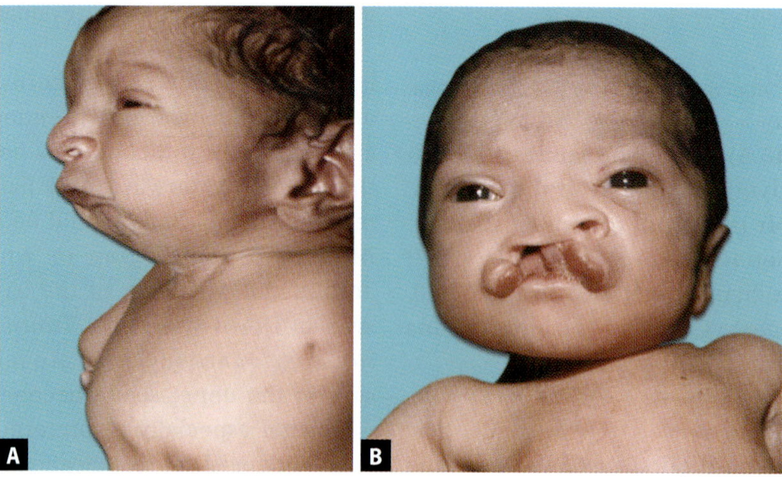

Figs. 15.8A and B: (A) Retrognathia; (B) Cleft lip, cleft palate, and hypertelorism.

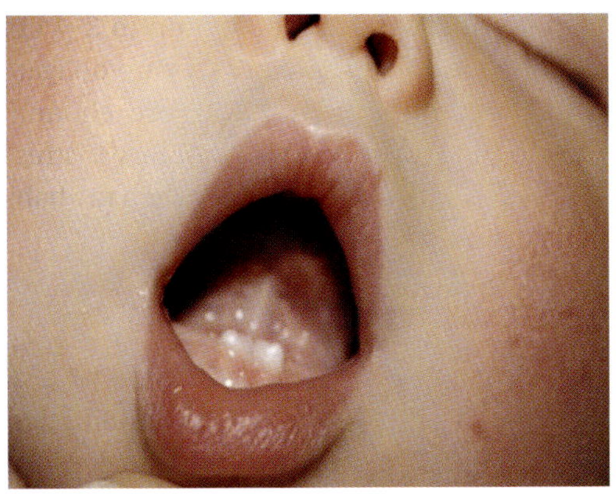

Fig. 15.9: Newborn with natal teeth.

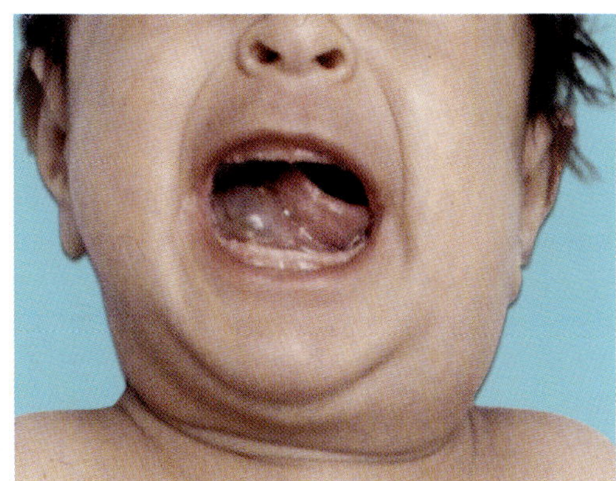

Fig. 15.10: Ranula in a newborn.

the under surface of the tongue caused by the obstruction in the sublingual gland duct **(Fig. 15.10)**. Patency of esophagus should be checked by introducing a nasogastric feeding tube in all *babies with frothiness and drooling of saliva*, and associated *polyhydramnios*.

Neck

Evaluate the length and look for webbing, hairlines, and evidence of fracture of the clavicle which may be associated with Erb's palsy and diaphragm paralysis. Palpate the sternonocleidomastoid muscles and assess the range of movement of the neck to rule out congenital torticollis.

Skin (Read Ch. 10)

Pallor may indicate hypothermia, hypothyroidism, anemia, and septicemia. Skin signs of dysmaturity should be assessed as in **Table 15.1**. Acrocyanosis is bluish discoloration of the peripheries due to benign vasomotor changes and is transient. Vernix caseosa is cheesy white material seen over the newborn skin at birth which has moisturizing, anti-infective and antioxidant properties. Erythema toxicum or urticaria neonatorum appear as erythematous rashes with central pallor, seen in term babies on the 2nd or 3rd day of life. Peeling of skin is seen in post-term babies. Cutis marmorata is a vascular pattern of skin, seen as an evanescent, lacy, reticulated red, or blue-marbled appearance of the extremities and trunk, especially when the baby is exposed to a cold environment. In hypothyroidism, it can persist longer. Harlequin color change is a vasomotor phenomenon characterized by blanched and pale appearance on one half of the body and pink color on the other half. Harlequin fetus is a type of icthyosis **(Fig. 15.11)** where the baby is pink, skin is very thick and armor-like, marked by deep red fissures. Milia are yellow white spots 1–2 mm in size seen over the nose and are retention cysts of pilosebaceous glands. Acne neonatorum appear on the forehead, nose, and cheeks in term babies due to the transplacental passage of maternal androgens. Nevus simplex are capillary hemangiomas seen as pink to red lesions on the nape of neck (Stork bites), upper eyelids, forehead, and root of nose (salmon patches). Mongolian spots are slate gray-colored or bluish patches, mostly seen over the sacral region and buttocks and the lower limbs but rarely over the body **(Fig. 15.12)**. These spots are produced by the dermal location of melanocytes due to their migration arrest

TABLE 15.1: Expanded New Ballard score to assess physical maturity.

Physical maturity	***–1***	***0***	***1***	***2***	***3***	***4***	***5***
Skin **(Fig. 15.21)**	Sticky friable, transparent	Gelatinous red, translucent	Smooth pink, visible veins	Superficial peeling and/or rash, few veins	Cracking, pale areas, rare veins	Parchment deep cracking no vessels	Leathery, cracked, wrinkled
Lanugo	None	Sparse	Abundant	Thinning	Bald areas	Mostly bald	
Plantar surface	Heel-toe 40–50 mm: –1 <40 mm: –2	50 mm no crease	Faint red marks **(Fig. 15.22)**	Anterior transverse crease only	Creases on anterior two-thirds of sole	Creases on entire sole **(Fig. 15.23)**	
Breast	Imperceptible	Barely perceptible **(Fig. 15.24)**	Flat areola no bud	Stripped areola 1–2 mm bud	Raised areola 3–4 mm bud	Full areola 5–10 mm bud **(Fig. 15.25)**	
Eye/ear	Lids fused Loosely (–1), Tightly (–2)	Lids open, pinna flat, stays folded	Slightly curved pinna, soft; recoils	Well curved pinna, soft show recoil	Formed and firm, instant recoil	Thick cartilage, ear stiff	
Genitals, male	Scrotum flat, smooth	Scrotum empty, faint rugae	Testes in upper canal, rare rugae	Testes descending few rugae	Testes down, good rugae	Testes pendulous, deep rugae	
Genitals, female	Clitoris prominent, labia flat	Clitoris prominent, small labia minora	Clitoris prominent, enlarging labia minora	Majora and minora equally prominent	Majora large, minora small	Majora cover clitoris and minora	

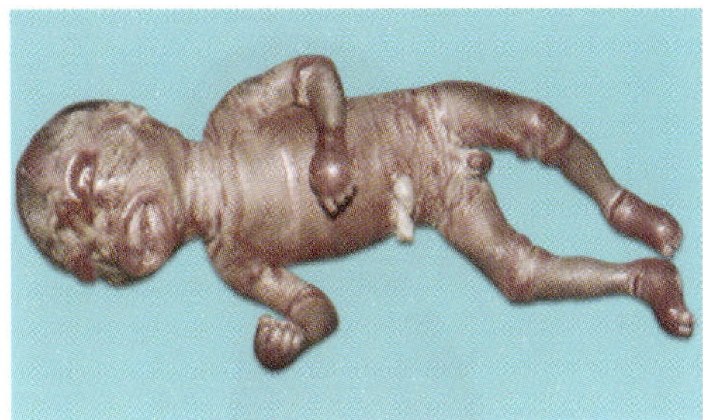

Fig. 15.11: Harlequin fetus.

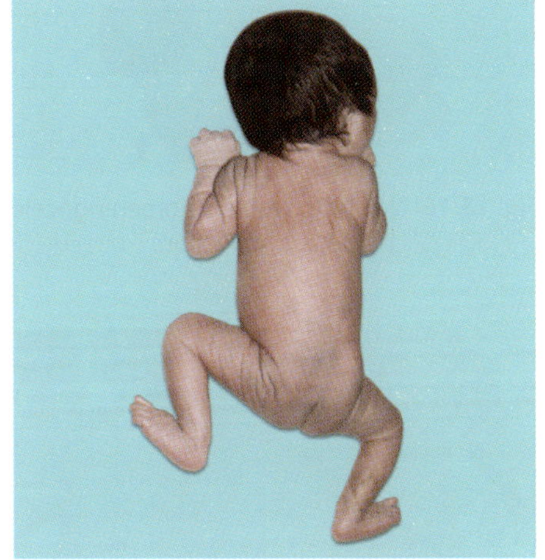

Fig. 15.12: Newborn with Mongolian spots.

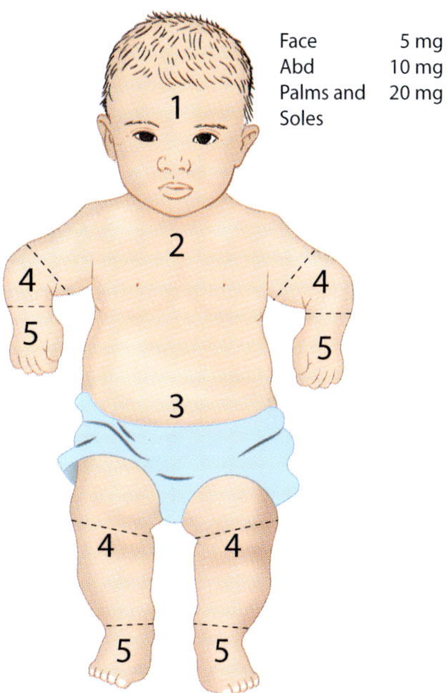

Fig. 15.13: Kramer index.

while traveling to the epidermis. Lanugo hairs are fine, soft, and nonpigmented hair in the fetus and newborn which are soon shed.

Jaundice in newborns progresses in the cephalocaudal direction as the severity increases.

Approximate value of serum bilirubin can be assessed by *Kramer's criteria* for yellow staining of body [face <5 mg/dL, upper chest 5-8 mg/dL, abdominal wall 10–15 mg/dL, extremities 15 mg/dL, palms and soles >15 mg/dL **(Fig. 15.13)**]. After phototherapy this visual estimation may not be reliable.

Subcutaneous fat necrosis (pseudo-sclerema) are localized areas of induration without any inflammatory changes seen over the buttocks, back, cheek, and extremities; may be associated with hypercalcemia. The skin over these lesions is stretched and not pinchable. It is usually benign.

Chest

The Chest in newborns is barrel shaped. Observe for any abnormalities. There may be asymmetry of the chest wall. In POLAND syndrome anterior axillary wall is not well formed since the pectoralis major muscle is absent. Engorgement of the breast (*mastitis neonatorum*) on one or both sides from the 3rd or 4th day may occur due to circulating maternal hormones not inactivated by the immature neonatal liver **(Fig. 15.14)**. It can persist for months.

Abdomen

The abdomen is usually distended in the newborn. Abdominal wall may be weak especially in preterm babies and diastasis recti and umbilical hernia are common. *Scaphoid* abdomen indicates diaphragmatic hernia.

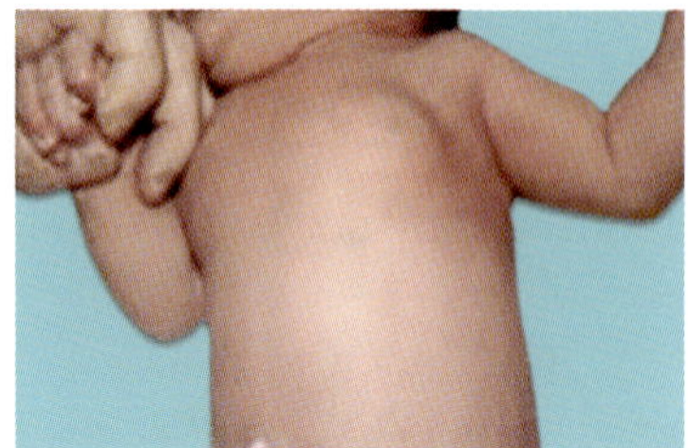

Fig. 15.14: Newborn with mastitis neonatorum.

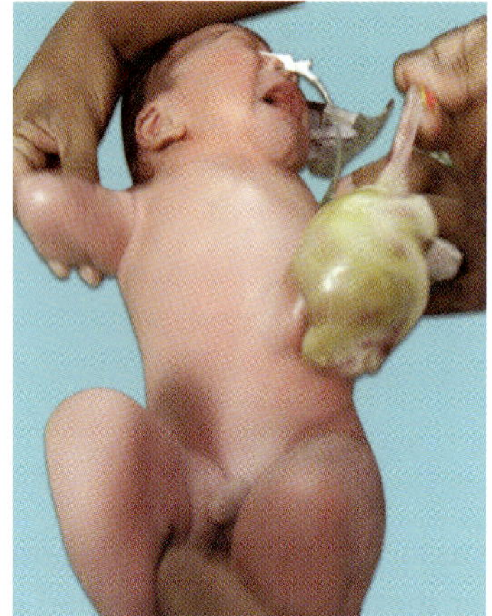

Fig. 15.15: Newborn with omphalocele.

Observe for distended bowel loops and visible peristalsis. Examine the umbilical cord for bleeding, granuloma, evidence of infection, and anomalies such as umbilical hernia (most common) or omphalocele **(Fig. 15.15)**.

Purulent discharge, foul smell, and periumbilical redness indicate infection. Large or irreducible umbilical hernias require surgical intervention **(Fig. 12.3)**. Inguinal region may reveal hernia **(Fig. 12.4)**. Inguinal hernias may be seen in preterm babies and should be repaired early to avoid incarceration. Examine the genitals for any anomaly (**Fig. 7.41** ambiguous genitalia). Scrotum may reveal small hydrocele which is transilluminable and gets absorbed within a few weeks. Female babies may have white vaginal discharge or sometimes pseudomenses in the initial days. Back should be examined for anomaly or deformity of spine, myelomeningocele **(Fig. 15.16)**, lipomas, tufts of hair, spina bifida, sacral dimple, and pilonidal sinus. Sacral agenesis can occur in infants of diabetic mothers. Sacral pit >5 mm in dimension or >2.5 cm above anus needs investigation. Sore buttocks and napkin rashes are characterized by redness, excoriation of skin, and sometimes induration **(Fig. 15.17)**. The changes are due to ammoniacal dermatitis or true candidal infection.

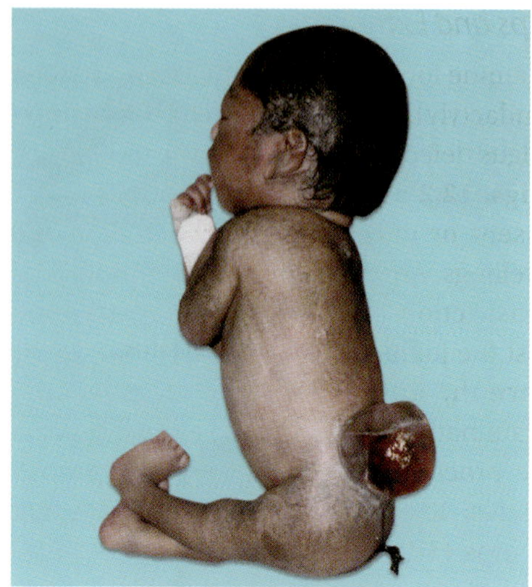

Fig. 15.16: Newborn with myelomeningocele, paraplegia in flexion.

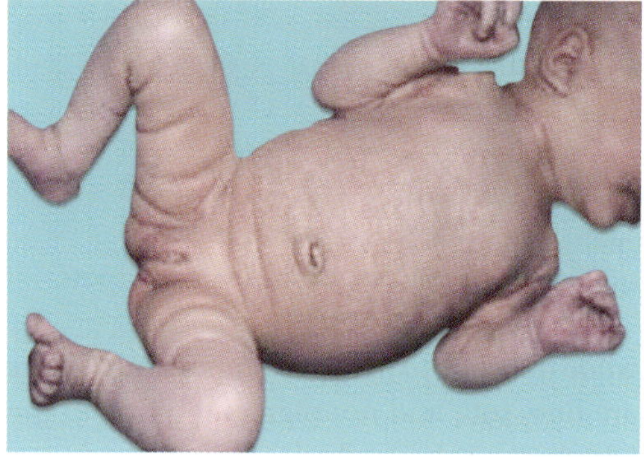

Fig. 15.17: Diaper dermatitis in the newborn.

Hips and Extremities

Examine for anomalies of digits (polydactyly, syndactyly), hands and feet [club foot, varus or valgus defects, talipes equinovarus deformity **(Figs. 12.2 and 12.6)**]. Long bones may be absent or may have anomalies or painful swellings. Amniotic bands may produce ring constriction or amputation of extremities. Test the joints for pain, tenderness, swelling warmth, and restriction of movement. Examination of hips must be the last part as the procedure may induce crying in most babies. Exclude developmental dysplasia of hips (*DDH*) in all newborns and up to 2 m of age. After this age, clinical examination for DDH is difficult since soft tissue contractures develop around the joint. DDH is more frequent on the left side and in breech presentation, postmature babies, oligohydramnios, arthrogryposis, and chromosomal anomalies. On inspection the affected limb reveals increase in the number of skin folds on the medial aspect of the thigh, apparent shortening, and limitation of abduction. When the supine infant's feet are placed together on the examining table with the hips and knees flexed, the knee on the affected side will be at a lower level [*Galeazzi's or Allis sign* **(Fig. 15.18)**].

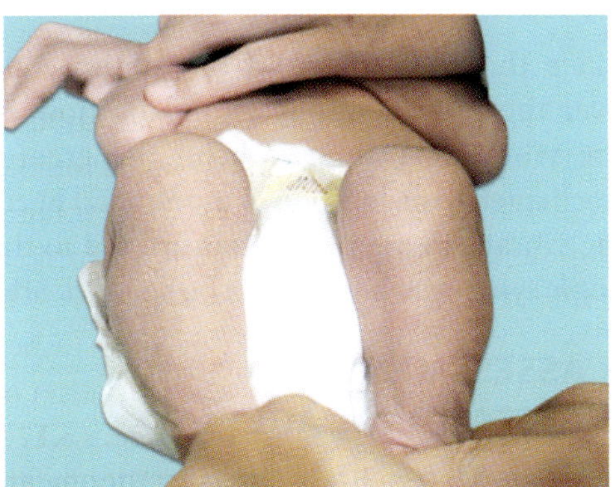

Fig. 15.18: Positive Galeazzi's sign in DDH (L) side.

Evaluation of DDH: Place the baby supine after undressing below the waist. Examine the hips one at a time. Stabilize the pelvis with the examiner's thumb on symphysis pubis and fingers under the sacrum (for the left hip evaluation, the examiner should use the left hand to stabilize the baby's pelvis from the right side and right hand to examine the hip). Flex the hip and knee to 90°. Grasp the thigh keeping the middle finger on the greater trochanter and thumb over the lesser trochanter.

Barlow test **(Fig. 15.19)** is a provocative test to dislocate an unstable hip. The flexed thigh is adducted and a posterior force (backward and outward) is applied to dislocate the femoral head. The dislocatable femoral head moves backward over the acetabular rim with or without a palpable or audible "clunk". The test should not be done repeatedly and forcefully.

Ortolani test **(Fig. 15.20)** is applicable in infants of 1–2 m to reduce a recently dislocated hip. The flexed thigh is abducted and the femoral head is lifted anteriorly into the acetabulum by applying pressure over the greater trochanter by the middle

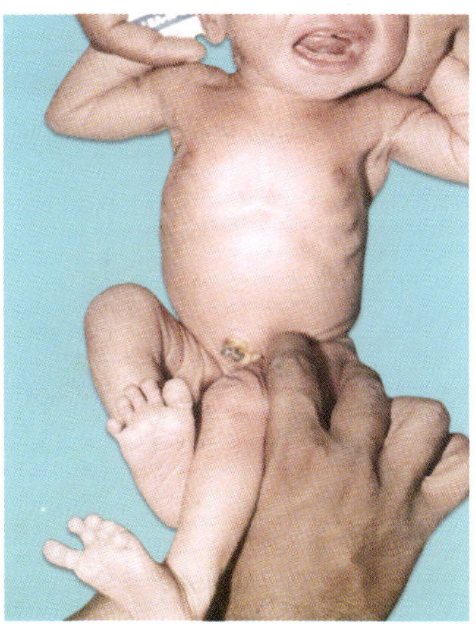

Fig. 15.19: Barlow test.

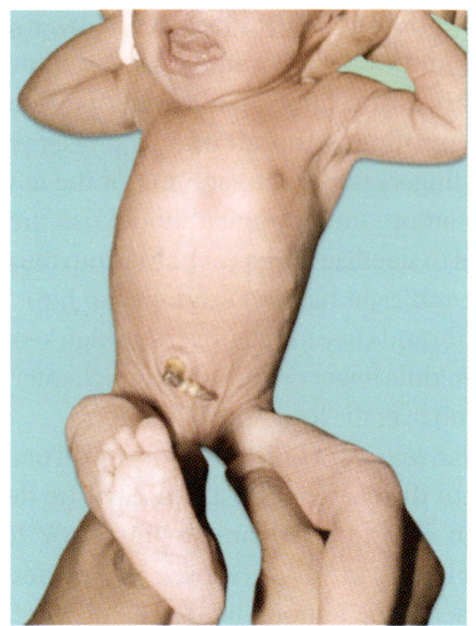

Fig. 15.20: Ortolani test.

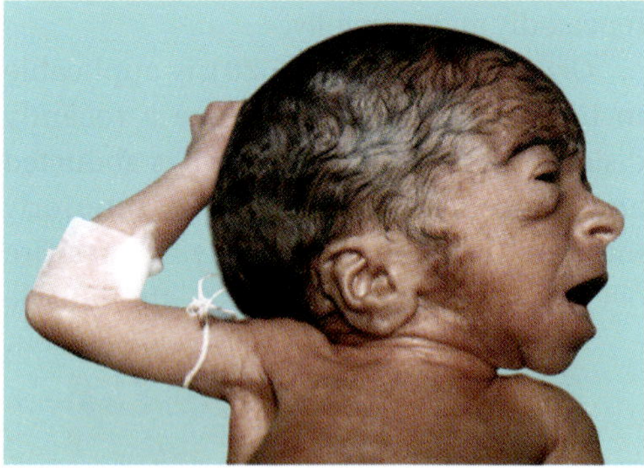

Fig. 15.21: Preterm skin—sticky, friable.

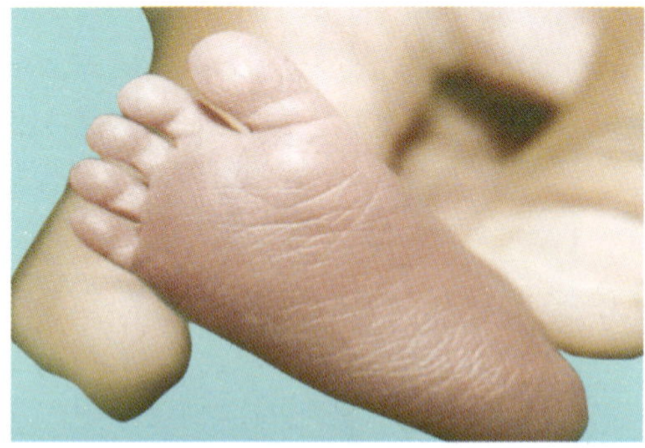

Fig. 15.22: Preterm sole creases—faint.

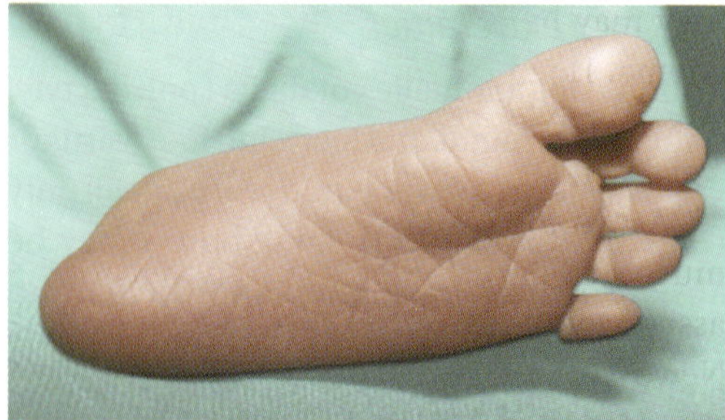

Fig. 15.23: Term baby—sole creases deep—prominent, entirely distributed.

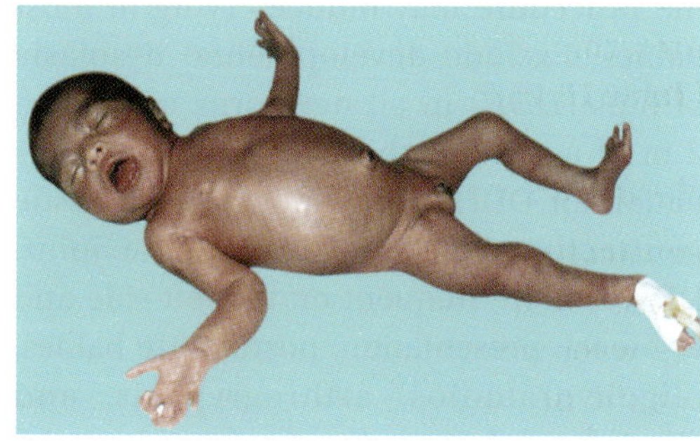

Fig. 15.24: Preterm baby—underdeveloped breast nodule, pithed frog posture due to hypotonia.

finger. The dislocated femoral head comes back into the acetabulum with a palpable or audible clunk. The right hip is examined similarly using the left hand. Ligamentous clicks may be appreciated in 5–10% of hips without any movement of the femoral head.

Auscultatory Method

Place the chest piece of the stethoscope over the pubic symphysis and the foot of the vibrating tuning fork on the greater trochanter. In dislocation of the femoral head, the vibrations are poorly transmitted to the pubic symphysis and will not be heard clearly.

ASSESSMENT OF GESTATIONAL AGE

Anthropometry: Body measurements are not reliable parameters of maturity, since they may be adversely affected by IUGR or edema. Head circumference and length are less affected in IUGR babies as compared to weight and chest circumference.

A combination of physical and neuromuscular criteria is used for the correct assessment of gestational age. The expanded New Ballard scoring system (1991) is widely accepted.

Physical Criteria

Six criteria are applied to differentiate a preterm baby <37 w of gestational age **(Table 15.1)**.

Neuromuscular Criteria

Physical criteria are of limited value to assess the precise gestational age of babies <36 w for which neuromuscular parameters should be applied. Six criteria are used to assess muscle tone and joint mobility **(Fig. 15.26)**.

Muscle tone: Assess by posture, passive tone (popliteal angle and scarf sign) and active tone by arm recoil. The tone progressively increases in utero as the maturity proceeds.

Joint mobility: The degree of flexion at ankle and wrist (square window) is limited in preterm babies because of the stiffness of joints. As the baby matures, the joints become more flexible and relaxed to allow for easy molding during delivery.

Time of appearance of some of the newborn reflexes are helpful to assess gestational age of the baby. Most important is the Moro reflex which appears at 28 w of gestational age. In neurologically damaged, very sick or IUGR babies, assessment of gestational age by the above parameters can be applied only if Moro reflex is present. **Table 15.2** reveals the relationship between combined total score with gestational age.

SYSTEM EXAMINATION

Nervous System (Ref. Ch. 21 for more details)

Careful observation without disturbing the baby will provide sufficient information. The neurodevelopmental examination should be done when the baby is active and alert, preferably 2 hr after feeding, in a well-lit warm room and completely undressed. The examiner should be relaxed, not in a hurry, and should be with warm and clean hands. Detailed neurological examination is not

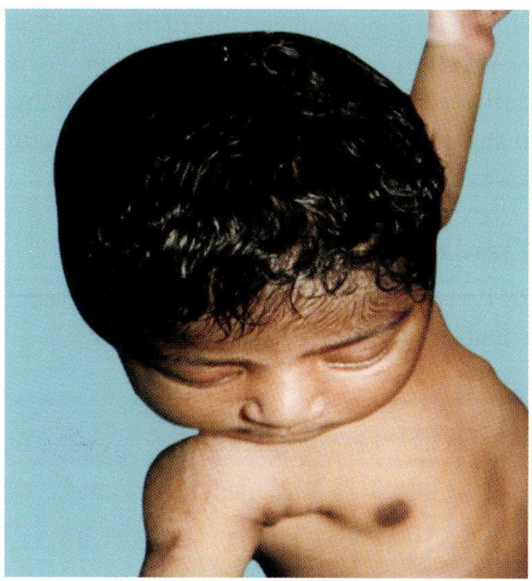

Fig. 15.25: Term baby—well developed breast nodule.

TABLE 15.2: Maturity rating–New Ballard score.

Score	−10	−5	0	5	10	15	20	25	30	35	40	45	50
Weeks	20	22	24	26	28	30	32	34	36	38	40	42	44

Note: The physical and neurologic scores are added to calculate gestational age.

essential if the newborn is active, feeding well, spontaneously moving all limbs, and does not have any external anomalies of the skull or spine.

Indications of detailed neurological examination in newborns are to diagnose neurological illness when the baby has symptoms suggestive of nervous system diseases, prognosticate future psychomotor development of babies with perinatal insults or neurological illness, assess gestational age of the baby and for adoption purposes.

Examine under the following headlines:

- Higher mental functions
- Cranial nerves
- Motor functions
- Sensory functions
- Skull and spine.

Higher mental functions: Assessment should be done in stage 3 or 4 of the *Brazelton Scale* as shown in **Table 15.3**. Observe the activity and general behavior of the baby. If the sensorium appears dull, GCS (infant assessment) should be done (Ch. 9).

Cranial Nerves

Ist nerve: Grimacing is seen with unpleasant smell around (cannot be used as a test).

TABLE 15.3: Brazelton scale—stages of wakefulness in the neonate.

Stages	*Nature of wakefulness in the baby*
I	Deep sleep with regular respirations
II	Light sleep with eyes closed, occasional movements of eyelids, lips, fingers, irregular respirations (REM sleep)
III	Eyes open with no gross body movements (quiet wakefulness)
IV	Eyes open with gross body movements
V	Eyes open or closed and crying

(REM: rapid eye movement)

IInd nerve: Test materials needed are moderately bright torch light, bright red ball, and ophthalmoscope. Examine the visual fixation, visual attention (following the moving red ball), pupillary size and reaction, and optic fundi. Observe the size and reaction of pupils and the blinking response (both appear *at 28 w of gestation*) on focusing the bright light. Baby turns toward light by 32 w and follows the moving red ball by 34 w of gestation. By term, visual fixation and the ability to follow bright light for a few degrees are attained. Instil 1% neosynephrine eye drops to dilate the pupils for visualizing the optic fundi. The disc is usually pale and foveal reflex is absent. Retinal hemorrhages can be considered normal. Chorioretinitis indicates intrauterine infections. More sophisticated test is detection of optokinetic nystagmus when the alert baby watches the rotating striped drum. Visual acuity in a term baby is 20/150.

IIIrd, IVth, VIth nerves: Look for ptosis, inability to close the eyes, squint, and nystagmus.

Doll's eye maneuver can be applied as early as at 25 w of gestation to demonstrate complete ocular movements. Baby in supine position, grasp the head of the baby with both hands, and using the thumbs gently open the eyelids. When the head is suddenly turned to one side (through 70°) the eyes look to the opposite direction normally. Vertical movements of the eyes can be observed by rapid flexion and extension of the neck. Failure of the doll's eye movements indicates paralysis of ocular muscles or extensive brain stem damage.

Vth nerve: Sensory part is assessed by the corneal reflex. It is best documented by facial grimacing to touching the nostril with a wisp of cotton (or by a pin prick over the face—less accepted). Motor paralysis is indicated by

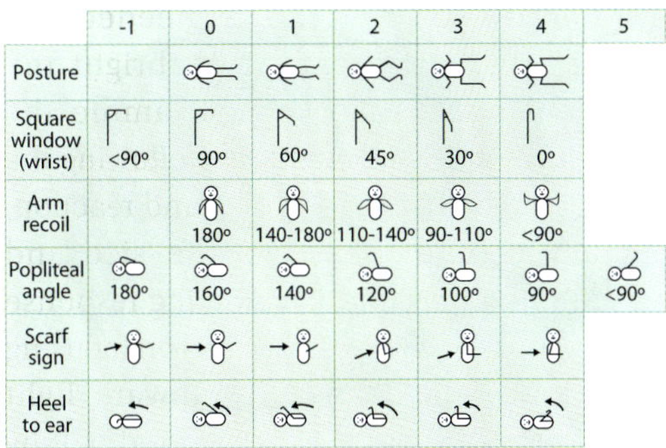

Fig. 15.26: Neuromuscular criteria for maturity—New Ballard score.

the deviation of angle of mouth to affected side as the baby opens the mouth, being pushed over by the healthy lateral pterygoid muscles.

VIIth nerve: Asymmetry on the face is observed especially when the baby cries. Closure of the eyes is incomplete and the nasolabial fold is less prominent on the affected side.

VIIIth nerve: Sound stimulus (500–1,000 cycles per second) with a cup and spoon or rattle in level with the ears, 18 inches away (to avoid air current) is advised. The hearing response is revealed by a startle reflex, blinking, crying, quieting if crying, momentary catch in respiration, or changes in the heart rate. Positive response confirms intact hearing but negative response does not rule out the same.

IXth and Xth nerves: Nasal regurgitation during feeding is suggestive of paralysis. Negative gag reflex confirms paralysis.

XIth nerve: Observe asymmetry in Moro reflex. Shrugging can be observed by cutaneous stimulation.

XIIth nerve: Asymmetry of the tongue is suggestive of weakness on one side. Sucking will be difficult when there is complete paralysis and tongue movements will be less. Fasciculations of the tongue are seen in Werdnig-Hoffmann disease.

In general, if the baby cries well and is consolable, the higher functions are normal. Good suck and swallow reveal that cranial nerves V, VII, IX, X, and XII are intact.

Motor Functions

Motor functions are assessed under the following aspects:

- Bulk of muscle
- Strength
- Muscle tone
- Reflexes
- Involuntary movements

Bulk of Muscle and Strength

Bulk of muscle is reduced in congenital absence, myopathies, and IUGR.

Strength is assessed by observing spontaneous movements and ventral suspension.

Spontaneous movements: Normally there are active movements of limbs when the baby is awake. Paucity of movements on any limb suggests weakness. Giving resistance to the different movements will help to assess the power of muscles around joints.

Ventral suspension is done to detect the ability to hold the head and flex the limbs against gravity. Hold the baby in the air in prone position with the examiner's hands under the chest. Observe whether the head is in line with the body for a few seconds and limbs show flexion against gravity **(Fig. 15.27)**.

Muscle Tone

Muscle tone is assessed by (1) Observation of posture, (2) feeling the tone of muscles, (3) assessing the range of active movements, (4) assessing the resistance to passive

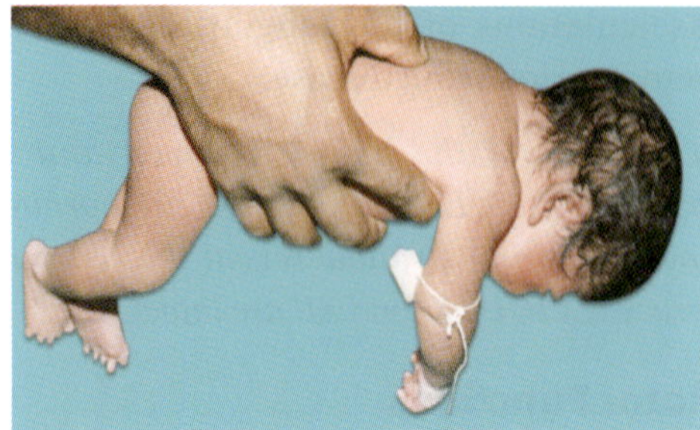

Fig. 15.27: Term baby-ventral suspension—head in line with body, limbs in flexion against gravity.

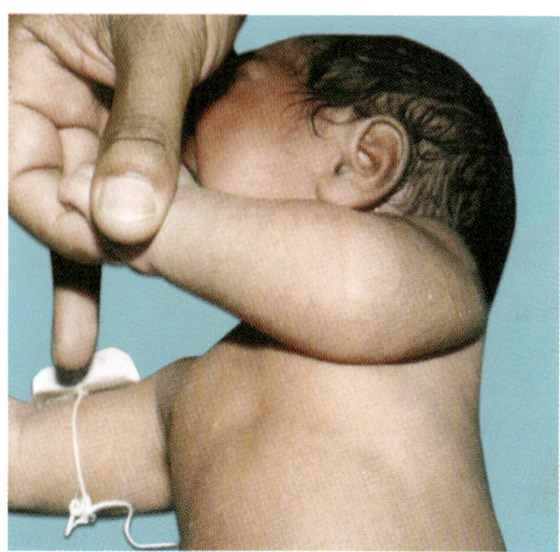

Fig. 15.28: Scarf sign—term baby— elbow does not cross midline.

movements, and (5) indirect assessment by deep tendon jerks.

Normal term newborns reveal increased muscle tone than preterms. Differences in muscle tone in different limbs is abnormal. One can differentiate between hypo (flabby muscles) and hypertonia by feel of the muscles, dangling movements of extremities, and range of movements at various joints.

Posture: Newborns with normal muscle tone usually remain in partial flexion of all limb joints **(Fig. 15.3)**. Reduced muscle tone leads to extension of joints or "pithed frog posture" as shown in **Figure 15.24**.

Assessing range of active movement: Bring the baby's head to the midline prior to assessment of muscle tone (active and passive). Otherwise tonic neck reflex will influence the muscle tone unequally on the two sides—reduced tone on the side to which the face is turned and increased tone on the side of the occiput. The following tests are advised.

- *Arm recoil:* Baby in supine position, the forearm is extended by pulling at hands and then released. If the muscle tone is adequate the arm briskly returns to full flexion. Arms will not return to full flexion in hypotonia.
- *Pull to sit maneuver* demonstrates the tone of the neck muscles and trunk. From the supine position, the baby is pulled to sit by holding the wrists. In normal term newborns, the head comes up in line with the body initially and thereafter shows some lag. Hypotonia is revealed by complete head lag **(Fig. 12.8A)**. In hypertonia, the head comes with the body and remains in that position even when the baby is sitting.

Assessing resistance to passive movement

- *Scarf sign* tests the muscle tone in upper limbs. Baby in supine position, with back flat against a hard surface, the wrist is grasped and swept across the chest until resistance is felt. The upper limb should be flexed at the elbow. The position of the elbow in relation to the midline of the body is noted. In term newborns, the elbow does not cross the midline. In preterms and conditions associated with hypotonia, the elbow crosses midline, the extent being directly proportional to the degree of hypotonia **(Figs. 15.26, 15.28, and 15.29)**.
- *Adductor angle* reveals the tone of hip adductors. Baby in supine position, the examiner's index fingers are kept in line

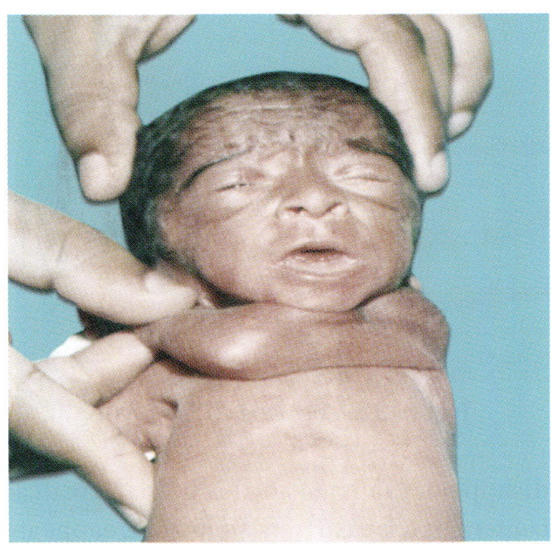

Fig. 15.29: Scarf sign—preterm baby—elbow crosses the midline.

with the long axis of the thighs which are maximally abducted by holding at both knees **(Figs. 15.30A and B)**. The angle between the two index fingers with the vertex at symphysis pubis is the adductor angle. Normal value for the term newborn is 40–80°. It is increased in preterm babies and babies with hypotonia.

- *Popliteal angle* detects the tone of hamstring muscles. Baby in supine position, the buttocks touching the table, both hips are fully flexed on the abdomen by holding the knees. The legs are then extended with the examiner's thumbs placed behind the legs until resistance is felt. The popliteal angle is measured between thigh and calf. Normal angle is 80–100° in term newborn **(Fig. 15.26)**. Simultaneous evaluation of both sides is needed to recognize any disparity.
- *Heel to ear maneuver* tests muscle tone in lower limbs. Baby in supine position, the buttocks touching the table (fixed by one hand), the leg is extended and feet moved toward the ear until resistance is felt. The angle between the table surface and the back of the leg is measured. In the normal full-term baby the value is 80–100°. Complete extension allowing feet to touch the ears indicates hypotonia, whereas in hypertonia the value is below 80° **(Fig. 15.31)**.
- *Dorsiflexion angle of foot:* Baby in supine position foot is passively dorsiflexed

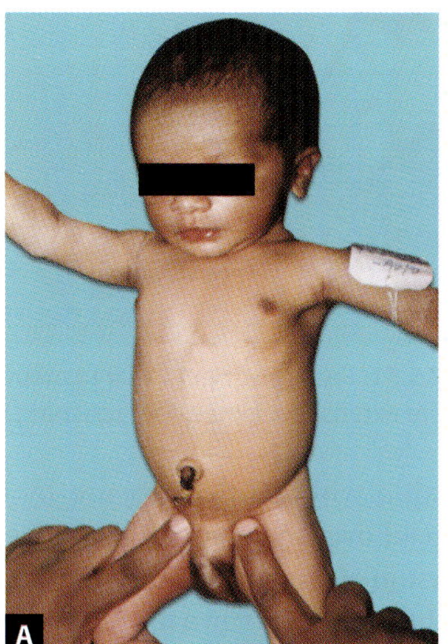

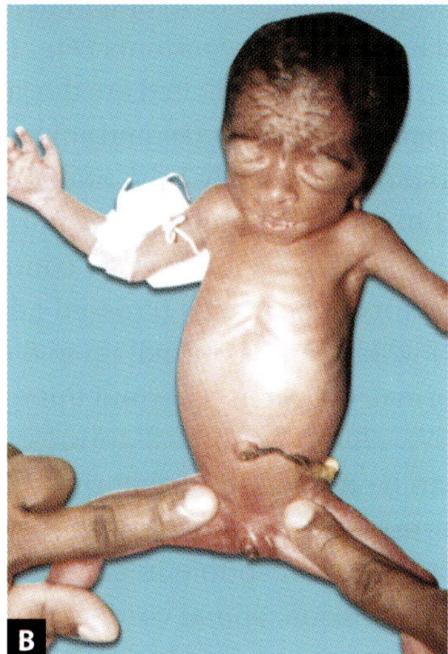

Figs. 15.30A and B: (A) Adductor angle–term baby <80°; (B) Adductor angle—preterm baby >120°.

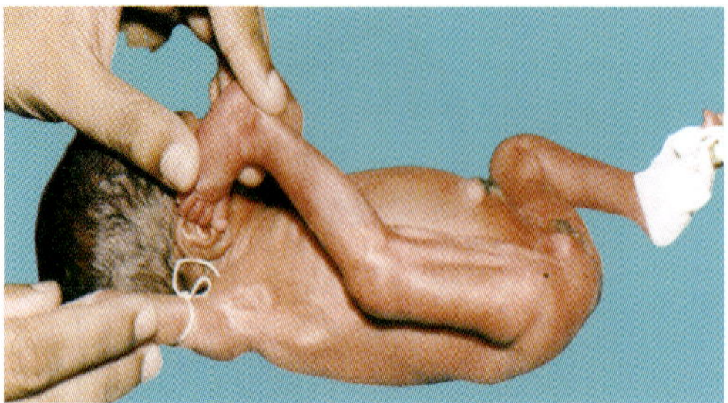

Fig. 15.31: Preterm—Heel to ear maneuver—complete extension of knee, foot touching the ear.

to shin with gentle pressure by thumb placed over the sole. Angle between the dorsum of the foot and the anterior aspect of the leg is *60–70°* in a normal newborn. It is decreased in preterm and in hypotonia and increased in hypertonia **(Fig. 15.26)**.

Deep tendon jerks elicited are the jaw jerk, biceps, knee and ankle jerks, and ankle clonus. Tendon jerks are usually brisk and are better elicited in the lower limbs in newborns. The knee jerk is normally followed by contraction of adductors of both hips (crossed adductor spread) which can be normal up to 6 m, and is abnormal, if it persists beyond this age.

Ankle clonus with 6–8 uninterrupted jerks can be normal for newborns; >12 jerks is abnormal. The deep tendon jerks become sluggish or imperceptible in general neurological depression, spinal cord lesions, peripheral nerve injuries, and hypotonia, and are exaggerated in hyperexcitability.

Reflexes

Reflexes are the sum total of an involuntary activity in response to a stimulus. They are grouped into cranial nerve, cutaneous, extensor progression, and tendon reflexes. A large number of them are primitive reflexes.

Primitive reflexes develop during intrauterine life and get gradually suppressed (but never get abolished) as the higher cortical centers become functional. By 4 m they disappear. Damage to the higher cortical centers may cause persistence or reappearance of such reflexes. Total 73 reflexes are described but the following four are important in routine evaluation:

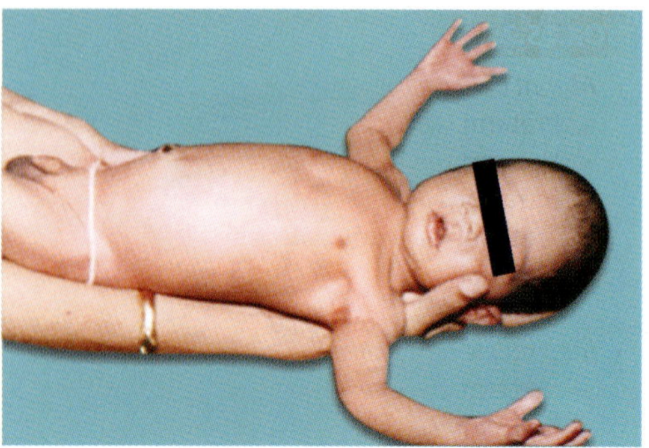

Fig. 15.32: Moro reflex—2nd phase.

1. *Moro reflex* is a vestibular reflex.

   Preferred method for eliciting: Hold the baby in semi upright posture at 45° angle (head in midline), with shoulders and back supported on left hand, and arm and occiput on the right hand of the examiner. Allow the head to fall back approximately to *30° momentarily*, with immediate support with the right hand, while the rest of the body remains supported as such. Rapid release of the hand causes sudden movement of the cervical region, which initiates the reflex revealed by abduction and extension of the upper limbs followed by flexion and adduction [embracing movement **(Fig. 15.32)**]. Hands open, thumbs remain flexed, a shrill cry may occur, followed by extension of the trunk and head and flexion of legs. See **Box 15.2** for the abnormalities in Moro reflex. In preterm >28–34 w, the adduction phase is incomplete because of the weakness of antigravity muscles. Persistence of the reflex beyond 4 m indicates cerebral dysfunction.

BOX 15.2: Abnormalities in Moro reflex.

- *Absent or sluggish:*
  - Preterm <28 w
  - Hypoxic ischemic encephalopathy
  - Intracranial hemorrhage
  - Metabolic encephalopathy
  - Sedation
  - Hypotonia
- *Incomplete adduction:*
  - Preterm 28–34 w
  - Early kernicterus
  - Hypertonia
- *Asymmetric:*
  - *Brachial* palsy
  - Fracture clavicle, humerus
  - Hemiplegia
- *Exaggerated or jumpy:*
  - Cerebral irritation
- *Extensor Moro:*
  - Kernicterus

Startle reflex is less important and differs from the Moro reflex. It is elicited by sudden loud noise or by tapping the sternum. The elbow is flexed and hands remain closed. The outward and inward movements are less intense, less simultaneous, and less symmetrical. The reflex is exaggerated in conditions with hyperacusis (Tay-Sachs disease, GM1 gangliosidosis, and Sandhoff disease), progressive degeneration of the brain, and blindness.

2. *Grasp reflex* includes palmar and plantar grasps. Palmar grasp is elicited by introducing the examiner's finger across the baby's palm from the ulnar side. The reflex consists of grasp [the baby's fingers flex and grip the examiner's finger-phase 1 **(Fig. 15.33A)**] and response to traction [grip is reinforced when the grasped finger is gently drawn upward until the baby hangs from the examiner's finger momentarily-phase 2 **(Fig. 15.33B)**]. The intensity, symmetry, and persistence of the reflex are assessed. It is less intense in preterm (grip opens on traction) and sick babies. Asymmetry indicates focal neurologic deficit. Exceptionally strong grasp reflex occurs in spastic cerebral palsy and kernicterus. The reflex normally disappears by 2–3 m. Persistence occurs in spastic cerebral palsy and it reappears in frontal lobe lesions.

   The *plantar grasp* is elicited in a similar way by introducing the examiner's finger from the lateral aspect of the plantar surface of the sole anteriorly. The toes go into flexion.

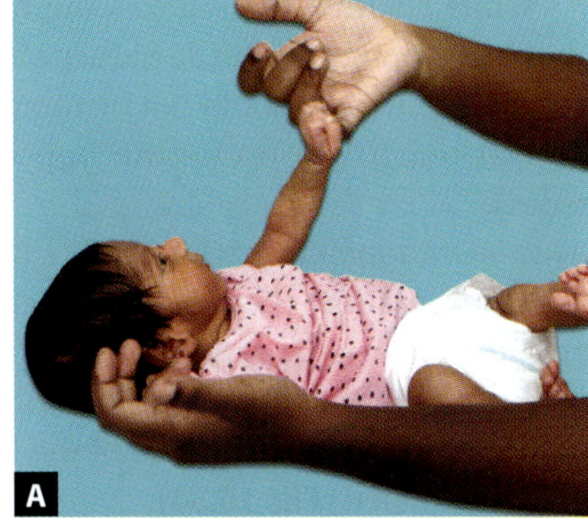

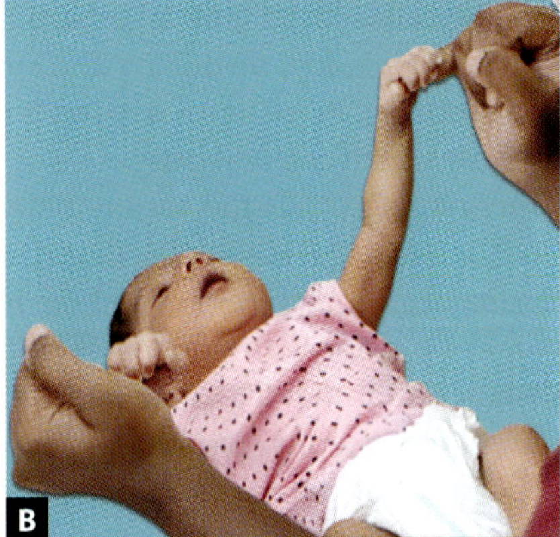

Figs. 15.33A and B: (A) Normal grasp reflex-phase 1 grasp; (B) Normal grasp reflex-phase 2 response to traction.

Courtesy: Dr. Bini Mariam Chandy, Assistant professor Pediatrics, Govt. Medical College, Kottayam.

While eliciting the reflexes the baby should be supine and the dorsal aspects of the hand and foot should not be touched (dorsal touch will excite the opposite reflex).

3. *Asymmetric tonic neck reflex (ATNR):* Baby in supine posture, the head is turned to one side to elicit the reflex. The arm and the leg on the side of the occiput will be flexed while those on the side of the face will be extended **(Fig. 15.34)**.

   The reflex is absent in generalized central depression, medullary and spinal cord damage. Persistence beyond 3 m is an early sign of cerebral palsy.
4. *Traction reflex:* Lift the supine baby by both wrists. The neck gets flexed with flexion of arms at the elbow and the head comes up along with the body for some distance and then lags. The response is absent in preterms, cerebral insult, and generalized hypotonia.

   Of the remaining reflexes the following are worth mentioning and may be elicited, when indicated.

Glabellar tap (Ref. Ch. 21): A sharp tap on the glabella (the point between eyebrows in the mid sagittal plane) produces momentary tight closure of the eyes. Reflex indicates intact functioning of cranial nerves V and VII. It is absent in paralysis of these nerves and in central depression. Repeated tapping 3–4 times elicits blinks, after which conditioning occurs. In hyperexcitability, reflex blinking occurs with each tap.

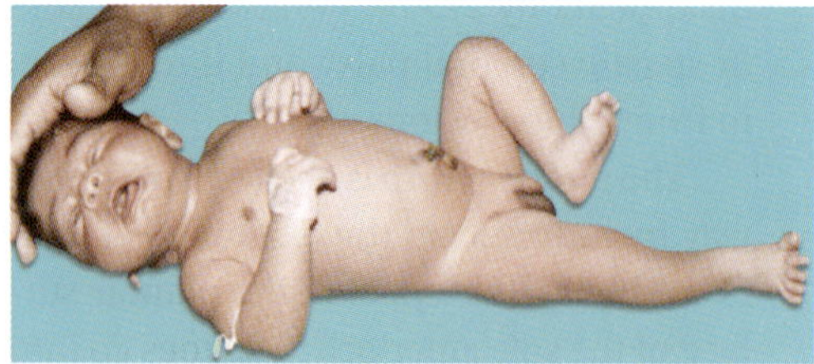

Fig. 15.34: Asymmetric tonic neck reflex.

Blink reflexes appear as blinking of the eyes due to different stimuli. If the eyes are closed there is tensing of the eyelids instead of blinking. Stimulation of the circumoral region can cause eye opening and the reflexes can be well demonstrated. Most important are:

- *Optic blink (cranial nerves II and VII):* Shine a bright light suddenly at the eyes which produces blinking. Reflex is absent in general neurological depression and impaired vision (both central and optic nerve damage).
- *Acoustic blink or cochleopalpebral reflex (cranial nerves VIII and VII):* Clap the hands 10–18 inches away from the infant's head (avoiding air stream across the face) to obtain blink response. Absence indicates central depression or impaired hearing.

Doll's eye reflex (cranial nerves III, IV, and VI): Turn head to right or left, watching the position of eyes which normally deviate to the opposite side. Absence indicates ophthalmoplegia or severe brain stem damage.

Labyrinthine reflex (cranial nerves VIII, III, IV, and VI) is the response seen to rotation. Hold the baby upright facing the examiner, keeping the hands under the baby's arms, the head being supported on each side with forefinger and middle finger, tilt forward for about 30°. Spin around two to three times. The eyes move in the direction of rotation. On stopping, the eyes move in the opposite direction and coarse nystagmus occurs. Test is negative in vestibular dysfunction and ocular palsy.

Mouth cardinal reflexes are at least ten, of which rooting, sucking, swallowing, and snout reflex are the important ones.

Rooting reflex (cranial nerve V): On light contact over the infant's cheek, the baby turns toward the point of contact. Reflex disappears after 9 m of age. It is pathologically absent in general neurological depression, prematurity, bulbar palsy, and hypotonia.

Sucking reflex (*cranial nerves IX, X, and XII*): Touch the dorsum of the tongue. Baby tries to suck. The reflex may follow the rooting reflex. Time of disappearance and abnormalities are as in rooting reflex.

Snout reflex (cranial nerves V and VII): Gentle pressure with the examiner's finger or knuckle against the baby's lips causes reflex puckering of the orbicularis oris. Time of appearance and abnormalities are as in rooting reflex.

Involuntary Movements

Involuntary movements usually seen in the newborn are tremor, jitteriness, and convulsions.

Sensory Functions

Assessment of sensations is difficult in a newborn, since the examiner has to depend on the infant's response of crying or movement to touch or to pin prick. Loss of sensation occurs in damage or injury to the spinal cord and peripheral nerves as in spina bifida, myelomeningocele, and birth injuries.

Trunk incurvation reflex (Galant reflex): Place the infant prone on a flat surface, scratch the paraspinal region (3 cm lateral to the spine) from shoulder to buttocks. Trunk curves toward the side of stimulation. Absence indicates spinal cord injury or anomaly. Persistence after 6 m indicates cerebral palsy.

Skull and Spine (Ref. Ch. 21 also)

Newborns with fetal or neonatal hypoxic insult require monitoring for 4 days for evidence of hypoxic ischemic encephalopathy (HIE). *Sarnat staging system* is widely accepted for severity assessment **(Table 15.4)**.

Levene staging is a simpler clinical staging system requiring only four clinical parameters which can be advised in resource poor settings **(Table 15.5)**.

Brainstem involvement is ominous, revealed by irregular breathing, apneic

TABLE 15.4: Sarnat staging.

Features	***Stage I***	***Stage II***	***Stage III***
Consciousness	Hyper alert	Lethargic	Stupor, coma
Muscle tone	Normal	Hypotonic	Flaccid
Posture	Normal	Flexion	Decerebrate
Tendon reflexes/Clonus	Hyperactive	Hyperactive	Absent
Myoclonus	Present	Present	Absent
Moro reflex	Strong	Weak	Absent
Pupils	Mydriasis	Miosis	Unequal, poor light reflex
Seizures	Absent	Common	Decerebration
EEG	Normal	Low voltage changing to seizure activity	Burst suppression to isoelectric
Duration of seizures	<24 hours	Seizure activity 24 hr–2 w	Days to weeks
Outcome	Good	Variable	Death, severe deficit

(EEG: electroencephalogram)

TABLE 15.5: Levene staging for hypoxic ischemic encephalopathy (HIE).

Features	***Mild***	***Moderate***	***Severe***
Sensorium	Irritable	Lethargic	Comatose
Tone	Hypotonia	Marked hypotonia	Severe hypotonia
Seizures	No	Yes	Prolonged
Sucking/respiration	Poor suck	Unable to suck	Unable to sustain spontaneous respiration

BOX 15.3: Neurologic alarm signs in the newborn.

- Persistent irritability
- Difficulty in feeding
- Persistent deviation of head or eyes
- Persistent asymmetry in posture and spontaneous movements
- Opisthotonus, excessive fisting
- Apathy, immobility
- Floppiness, persistent hypotonia
- Hyperexcitability, jitteriness
- Convulsions
- Abnormal crying
- Sunset sign, vomiting, wide sutures, abnormal increase in OFC
- Occurrence and recurrence of respiratory difficulties, apneic episodes
- Loss of variability in respiration, heart rate, and oxygen tension
- Midline lesions of the spine

(OFC: occipitofrontal circumference)

attacks, changes in pupil size and disconjugate eye movements, poor sucking and swallowing, and pooling of secretions in the mouth. **Box 15.3** reveals the neurological alarm signs in newborns.

GASTROINTESTINAL SYSTEM AND ABDOMEN

Gastrointestinal system and abdomen (Ref. Ch. 20): Examine the mouth and oral cavity, when the baby is relaxed. Abdomen shows minimal distension due to aerophagia during feeding and crying. Scaphoid abdomen may indicate diaphragmatic hernia (Ref. **Fig. 20.19**). In Prune Belly syndrome, abdominal wall muscles are absent revealing wrinkled hypotonic picture **(Fig. 15.35)**. Observe the movements of the diaphragm to exclude paralysis.

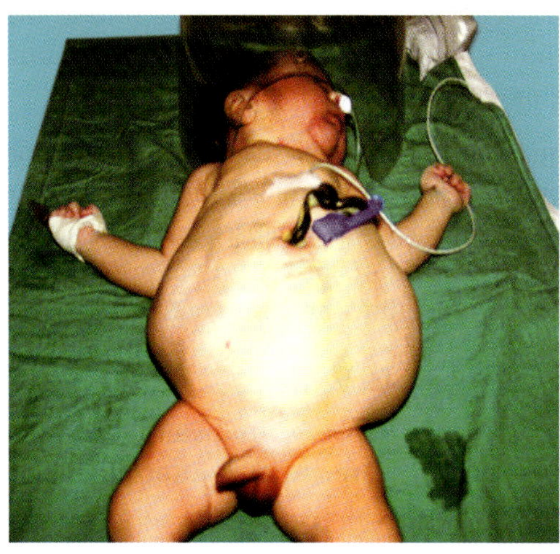

Fig. 15.35: Prune Belly syndrome.

Umbilical cord may be yellow in color, if the amniotic fluid is meconium stained. The cord separates by 5–7 days leaving a raw area for few days before it heals. Umbilical hernia may be seen in some newborns and is often associated with diastasis recti (Ref. **Fig. 7.40**) (a midline defect in abdominal muscles).

Umbilical granuloma is dull red or pink granulation tissue, soft in consistency with slight mucoid or mucopurulent discharge. It must be differentiated from umbilical polyp which is firm and resistant, is bright red, and may reveal mucoid, fecal, or urine discharge. Features of pyogenic infections of the umbilicus are pus discharge, foul smell, and/or periumbilical erythema **(Fig. 15.36)**.

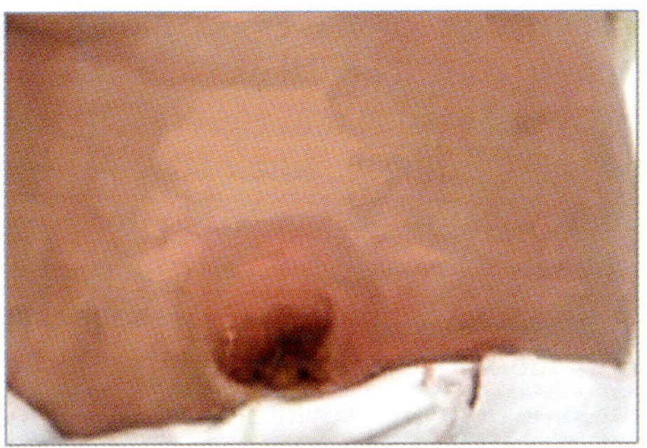

Fig. 15.36: Umbilical infection.

Bleeding from the umbilical cut end is usually due to inadequate ligation. Trauma, failure of normal thrombus formation, hemorrhagic disease of the newborn, other coagulopathies (factor XIII deficiency), septicemia, local infection, and disseminated intravascular coagulation are other causes of umbilical bleeding.

Inguinal hernia appears mostly on the right side since the processus vaginalis closes earlier on the left side. The liver is usually palpable 2 cm below the costal margin; liver span is normally <6 cm. Abdominal distension, prominent visible peristalsis, and bilious vomiting indicate anomalies of the intestine leading to obstruction. In most newborns the spleen is palpable just below the costal margin and kidneys are normally palpable.

Bimanual palpation of kidneys is done with the thumb on the lumbar quadrant of the abdomen and other fingers on the lumbar region on the back. Evaluate other masses in the abdomen by palpation. Elicit shifting dullness and fluid thrill, if the abdomen is distended. Bowel sounds should be auscultated.

Examine the *genitalia* (Ref. Ch. 7 for more details) for any abnormality. In a term infant, scrotum is large, pendulous and darkly pigmented, and testes are easily palpable. Measure the stretched penile length *(SPL)* (Ref. Ch. 7, 24) to exclude *micropenis* which is a diagnostic sign of *hypopituitarism*. Prepuce is not retractable in the newborn. Hymenal tags are mucosal tags seen at the margin of the hymen in some babies. Grayish white mucoid discharge from vagina can be seen in normal babies. Vaginal bleeding, if profuse or lasts longer than 5 days, other causes for bleeding should be excluded.

CARDIOVASCULAR SYSTEM (REF. CH. 17 ALSO)

Pulse

Palpate the femoral and brachial pulses on both sides simultaneously, since the difference in volume may indicate coarctation of the aorta (COA) and anomalous origin of the subclavian artery. The femoral pulses are feeble or absent and upper limb pulses are of higher volume in COA. All the pulses will be of low volume and feeble when the baby is collapsed due to any reason. CHDs presenting as collapse in early neonatal life are *hypoplastic left heart syndrome, severe aortic stenosis, and some cases of COA*. High volume pulses in all peripheral vessels suggest patent ductus arteriosus (PDA), truncus arteriosus, large arteriovenous fistulae, and aortopulmonary septal defect and communications.

Blood Pressure

Indirect measurement by conventional auscultatory method using sphygmomanometer, gives more accurate values but is difficult in newborns because of the difficulty in palpating and auscultating the vessels properly. The *flush method* is easier to apply. The limb is raised and squeezed till the hand becomes pale. The manometer cuff (size 2.5–4 cm) is applied over the arm and is

TABLE 15.6: BP in newborns at 12 hr of life.

	BP (mm Hg)		
Birth weight (g)	***Systolic***	***Diastolic***	***Mean***
1,001–2,000	50	30	38
2,001–3,000	59	35	42
>3,000	60	41	50

inflated to a pressure above 110 mm Hg. The limb is then lowered and placed on the baby's side. Release the pressure by 5 mm Hg. The point at which the limb becomes pink and flushed is the systolic blood pressure (SBP), which is a little lower than the reading obtained by the auscultatory method **(Table 15.6)**. The diastolic pressure cannot be measured using this technique. SBP persistently above 100 mm Hg in a relaxed newborn is suggestive of hypertension.

Normally babies are pink. Cold environment can cause peripheral cyanosis which has to be differentiated from ecchymosis (the latter will not blanch to pressure). The differentiation between central and peripheral cyanosis is essential. In a collapsed baby (due to any reason) even the tongue will be cyanosed. In the absence of cardiac disease, central cyanosis may be seen in a crying newborn due to right to left shunt across the patent foramen ovale (PFO) or PDA and with high levels of hemoglobin causing hyperviscosity. Central cyanosis in a neonate may be due to cardiac and respiratory disorders, central depression or methemoglobinemia. In babies with cardiac or pulmonary problems breathing effort will be vigorous whereas the effort is normal in methemoglobinemia. In central depression breathing will be weak and irregular.

Hyperoxia test: Administering 100% oxygen to the baby is an effective and simple method to differentiate between cardiac and pulmonary causes of cyanosis. After oxygen administration, if partial pressure of oxygen (PaO_2) exceeds 100 mm Hg, cyanotic heart disease is unlikely, whereas remarkable improvement in oxygen tension occurs in respiratory disease. Intensity of cyanosis can be appreciated clinically and SpO_2 can be documented by pulse oximetry. This test should be done in all cyanotic babies without clinical evidence of cardiac disease, if the cause of central cyanosis is not clear.

Noncardiac malformations are seen in 20% of newborns with CHDs, the common associations being ear, limb, and vertebral anomalies. Tracheoesophageal malformations associated with vertebral, anorectal, cardiac, renal, radial, and limb anomalies form the VATER or VACTERL syndromes. Since CHDs are common in chromosomal anomalies, intrauterine infections, and genetic syndromes, physical features of these clinical conditions should be evaluated.

Jugular venous pressure is difficult to assess in newborns since the neck is short. Extension of the neck and turning to either side will help to visualize abnormal arterial and venous pulsations.

Precordium: Cardiac apex in the newborn lies usually at the 4th left intercostal space in the midclavicular line. If not located on the left side, scrutinize on the right side. Apical impulse is obtained on the right side in dextrocardia (heart on the right chest) and dextroposition (displacement of heart to the right) due to many causes as given in **Box 15.4**.

Shift of the apical impulse further to the left may occur due to the same etiological factors on the opposite side. Consider cardiomegaly, if the apical impulse is perceived 1 cm outside the midclavicular line on the left side, with the right border of heart normally located. If the impulse is not obtained on either sides

BOX 15.4: Causes of dextroposition of heart.

- *Left side:*
  - Pneumothorax
  - Pleural effusion
  - Congenital lobar emphysema
  - Diaphragmatic hernia
  - Eventration of diaphragm
- *Right side:*
  - Agenesis of lung
  - Atelectasis of lung
- *Thoracic cage:*
  - Congenital anomalies (vertebrae, ribs)
  - Birth trauma

suspect pericardial effusion or myocardial disease; care fully assess cardiac size by light percussion.

Auscultation of the heart in newborns should be with small-sized chest piece. In the initial 48 hr of life, both heart sounds appear single. Normal splitting of the second heart sound (develops after 48 hr), and is difficult to detect because of the physiologic tachycardia. Soft early systolic clicks can be normal in newborns. Cardiac murmurs are often associated with thrills in neonates. Transient cardiac murmurs, mostly systolic, may be revealed in 10% of newborns in the initial 48 hours of life.

Significant cardiac murmurs are often loud (*grade III or more in intensity*) associated with ejection clicks and abnormal second heart sound. Absence of cardiac murmur does not exclude the possibility of heart disease. In a severely symptomatic baby, serious underlying heart disease should be suspected with insignificant cardiac murmur or even without any murmur. Murmurless heart diseases in newborns are given in **Box 15.5**. In conditions with left to right shunt, murmurs usually appear by the end of 1 month, when the pulmonary artery pressure falls; the baby becomes symptomatic by this period.

BOX 15.5: Cardiac diseases without murmur in newborns (murmurless heart diseases).

- *With cardiomegaly*
  - *Acyanotic*
    - Anomalous origin of left coronary artery from pulmonary artery
    - Coarctation of aorta
    - Endocardial fibroelastosis
    - Primary cardiomyopathies
    - Pompe disease
    - Pericardial cyst/effusion
    - Arrhythmias (supraventricular and ventricualr tachycardias, complete heart block)
    - Hypertension
  - *Cyanotic*
    - Hypoplastic left heart syndrome
    - Persistent fetal circulation
    - Transposition of the great arteries with intact ventricular septum
- *Without Cardiomegaly (cyanotic only)*
  - *Ebstein anomaly*
  - *Hypoplastic right heart syndrome*

Babies with cardiopulmonary distress may develop flow murmurs like tricuspid regurgitation murmurs due to right ventricular dilatation. The murmur disappears as the clinical condition improves. Continuous murmurs with severe cyanosis indicate pulmonary atresia with collaterals in the lung.

Dyspnea, tachypnea, excessive scalp sweating, feeble cry, interrupted feeding, refusal of feeds, listlessness, interrupted sleep, and poor weight gain are the usual symptoms of congestive cardiac failure (CCF). Signs of CCF are tachycardia (>180/min), tachypnea (RR >60/min), increased chest excursion, sudden weight gain, puffiness of eyelids, presacral edema, generalized edema, cardiomegaly, abnormalities in heart sounds, presence of murmurs, tender hepatomegaly, and crackles and wheezes in lungs.

RESPIRATORY SYSTEM (REF. CH. 19 ALSO)

Examine the nostrils for any block due to secretions which are relieved by sneezing. Congenital obstructions like bilateral choanal atresia produce severe respiratory distress. Persistent rhinitis with serosanguinous discharge indicate congenital syphilis; detailed examination will reveal other features of syphilis.

Stridor (Ch. 19) may manifest immediately after birth, within a few hr or after some days. The most common condition presenting with stridor after a few days of life is laryngomalacia; The causes of early stridor in newborns are given in **Box 15.6**.

Examination of the lower respiratory tract includes the rate, rhythm, type of breathing (diaphragmatic in newborns) and chest retractions. Upper airway obstructions are characterized by suprasternal, supraclavicular, and lower sternal retractions whereas subcostal and intercostal retractions, fast breathing (>60/min), flaring of alae nasi, cyanosis, and grunting indicate severe lower respiratory disease. Clinical scoring systems for respiratory distress can be used for assessing the severity of the disease. See **Tables 15.7 and 15.8** for the details of scoring systems.

BOX 15.6: Causes of early onset stridor in newborns.

- *Laryngeal*
  - *Congenital:*
    - Laryngomalacia
    - Atresia, stenosis, webs
    - Cysts
    - Chondromalacia (severe form)
    - Hemangiomas
    - Lymphangiomas
    - Neoplasia
  - *Acquired:*
    - Aspiration (meconium, mucus)
    - Edema larynx
    - Paralysis of vocal cords
    - Tetany
- *Extralaryngeal:*
  - *Congenital*
    - Glossoptosis (due to various causes)
    - Macroglossia
    - Aberrant blood vessels
    - Tumors, cysts of neck
  - *Acquired:*
    - Bleeding around larynx
    - Cellulitis of neck

TABLE 15.7: Clinical scoring system for respiratory distress—Downe's score.

Findings	***Score 0***	***1***	***2***
Air entry	Good	Decreased	Not audible
Cyanosis	Nil in room air	Nil with 40% oxygen	Present with 40% oxygen
Grunting	None	Audible with stethoscope	Audible without stethoscope
RR*/min	<60	60–80	>80
Retraction	Nil	Mild	Moderate-to-severe

*Respiratory rate.
Note: Score >3 indicates serious illness.

TABLE 15.8: Silverman Andersen score.

Feature	***0***	***1***	***2***
Upper chest movement	None	Respiratory lag	See-saw respiration
Lower chest retractions	None	Minimal	Marked
Xiphoid retractions	None	Minimal	Marked
Nasal flaring	None	Minimal	Marked
Grunting	None	Audible with stethoscope	Audible without stethoscope

Note: Score >7 = Impending respiratory failure.

Palpation of the chest is not much helpful to confirm the position of mediastinum. Vocal fremitus may be felt when the baby is crying. Light percussion helps to assess the upper border of liver dullness and to diagnose pneumothorax. Auscultation of the chest should be by using a stethoscope with small chest piece as in older children. In the absence of any clinical signs of respiratory illness, the possibility of metabolic disorders should be considered as the cause.

SUGGESTED READING

1. Illingworth's: The Development of the Infant and Young Child: Normal and Abnormal 11e, 2021, Illingworth (Author) Publisher: Elsevier.
2. Manual of Neonatal Care, 2nd South Asian Edition (Paperback) 2023, Navee Jain (Author) Wolters Kluwer India Pvt.Ltd.
3. Rees EP. Evaluating the Newborn Infant: Diagnostic Approach in Pediatric Clinical Skills 2/e, 1997. Ed Goldbloom RG; Churchill-Livingstone, USA. pp. 49-75

16 CHAPTER

Daily Examination of the Newborn

L Rajam, S Radhika

Chapter Outline

INTRODUCTION

Detailed examination of the baby is not needed daily unless the baby is critically ill; frequent handling of the baby is harmful due to transmission of infections. Mother's presence is ideally needed while examining the healthy baby also to clarify her minor doubts and to improve her confidence especially in feeding the baby. Proceed asunder the following headlines:

- Physiology of the newborn
- Danger signs in the newborn
- Evaluation of jaundice, infections
- Evaluation of the sick baby
- Assessment of breastfeeding
- Examination at discharge

PHYSIOLOGY OF THE NEWBORN

- A term healthy baby should be active revealing periodic limb movements and episodes of wakefulness, interspersed with sleep; should feed well and cry vigorously when wet or hungry.
- Persistent crying in a newborn indicates illness or pain.
- The newborn should sleep at least 18 hr/day with periods of wakefulness in-between. Excessive sleepiness may be observed in some babies in the initial 48 hr, but the baby should be arousable.
- Meconium may be passed immediately after labor and should be passed within 24 hr after delivery. Urine should be passed within 48 hr after delivery.
- Baby should be sucking the breast actively, pass urine at least 6 times daily, and pass stools everyday (usually after each feed).
- Repeated vomiting is abnormal and needs evaluation.
- Assess whether the body is pink and warm. Cyanosis requires detailed evaluation. Mild jaundice (Kramer index **Fig. 15.13** or <10 mg/dL) can be ignored. Infections of the conjunctiva, skin, umbilicus, or oral thrush are often nosocomial. Recheck for undetected minor anomalies and birth injuries.
- Difficulties encountered in breastfeeding should be checked daily and must be corrected. Assess Latch score for the adequacy of breastfeeding; correct the maternal breast problems **(Table 16.1)**. Score ≥8 indicates good attachment.

DANGER SIGNS IN THE NEWBORN

Ask and look for danger signs in the newborn as given in **Box 16.1**.

Neonates with danger signs should be categorized as sick babies; their further evaluation should be that of sick babies.

TABLE 16.1: Latch scoring.

	0	*1*	*2*
L—Latch	• Too sleepy or reluctant • No latch achieved	• Repeated attempts • Hold nipple in mouth • Stimulate to suck	• Grasps breast • Tongue down • Lips flanged • Rhythmic sucking
A—Audible swallowing	None	A few with stimulation	• Spontaneous and intermittent <24 hr old • Spontaneous and frequent • >24 hr old
T—Type of nipple	Inverted	Flat	Everted (after stimulation)
C—Comfort (breast/nipple)	• Engorged • Cracked, bleeding, large blisters or bruises • Severe discomfort	• Filling • Reddened/small blisters or bruises • Mild/moderate discomfort	• Soft • Nontender
H—Hold (positioning)	Full assist (staff holds infant at breast)	• Minimal assist (i.e., elevate head of bed, place pillows for support) • Teach one side; mother does other • Staff holds and then mother takes over	• No assist from staff • Mother able to position/hold infant

BOX 16.1: Danger signs in the newborn.

- Lethargy
- Drowsiness
- Pallor
- Poor feeding
- Excessive cry
- Abdominal distension
- Convulsions
- Apneic episodes
- Bleeding
- Breathing difficulty
- Choking at feeds
- Cyanosis
- Vomiting/diarrhea
- Drooling
- Edema
- Skin changes—mottling, sclerema
- Superficial infections **(Fig. 16.1)**
- Failure to pass meconium and urine (<24 hr), urine (<48 hr)
- Grunting
- Hypo-/hyperthermia
- Jaundice <24 hr or deep jaundice **(Fig. 16.2)**

Evaluation of sick babies should be done daily or more frequently as the situation demands. The approach should be systematic **(Box 16.2)**. A multichannel vital signs monitor including sensor for arterial oxygen saturation is ideally needed for monitoring.

Rapid evaluation of the sick neonate can be done by the acronym *"STOPS"* (S—Skin and sensorium, T—Temperature, O—Oxygenation, P—Perfusion, S—Sugar).

Skin: Look for peripheral cyanosis (cold stress), plethora, pallor, or central cyanosis.

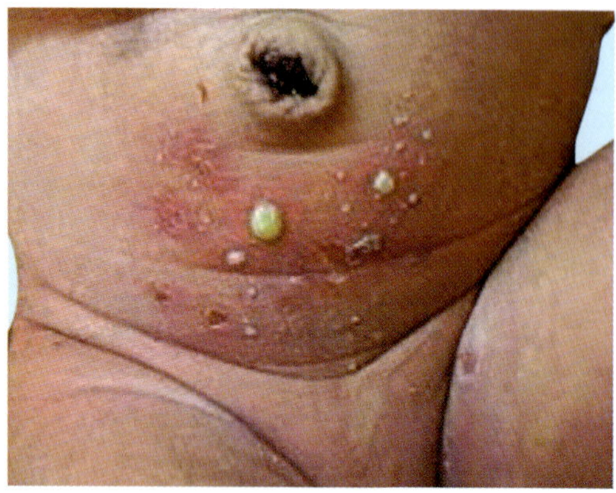

Fig. 16.1: Neonatal impetigo.

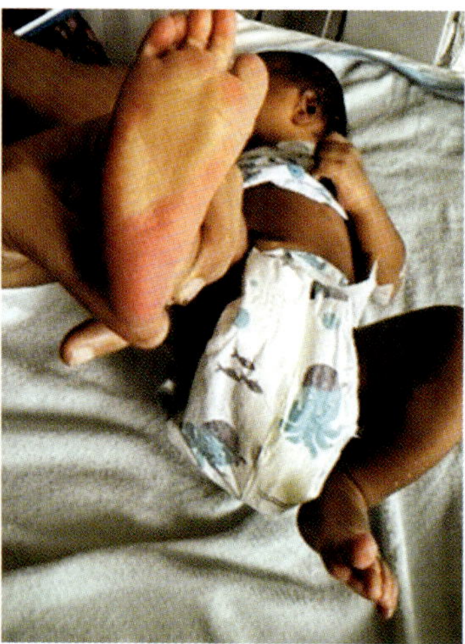

Fig. 16.2: Neonate with deep jaundice revealing yellow staining of the sole.

Courtesy: Dr Bini Mariam Chandy, Assistant Professor of Pediatrics, Govt Medial College, Kottayam, Kerala, India.

Sensorium:

- Active (normal tone, respiration, good cry spontaneous movements)
- Lethargic (floppy, hypotonic with poor responsiveness, weak cry and requires constant observation and investigations)

Temperature: Cool hands and feet indicate hypothermia (<36°C—perceived by the dorsum of the examiner's hand).

BOX 16.2: Evaluation of sick baby.

- Appearance, posture, alertness, abnormal movements, GCS, and Moro reflex
- *Vitals:* BP, HR, RR, temperature, pulse oximetry status
- Head to foot examination—AF, bleeding, CRT, color, hydration, stomach aspirate (quantity and color), stools, urine output (monitor every 3 hours)
- Fluid intake—output, weight recording daily
- Systemic examination
- Evaluation of investigations

(AF: Anterior fontanelle; CRT: Capillary refill time; GCS: Glasgow coma scale; HR: heart rate; RR: respiratory rate)

Oxygenation: Respiratory rate >60 breaths/min or chest indrawing indicates respiratory distress. Assess the severity by the clinical scoring systems for respiratory distress as given in **Tables 15.6 and 15.7**.

Perfusion: Early signs of impaired perfusion (compensated shock) are cool peripheries despite proper covering or using radiant warmer and CRT >3 seconds. Late signs of poor perfusion (decompensated shock) are altered sensorium, poor pulses, low BP and signs of organ dysfunction like mottled skin, oliguria, feed intolerance, abdominal distension, and vomiting.

Blood sugar: Hypoglycemia (<40 mg/dL) should be anticipated in preterm and intrauterine growth restricted babies, infants of diabetic mothers and any sick neonate.

Scoring systems available to assess the disease severity and to predict morbidity and mortality in sick newborns are the CRIB (clinical risk index for babies—developed in UK) and the SNAP (score for neonatal acute physiology—USA).

Musculoskeletal system: Detailed examination of skull, all flat bones, vertebrae, and long bones is mandatory as a part of routine examination of newborns to detect musculoskeletal anomalies such as developmental dysplasia of hip, septic arthritis, and osteomyelitis.

Examination of the baby at discharge: Detailed examination is a must at discharge (ideally at 1 week of age) especially to detect minor congenital anomalies, posterior cleft palate, birth injuries, cephalohematoma, new heart murmurs and umbilical sepsis and to assess breastfeeding adequacy. Hearing and vision assessment are to be arranged by 2 w of age especially for preterm babies. Mother should be medically stable, confident to look after the baby and breastfeed without any cracked nipple. Feeding technique would have been adequately verified prior to discharge. High-risk babies should be advised for follow-up at 2 w for growth monitoring and neurodevelopmental evaluation.

Ref. Appendix 1, Fig. 11.5: Growth charts for Preterm babies No. 11–16; Intrauterine Growth chart No. 17.

SUGGESTED READING

1. Agarwal R, Sethi A. Newborn Care. In: Paul VK, Bagga A (Eds). Ghai Essenial Pediatrics 10th edition, 2023 BS Publishers and distributors, Pvt Ltd, New Delhi 110002, India pp. 119-184.
2. Bernstein S, Heimler R, Sasidharan P. Approaching the management of the neonatal intensive care unit graduate through history and physical assessment. Pediatr Clin North Am. 1998;45:79-105.
3. Cloherty JP, Stark AR. Manual of Neonatal Care, 4th edition. Philadelphia: Lippincott-Raven. 1997.
4. Day RE, Baird G, Salt A. Developmental Pediatrics. In: Mc Intosh, Helms, Smyth (Eds). Forfar and Arneil's Textbook of Pediatrics, 6th edition. Philadelphia USA: Elsevier Ltd.; 2003.
5. Fenton TR, Kim JH. A systematic review and meta-analysis to revise the Fenton growth chart for preterm infants. BMC Pediatr. 2013; 13:59.
6. Gondy GM. Examination of the neonate including gestational age assessment. In: Roberton NRC II (Ed). Text book of Neonatology. Edinburgh. Churchill Livingston; 1992.
7. Illingworth RS. Development of the infant and young child. Normal and Abnormal 8th edition. Edinburgh: Churchill Livingston; 1985.
8. Jain N. Cloherty and Stark's Manual of Neonatal Care, 2nd South Asian Edition 2023, Wolters Kluwer India (Publisher), Pvt Ltd.
9. Jensen D, Wallace S, Kelsay P. LATCH—a breastfeeding charting system and documentation tool. J Obstet Gynecol Neonatal Nurs. 1994;23(1):27-32.
10. Liptak GS. The child who has severe neurologic impairment. Pediatr Clin North Am. 1998;45:123-43.

SECTION

Basic System Examination

CHAPTER

Cardiovascular System

S Letha, M Zulfikar Ahamed

Chapter Outline

INTRODUCTION

Please read chapters 6, 7, 11, 12, and 15 before you proceed.

Technological advances in the past few decades have brought tremendous progress in the early diagnosis of childhood cardiovascular diseases and their timely correction. Still cardiac diseases continue to remain as one of the common concerns for the primary care pediatrician. Along with the infants with congenital heart diseases (CHDs) of various types and subsequent complications, a group of survivors of newborn and infant cardiac interventions with differing problems are added. Innocent cardiac murmurs, chest pain, syncope and palpitation, and CHD becoming clinically evident later are increasingly observed. Rheumatic heart disease has been replaced by Kawasaki disease (KD), myocarditis, long QTc syndrome, drug-induced heart diseases, childhood hypertension and arrhythmias. Thus, the cardiovascular system (CVS) examination continues to be challenging to the students and residents in pediatrics which can be overcome only by methodical clinical approach and mastering the auscultatory skills.

CARDIAC HISTORY

History should include family details, antenatal, natal, and postnatal problems, and symptoms of cardiovascular disease. Family history of sudden death, rheumatic fever, sudden infant death syndrome, and structural cardiac abnormality in a first-degree relative, all have diagnostic relevance. Hypertrophic cardiomyopathy (HCM) in a first-degree relative has a 50% inheritance pattern. Gestational diabetes mellitus is commonly associated with the transposition of great arteries (TGAs) and neonatal transient HCM apart from other congenital structural abnormalities. Ask for acute or chronic maternal diseases, congenital infections, and drug use. Perinatal asphyxia in a baby may produce persistence of fetal circulation. Neonatal sepsis may lead to cardiac failure.

- *Symptoms and signs of heart disease*: Physical growth, development, and history of past illnesses are relevant. Failure to thrive (weight gain of <15 g/day) in an infant or child with heart disease may reflect the duration and severity of the disease and the poor effectiveness of treatment.

- *Pulsus alternans* is strong and weak pulses occurring alternatively, encountered in left ventricular failure (LVF) and myocarditis due to severe damage of the ventricular muscle.
- *Pulsus paradoxus:* Normal peak fall in arterial pressure (5–10 mm Hg) during inspiration is exaggerated [large pericardial effusion (PE)] or severe asthma) as inspiratory fall in SBP occurs to >10 mm Hg. In large PE, the pericardial fluid restricts the cardiac volume. When the right ventricular (RV) volume increases during inspiration, the left ventricular (LV) volume falls, decreasing the arterial pulse volume. The paradox is that the heart sounds are heard without a palpable pulse. Pulsus paradoxus and pulsus alternans are assessed more reliably from BP recording.
- *Pulse pressure (PP)* is the difference between SBP and DBP (normal 30–40 mm Hg). Wide PP (>50 mm Hg in children and >60 mm Hg in adults) is seen in collapsing pulse; it is narrow (PP <30 mm Hg) in low cardiac output (CHF, cardiomyopathy, and shock), mitral stenosis (MS), AS, pericardial tamponade, and constrictive pericarditis.
- *Pulse volume (PV)* by palpation is a rough guide to the PP; BP measurement is superior.
- Check all the visible pulsations over the neck and other arteries. All pulses routinely described are peripheral pulses. Carotid pulse is the central pulse. A comment on carotid pulse should be made always at the end of the pulse description.

Example

Baby girl, 1 yr with PDA, pulse can be described as rate 120/min, regular rhythm, high volume, collapsing in character, all peripheral pulsations are equally felt and there is no radiofemoral delay; the carotid pulse is prominently felt and seen.

VENOUS EXAMINATION

The *internal jugular venous* pulse indicates right atrial pressure (RAP) but is difficult to assess in infants and young children. Assess the waveforms and venous pressure. The venous pulse has three positive waves (a, c, and v) and two negative waves (x and y). The "a" wave is due to atrial contraction, and is followed by the "x" descent which is interrupted by a small "c" wave (rarely visible). The "c" wave coincides with the onset of ventricular systole. The "v" wave is the result of right atrial filling when the tricuspid valve is still closed. When the tricuspid valve opens, blood enters the RV and the resultant lowering of RAP is the "y" descent.

Internal jugular venous pulsations are not seen normally since the pulsation level in the vein is at the level of the sternal angle. Reclining at an angle of 45°, the waves are just below the clavicle but the a, c, and v waves may appear above the clavicle. When the RAP is raised, the mean level of pulsations reaches above the clavicle; the jugular venous pressure (JVP) is measured by the vertical distance from the sternal angle to the imaginary line at the upper end of the jugular venous column (Ref. **Fig. 17.5A, B**). JVP is elevated if this vertical distance from the sternal angle is >3 cm in children and >4 cm in adults.

JVP observation is useful in older children having CHF, CHD, PE, constrictive pericarditis, and mediastinal mass. Prominent "a" waves occur in right ventricular hypertrophy (RVH) with increased resistance to atrial filling (TA and stenosis, PH, and PS). Absent "a" waves occur in AF. Giant "a" waves (Cannon waves) are seen when the atrium contracts against a closed AV valve as in AV junctional rhythm, complete heart block, ectopic beats, and VT.

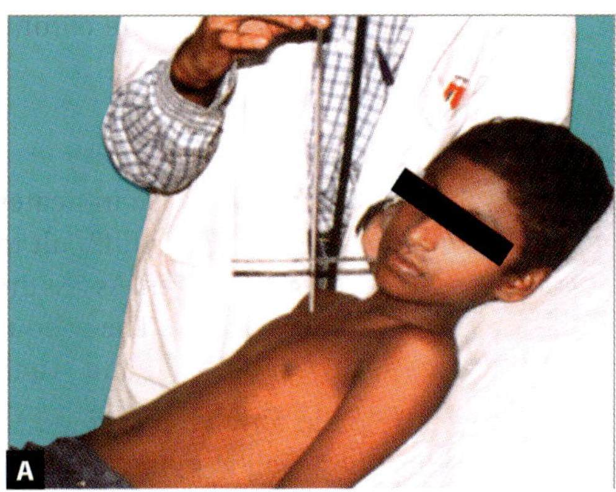

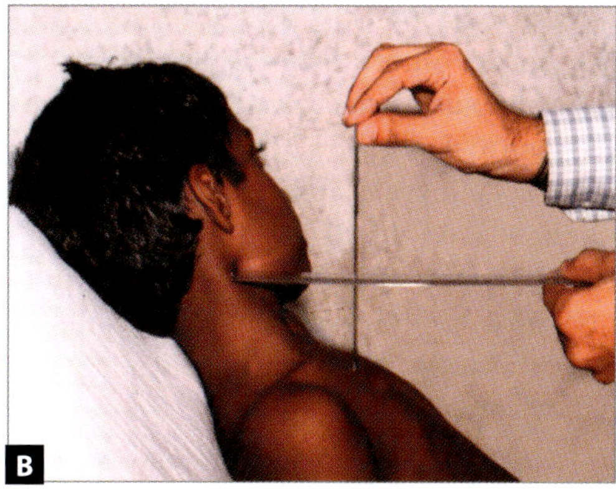

Figs. 17.5A and B: (A) Measuring the JVP; (B) Measuring the JVP Level.

Prominent "v" wave is seen in tricuspid regurgitation (TR) due to the regurgitation of blood into the right atrium during right ventricular systole. This systolic "v" wave is followed by a prominent "y" descent.

THE LIVER

In infants and small children, the character and size of the liver is a reliable indicator of systemic venous congestion. Assess the position, size, and consistency of the liver in an unhurried manner. Locate the liver edge at the lateral margin of the rectus muscle and measure the span (Ref. Ch. 20). The margin normally feels like the cartilage of the external auricular pinna and is sharp and angulated. In CHF liver enlarges, becomes tender with rounded and firm margins, and is more difficult to feel. In storage disorders involving the myocardium and in long-standing CHF, the liver enlarges with firm-to-hard consistency. In TA liver becomes elnlarged, is tender and is pulsatile which can be perceived at the epigastrium.

PRECORDIAL EXAMINATION

Precordium is the area of the chest overlying the heart. Describe the clinical findings in relation to the landmarks on the precordium. The ribs and intercostal spaces on either side form the horizontal landmarks. Locate the sternal angle (angle of Louis) and run the finger outward to reach the second costal cartilage. The space above this is the first intercostal space. Count the spaces down away from the sternum. The vertical landmarks are formed by some artificial lines. The midpoint of the space between the suprasternal notch and tip of the acromion when projected down forms the midclavicular line (MCL). The anterior, posterior, and midaxillary lines descend from the anterior and posterior borders and the middle of the axilla, respectively.

Systematic examination of the heart is done by inspection, palpation, percussion, and auscultation.

Inspection

Keep the child in a supine lying position; young babies will be comfortable on the mother's lap. The examiner's eyes should be at the level of the patient's precordium. Look for *precordial bulge* (indicates long-standing cardiac problems with cardiomegaly) by standing at the foot end of the patient. Then stand at the right side of the patient and look for *bulging of the intercostal spaces* (seen in PE).

Next look for *cardiac pulsations*. The lowest and outermost point of definite cardiac impulse is the *apical impulse*, noted in relation to the nipple and midclavicular line. If cardiac impulse is absent on the left side, search for it on the right side (dextrocardia and dextroposition). Look for other pulsations over the precordium, epigastrium, and suprasternal and parasternal regions and on the right side.

A wave of pulsations on the left, toward the apical impulse is seen in left ventricular hypertrophy (LVH) or volume overload, left atrial enlargement, and aortic aneurysm. Prominent epigastric pulsations are suggestive of RVH, aortic aneurysm and a pulsatile liver in TA. Pulsations in the second left intercostal space (LICS) may be from a dilated pulmonary artery, enlarged left atrium, or due to hyperkinetic circulation. Suprasternal pulsations are prominent in AR, carotid aneurysms, and hyperkinetic states.

Look for surgical scars which can be median sternotomy scar (open heart surgery), left posterolateral thoracotomy scar (in PDA ligation, COA repair, closed mitral valvotomy, BT-shunt), and right posterolateral thoracotomy scar of right Blalock–Taussig (BT) shunt.

Precordium is described as hyperkinetic or hyperdynamic when pulsations are prominent, seen in left to right shunt, mitral regurgitation (MR), AR, anemia, thyrotoxicosis, etc. Precordium is quiet or silent in PE, Ebstein anomaly (EA), TOF, and endomyocardial fibrosis.

Palpation

Apply the entire palm and hand (should be warm) over the chest wall to detect thrills or heaves. The palmar surface of the metacarpals and first phalanges are more sensitive for detecting low-frequency events but fingertips are best to localize an abnormality (Ref. **Fig. 17.6A, B**).

Palpate the apical impulse to confirm the position and character; start searching from the axilla with the palm. Localize the impulse with fingertip (better appreciated on sitting and leaning forward). The apex should be confined to one intercostal space at all ages; describe it as diffuse if equally dynamic in more than one interspace.

Age-wise change in the position of the apical impulse is shown in **Table 17.4**.

Always search for the apical impulse on the right side and other areas if not felt in the normal position.

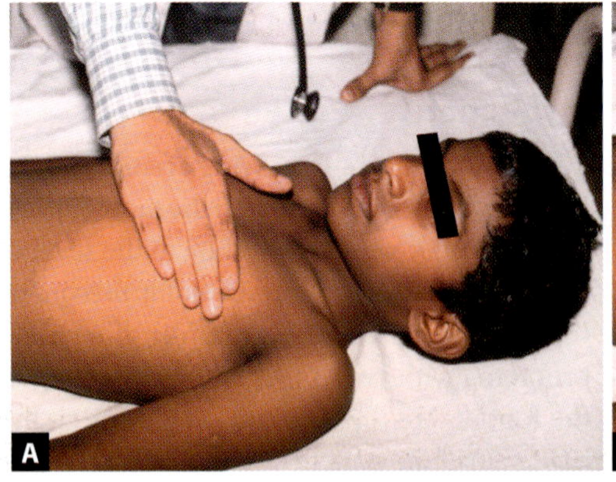

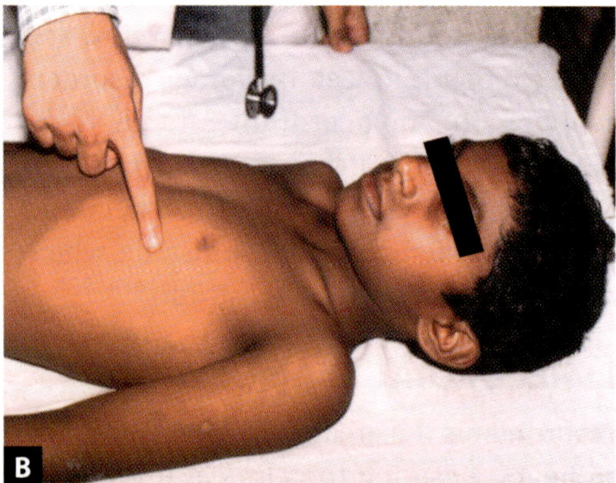

Figs. 17.6A and B: (A) Palpation to locate the apex beat; (B) Locating the apical impulse.

TABLE 17.4: Age-wise change in location of apical impulse.

Age in years	*Location*
>7 yrs	Fifth LICS 1 cm inside MCL
4–7 yr	Fifth LICS in the MCL
<4 yr	Fourth LICS up to 1 cm outside MCL

(LICS: left intercostal space; MCL: midclavicular line)

See **Box 15.5** for the causes of cardiomegaly in newborns.

The apical impulse is felt forceful but less sustained (forceful or hyperkinetic apex) in left ventricular dilatation due to volume overload as in AR, MR, and large left to right shunts. In the *heaving apex*, the impulse is sustained for some time (no displacement). It is characteristic of raised left ventricular pressure (LVP) without dilatation seen in AS and systemic hypertension (SH). *Tapping apex* (just taps the palpating fingers) occurs in RVH as in MS and also in fever and anxiety.

Parasternal heave is perceived as the lift of the examining hand placed over the left parasternal area and is better demonstrated by placing a pen or a pencil over the area. The upward lift of the pen with each heartbeat is well visualized and indicates RVH **(Fig. 17.7)**.

Heart sounds can be palpable as the apical filling impulse (S3) in adolescents, a pulmonary component of S2 (P2) in pulmonary hypertension (PH), and an aortic component of S2 (A2) in SH. Palpable third and fourth heart sounds together give a double thrust to the apical impulse.

Thrills are palpable vibrations felt better with the palm, as the purring of a cat, over the precordium and suprasternal area in VSD, PDA, and AS. They can be timed with the cardiac cycle by palpating the carotid pulse simultaneously with the other hand.

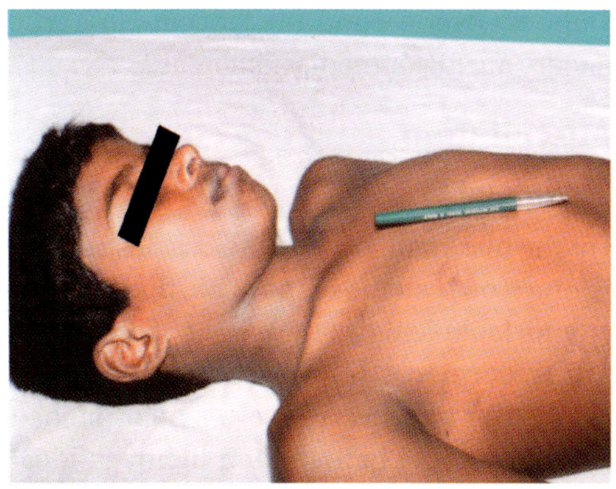

Fig. 17.7: Demonstration of L parasternal heave.

Percussion

Percussion helps to detect cardiomegaly and to differentiate it from PE.

Left Border

Percuss medially from the midaxillary line in the interspace corresponding to the apical impulse. The impaired resonance normally corresponds with apical impulse. A dull percussion note elicited lateral to the apex suggests PE. Next, percuss the second and third LICS. Normally, the second LICS is resonant and the third space is dull. Dullness of the second LICS occurs in PH, PE, left atrial enlargement, and aortic aneurysm. In PE since the dullness is shifting in nature, second LICS becomes resonant when percussed in the sitting position.

Right Border

The right side of the chest is percussed in the MCL from first the right intercostal space (RICS) downward until liver dullness is reached. Percussion to the heart border is done one space higher, toward the right sternal border which flushes with the right cardiac border. If dullness extends laterally, it suggests PE or right atrial enlargement.

Dullness over second RICS occurs in aortic aneurysm, PE, or mediastinal mass.

Auscultation

Technique

For the maximum benefit, the best instrument is one's own stethoscope with the shortest comfortable length (18") and soft correctly fitting earpieces. The diaphragm applied firmly over the chest perceives high-pitched sounds and the bell applied lightly is ideal for low-pitched sounds. Assess the heart sounds first in sequence, next the effects of inspiration and expiration on them followed by the additional heart sounds and lastly the murmurs. The variability that occurs with a change of body position, exercise, and Valsalva technique (Ref. Ch. 21) should be evaluated lastly.

Auscultatory skills and confidence are acquired through knowing cardiac mechanics, using correct techniques, and repeated training, and sustained through continued application. Supine, sitting, and standing positions are needed for auscultation in different areas. Always follow the four conventional areas sequentially for auscultation **(Fig. 17.8)**.

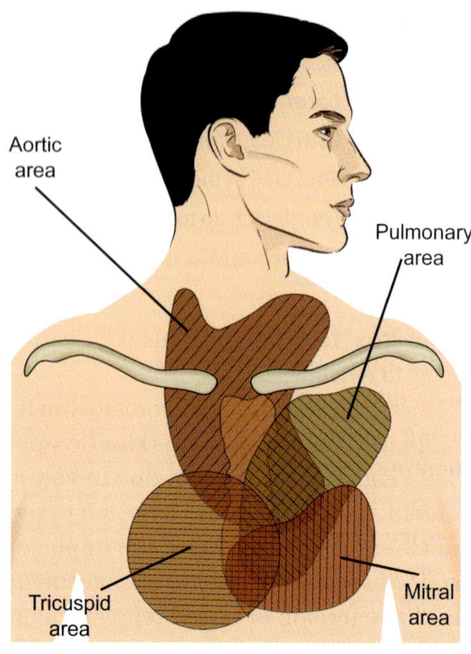

Fig. 17.8: Conventional areas for auscultation.

1. *Mitral area (MA)* is the region of the apex and the fifth LICS in the MCL, extends medially to the left sternal edge and laterally to the axilla. The well-perceived events are the MR and stenosis (MS) murmurs. Use diaphragm and bell respectively for the events; auscultate first in supine and then in left lateral positions.
2. *Tricuspid area* involves the fourth and fifth LICS along the left sternal edge, and can extend to the right of the sternum and the subxiphisternal area; choose diaphragm for murmurs of TR, TS, and VSD.
3. *Pulmonary area (PA)* is on the second LICS along the left parasternal area to the infraclavicular region up to the third LICS. Auscultation with the diaphragm well perceives the murmurs of PDA, PS, and PR.
4. *Aortic area (AA)* is the second RICS at the right parasternal line, reaching the right suprasternal area, neck, and down to the third RICS. Use diaphragm for AS and HCM murmurs.

HEART SOUNDS

First Heart Sound (S1)

Closure of AV-mitral and tricuspid valves produces S1 which is best appreciated in the MA and TA as a single sound. The mitral valve may close earlier to the tricuspid valve, hence occasionally at the lower left sternal edge, two components (splitting) may occur. S1 makes the beginning of systole and is heard well with diaphragm. It is loud in atrial septal defect (ASD), MS, EA, and in fever. S1 is soft in myocarditis, primary myocardial diseases, AR, and MR.

Second Heart Sound (S2)

The closure of the semilunar valves generates the S2. Normally, the S2 consists of a louder and earlier aortic valve (AV) closure followed by a later and quieter PV closure—A2 and P2 sounds. This normal physiologic splitting is best appreciated with the diaphragm in the PA during or near the end of inspiration. During expiration, the AV and PV close synchronously producing a single or narrowly split S2. If the PV closes earlier than the AV, it is reverse split S2. *Evaluation of S2 is important in the diagnosis of heart diseases, especially ASD. P2 and A2 are loud in PH and SH, respectively.*

The abnormalities in S2 are the following:

- *No split—single S2 occurs if there is*:
  - Single semilunar valve, e.g., aortic atresia and pulmonary atresia.
  - *PAH*: Pulmonary pressure equals the systemic so that both valves close together.
  - Both ventricles eject simultaneously as in a large VSD or single ventricle.
  - TGA—split may not be heard due to the anterior position of the aorta.
  - *PV closure soft*: TOF and critical PS
  - *Only one valve*: Truncus arteriosus
- *Wide split (>0.04 seconds)*: Heard when P2 closure is delayed than normal, e.g., right bundle branch block, ASD, PS, VSD, MR, and right ventricular failure (RVF).
- *Paradoxical split*: Occurs when the pulmonary valve closes earlier than the AV as in the left bundle branch block, AS, PDA, LVF, COA, and SH.
- *Wide and fixed split:* With open communication between two atria, the effect of respiration on the splitting of the S2 is diminished. The atrial left to right shunt increases the right ventricular stroke volume accentuating the split; a widely split S2 with no variation with respiration is almost diagnostic of ASD.

Third Heart Sound (S3)

S3 heard during diastole is due to rapid inflow into the ventricle and is normal in children. It is best heard at the apex with the bell. In the presence of tachycardia, it produces the "gallop rhythm" which suggests CHF, particularly in those with myocardial disease.

Fourth Heart Sound (S4)

S4 is rarely a normal finding and is due to atrial contraction when there is excessive stiffness or noncompliance of ventricles; heard best with the bell, the patient lying slightly turned to the left side. S4 is not audible in rhythm abnormalities, such as AF and junctional tachycardia. In tachycardia, diastole is shortened and S3 and S4 coincide to produce the *summation gallop*.

Clicks

These are high-frequency sounds best heard with a diaphragm, in standing posture or doing the Valsalva maneuver. Early systolic clicks are heard in semilunar valve lesions (PS, AS, and bicuspid AV), dilatation of great arteries, and PAH. Midsystolic clicks occur in MVP.

Opening Snap

Opening snap (OS) is a high-pitched sound produced by sudden tensing of cusps of the mitral or tricuspid valve on opening during diastole and occurs before S3. The more severe the valve stenosis, the shorter will be the interval between OS and S2. The presence of OS indicates thickened but mobile valve leaflets. Calcification and fibrotic thickening of valve leaflets reduce the intensity of OS.

Pericardial Rub

The leathery scratchy sound in pericarditis occurs in systole and diastole due to the rubbing of the inflamed pericardial surfaces. Occasionally, it can be triphasic. It is best heard in the upright position, and increases in intensity on bending forward and on pressing with the diaphragm, firmly to the chest wall. The sound may vary from time to time and disappear when effusion develops.

MURMURS

They are abnormal sounds heard when blood passes through a narrow orifice, but all of them do not indicate structural or physiologic cardiac problems (organic murmurs). The sequence of auscultation for murmurs is upper precordium, left and right sternal borders, the apex, left and right axillae, and both sides of the back. Describe the following features of the murmur:

- *Timing:* Timing is the relation between systole and diastole or to S1 and S2—assess by palpating the right carotid pulse simultaneously with auscultation **(Fig. 17.9)**. Can be systolic, diastolic, systolic-diastolic, and continuous.
- *Intensity:* There are six grades as per Levine grading for systolic murmurs:
  - I: Heard with intense concentration
  - II: Faint but heard immediately
  - III: Easily heard of intermediate intensity
  - IV: Easily heard and associated with thrill
  - V: Loud, thrill present, audible with an edge of the stethoscope on the chest wall
  - VI: Audible with a stethoscope of the chest wall

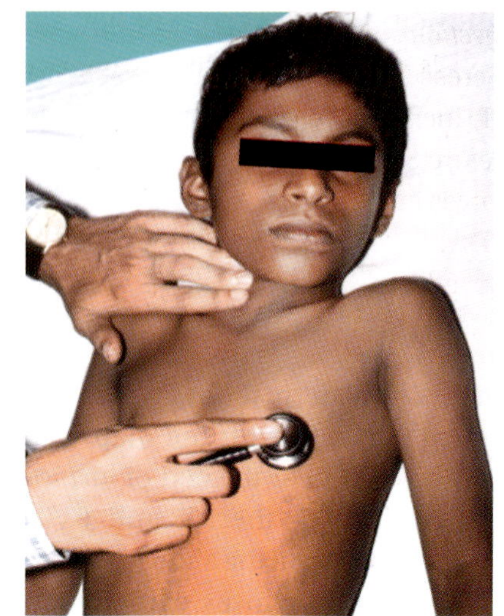

Fig. 17. 9: Evaluating the timing the murmur with the cardiac cycle.

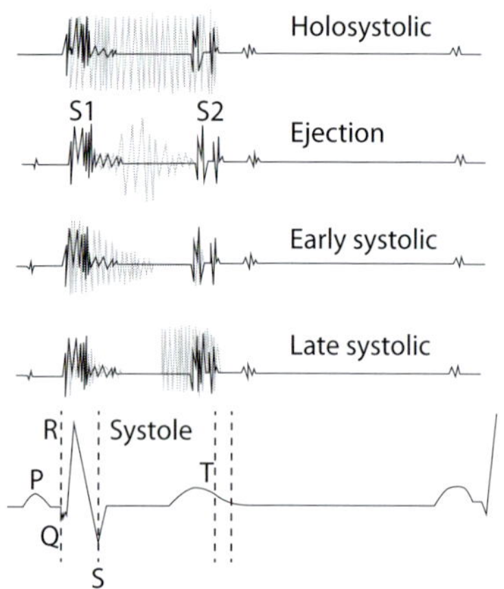

Fig. 17.10: Four types of systolic murmurs.

- *Duration*: Duration tells the beginning to end of the murmur. **Figure 17.10** reveals the duration of systolic murmurs.
- *Holo/pansystolic murmur*: It begins abruptly with S1 and continues throughout the systole at the same intensity up to S2, heard best with the diaphragm, and can be graphically depicted as a rectangle. Heard in regurgitant valves (MR and TR) or VSD.

- *Ejection systolic (midsystolic) murmur:* It is a crescendo decrescendo, that starts after S1, increases in intensity, and disappears before S2. Arise from narrowed semilunar valves or outflow tracts as in AS, PS, COA PDA, TOF, ASD, and PAH. Best heard with the diaphragm while the patient sits leaning forward.
- *Early systolic murmur*: It starts with S1, tapers and disappears before S2. It is exclusive of small muscular VSD.
- *Mid-to-late systolic murmur:* It begins midway through systole and ends with S2; heard in association with midsystolic clicks and insufficiency of MVP. Intensity increases from sitting to standing position.
- *Diastolic murmurs*: Diastole, the period between the closure of semilunar valves (S2) and AV valves (S1), is normally silent because of low-pressure flow through large valve orifices. The murmurs are graded I–IV.
- *Early diastolic murmur* is decrescendo in nature, characteristic of AR or pulmonary valve regurgitation; starts with S2 and fades by mid diastole, heard best with the diaphragm of the stethoscope. Graham Steell murmur is the early diastolic murmur of PAH.
- *Mid-diastolic murmur (MDM)* is a diamond-shaped murmur in the mid-diastole (starts well after S2 and fades before S1) due to increased flow across a normal mitral or tricuspid valve (flow murmurs) or normal flow across a stenotic or obstructed valve [e.g., Carey Coombs murmur (soft flow murmur in mitral valvulitis), Austin Flint murmur in AR]. Best heard with the bell of the stethoscope. MDM observed in ASD, VSD, and PDA indicate that the shunt is large.
- *Late diastolic or presystolic murmur* is heard immediately before S1, due to atrial systole, and may be perceived as an accentuation of the MDM associated with MS/TS/atrial myxoma; it will be lost in AF.
- *The point of maximum intensity* is the area where the murmur is heard best in supine posture.
- *Selective propagation* is the site where the murmur radiates (usually to the direction of the blood flow), e.g., murmurs of MR to the axilla, VSD to the left sternal area and back, PS to the left clavicle, AS to the carotids.
- *Configuration* reveals the dynamic shape of the murmur, i.e., the intensity over time. Crescendo decrescendo is progressively increasing followed by decreasing intensity (diamond or kite shaped) murmur, e.g., ejection systolic murmur (ESM) of AS and PS; AR murmur is decrescendo.
- *Pitch* is the frequency range of the murmur. Low-pitched murmur is heard with the bell of the stethoscope, e.g., murmur of MS. High-pitched murmur is heard better with the diaphragm.
- *Relation with respiration*: During inspiration, the venous blood flow to the RA and RV increases and so does the systolic stroke volume of RV. Blood leak from RV to RA increases leading to louder TR murmur.
- *Quality of the murmur*: It denotes the unusual descriptive character of the murmur, e.g., blowing pansystolic murmur of MR, a harsh rumbling murmur of MS, and a machinery murmur of PDA.
- *Systolo, diastolic murmur:* It is a to-and-fro murmur heard in systole and diastole, not obscuring S2; heard in AS with AR, PS with PR, VSD with AR.
- *Continuous murmur (CM):* It is a systolic murmur that starts with S1, continues, or spills into diastole *obscuring S2* in contrast

to to-and-fro murmur. Indicates continuous flow as in PDA or aortopulmonary (AP) communication. All CMs are pathologic except venous hum (VH). The diseases with CMs are PDA, AP window, rupture of the sinus of Valsalva, and coronary AV fistula. CMs can occur in CCHDs, such as PA with collaterals, pulmonary AV fistula, supracardiac total anomalous pulmonary venous connection (TAPVC), and truncus arteriosus. VH can be differentiated from CM, having incidentally detected, without any associated cardiac findings, its disappearance by applying mild pressure to the lower part of the neck and changing the position of the neck.

- *Maneuvers:* They can change the intensity of the murmurs and help in their differentiation as detailed below:
  - *Handgrip*—increases the afterload and thus the intensity of the murmurs of AR, MR, and VSD and decreases the murmurs of HOCM and MVP.
  - *Squatting*—increases the preload and the intensity of the murmur of AS, MS, AR, and MR.
  - *Valsalva*—decreases the preload and so increases the murmur of HOCM and MVP and decreases the murmur of AS, MS, MR, and VSD.
  - *Abrupt standing from sitting*—decreases the preload, so increases the murmur of HOCM and MVP and decreases the murmur of AS, MS, AR, MR, and VSD.

Innocent/Functional Cardiac Murmurs

Up to 30% of children (6 m to 6 yrs of age), reveal murmurs without symptoms or cardiac lesions, but are a concern to the parents and physicians. They are presently termed *normal murmurs*. The features are asymptomatic short, soft (intensity less than grade 3), often systolic, and of low intensity on sitting or standing. It can be continuous but never solely diastolic, accentuated by fever (being first detected by a practicing pediatrician), anemia, and increased cardiac output. Five systolic and two continuous types are described as innocent murmurs. Systolic types are vibratory Still's murmur, pulmonary flow murmur, peripheral pulmonary arterial stenosis murmur, supraclavicular systolic murmur, and aortic systolic murmur. Continuous murmurs are VH and mammary arterial souffle. VH is produced by the turbulence of blood in the jugular venous system, heard as a soft humming sound in the anterior chest or neck, and can be reduced or made to disappear by changing the position of the neck or gently pressing the jugular veins of the neck. The main differential diagnosis is PDA.

OTHER POINTS

Presence of capillary pulsations (over uvula, ear lobule, lips, and nail beds), pistol shot sounds (sounds heard over brachial or femoral artery through the stethoscope) and Duroziez's sign (systolic murmur heard on applying pressure to partially occlude the artery proximal to the chest piece of a stethoscope and diastolic murmur when pressure is applied distally) and visible arterial pulsations over the extremity vessels (dancing peripheral arteries) are features of AR. Abdominal examination for hepatomegaly (in CHF), splenomegaly (in SABE), renal anomaly (in systemic HT), prominent pulsations (in aortic aneurysm), and lung crackles (in CHF) are mandatory in completing CVS examination in all age groups.

All steps in the CVS examination should be carried out systematically under the headlines as described. If the baby/child is irritable, a safe sedative (chloral hydrate) for clinical examination, can be administered after getting the parent's permission. In most patients, an idea of the expected auscultatory findings can be guessed from the preliminary steps if done methodically.

The format of stating the final diagnosis should be in the order of clinical diagnosis (in view of the physiologic impairment), functional impairment followed by etiology.

For example, MR (moderate degree), congestive heart failure, no PAH, normal sinus rhythm; etiology—rheumatic carditis.

SUGGESTED READING

1. Bernstein D. The Cardiovascular System. In: Kliegman R, St Geme III JW (Eds). Nelson Textbook of Pediatrics, 21st edition. Amsterdam: Elsevier; 2020.
2. In: Davies C (Ed). Cardiovascular system. Hutchison's Clinical Methods: An Integrated Approach to Clinical Practice, 24th edition. Philadelphia: Saunders; 2018.
3. Pelech AN. Evaluation of the pediatric patient with a cardiac murmur. Pediatr Clin North Am. 1999;46(2):167-88.
4. Pickering D. Precordial catch syndrome. Arch Dis Child. 1981;56(5):401-3.
5. Sinha R, Saha A, Samuel J. American Academy of Pediatrics Clinical Practice Guidelines for Screening and Management of High Blood Pressure in Children and Adolescents: What is New? Indian Pediatr. 2019;56(4):317-21.
6. Weeks B, Friedman HA. Training pediatric residents to evaluate congenital heart disease in the current era. Pediatr Clin North Am. 2004;51(6):1641-51, ix.

CHAPTER

The Electrocardiogram

M Veerendra Kumar, M Zulfikar Ahamed

Chapter Outline

INTRODUCTION

Systematic evaluation of electrocardiogram (ECG) is an important aid in the diagnosis of heart diseases, especially the congenital group. Being the surface recording of the electrical activity of cardiac muscle mass it helps in determining the position of the heart and chambers, bulk of ventricular muscle mass, volume or pressure overload of ventricles, ischemic or inflammatory changes of the myocardium, pericarditis, electrolyte changes in serum, and rhythm abnormalities.

ECG LEADS

In children, 14 leads ECG is advised.

- *Three bipolar limb leads:* LI, LII, and LIII.
- *Three unipolar limb leads:* Augmented vector right (aVR), augmented vector left (aVL), and augmented vector foot (aVF).
- *Six usual chest leads:* V_1 to V_6
- *Two right chest leads:* V_3R and V_4R

ECG PAPER

Electrocardiogram paper has 1 × 1 mm small squares **(Fig. 18.1)**. The horizontal limb of each small square represents 40 milliseconds (ms) and the vertical limb is 0.1 millivolts (mV). The usual paper speed is 25 mm/s. Paper speed may be increased to 50 mm/s for definite assessment of certain intervals and detection of certain arrhythmias like atrial fibrillation.

ANATOMY OF IMPULSE ORIGIN AND CONDUCTION

As shown in **Figures 18.2 and 18.3,** impulses originate in the SA node, situated just right

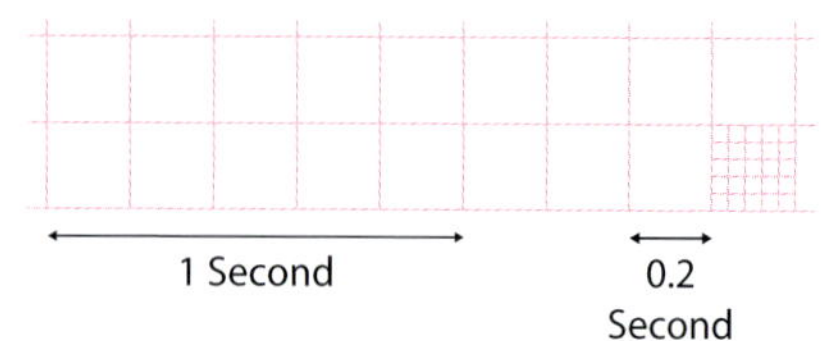

Fig. 18.1: ECG paper.

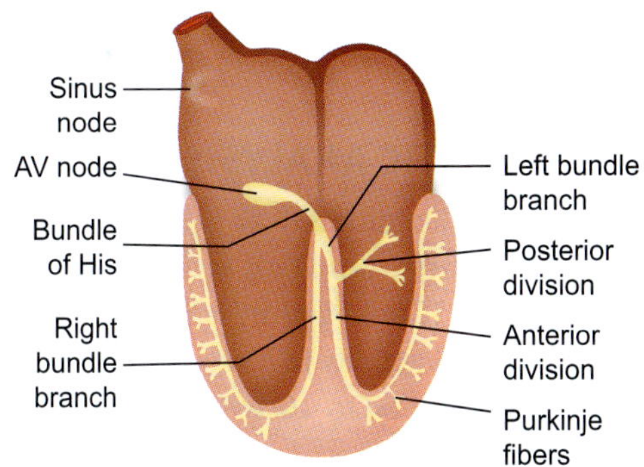

Fig. 18.2: Anatomy of impulse origin and conduction.

to the superior vena cava (SVC) in the right atrium (RA). From the SA node impulses reach the atrioventricular (AV) node and activate the RA through three internodal pathways and the left atrium (LA) through the tract "Bachmann's" bundle.

From the AV node impulse passes through "bundle of His," which travels anteroinferiorly, and then divides into right and left bundle branches. The left bundle branch (LBB) again divides into anterosuperior and postero-inferior Hemi branches. These bundles branch into the Purkinje network of fibers, which travel vertically from the endocardial to the epicardial surface. Impulses travel between atria and ventricles only through a bundle of His or accessory tract if any, since the fibrous tissue between atria and ventricles acts as an insulator.

PHYSIOLOGY OF ECG

Figure 18.4 shows the waves of ECG. Each wave and interval represent the following:

- *P-wave:* Atrial depolarization
- *PR segment:* Conduction through the AV node and His bundle
- *QRS:* Ventricular depolarization
- *ST and T:* Ventricular repolarization
- *U-wave:* Repolarization of Purkinje system and papillary muscles

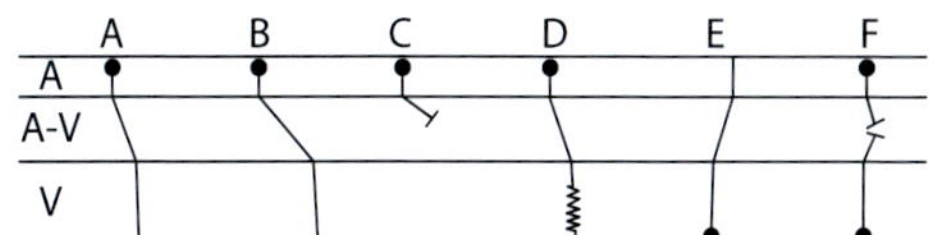

Fig. 18.3: Diagrammatic representation of impulse conduction.

Note: Graphic representation of the use of the "ladder" diagram in depicting arrhythmias. The ordinate reflects the anatomical levels. The abscissa reflects time. The black dot reflects impulse origin. (A = normal conduction. B = delayed A-V conduction; C = A-V block; D = aberrant ventricular conduction; E = ectopic ventricular impulse with retrograde A-V conduction to the atria; F = interference between a sinus impulse and an ectopic ventricular impulse within the A-V junction).

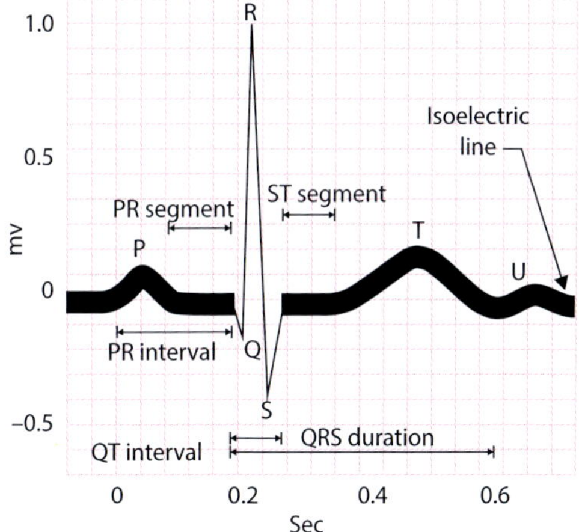

Fig. 18.4: Waves of ECG.

Note: Atrial repolarization is submerged in QRS and hence not picked up.

Any electrical activity moving towards a surface lead will be picked up as positive deflection (i.e., upward tracing) and reversed as negative (downward). **Figure 18.5** depicts the activation of the ventricles.

Ventricular depolarization starts first in the interventricular septum from left to right. Thus, leads over the right ventricle (RV), i.e., V_1 and V_2 pick-up a small positive ("r" wave), and leads over the left ventricle (LV), i.e., V_5 and V_6 pick up the initial negative "q" wave. Small deflection is denoted by a small letter and large deflection by a capital letter. Subsequently, ventricular muscles get activated from the apex to the base. Since muscle mass is more in LV, surface leads pick-up deep negative waves in V_1, and V_2 and tall positive waves in V_5 and V_6 **(Figs. 18.6A and B)**.

Of the chest leads, V_1, V_2, V_3R, and V_4R show RV activity and V5 and V6 reveal LV activity. If the interventricular septum is absent no "q" wave will be seen in V_5, V_6 and if ventricles are reversed [l-transposition of the great arteries (TGA)] "q" wave will be seen in V_1, V_2.

In intraventricular conduction defect or bundle branch block, since the ventricular activation takes more time, QRS will be wide, and the wave pattern depends on the site of the block.

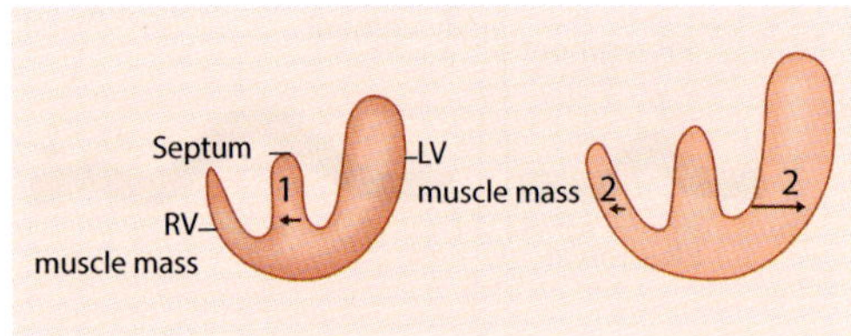

Fig. 18.5: Activation of ventricles.
Note: The direction of impulses is shown by arrows. The number represents the sequence of activation of each area.

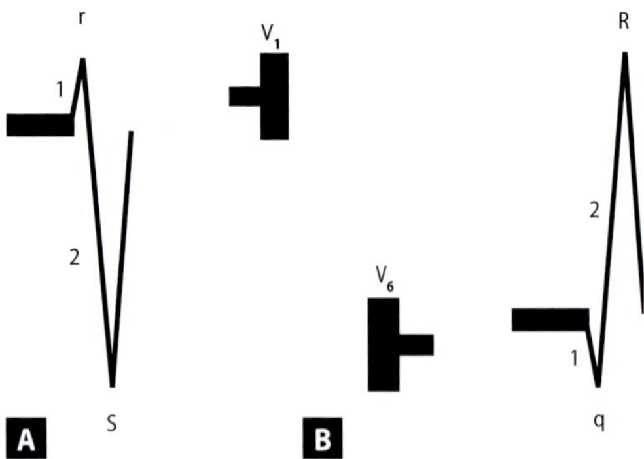

Figs. 18.6A and B: (A) Normal ECG record in V_1; (B) Normal ECG record in V_6.

SYSTEMATIC ANALYSIS OF ECG

Heart rate is calculated as 1,500/number of small squares between two "R" waves (RR interval). If the rhythm is irregular, the number of QRS activity in 6 seconds (30 large squares) multiplied by 10, will give the rate.

P-wave

P-wave is always positive in LI, LII, V_4, V_5, and V_6 and negative in aVR. If reversed, either not in sinus rhythm or the sinus node (RA) is on the left side. Amplitude (height) >3 mm (tall P-wave) is seen in RA enlargement. Width >3 mm (wide P-wave) is seen in LA enlargement. *Bifid P-wave* (with interspace distance >1 mm) and *biphasic P-wave* (negative deflection *>1 mm of width and depth*) are also indicative of *LA enlargement* **(Fig. 18.7)**. P-wave changes are best assessed in LII, V_3R, and V_1.

Normal P-wave axis is +30° to +60°. The P-wave axis is determined by P-waves in

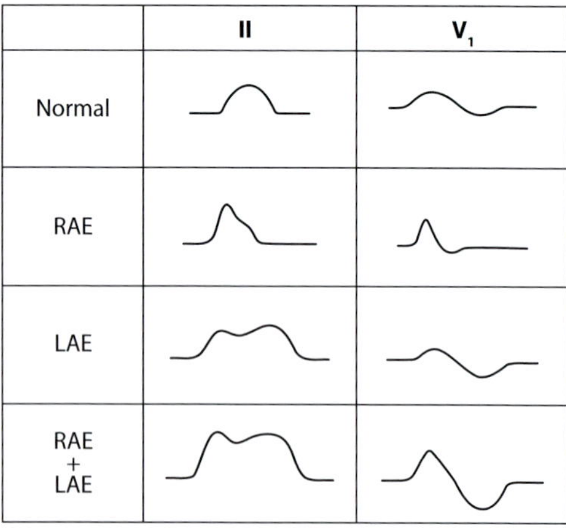

Fig. 18.7: P-wave changes. (LAE: left atrial enlargement; RAE: right atrial enlargement; RAE + LAE: biatrial enlargement)

lead 1 and aVF. If it is upright in both, the axis is normal. If in L1 negative and aVF positive, atrial inversion. L1 positive and aVF negative is ectopic atrial activity. Abnormal P-wave axis is seen in dextrocardia, nonsinus rhythm, ASD (sinus venosus type), and in single atrium.

PR Interval

PR interval is the time from the onset of the P-wave to the onset of QRS. The normal value in children is 110–160 milliseconds (2.5–4 divisions) and in neonates it is 100–140 msec (2.5–3.5 divisions). The longest PR interval is taken for measurement. Short PR interval (<80 milliseconds) is seen in small infants, Wolff-Parkinson-White (WPW) syndrome, Lown Ganong-Levine syndrome, and Pompe disease. Long PR interval is seen in 1° block, e.g., rheumatic carditis.

QRS Complex

Normal duration is 50–100 milliseconds (1.5–2.5 divisions). Longer duration (>100 milliseconds) is observed in intraventricular conduction defects or bundle branch blocks. Low amplitude (height) of QRS (<5 mm in limb leads and <10 mm chest leads) denotes incorrect standardization, thick chest wall, myocarditis, pericardial effusion, emphysema, hypothyroidism, and hypopituitarism. High voltage (>20 mm in limb leads and >30 mm in chest leads) can be normal.

Q-wave Changes

- Absent—absent interventricular septum
- q in V_1, V_2—right ventricular hypertrophy (RVH) (suprasystemic pressure). If no other evidence of RVH presence of q in V_1, V_2 and absence in V_5, V_6 is suggestive of levotransposition of the great arteries (L-TGA) (ventricular inversion).
- *Deep q in V_5, V_6:* >4 mm depth or >25% of R height is seen in LV volume overload.

Transition

Transition is the point at which dominant polarity changes from negative dominance of RV lead to positive dominance of LV leads (normally in V_3 and V_4). Early transition (in V_2) occurs in left ventricular hypertrophy (LVH) and late transition (in V_5) in RVH.

QRS Axis (Figs. 18.8 and 18.9)

- *Left Lower quadrant:* Normal axis (NA)
- *Right lower quadrant:* Right axis deviation (RAD)
- *Right upper quadrant:* Extreme right or left axis
- *Left upper quadrant:* Left axis deviation (LAD)

Method to Determine QRS Axis

Look for the predominant deflection in LI and aVF.

	NA:	LAD	RAD	Indeterminate
Lead I:	+	+	–	–
aVF:	+	–	+	–

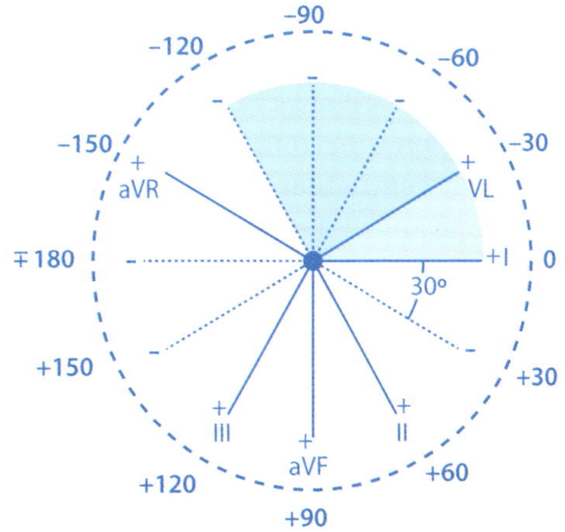

Fig. 18.8: Hexaxial representation of limb leads.

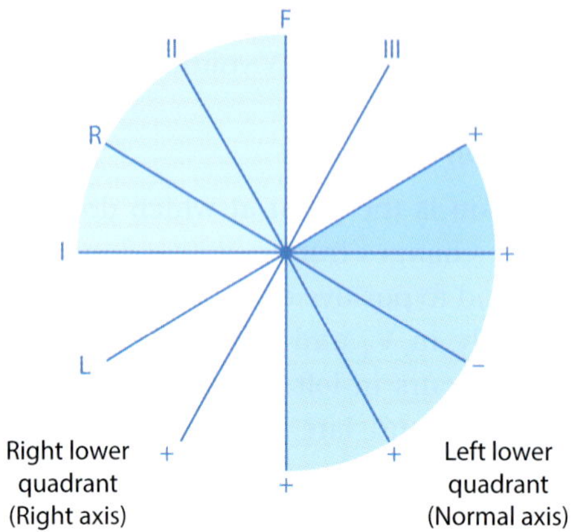

Fig. 18.9: Four quadrants of the QRS axis.

When the axis is indeterminate look for q in LI and aVL (extreme left axis) and in LII, LIII, and aVF (extreme right axis).

Determination of the QRS axis is important in diagnosing congenital heart diseases **(Box 18.1)**.

BOX 18.1: QRS axis in various congenital heart diseases.

- *LAD:**
  - *Cyanotic:*
    - AV canal defect
    - DORV with restrictive VSD
    - Single atrium
    - Single ventricle
    - Tricuspid atresia
  - *Acyanotic:*
    - Multiple muscular VSD
    - ASD primum
    - L-TGA
- *RAD:*
  - All RVH
  - Dextrocardia**
  - Left posterior hemiblock**
  - Reverse arm leads**
  - WPW syndrome (type B)

*Other conditions with LAD are left anterior hemiblock, WPW syndrome (type A), apical ectopic ventricular impulse, and apical pacing.

**In reverse arm, leads unlike in dextrocardia V_1 to V_6 progression of R-wave height is normal.

(AV: atrioventricular; DORV: double outlet right ventricle; L-TGA: levotransposition of the great arteries; RAD: right axis deviation; RVH: right ventricular hypertrophy; VSD: ventricular septal defect; WPW: Wolff–Parkinson–White)

ST segment: Look for deviation from the baseline (T-P segment). Deviation >1 mm is abnormal. Some ST elevation can be normal in V_1 to V_3.

ST depression: Any depression is abnormal. If the J point (junction of the end of "s" wave and beginning of ST segment) only is depressed and the rest part comes to baseline it is physiological. Horizontal depression and sagging depression **(Figs. 18.10A and B)** indicate myocardial ischemia and damage. ST depression with convexity up **(Fig. 18.11)** is seen in ventricular hypertrophy due to pressure overload, i.e., strain pattern in (V_1, V_2 in RVH and V_5, V_6 in LVH).

ST ELEVATION

ST elevation with concavity up occurs in pericarditis. Slope elevation of "ST" occurs in myocardial infarction **(Figs. 18.12 and 18.13)**.

T-wave polarity is the same as that of QRS in that lead. Up to three days of postnatal life T is upright in V_1, V_2, and V_3R. After that, it is normally negative up to V_3. T-wave is the unstable component of ECG and hence isolated T wave changes need not be abnormal. Normal T-waves are asymmetrical. T-waves are tall (>5 mm in limb leads or >10 mm in chest leads) in hyperkalemia, coronary insufficiency, and LVH with volume overload and flat in hypokalemia and hypothyroidism. T-inversion occurs in all forms of carditis, ischemia, ventricular hypertrophy, and digitalis toxicity.

The *QT interval* is the beginning of the "q" wave to the end of the "T" wave.

QTc (corrected QT to heart rate)

$$= \frac{\text{QT in milliseconds}}{\sqrt{\text{RR}}\text{ interval in sec}}$$

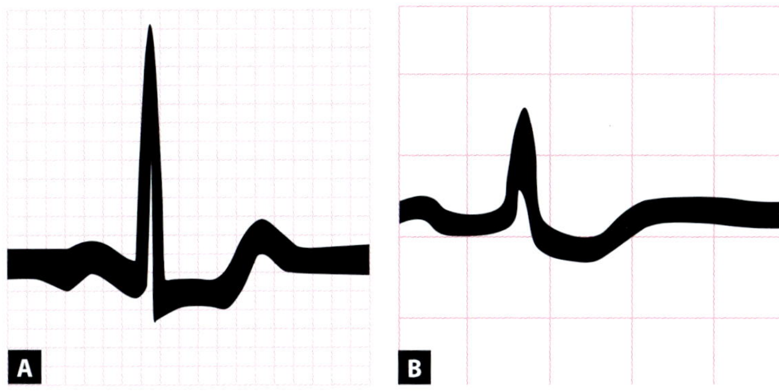

Figs. 18.10A and B: (A) ST horizontal depression; (B) "ST" sagging depression.

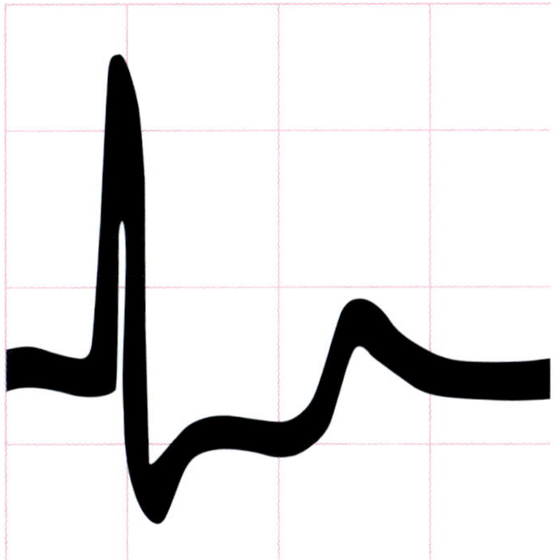

Fig. 18.11: ST depression with convexity up.

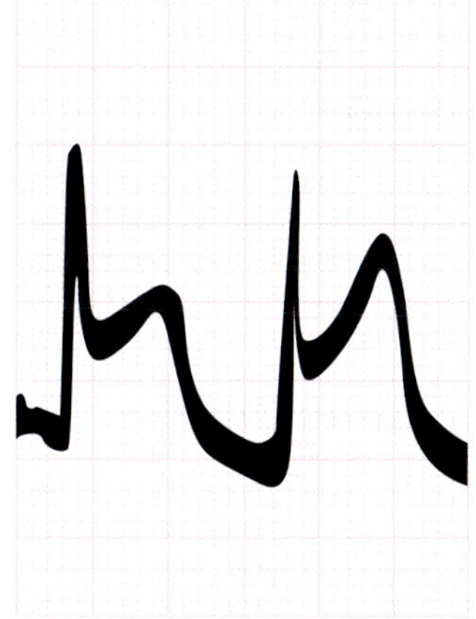

Fig. 18.12: ST elevation with concavity upward.

The normal value of QTc is <440 milliseconds. The borderline value is 440–460 milliseconds. Prolonged QTc is >460 milliseconds seen in rheumatic carditis, hypothermia, hypocalcemia, drug toxicity (quinidine), myocardial infarction, sympathetic stimulation as in head injury, cerebral hemorrhage and syncope, and long QT syndromes. Short QTc is seen in digitalis toxicity, hypercalcemia, hyperthermia, and vagal stimulation.

U-wave is the small round deflection just after the T-wave, best seen in V_2 to V_4, in the same direction as the T wave. *Normal amplitude is ¼ of the T-wave.* Prominent "U" waves are seen in hypokalemia and

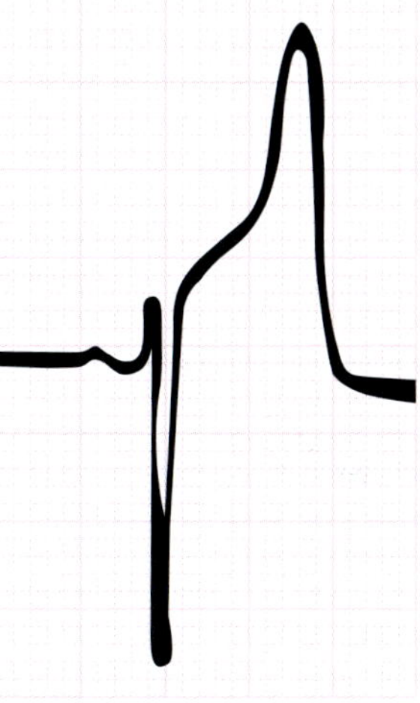

Fig. 18.13: ST slope elevation.

can be mistaken for T-waves. The "U" wave opposite in direction to the T-wave occurs in hypertension and coronary insufficiency.

Criteria for Chamber Enlargements

- *Left atrial enlargement*: Look in LII, V_1
  - Negative deflection of P in V_1 >1 mm depth and width
  - P-wave width >3 mm
  - In bifid P interpeak distance >1 mm
  - P axis <+30°
- *Right atrial enlargement*: Look in LII, V_1
  - Tall, peaked P >3 mm in LII
  - P axis >+ 60°
  - Initial force of P in V_1 >1.5 mm (horizontal interval between beginning and peak of P-wave)

NB: Terms P pulmonale and "P mitrale" are not used now.

LEFT VENTRICULAR HYPERTROPHY

- *R in V_5/ V_6 + S in V_1:* >45 mm
- *R in V_5/V_6:* >35 mm
- *R in aVL:* >20 mm
- Ventricular activation time (VAT)* >1 mm *(Horizontal distance from beginning of q to peak of 'R')
- Wide QRS ~ 100 milliseconds

Note: LVH may be volume overload or pressure overload.

Volume Overload

- Prominent q (>4 mm) in LI, aVL, V_5, V_6
- Tall R in V_5, V_6
- Tall upright T in V_5, V_6

Pressure Overload

- No significant q in V_5, V_6
- T inversion and ST depression with convexity upward (strain pattern)

RIGHT VENTRICULAR HYPERTROPHY

- Upright T in V_1/V_3R after 3 days of life
- *R/S ratio in V_1:*
  - *>5:* <6 m of age
  - *>3:* 6 m to 3 yr
  - *>1.5:* 3–6 yr
  - *>1:* After 6 yr
- qR in V_1 or V3R
- R in V_1 plus S in V_6 >11 mm
- R in aVR >5 mm
- Right axis of QRS >+110°

There are three types of RVH:

1. *Type a:* Monophasic R or qR in V1 (pressure overload)
2. *Type b:* rsR′ in V1 and V3R. Indicate volume overload of RV
3. *Type c:* rs pattern in V_5/V_6 (negative deflection predominant)

BIVENTRICULAR HYPERTROPHY

- Independently RVH + LVH by above criteria
- LVH + right axis of QRS
- RVH + left axis of QRS
- Katz-Wachtel phenomenon (tall R-wave and deep S-wave in V_3, V_4 measuring >40 mm full ECG paper width)

CRITERIA FOR RVH AND LVH IN NEWBORNS

- *RVH*:
  - R/S >5 in V_1
  - R in V_1>25 mm—first week
  - S in V_5 >15 mm—first week
  - R in V_1, S in V_5 >10 mm—after the first week up to 1 month
  - q in V_1 and V_3R
  - T upright in V_1 after the third day of life
- *LVH*:
  - Absence of normal right axis
  - *R/S <1 in V_1:*

- *R in V_5:*
  - *>15 mm:* First week
  - *>25 mm:* Thereafter up to 1 month
- *Inverted T in V_5:* After 3 days of life

COMMON ARRHYTHMIAS

Cardiac rhythm has three fundamental aspects: (1) Anatomical origin, (2) discharge sequence, and (3) conduction sequence. For determining rhythm look for:

- P-wave configuration and axis
- P-wave rate by PP interval
- PR interval whether normal or not
- Whether all P-waves are followed by QRS or missed or QRS and P totally chaotic.
- QRS width (wide QRS due to ventricular origin of impulse or due to ventricular conduction defect)
- Ventricular rate by RR interval

If sinus rhythm, P-wave configuration, and axis are normal, all P-waves will be followed by normal width QRS.

Sinus Arrhythmia

RR intervals vary with gradual increase and decrease in rate. PQRST normal. This can be due to *respiratory* and *nonrespiratory* causes. In respiratory sinus arrhythmia, the rate increases in inspiration and decreases in expiration. Nonrespiratory causes are vagotonic procedures like carotid compression and digitalis toxicity.

Atrial extrasystole is characterized by premature P (P-wave earlier than in expected position) with abnormal contour, variable PR, narrow QRS, and compensatory pause is incomplete **(Fig. 18.14)**.

The sum of the pre- and postextrasystole RR interval is less than the sum of two normal RR intervals.

Ventricular ectopics are characterized by premature wide and abnormal QRS without preceding P-wave. Secondary ST-T changes follow. Compensatory pause is complete [sum of pre- and postexcitation intervals is equal to the sum of 2 normal RR intervals **(Figs. 18.15A and B)**].

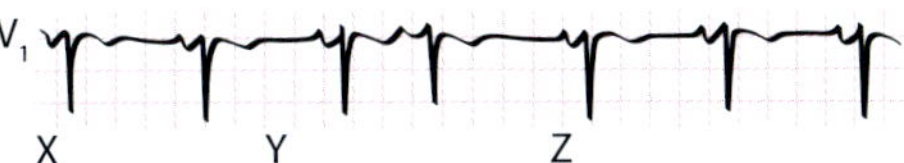

Fig. 18.14: *ECG changes in atrial extrasystole:* Lead V_1, normal sinus rhythm, atrial extrasystole at Y-Z interval.
Note: The fourth P-wave which is premature and bizarre: pointed, narrow, and entirely positive with incomplete compensatory pause, i.e., the sum of the pre- and postectopic intervals (interval Y-Z) is less than the sum of two consecutive sinus intervals (Interval X-Y).

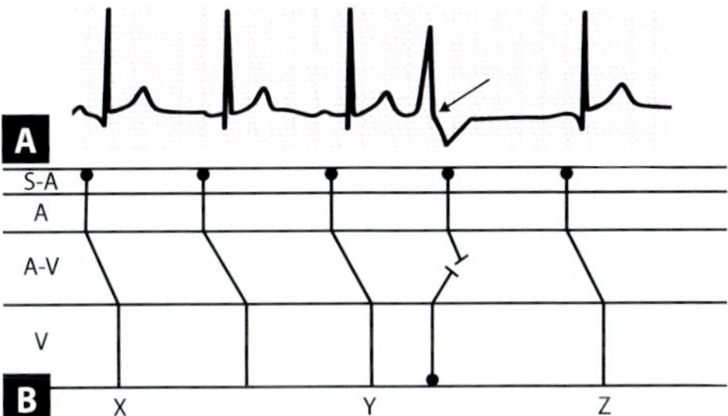

Figs. 18.15A and B: *ECG changes in ventricular extrasystole:* Lead II with a ventricular extrasystole at Y–Z interval.
Note: (A) The bizarre premature QRS complex of the extrasystole which occurs concomitantly with a sinus discharge; the P-wave of this sinus discharge is thus largely hidden within the QRST complex of the extrasystole but may just be seen (arrow); (B) The compensatory pause is complete, i.e., the sum of the pre- and postectopic intervals (Y–Z) is exactly equal to two consecutive sinus cycles (X–Y).

Supraventricular tachycardia (SVT) is an important rhythm abnormality in children. Ventricular rate is 180–300/min. Differentiation is from sinus tachycardia **(Table 18.1)**.

Wolff-Parkinson-White syndrome is due to an accessory tract between the atrium and ventricle (bundle of Kent). Features are short

TABLE 18.1: Differentiation between supraventricular tachycardia (SVT) and sinus tachycardia.

Parameters	***SVT***	***Sinus tachycardia***
• Heart rate	• >200/min	• <200/min
• P-wave	• Absent/retrograde	• Present
• P-wave axis	• Abnormal	• Normal
• RR interval	• No variation	• Variable
• Termination	• Abrupt	• Gradual

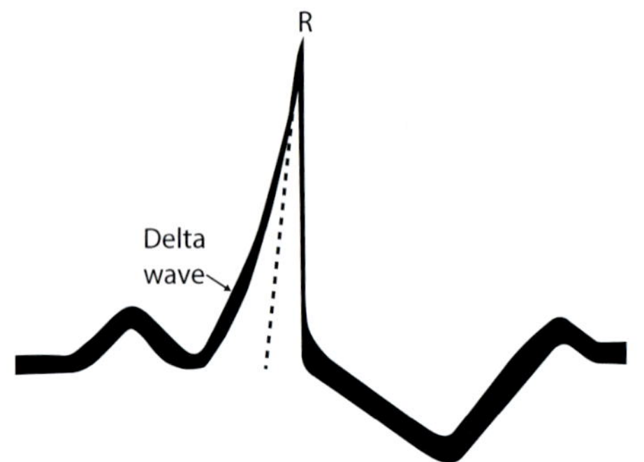

Fig. 18.16: ECG of Wolff–Parkinson–White (WPW) syndrome.

PR interval (<110 milliseconds), Delta-wave (a hump in the proximal part of R-wave), wide QRS (>110 milliseconds), and additional ST-T changes and may be associated with SVT at times **(Fig. 18.16)**. The first four features are seen in nontachycardia phase only. There are two types:

1. *Type A*: QRS—positive in V_1 and V_2 (bundle of Kent between LA and LV)
2. *Type B (access ory tract between RA and RV)*: QRS is negative in V_1, and V_2 and is typical of Ebstein anomaly.

Ventricular tachycardia is uncommon in children. May occur with "long QT syndromes" **(Fig. 18.17)**.

Ventricular fibrillation is revealed by irregular, chaotic low voltage ventricular activity **(Fig. 18.18)**.

Asystole: Absent electrical activity, flat tracing **(Fig. 18.19)**.

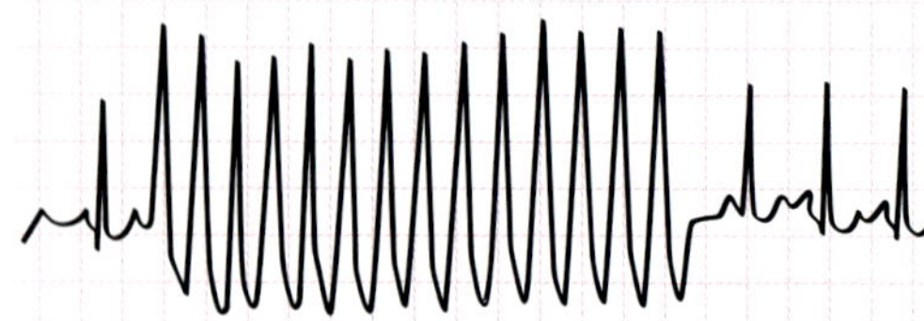

Fig. 18.17: Ventricular tachycardia.

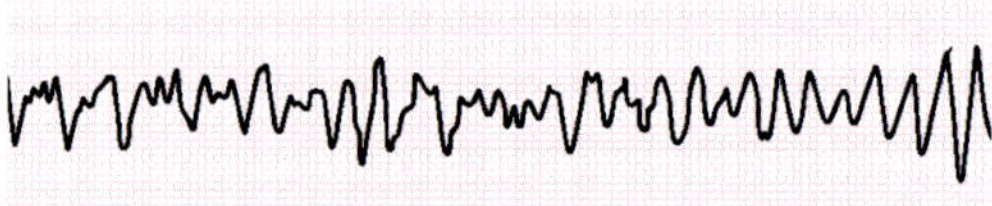

Fig. 18.18: Ventricular fibrillation.

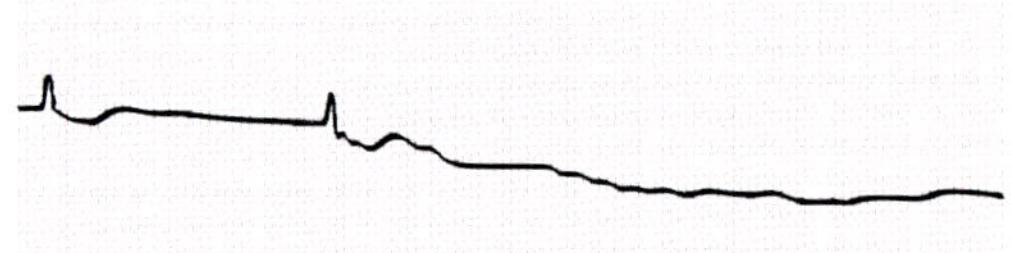

Fig. 18.19: Asystole.

HEART BLOCKS

A *sinoatrial block* is uncommon in children. Present as bradycardia or as escape beats from other sites (atria, AV node, His bundle, or ventricle).

Atrioventricular Block

There are three types of AV block:

1. *I AV block:* Prolonged PR interval >145 milliseconds in newborn; >180 milliseconds in Infants and young children; >200 milliseconds in adolescents and adults.
2. *II AV block:* Mobitz type I-gradual prolongation of the PR interval followed by dropping of QRS; can be physiological or pathological. In Mobitz type II there is no preceding PR prolongation and QRS is abruptly dropped. The ratio of P to QRS

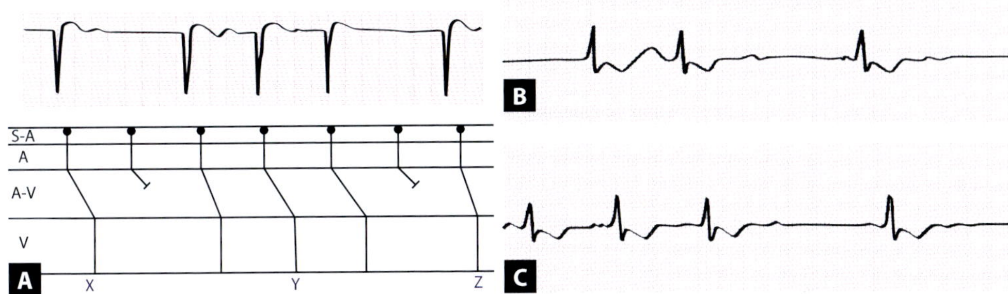

Figs. 18.20A to C: (A) ECG (lead V_3) showing sinus rhythm complicated by a 2° A-V block of the Wenckebach type. *Note:* (1) Following the 'dropped' beat occasioned by a blocked sinus impulse, the P-R interval becomes progressively longer until another sinus impulse is blocked and a further beat is "dropped"; (2) The atrial rhythm is regular and all the P-waves are present; it is thus the QRS complex that is "dropped"; (3) The fully evolved phase of anterior myocardial infarction; (B and C) Electrocardiogram (ECG) (Continuous strip of standard lead II) shows sinus rhythm complicated by type II second-degree A-V block. *Note:* (1) Beats are "dropped" irregularly as a result of successive 3:2, 2:1, 4:3, and 2:1 A-V block; (2) The P-R interval is prolonged (0.26 seconds) but is the same for all conducted beats; (3) The P-wave is broad and notched reflecting *P mitrale*.

may be 2:1 or 3:1. It is always pathological and carries a bad prognosis **(Figs. 18.20A to C)**.

II° AV block may be associated with fast atrial rates as in atrial flutter, fibrillation, or atrial tachycardia. Here the block is physiological and protective to ventricles. Mobitz type II block will not occur in digitalis toxicity.

III° AV block: P-waves bear no relation to the QRS complex. It is not seen in rheumatic carditis. QRS width depends on the site of ventricular focus. If close to the AV node, QRS is narrow and if peripheral ventricular focus, QRS is wide.

BUNDLE BRANCH BLOCK

Right Bundle Branch Block (Changes in V_1 and V_2)

- *QRS:* 120 milliseconds: >100 milliseconds in incomplete block
- rsR' pattern
- ST depression
- T inversion

Left Bundle Branch Block

- *QRS >120 milliseconds*: >100 milliseconds in incomplete block
- M pattern or monophasic wide R in V_5, V_6
- ST depression
- T inversion
- Absent q in V_5, V_6
- Broad negative deflection in V_1

NB: rsR' pattern in V_1 is also seen normally, and in pectus excavatum, straight back, RV volume overload, cor pulmonale and WPW syndrome.

How to read ECG?

Look at standardization **(Figs. 18.21 A to C)**. If standardization is correct, the height of standard waves will be 10 mm and corners will be at right angles to each other. If overdamping, ECG will be of pseudolow voltage and overshooting will result in pseudohigh voltage.

PATTERN OF REPORTING

(1) Rate; (2) rhythm; (3) P-wave (configuration, measurement, and axis); (4) PR interval;

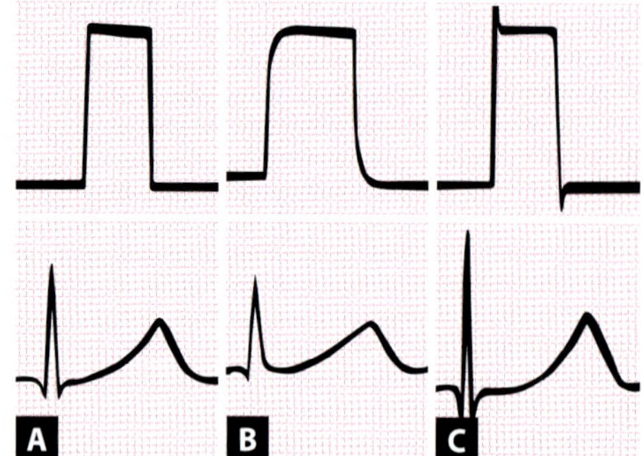

Figs. 18.21A to C: Diagrams of ECG standardization. (A) Correct normal standardization; (B) Overdamping; (C) Underdamping—"overshoot."

(5) QRS (configuration, measurement and axis); (6) ST segment; (7) T-wave; (8) QTc interval; (9) U-wave, and (10) conclusion.

ECG CHANGES IN SPECIFIC SITUATION

- *Hyperkalemia:* Tall, peaked T-waves, R-wave decrease in height, QRS widening, P-wave decrease in height and becoming flat.
- *Hypokalemia:* T-wave decreases in amplitude, becoming flat and later negative, U-wave increases in amplitude, ST depression, and PR prolongation.
- *Hypocalcemia:* QTc long >440 milliseconds.
- *Digitalis* has both effects and toxicity. The effects are sinus bradycardia, short QTc (<350 milliseconds), mirror image of "correction mark" such as ST depression and T inversion in V_4 to V_6. In *toxicity*, the most common abnormalities observed are ventricular extrasystole and paroxysmal SVT with varying Type II AV block. Other manifestations are atrial extrasystole, paroxysmal ventricular tachycardia, complete heart block, and ST, T-inversion in all leads where the R-wave is not tall.

CHANGES IN CONGENITAL HEART DISEASES

Ventricular Septal Defect

Normal sinus rhythm 1/3 has LA enlargement, biventricular hypertrophy, and LV volume overload changes. Similar findings are observed in PDA.

Atrial Septal Defect

- *I:* Left axis, RVH (rsR' pattern)
- *II:* Right axis, RVH (rsR' pattern)
    - *Sinus venosus type:* P-wave axis left (<+30°), RVH
    - *Single atrium:* P axis left, QRS axis left, and RVH

Pulmonary Stenosis

- Right axis, RA enlargement, and RVH (strain pattern).
- *Aortic stenosis and coarctation:* LVH (pressure overload).

Tetralogy of Fallot

Right axis, RVH, sudden early transition (V_1 shows tall R wave, but V_2 shows deep S wave).

Ebstein Anomaly

Normal sinus rhythm, SVT sometimes, tall P, long PR interval, right bundle branch block (RBBB), no RVH, type-B WPW.

Tricuspid Atresia

Left axis, LV forces, paucity of RV forces.

d-TGA

Right atrial enlargement, RVH, and right axis.

L-TGA

Left axis, q in V_1 V_2, no q in V_5 V_6, WPW syndrome (type A).

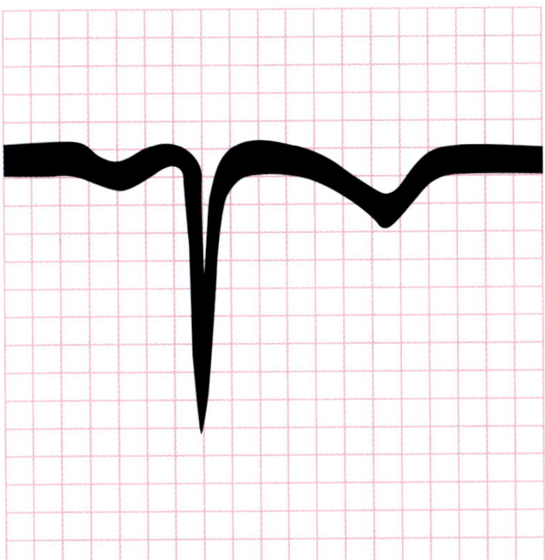

Fig 18.22: ECG in lead 1 in dextrocardia (mirror image of normal lead I dextrocardia), for example, if V_5R and V_6R reveal normal V_5, then V_6 pattern morphological LV is on the right side.

Dextrocardia

Lead I and aVR are just opposite to normal patterns (lead I negative and aVR positive). Chest leads show the absence of R progression form V_1 to V_6 **(Fig. 18.22)**. Position of ventricles can be made out from right-sided chest leads.

SUGGESTED READING

1. Evans WN1, Acherman RJ, Mayman GA, Rollins RC, Kip KT. Simplified pediatric electrocardiogram interpretation. Clin Pediatr (Phila). 2010;49(4):363-72.
2. Goodacre S, McLeod K. ABC of clinical electrocardiography: Paediatric electrocardiography. BMJ. 2002;324(7350):1382-5.
3. O'Connor M, McDaniel N, Brady WJ. The pediatric electrocardiogram. Part I: Age-related interpretation. Am J Emerg Med. 2008;26(2):221-8.

19 CHAPTER Respiratory System

MD Fiji, VT Ajith Kumar

Chapter Outline

- Introduction
- Clinical Anatomy
- History in Respiratory Illnesses
- General Assessment
- Upper Respiratory Tract
- Lower Respiratory Tract
- Points to Consider in Formulating Final Diagnosis
- Clinical Case Scenarios

INTRODUCTION

Please read Chapters 6 and 7 before you proceed.

Respiratory disorders contribute up to two-thirds of patients in the pediatric age group, leading to loss of school days and increased under-five mortality. Systematic history tailored to the patient's particular complaint and physical examination are helpful to arrive at the diagnosis and identify the gravity of the situation.

Symptoms may be trivial or extremely distressing but either may indicate serious and life-threatening disease. Complaints generally draw attention to the respiratory system (RS) but there are exceptions, e.g., a child with progressive pulmonary tuberculosis or lung abscess presenting with irregular fever, or a child with hypoxia presenting as seizures. Nonrespiratory disorders also present with respiratory symptoms such as children with metabolic acidosis (due to diabetic ketoacidosis, or inborn errors of metabolism), cardiac failure, or renal failure.

CLINICAL ANATOMY

The RS extends from the external nares to the terminal alveoli and includes the paranasal sinuses, middle ear, and pleura. For ease of clinical assessment, the system is divided into upper and lower respiratory tracts by an arbitrary line at the upper level of the larynx, though the anatomical division is at the bifurcation of the trachea. The trachea originates from the lower part of the larynx and bifurcates into two main bronchi. The right main bronchus has three divisions supplying the upper, middle, and lower lobes. The left main bronchus divides to supply the upper and lower lobes.

The bifurcation of trachea corresponds to the angle of Louis anteriorly (the lower border of manubrium sterni) and the disc between the 4th and 5th thoracic vertebrae posteriorly. The major interlobar or oblique fissure extends from the 2nd thoracic spine to the 6th costochondral junction anteriorly, and corresponds to the upper border of the lower lobe which is mainly represented posteriorly. A horizontal line on the right side from the sternum at the level of the 4th costal cartilage drawn to meet the major fissure forms the minor inter lobar fissure and marks the boundary between the upper and middle lobes. The middle and upper lobes on the right side and the upper lobe on left occupy

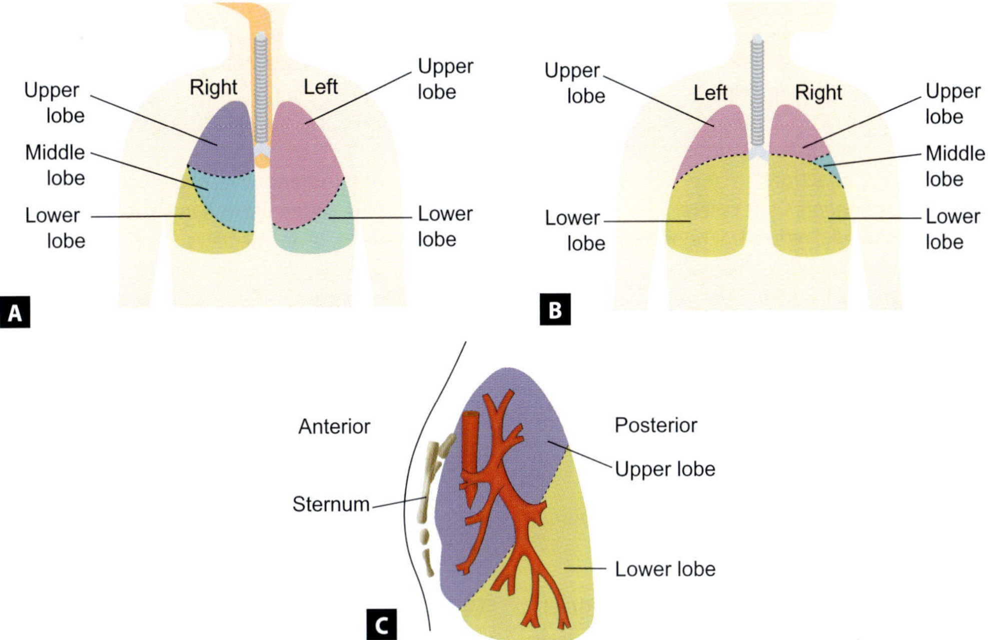

Figs. 19.1A to C: The lung segments: (A) Anterior view; (B) Posterior view; and (C) Lateral aspect of left lung.

most of the area in front. In the axillary region, all lobes are accessible **(Figs. 19.1A to C)**.

HISTORY IN RESPIRATORY ILLNESSES

Symptoms

In children the most common respiratory symptoms are cough, noisy breathing, and respiratory distress (dyspnea) with or without fever. Less common are chest pain, abdominal pain, hemoptysis, dysphagia, recurrent vomiting, headache, and disturbed sleep as the initial symptoms. Sputum production and halitosis are rare complaints.

Cough

Cough is the sudden release of air through a partially closed glottis after deep inspiration. Parents differ in considering how much cough is abnormal. The following aspects should be an analyzed.

Onset and duration: Sudden onset of coughing and choking usually indicates *foreign body aspiration*, the other causes being chemical injury, pulmonary edema, and embolism or pulmonary hemorrhage. Chronic cough (>8 w) occurs in a large number of conditions **(Box 19.1)**.

Intensity and nature of cough: Cough may be mild or intractable, paroxysmal, dry or productive, honky, or feeble. Mild dry cough is usually a presentation of cough variant asthma. In children with postnasal drip, cough appears like an attempt to clear the throat secretions described as hawking cough. Intractable cough occurs in severe asthma and pneumonia. Paroxysms of cough with vomiting followed by whoop (forceful inspiratory gasp through partially

BOX 19.1: Common causes of chronic cough in children.

- Hyperreactive airway disease
- Postnasal drip
- *Infections of the respiratory system:* Tuberculosis, pertussis, HIV infection
- *Recurrent aspiration:* Cleft palate, gastroesophageal reflux, tracheoesophageal fistula, bulbar/pseudobulbar palsy, velopharyngeal insufficiency
- *Developmental abnormalities of the lung:* Bronchiectasis, sequestration lung
- *Smoking:* Active, passive
- *Drug-induced:* ACE inhibitors
- Impacted foreign body airways
- Habit cough

(ACE: angiotensin-converting enzyme; HIV: human immunodeficiency virus)

BOX 19.2: Common causes of paroxysmal cough in children.

- Respiratory
  - Hyperreactive airway disease, postnasal drip
  - Infections (adenovirus, chlamydia, pertussis, tuberculosis, lung abscess, empyema, bronchiectasis, cystic fibrosis)
  - Foreign body impaction airway
- Gastroesophageal reflux (GER)
- *Mediastinal compression:* Cysts, enlarged lymph nodes, tumors, vascular rings
- *Drugs and irritants:* ACE inhibitors, cigarette smoking
- *Cardiac anomalies:* LVF, congenital MS
- Pseudobulbar palsy

(ACE: angiotensin converting enzyme; LVF: left ventricular failure; MS: mitral stenosis)

open larynx) are characteristics of pertussis. Common causes of paroxysmal cough in children are given in **Box 19.2**.

Cough on waking up in the morning with excessive production of tracheobronchial secretions occurs in asthma, bronchiectasis, chronic rhinopharyngitis, and cystic fibrosis. Exercise induced cough is characteristic of asthma. *Weak cough* suggests *vocal cord palsy* or a neuropathic condition (e.g., spinal muscular atrophy). Honky cough indicates psychogenic nature which should only be diagnosed after thorough assessment.

Note: Cough is not a common symptom in neonates, sick, and undernourished children.

Noisy Breathing

The most common respiratory noise is *wheeze* (continuous sound of musical quality, heard mainly during expiration due to intrathoracic airway narrowing). *Stridor* is loud, continuous, harsh, monophonic, and usually inspiratory sound due to upper airway obstruction. Expiratory stridor is the harsh sound that occurs in intrathoracic tracheal obstruction and may be indistinguishable from wheeze. In midtracheal obstruction, stridor and wheeze may coexist. Stridor follows a large number of causes in newborns and young babies **(Box 15.6)**. The most common cause of acute stridor in infants and young children is the croup syndrome which includes acute laryngotracheobronchitis, acute epiglottitis, spasmodic laryngitis, and bacterial tracheitis. Foreign body impaction of the upper respiratory tract, chemical injuries, and angioedema of the larynx are less common causes of acute stridor and can cause sudden death unless timely intervention is done. Associated high fever and toxicity suggest acute epiglottitis and bacterial tracheitis. Repeated episodes of stridor are characteristic of spasmodic laryngitis.

Grunting is episodic short early expiratory sound caused by partial closure of the larynx, so as to increase the functional residual capacity of the lungs. It is a pathognomonic sign of pneumonia in children, can occur in pulmonary edema also and indicates hypoxia. *Snoring* is inspiratory noise of irregular quality caused by partial obstruction of the upper respiratory tract, usually in the region of nasopharynx. The causes are adenoid hypertrophy, foreign body in the nostril, Down syndrome, severe obesity and unilateral choanal atresia. Minimal snoring in newborns is not pathological. *Rattling* is coarse irregular sound heard mainly during inspiration indicating secretions in trachea or major bronchus. They can be felt by hands placed on the chest.

Respiratory Distress

Older children will be able to report dyspnea (subjective feeling of difficult breathing) as "cannot get enough air." Parents perceive respiratory distress in infants and young children from the rapid respiratory rate (RR) or *fast breathing*, exaggerated chest movements *(chest indrawing)*, and *noisy breathing*.

Tracheal tug is the indrawing of suprasternal region in severe respiratory distess.

Chest pain due to respiratory problems is not uncommon. As an isolated complaint, it rarely indicates pathology. Excruciating chest pain following a bout of cough in asthma or pertussis can indicate pneumothorax. Chest pain along with cough and fever indicates pleural involvement in pneumonia. Common respiratory conditions causing chest pain are pneumonia, pneumothorax, trauma, pleurodynia, sickle cell anemia, pulmonary embolism, and pleural or lung tumors.

The sudden recurrent chest pain lasting only seconds to minutes, experienced by most children, is due to transient involuntary spasm of intercostal muscles. Localized chest pain is a common complaint in costochondritis *(Teitze syndrome)*. A teenager's chest pain without any associated symptom is often psychosomatic, but sports injuries must be kept in mind and relevant questions to be asked to clarify the symptom. Mastalgia is another cause of chest pain in early puberty.

Hemoptysis is spitting or coughing of blood arising from a lesion in the respiratory tract. Very often it is streaks of blood mixed with sputum indicating trivial superficial erosion. Massive bleeding points to serious respiratory illness. It should be differentiated from hematemesis by detailed history of associated respiratory or gastrointestinal symptoms and concerned system examination. Oozing of blood from the *gums* can also cause hemoptysis which should be verified. Hemoptysis is preceded by bouts of cough and blood is bright red. In hematemesis blood is usually coffee colored due to gastric acid contact. Common causes of hemoptysis in children are given in **Box 19.3**.

Dysphagia is a feature of pharyngitis and tonsillitis and is a prominent complaint in *impacted foreign bodies* in pharynx, retropharyngeal and lateral pharyngeal abscesses, and acute epiglottitis.

Recurrent vomiting is very often an associated complaint. Vomiting after paroxysmal cough (posttussive vomiting) is seen in pertussis asthma and foreign body impaction of airways.

Sputum production as an isolated complaint is uncommon in children. At times vomiting of mucus from gastric contents and

BOX 19.3: Common causes of hemoptysis in children.

- Pneumonia [bacterial (tuberculosis), fungal (aspergillosis)]
- Bronchiectasis, lung abscess
- Trauma (contusion, rib fracture)
- Infected lung cyst
- Congestive heart failure
- Foreign body aspiration
- Pulmonary embolism
- Others
  - Arteriovenous malformations
  - Coagulation disorders (congenital, acquired)
  - Anticoagulant therapy
  - Drug-induced—cocaine intake

thick saliva may be reported as sputum. Most children below 4 yr swallow sputum. When spitted out, the quantity and color should be enquired. Purulent sputum though indicates pulmonary infection, may occasionally be produced in allergic airway diseases without superadded infection. Spitting large amounts of sputum with postural variation indicates suppurative lung diseases (bronchiectasis, lung abscess). Purulent nasal secretion may be spitted out in sinusitis.

Acute abdominal pain (upper) may be the single symptom reported occasionally in children with lower lobe pneumonia and may cause mistaken diagnosis of hepatitis, biliary colic, pancreatitis, appendicitis or renal pain.

Radiating pain to shoulder with lower lobe pneumonia and also pain over the neck and stiffness are not unusual in upper lobe pneumonia.

Halitosis (offensive breath) as a respiratory symptom occurs secondary to anaerobic bacterial infections in suppurative lung disease. It is commonly due to poor oral and dental hygiene.

Sleep disturbances are usual with any respiratory problem—can be upper airway obstruction (as upper respiratory infection and adenoids) and reactive airway disease with aggravated cough and respiratory distress in the night. Primary hypoventilation is a rare problem in Leigh's encephalopathy and Ondine's curse (congenital central hypoventilation due to generalized impairment of autonomic nervous system).

Headache is a common symptom in most respiratory diseases. It can be localized headache over the paranasal sinuses in sinusitis. Generalized headache due to chronic hypoxia can occur in severe persistent asthma, obstructive sleep apnea, and in persistent or repeated infections of paranasal sinuses and lung parenchyma. In acute asthma exacerbation transient hypoxia can be the cause for headache.

Recurrent or chronic respiratory problems with frequent or *chronic diarrhea* indicate immune deficiency disorders (congenital and acquired) or cystic fibrosis. Persistent candidiasis, resistant/atypical tuberculosis, recurrent pneumonia, sinusitis, and otitis are suggestive of immune deficiency disorders. Eczema associated with recurrent cough denotes atopy.

Severity of respiratory illness in the patient can be evaluated by asking about the child's physical activity at home and school, sleep disturbances, frequency of hospitalization, and loss of school days, details of medicine intake, academic performance, and enquiring the degree of growth retardation.

Personal habits: Details of diet, and the adequacy of food intake, food faddism, schooling, play activities, extracurricular activities, peer relations (especially smoking habits and substance abuse in adolescents) should be enquired in detail. Chronic/recurrent respiratory problems lead to frequent school absenteeism, poor scholastic performance, and very low self-esteem keeping them aloof. Most patients will be consuming deficient diets due to poor appetite, food faddism, and added food restriction implemented by the family. Enquire the participation of the patient in sports and recreational activities. Children and adolescents with poor health and respiratory stamina will be reluctant in sports and games.

Family history of hyperreactive airway disease and atopy can be elicited in most children. Occupational history of parents should be clarified. Children whose parents are involved in woodworks, carpentry, spray painting, and rubber and plastic industries do have the hazard of aggravation of airway hyperreactivity from the dust transmission by body contact.

Social and environmental history should be elicited in detail. Poor socioeconomic and educational status of the family predisposes to undernutrition, lack of parental interest in proper immunization, internal air pollution from poor housing with defective ventilation, pets and pests infestation, and overcrowding; all produce internal pollution resulting in frequent respiratory infections and exacerbation of airway hyperreactivity. Also the diseases may not be treated properly and in time due to ignorance and financial constraints. External environmental pollution from rearing domestic animals, unscientific public waste disposal and waste dumping from factories, small scale industries, markets, and slaughterhouses are the other predisposing factors to respiratory illnesses.

GENERAL ASSESSMENT

The schema of examination should be as given in **Box 7.1**, but the first step is to detect the danger signs related to the RS so as to provide urgent life support. These are apnea, abnormal breathing patterns, increased work of breathing, altered sensorium, convulsions, cyanosis, poor feeding, sweating, weak or absent cry, hypotonia, repeated vomiting, dehydration, paralysis, and undernutrition. Proceed as in Ch. 8 for rapid assessment and urgent lifesaving support to the sick child.

Abnormal Breathing (Figs. 19.2A to D)

- *Apnea* is cessation of breathing for >20 seconds associated with bradycardia or neurologic impairment. Duration <20 seconds but if associated with pallor, limpness, cyanosis, or convulsions, should be a cause for alarm. Immediate resuscitation should be done, if the patient is apneic.
- *Cheyne stokes breathing* is characterized by rhythmic waxing and waning of the depth of respiration, with regularly recurring periods of apnea. It is seen in congestive heart failure and raised intracranial pressure with cerebral cortical impairment.

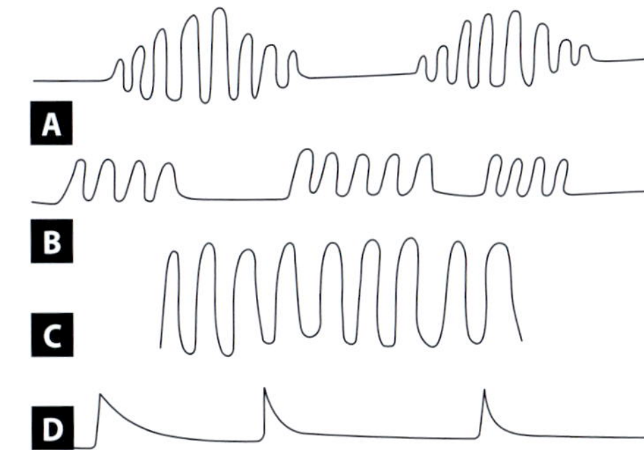

Figs. 19.2A to D: Patterns of abnormal breathing: (A) Cheyne Stokes; (B) Biot's; (C) Kussmaul; and (D) Gasping.

- *Biot's breathing* is characterized by irregular periods of apnea, alternating with periods of four or five breaths of identical depth, and indicates severe brain stem damage.
- *Kussmaul breathing* is rapid deep breathing of metabolic acidosis—may indicate diabetic ketoacidosis.
- *Gasping or jaw breathing* is of slow rate with rapid inspiration, prominent jaw movement, and slow expiration. Indicates severe hypoxia due to any cause.

Work of breathing: Overactivity of accessory muscles of respiration indicates increased work of breathing. This includes flaring of ala nasi, head nodding (sternomastoids and scalenes overactivity), tracheal tug and chest retractions (intercostal, subcostal, suprasternal, and infrasternal).

Chest-abdominal movements: Observe the chest movements from the child's side in supine and standing positions to confirm that both sides are moving equally and to assess the relative contributions of chest and abdomen. In normal inspiration, lower chest flares out and abdomen moves forward by the action of lower intercostal muscles and diaphragm, respectively. When the intercostals are paralyzed, as in spinal muscular atrophy, the lower chest is drawn inward by the diaphragm and abdominal wall movement is prominent during inspiration. Such movements can occur in upper airway occlusion also due to the violent action of diaphragm. Reverse movement is seen in diaphragm weakness when the abdomen is drawn in during inspiration—*paradoxical breathing*. In unilateral phrenic nerve paralysis, the abdomen is drawn in on the paralyzed side during inspiration whereas the movement is normal (i.e., moves out) on the other side.

Altered sensorium and convulsions indicate hypoxemia but underlying meningitis, brain abscess, metabolic disorders, or drug toxicity should be suspected.

Cyanosis in respiratory diseases indicates serious degree of hypoxia. Associated circulatory failure or underlying cardiac lesions should be ruled out. It can be differentiated from cyanotic heart disease by hyperoxia test (Ch. 15). Refer **Box 7.2** for the causes of cyanosis in children.

Clubbing in respiratory diseases manifests early in lung abscess, empyema, and malignancies. **Box 7.3** reveals the causes of clubbing in children. In bronchiectasis it may take at least 1 yr for clubbing to manifest.

Indicators of serious chronic respiratory illness as given in **Box 19.4** should be looked for.

BOX 19.4: Indicators of serious chronic respiratory illness in children.

- Persistent fever
- Limitation of physical activity
- Chronic purulent sputum
- Cyanosis
- Clubbing
- Persistent tachypnea
- Labored breathing
- Growth retardation
- Persistent chest hyperinflation
- Family history of heritable lung diseases

Vital Signs (Tables 7.2, 7.3)

Tables 7.2 and 7.3 reveal agewise normal respiratory rate and the values for tachypnea in children. *Tachypnea (fast breathing)* is a reliable indicator of pneumonia in children but can occur in anxiety, nasal block (young babies), bronchiolitis, asthma, collapse lung, cardiac failure, pulmonary edema, pneumothorax, and pleural effusion. The rate should be counted by inspection for one complete minute in a quiet child and should be repeated in doubtful situations. Rapid shallow breathing indicates respiratory muscle paralysis. Metabolic acidosis of any etiology is characterized by increased rate and depth of breathing (**Fig. 19.2C** *Kussmaul breathing in diabetic ketoacidosis*). Happy tachypnea (tachypnea without retractions) is a feature of cardiac failure.

Tachycardia: Sinus tachycardia may be due to respiratory tract infection. Anxiety, cardiac failure, respiratory failure, simultaneous intake of sympathomimetic drugs, and salbutamol therapy are causes of tachycardia in respiratory diseases. Suspect salbutamol hypersensitivity if heart rate is >200/min and/or irregular.

Temperature >102°F indicates upper (sinusitis, otitis media, tonsillopharyngitis, and mastoiditis) and/or lower respiratory tract bacterial infections. Typical pattern of temperature in pneumococcal pneumonia of olden days is now rare due to the widespread early use of antibiotics. Common causes of high fever in lower respiratory illnesses are pneumonia, bacterial tracheitis (always suspect serious staphylococcal tracheitis in infants with stridor and high fever), empyema, lung abscess, and bronchiectasis. Low grade pyrexia in reactive airway disease may not indicate underlying bacterial infection. In viral and mycoplasmal infections and tuberculosis fever is usually low grade.

Blood pressure should always be recorded. Hypotension and pulsus paradoxus indicate serious respiratory impairment (Ch. 17).

Pulse oximetry: Pulse oximetry (indicates the percentage of hemoglobin saturated with oxygen) is a noninvasive method of monitoring the patient's oxygen saturation measured by pulse oximeter (Ref. **Fig. 7.8**). Normal oxygen saturation (SpO_2) values range from 95 to 100%. Value <92% indicates hypoxia. Values may be low in patients in shock, with cold extremities, cyanotic heart disease, and chronic airway diseases. Appropriate finger probes should be correctly applied in infants and young children so that erroneous values can be avoided.

Head to foot examination: Proceed as detailed in Ch. 7. Resting tremor and tachycardia and/or irregular heartbeats in a patient with respiratory distress indicate overuse of salbutamol or drug hypersensitivity. Oropharyngeal candidiasis and/or hoarseness of voice can be due to inhaled steroids of long duration or immunodeficiency. Congenital/acquired immune deficiency or cystic fibrosis must be suspected in grossly undernourished children with chronic or recurrent respiratory illness. Severe food restriction by parents is also a factor to be enquired in such cases. Obesity (predominantly truncal) with striae and cushingoid appearance indicate prolonged or repeated steroid therapy (especially if on alternate system prolonged drug therapy) in children with hyperreactive airway disease.

UPPER RESPIRATORY TRACT

Use a bright torch to examine the *nose, ears, and throat* (to be reserved as the last part if the child is young or noncooperative). Children with inhalant allergies frequently develop a transverse nasal crease due to the repeated nose rubbing *(allergic salute)* to relieve itching (Ref. **Fig. 7.28**). Dark pigmentation of skin below the eyes, the "allergic shiners" and "Dennie's sign" (or the Dennie–Morgan fold) skin crease radiating from the inner canthus of eyes to two-thirds of the length of lower eyelids are other features of nasopharyngeal allergy.

Adenoid facies, characterized by open mouth with protruding upper incisors, narrow pinched nose, and long face is seen in adenoid hypertrophy (Ref. **Fig. 7.29**). The nasal passages may be narrow as in midface hypoplasia associated with various syndromes. Look for congenital anomalies such as choanal atresia and deviated nasal septum. Extensive nasal polyps cause widening of the nasal bridge. Ulceration, crusting, purulent or blood stained discharge, presence of foreign bodies, trauma and tumors (vascular and nonvascular), etc., should be looked for. Persistent blood stained and foul smelling discharge from one side usually indicates foreign body in that nostril. *Leech invasion of nostrils* has to be suspected in children with persistent epistaxis in certain areas of the world (especially in children living in areas near forests) with leech infestation. Sinus tenderness can be elicited in older children >2 yr.

Examine the ears for congenital anomalies, infections, foreign bodies, and impacted wax. Gently move the pinna and tragus; tragus pain suggests otitis externa. Examine the mastoids and retroauricular areas for eczema, tenderness, and lymph node enlargement. For better visualization of external ear canal and tympanic membrane pull the pinna with thumb and index finger, up and posteriorly in older children, and down and lateral in young infants.

Otoscopic evaluation is a must in febrile young patients without obvious cause and also for those with ear symptoms. In the latter group, evaluate the healthy side first. The otoscope should be well lighted; use the largest speculum that fits comfortably into the ear canal. Older children cooperate, if the procedure is explained and the instrument is allowed to handle without damage. Young babies may be restrained on the mother's (parent's) shoulder. Instruct the parent to restrain the child's hands with one hand and head with the other hand. The testing may also be done with the baby restrained over the examination table. Gently place the otoscope over the external auditory meatus and observe the external ear canal. Carefully advance it to observe the tympanic membrane. Observe the absence of normal light reflex, dull appearance, bulge, retraction, and perforation—all are features of middle ear infection.

Throat (examination should be the last): *Young babies* are examined by placing over the cot as the mother restrains the baby. *Infants and toddlers* are allowed to sit on mother's lap. The child's legs should be restrained in between the mother's thighs, the arms and trunk by one hand, and head by the other hand of the mother.

The tonsils should be examined for size (*hypoplastic in X-linked agammaglobulinemia*, enlarged in infections and tumors), congestion, follicles, or membranes. Other evidence of pharyngeal infection are redness and mottling over soft palate and uvula. In *retropharyngeal abscess* the neck is hyperextended and respirations become noisy and gurgling with pooling of secretions. In *lateral pharyngeal abscess* the features are torticollis toward the same side, trismus

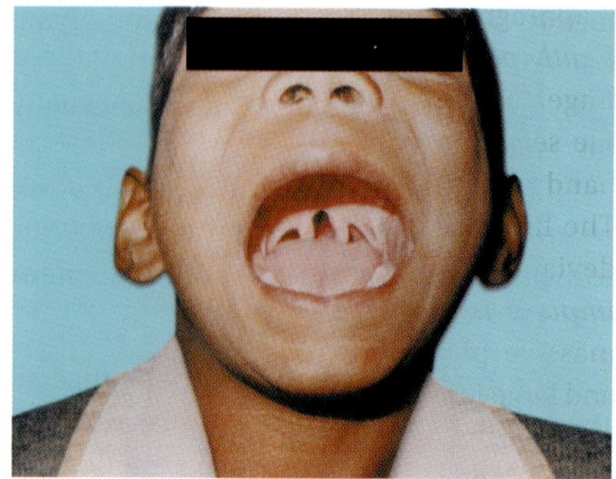

Fig. 19.3: Boy with bifid uvula.

and bulging in of the lateral pharyngeal wall. *Peritonsillar abscess* also is characterized by trismus, torticollis, and hot potato voice. Adenoidal tissue hypertrophy on the posterior pharyngeal wall may reveal "cobblestoning."

The *integrity of the palate* should be made out by palpation to exclude submucous cleft. Bifid uvula is a clue to occult submucous cleft palate **(Fig. 19.3)**.

LOWER RESPIRATORY TRACT

Neck

The important body parts to be assessed in relation to the respiratory tract are the trachea, neck veins, and the presence of surgical emphysema (Ref. Ch.7 for details on lymphadenopathy).

Trachea

Trachea is to be inspected and palpated for deviation in cooperative children (in standing or sitting position), the examiner facing the child. Lying position may be adapted in a sick child. *Tracheal deviation* causes the clavicular head of sternomastoid muscle on that side to appear prominent *(Trail sign)*. In severe respiratory distress, "*tracheal tug*," i.e., pulling in of trachea toward the chest occurs due to the vigorous contraction of diaphragm pulling down the mediastinum. *Gently palpate* the trachea with the middle finger at the suprasternal notch, keeping the second and fourth fingers of the same hand on either edges of the sternal notch. The finger will slip to the opposite side of deviation. *Trachea along with the cardiac impulse is pushed to the opposite side* in massive pleural effusion, pneumothorax, and large intrathoracic cysts and tumors. It is *pulled* to the *same side* in upper lobe collapse, fibrosis, and pleural adhesions.

Signs of superior mediastinal obstruction are edema of head and neck, cyanosis, proptosis, Horner's syndrome (Ref. Ch. 21) and distended nonpulsatile neck veins. The common cause is mediastinal mass especially due to lymphoma.

Subcutaneous emphysema: Patient should be palpated for crepitus over the supraclavicular regions. Common cause is exacerbation of asthma leading to pneumomediastinum or pneumothorax (Ref. Ch. 7 for more details).

Chest

The format for presentation is inspection, palpation, percussion, and auscultation, but the order of examination may be according to the age and cooperation of the patient but final documentation should be according to the format.

Inspection

Maximally expose the chest as the custom permits avoiding cold injury; keep the eyes at the level of chest, from head and foot ends and from front and lateral aspects observe the chest. Evaluate the overall shape and appearance of the chest. Normal chest is bilaterally symmetrical, is oval in shape in horizontal cross section with narrow anteroposterior (AP) diameter. Observe the chest for any drooping of the shoulders which occurs in painful conditions of the chest as given in **Box 19.5**.

BOX 19.5: Causes of drooping of shoulders.

- Painful conditions of the chest wall on same side—(injury chest wall, myalgia, cellulitis, herpes zoster, abscess, osteomyelitis, and fracture of ribs)
- Pleurisy
- Pneumonia
- Collapse
- Fibrosis

Inspect the spine for kyphosis (forward bending) or scoliosis (lateral bending); both can cause asymmetry and pain over the chest and progressive restriction of chest expansion. In children with long standing obstructive airway disease without proper treatment, the AP diameter of the chest increases due to air trap and hyperinflation of the lung revealing *barrel-shaped chest*.

Inspect the position of cardiac apical impulse, precordial shape, and overall shape of the chest. Localized bulge indicates parietal wall inflammatory swellings, hematoma, or tumors. In pleural effusion or pneumothorax, intercostal spaces (ICS) appear bulging. Localized indrawing may be due to congenital deformities or underlying collapse. Look at the chest movements. Localized paucity of movements occur in trauma, painful conditions of chest wall and pleura, pleural effusion, pneumothorax, pneumonia, collapse, and tumors of the lung.

Palpation

Confirm the inspection findings. Shifting of the cardiac impulse without tracheal deviation can occur in scoliosis, funnel chest, and with an enlarged left ventricle. Look for any tenderness and crepitus. Measure the chest expansion at the level of nipples after deep inspiration and expiration. Assess the expansion of identical sides of the chest in the order of supraclavicular, upper interscapular, and lower interscapular areas from the back and infraclavicular and mammary areas from the front. For this, encircle the chest from both sides with four fingers and palm, with the thumbs meeting in the midline, but not touching the chest wall. On inspiration, if one thumb remains closer to the midline it indicates reduced chest movements on that side. Tactile vocal fremitus is compared for spoken words or cry (in infants), over identical areas on both sides of the chest with the ulnar border of the right palm.

Percussion

The examiner should master the technique of percussion to feel, rather than hear the normal and abnormal lung resonance. Young children should be percussed lightly. The left middle finger (the pleximeter) is placed parallel to the area to be percussed, taking care to avoid any air column between the finger and the chest wall. With the tip of the plexor finger (right middle finger), the back of the pleximeter finger is struck at the distal interphalangeal joint, as a tapping movement arising from the wrist. The plexor finger should immediately be raised after the blow. The terminal phalanx of the plexor finger should be at right angles to the metacarpal bone and the pleximeter finger while the blow is delivered. The child should be in a comfortable position—sitting, lying, or placed over the parent's shoulders.

Start percussing the clavicles directly, which will enable the examiner to detect only the gross difference in the note in diseases of the upper chest. Proceed down the ICS in the MCL, each blow being compared with the other side. The upper border of liver dullness reaches the 5th right ICS in the MCL and will shift to one space lower down on deep inspiration (Ref. Ch. 20 for Tidal percussion). On the left side the normal resonance is replaced by the tympanitic note of the stomach at the same level. The cardiac dullness should be verified on the left side which will be more resonant in emphysema and dull in pericardial effusion.

To percuss the lateral side of the chest, the child's upper limbs should be raised above the shoulders with the hands resting over the vertex one over the other. For young children the arms should be raised by the parent. Each intercostal space is percussed and compared with the opposite side, the examiner standing or sitting on the side to be percussed. The normal resonance of the lung on the right side is replaced by liver dullness in the 7th space in mid axillary line, and on the left side by the tympanitic note of stomach almost at the same level.

For percussing the posterior part of the chest, the examiner should stand or sit behind the patient. Percussion should start from the supraclavicular area from medial to lateral side, the pleximeter finger being placed across the area with the tip directed forward. A band of lung resonance normally present in the central area *(Kronig isthmus)* will be replaced by dull notes in massive pleural effusion, consolidation, neoplasms, or collapse of the apical part of the lung. Subsequently, the upper and lower interscapular and the infrascapular spaces should be percussed. The resonance is replaced by the dullness of liver and spleen at the 9th and 10th ICS in the infrascapular area on the right and left sides, respectively.

The *abnormalities perceived from percussion are pain, tenderness, and changes in resonance*. Resonance is the normal feel and sound due to air being set into vibration. Lung resonance is increased in airway obstruction and pneumothorax, in the latter situation reaching up to tympanitic note, i.e., highest resonance. *Localized obstruction* occurs in congenital lobar emphysema or in partial obstruction by foreign body in the bronchus (check valve or ball valve). Overall hyperinflation occurs in obstructive airway disease as in asthma and bronchiolitis pushing down the liver dullness. *Percussion note is impaired or dull* when the lung becomes more solid (pneumonia, consolidation, collapse, fibrosis, sequestration, abscess, and infarction), or if the pleura becomes thickened or contains fluid (pleural effusion, empyema, and hemothorax), or becomes solid (mesothelioma). A *feel of resistance* below the pleximeter finger is perceived in pleural effusion as if percussed against a wall and is stated as *stony dullness.*

In *hydropneumothorax, shifting dullness* can be revealed by percussing the chest (from anterior to posterior) in supine lying position of the patient. As the fluid shifts to the posterior part of chest in lying position, the dull lower chest in sitting position becomes resonant anteriorly and a definite level below which there is complete dullness can be demonstrated.

Auscultatory percussion is helpful to detect mediastinal masses. The patient sits with arms resting on both thighs while the examiner sits facing the child. With the tip of the terminal phalanx of the middle finger of dominant side light percussion is directly applied over the sternum from center to either side, while the note is auscultated from behind over the corresponding areas. Area of impaired resonance on auscultation reveals the size of mediastinal mass.

Auscultation

The best instrument is one's own stethoscope which should be correctly selected (Ch. 17). Listen with the *diaphragm* since the respiratory sounds are relatively high pitched. Breath sounds are well heard in infants; older children should be demonstrated how to take deep breaths through an open mouth.

Developing expertise in interpreting auscultatory findings is very much an experimental process, and as such there is no substitute for having listened to a large number of patients, both with and without lung disease. Follow a consistent pattern for auscultation to avoid missing any area. Start from the infraclavicular area, proceed to mammary, axillary, and infraaxillary areas, each time comparing with the opposite side. Segmental auscultation is the technique of comparing breath sounds of homologous segments. The examiner should sit facing the child to auscultate the anterior aspect of the chest. The lateral side of the chest can be auscultated from front as well as from behind the patient. Posteriorly, auscultation is performed as in the order of percussion, the examiner sitting behind the child. The parameters to be assessed are the breath sounds, added sounds, and vocal resonance.

Breath sounds originate from turbulent airflow in the larger airways and are modified by the lung tissue as they reach the stethoscope diaphragm. Assess the intensity and quality of the breath sounds. Intensity may be normal, reduced, or increased. It is normal when the lung tissue is inflating normally and *reduced in airway obstruction, lung damage, and pleural thickening.* It is *absent in pleural effusion and pneumothorax.* Intensity is increased in young infants and thin children as well as *over the normal lung when the other side is diseased.*

The normal breath sounds are *vesicular* **(Fig. 19.4A)**. The inspiration is loud and high pitched followed by harsh low pitched expiration (without a pause in between)

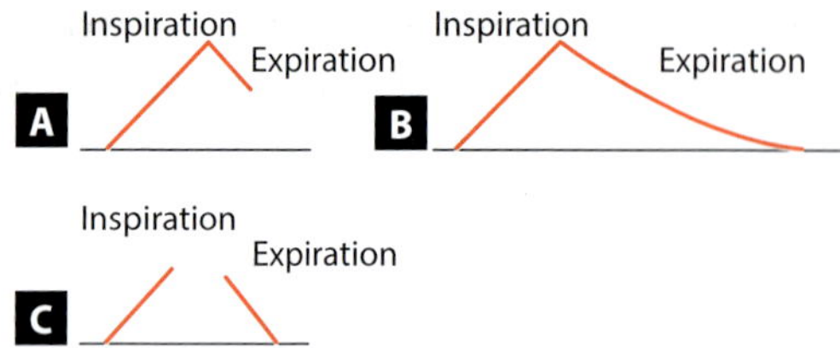

Figs. 19.4A to C: Three types of breath sounds: (A) Vesicular; (B) Bronchovesicular; and (C) Bronchial.

which is of short duration almost up to half of inspiration. The cycle is followed by a pause. In *bronchovesicular* breathing the expiration is prolonged up to or more than inspiration, and there is no pause in between **(Fig. 19.4B)**. It is heard in *normal infants, in bronchiolitis and asthma.*

Bronchial breathing is louder in intensity. Expiration is high pitched, loud, and prolonged (equal to or more than the duration of inspiration). There will be a pause in between **(Fig. 19.4C)**.

The normal vesicular breathing is replaced by *bronchial breathing* when the lung becomes more solid *(consolidation, collapse consolidation, fibrosis, abscess lung, and neoplastic growth)* or *contains a cavity*. In these situations, the sounds generated in large airways are transmitted more efficiently and resemble those obtained by listening over the trachea.

Added sounds are abnormal sounds which arise in airways, lung parenchyma, pleura, mediastinum, intestines, and soft tissues. They are wheezes, crackles, pleural rub, mediastinal crunch, peristaltic sounds, and crepitus.

Wheezes arise from narrowed intrathoracic airways and can be *high pitched* or *low pitched* and can be expiratory or inspiratory. The former occurs in smaller airway narrowing and the latter arise from larger airways. *Monophonic wheeze* is due to localized narrowing of a single bronchus as in *foreign body impaction*. Widespread *polyphonic wheezes* (with differing intensity) usually heard in expiration indicate diffuse airway obstruction as in *asthma* and *bronchiolitis*.

Crackles are *short bubbling* or clicking *noises* which arise from large airways with *secretions (coarse)* or from small airways *(fine)* and from alveoli containing exudates *(fine)*. These sounds are produced by sudden changes in gas pressure from rapid opening of previously closed small airways or alveoli. Crackles are heard in *obstructive airway disease*, pneumonia, and pulmonary edema. *Localized loud, coarse crackles* indicate *bronchiectasis*. *Rattling* indicates moist sounds heard while breathing due to secretions in the pharynx and tracheobronchial tree.

The *added sounds* can be differentiated from conducted sounds (from throat and pharynx.) as the latter disappear after suction, coughing, and change in position; are heard in equal intensity over equidistant parts of the chest and better heard by the stethoscope kept in front of the mouth and neck.

Pleural rub has a rubbing superficial leathery character, heard during identical phases of inspiration and expiration, and does not change after coughing as compared to crackles. Intensity increases as the chest piece is firmly pressed and can be felt with the palpating hand also. It is a sign of pleurisy and disappears when the patient develops pleural effusion.

Mediastinal crunch (Hamman Sign) is heard in children with mediastinal emphysema and left-sided pneumothorax. Crunching sound will be heard over the left sternal border during systole.

Peristaltic sounds are gurgling sounds occasionally heard over the lower part of the left side of the chest. Frequent peristaltic sounds with other clinical signs indicate *diaphragmatic hernia*. Suspect diaphragmatic hernia, if a newborn has scaphoid abdomen, respiratory distress, and bowel sounds heard on the left side of the chest.

Crepitus sounds may occur over the region of a *broken rib* or *surgical emphysema*. *False added sounds* arise by the movement of the stethoscope on the patient's skin and should be differentiated. They are common while auscultating malnourished children with prominent ribs and grooved intercostals spaces. Skin will lose contact with stethoscope intermittently and that detachment will produce a false added sound.

Vocal resonance is the sound perceived by the chest piece as the voice is transmitted through the lungs. The child is auscultated while saying one-one, or the name, or if crying, in the same order of auscultation and both sides are compared. The intensity will be decreased in airway obstruction, collapse, pleural effusion, or pneumothorax (except when bronchial breathing is present). Intensity is increased over areas of consolidation, cavity, infarction, and collapse consolidation. If the child is asked to whisper the same words, it will be heard clearly into the examiner's ears *(whispering pectoriloquy)* over massive consolidation and bronchopleural fistula.

Tips for auscultation: Concentrate on one aspect at a time during auscultation, i.e., intensity of breath sounds on same segmental areas, length of expiration, pause, type of added sounds, their relation to inspiration, expiration, and cardiac cycle, and whether conducted or true added sounds are there.

POINTS TO CONSIDER IN FORMULATING FINAL DIAGNOSIS

Make a mental note of the clinical features and answer the following questions:

- Is the child having respiratory illness?
- Is it acute or chronic?
- Is it a lower respiratory infection? Substantiate your opinion.
- Is it mild or severe? Substantiate.
- Which part of the lower RS is involved, (larynx, airways, parenchyma, or pleura)? Narrate the points in favor of your opinion.
- Is there involvement of more than one part of the RS or generalized involvement? Explain the points.
- Are there any contradictory findings? Are there involvement of nearby organs or other systems?
- Is the child having any life-threatening complications? Narrate and explain.
- Are there any underlying congenital lesions or atopy?
- What is the final diagnosis and probable etiology?
- Should you do any immediate life-saving intervention? Substantiate your opinion.

The final diagnosis should be stated as: Acute lower respiratory infection, severe illness, consolidation of right lower lobe with encysted empyema on the right side. Probable etiology—staphylococcal infection. Include the additional problems also which may be poor nutritional status, anemia, dental caries, etc.

CLINICAL CASE SCENARIOS

Case Scenario 1

Elna, 3 yr old, baby girl, is brought at 10 AM, in the emergency department (ED) with history of fever for 4 days and one episode of seizure 1 hr back. She had cough, breathing difficulty, and vomiting on these days for which she was on medicines prescribed by the local doctor. Elna was brought by her grandmother with a helping neighbor, as the lady had defective vision; the child's parents had gone for work. Elna was

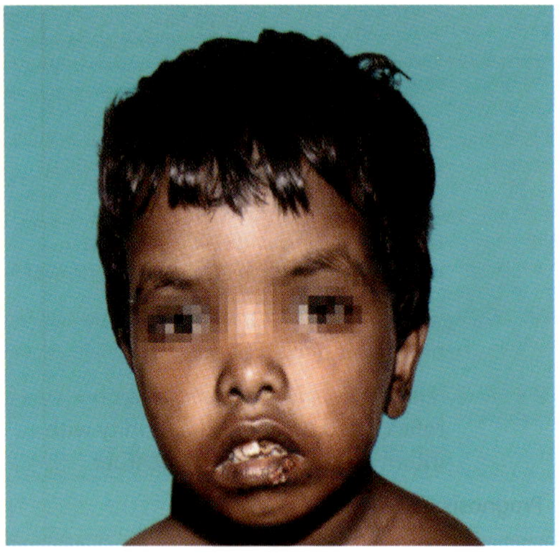

Fig. 20.7: Cheilosis-riboflavin deficiency.

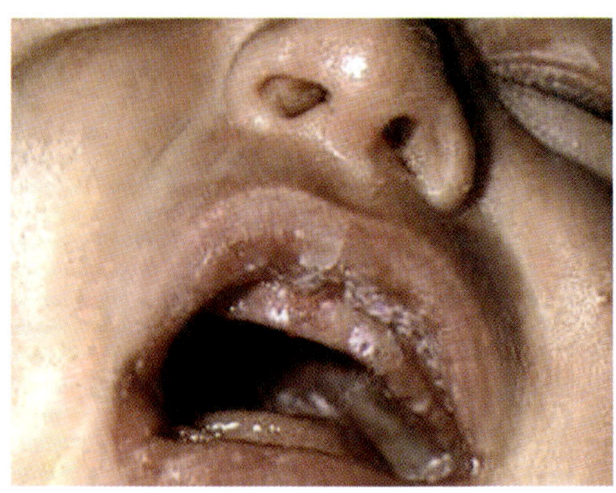

Fig. 20.9: Oral candidiasis—milk curd like lesions. *Courtesy:* www.nhs.uk/conditions/oral-thrush-mouth-Thrush/

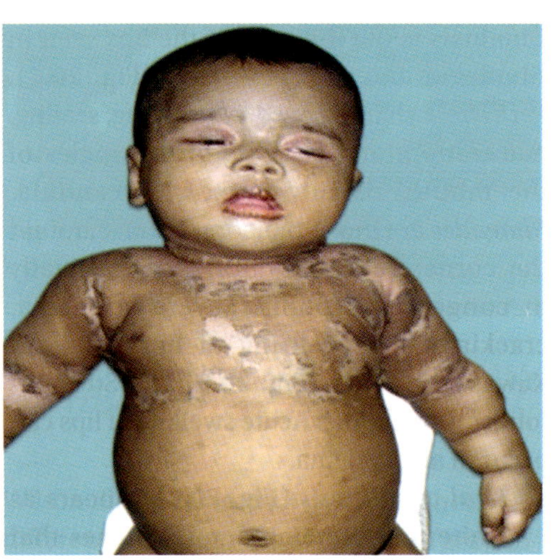

Fig. 20.8: Infant with Kawasaki disease—erythema, fissuring and cracking of lips.

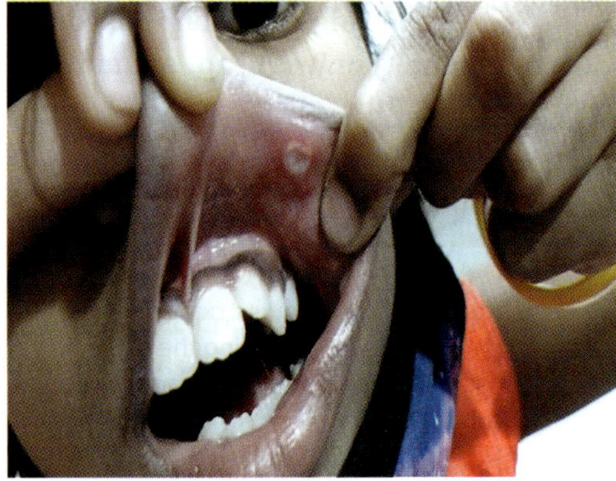

Fig. 20.10: Aphthous ulcer upper lip.

gingivostomatitis caused by fusiform spirochaetes, interdental papillae are ulcerated producing halitosis. Recurrent aphthous ulcers **(Fig. 20.10)** appear in children with undernutrition (iron and zinc deficiency), inflammatory bowel disease, and celiac disease. In Behcet syndrome recurrent oral, palatal, and pharyngeal ulcers occur. *Koplik's spots* are grayish or white dots resembling small grains of sand surrounded by red areola and appear first on the buccal mucosa opposite the lower molars. They are pathognomonic of measles. *Enanthems* are small red or purplish rashes seen on the palate in exanthematous fevers. Brown or blue-black *buccal pigmentation* is seen in Addison disease and Peutz-Jeghers syndrome **(Fig. 20.11)**.

Mucus retention cysts are bluish translucent cysts usually labial and rarely seen on the undersurface of the tongue.

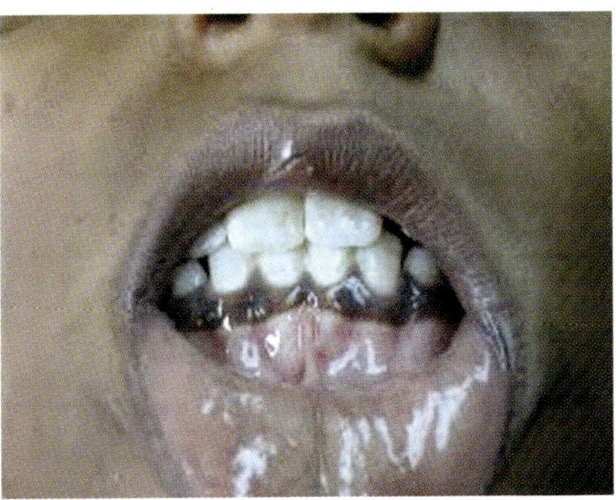

Fig. 20.11: Addison disease—pigmentation of lips and gums.

Spongy bleeding gum of scurvy is a rare finding in this era. Examine the gums for hypertrophy **(Fig. 7.32)**, and lead lines (Burton's line—thin black-blue line between the margin of the gums and the base of teeth, due to chronic lead poisoning) in children with pica.

- *Palate:* Observe for high arch, groove, or cleft (See **Fig. 19.3**: Bifid uvula). Such anomalies appear in association with various syndromes or as isolated defects **(Fig. 15.8B)**.
- *Tongue: Strawberry tongue* is due to desquamation of the white coating and loss of filiform papillae leading to raw-beefy red appearance (seen in vitamin B_{12}, riboflavin and iron deficiencies, celiac disease, chronic diarrhea, Kawasaki disease, scarlet fever, and severe febrile illness **(Fig. 20.12)**. *Glossoptosis* is the posterior positioning of the tongue due to a small lower jaw and may cause breathing difficulty in neonates. *Macroglossia* is big tongue that protrudes out from the mouth **(Fig. 20.13)**. Congenital hypothyroidism, glycogen storage disease, mucopolysaccharidosis, gangliosidosis, Beckwith-Wiedemann syndrome, and tumors of

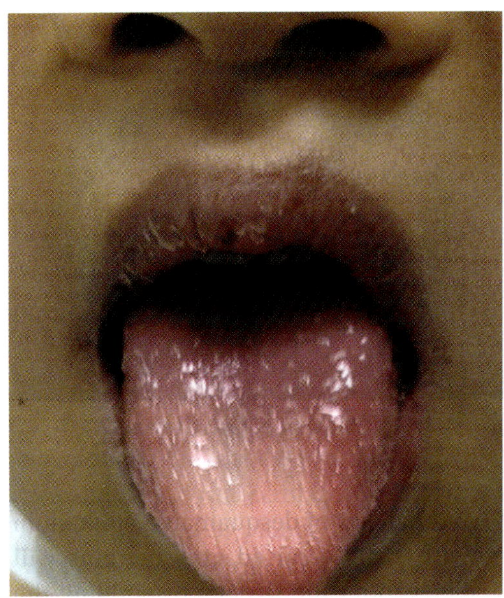

Fig. 20.12: Red cracked lips and strawberry tongue, lips, and gums in Kawasaki disease.

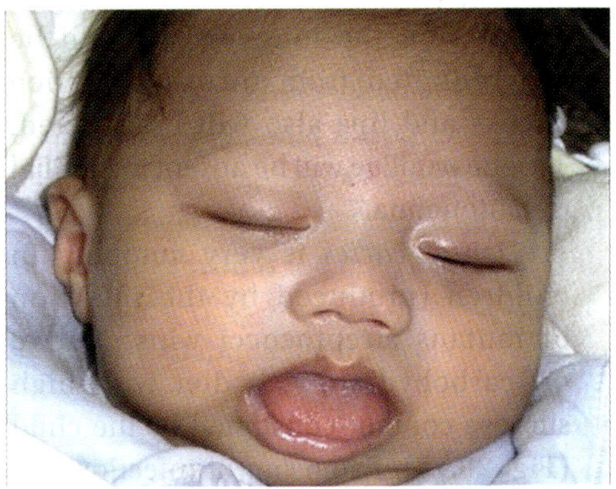

Fig. 20.13: Macroglossia in Beckwith–Wiedemann syndrome.

the tongue are diseases with big tongue. *Ranula* is a translucent bluish retention cyst of the sublingual glands, usually seen on one side of the frenulum beneath the tongue **(Fig. 15.10)**. The tongue reveals white coating in any fever due to desquamated cells, food debris, and bacteria. *In geographic tongue* (a benign condition), annular smooth

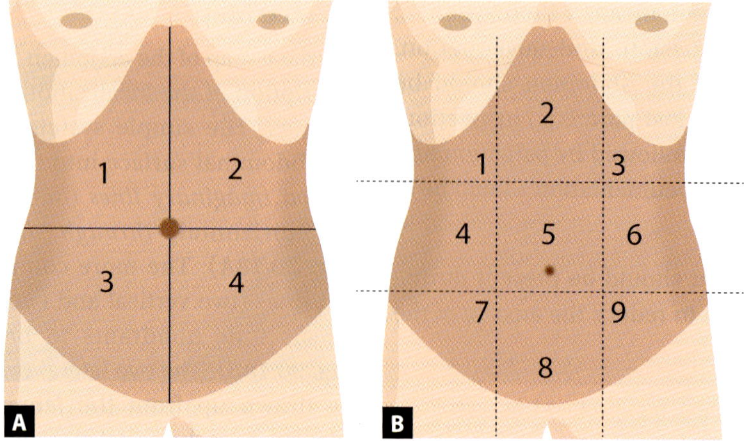

Figs. 20.18A and B: Surface map of the abdomen. (A) 1. RUQ, 2. LUQ, 3. RLQ, 4. LLQ; (B) Regions of the abdomen. 1. and 3. Right and left hypochondria, 2. Epigastrium, 4. and 6. Right and left lumbar, 5. Umbilical; 7 and 9: Right and left iliac; 8. Hypogastrium or suprapubic. (LLQ: left lower quadrant; LUQ: left upper quadrant; RUQ: right upper quadrant; RLQ: right lower quadrant)

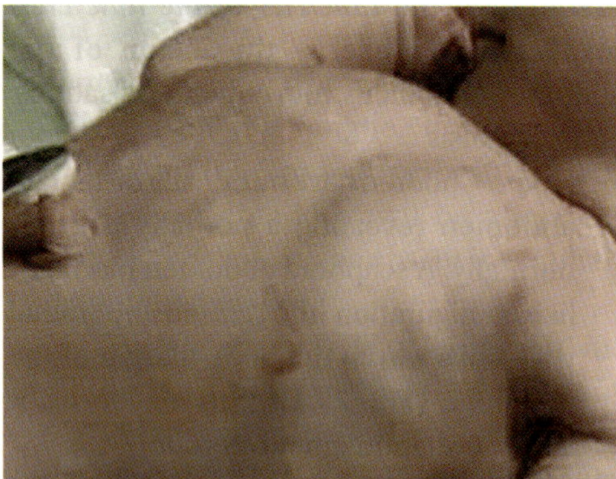

Fig. 20.19: Newborn with diaphragmatic hernia revealing scaphoid abdomen.

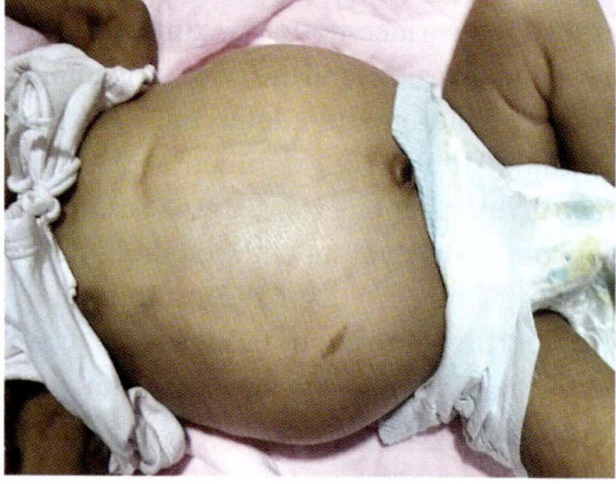

Fig. 20.20: Infant with Hirschsprung's disease revealing severe abdominal distension.

In infants and older children, the scaphoid abdomen indicates severe dehydration and cachexia **(Fig. 7.7)**. Retraction of the abdomen may occur in chorea (Czerny sign). Look for any scars and their location since they indicate previous abdominal surgery. Abdominal distension may be localized or generalized, symmetrical or asymmetrical, and is better appreciated with an oblique source of light. Make a mental note of the site of the bulge from the surface map and the intra-abdominal organs in that region. Common causes of abdominal distension in children are Hirschsprung's disease **(Fig. 20.20)**, ascites, organomegaly, tumor masses (Wilms tumor), and pregnancy in the teenage group.

The umbilicus has a "sprouted appearance" when the intra-abdominal pressure is raised. Atonic musculature occurs in anemia, Down syndrome, hypokalemia, hypothyroidism, and various syndromes [Prune Belly syndrome **(Fig. 15.35)**]. Localized distension occurs in segmental hypoplasia or parietal wall swelling which should be differentiated from intraabdominal masses; the latter becomes less prominent while the child cries or coughs. A linear bulge in the midline from the xiphisternum to the umbilicus is due to the divarication of the rectus abdominis muscle **(Fig. 20.21)**. Central linear bulge in the lower abdomen is usually produced by a distended or *hypertrophic urinary bladder* typically seen in posterior urethral valve.

- *Umbilicus* is everted in umbilical hernia **(Fig. 7.40)**, which can be confirmed by the expansile impulse on palpation when the patient coughs or cries. *Striae* are pink (later become white) wrinkled linear marks on the abdominal wall seen in obese children and following ascites and steroid therapy. The abdominal wall veins are visible in thin and marasmic children and in newborns. Distended veins around the umbilicus (caput medusae) indicate PHT with exaggerated portal systemic flow **(Fig. 20.22)**. Other causes for dilated veins over the abdominal wall are superior and inferior vena caval obstruction. The concerned vein can be diagnosed by assessing the direction of blood flow (see palpation). *Abdominal wall movement* will be absent in generalized peritonitis (the silent/still abdomen). In *diaphragmatic paralysis paradoxical abdominal wall movements* (indrawing of the abdominal wall on inspiration) become obvious, best in the standing posture. Intra-abdominal movements are better appreciated by shining a torch across the patient's abdomen, revealing alterations in the pattern of shadows. *Visible peristalsis* usually indicates intestinal obstruction. In pyloric stenosis and duodenal atresia, it is from left to right, seen in the epigastrium **(Fig. 20.23)**. In small intestinal obstruction "stepladder pattern" is found over the middle of the abdomen. Visible pulsations over the epigastrium may indicate aneurysm of the abdominal aorta or right ventricular hypertrophy.

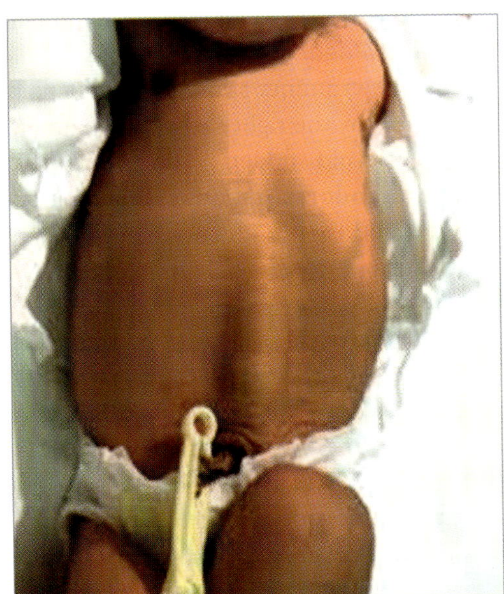

Fig. 20.21: Divarication of recti.

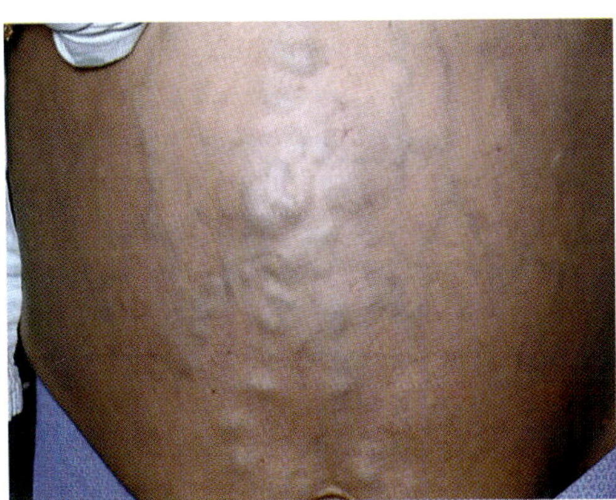

Fig. 20.22: Caput medusae.

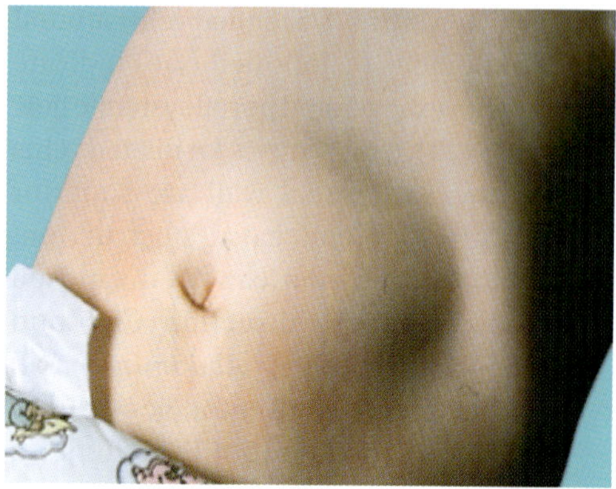

Fig. 20.23: Visible peristalsis in pyloric stenosis.

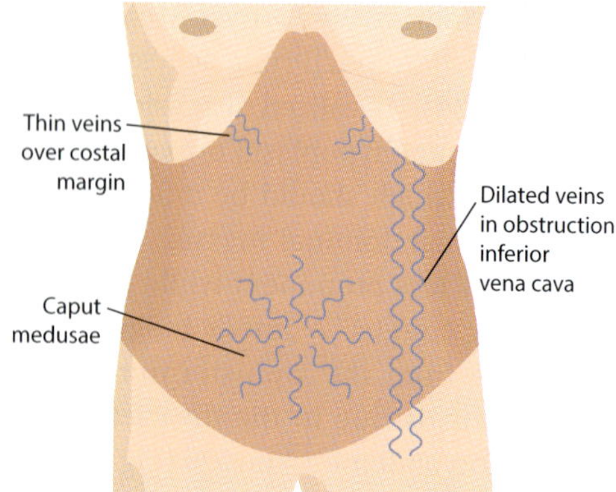

Fig. 20.24: Direction of blood flow in abdominal veins.

- *Palpation:* The examiner should see that the fingernails are trimmed, and the hands are warm before palpating the patient. Observe the child's face for pain expression and compare with the *pain rating scale* **(Fig. 7.20)**. Assess the direction of blood flow (in dilated veins) by tripping the veins. For this, place the two index fingers side by side across the engorged vein. Move the lower finger downward to empty that part of the vein and then withdraw the hand. Assess whether there is filling of the lower part of the vein from below upward. Replace the lower finger and remove the upper finger, pushing the finger upward along the course of the vein and observing the flow.

  Direction of the venous blood flow is away from the umbilicus normally and in portal venous system. In portal venous obstruction the veins are distended, and the flow is exaggerated. In inferior vena caval obstruction, direction of flow is from below upwards (from the long saphenous vein to the axillary vein) and in superior vena caval obstruction blood flows towards the umbilicus **(Fig. 20.24)**.

  Palpate lightly with *finger cushions* to detect tender areas initially. To get relaxation of the abdominal wall, flex the patient's knees and place a pillow behind the head. Distraction of the child by friendly conversation will greatly facilitate palpation of the abdomen. Use the right hand (except for the pyloric tumor), which should be relaxed, flexed minimally at the metacarpophalangeal joint, and placed parallel to the abdomen as if molded over the abdomen. For this, the examiner should sit on a chair or kneel by the right side of the patient. Always avoid sudden poking. Each part of the abdomen should be palpated recollecting the normal anatomical structures beneath the hand.
- *Tenderness* may be localized in acute appendicitis at right lower quadrant (RLQ), in acute hepatitis and acute cholecystitis at the right upper quadrant (RUQ), and in pyelonephritis it is perceived at the flanks. Generalized tenderness is observed in peritonitis.
- *Guarding* occurs when the child has pain while coughing, moving, walking, or jumping. If the child is *stooping forward*

while walking, it indicates *psoas irritation* typically seen in acute appendicitis. Also the patient also will experience pain at RLQ in acute appendicitis if asked to jump up and down. Palpate nontender areas first as perceived from a complaint or facial expression. Infants are best examined on mother's lap while breastfeeding.

Routine palpation in the sequence described here, will enable the examiner not to miss important points.

- Begin from the left iliac fossa **(Fig. 20.25)**, palpate lightly proceeding anticlockwise to end in the suprapubic region; repeat the sequence using deeper palpation with both hands if necessary, especially in obese children, so as to assess the feel of the abdomen—soft, tense, doughy, or rigid.
- Subsequent steps are palpation of the left kidney, spleen, right kidney, liver, urinary bladder, aorta, para-aortic glands, common femoral vessels, and abnormal swellings if detected. Palpate the groins and external genitalia at the end.
- Do not forget to replace the cloth after completion of examination and compliment the patient for the cooperation.

- *Left kidney:* Kidneys are not usually palpable beyond the newborn period unless enlarged or the abdominal wall muscles are hypotonic. The examiner's right hand is placed anteriorly over the left lumbar region while the left hand is placed posteriorly over the left loin **(Fig. 20.26)**. Press the left hand forward and the right hand backward, upward, and inward. The kidney is palpable in visceroptosis and when enlarged (normally palpable in newborns) and *is bimanually palpable* (both hands can feel it) and *ballotable* (can be pushed from one hand to the other). The most common renal mass in children is hydronephrosis. Other causes are renal vein thrombosis (tender nephromegaly), cysts, tumors (Wilms tumor), and malignant infiltrations.
- *Spleen:* In infants and young children, the spleen is palpated in a reclining posture on mother's lap. Older children are examined as in adults. The organ should be at least

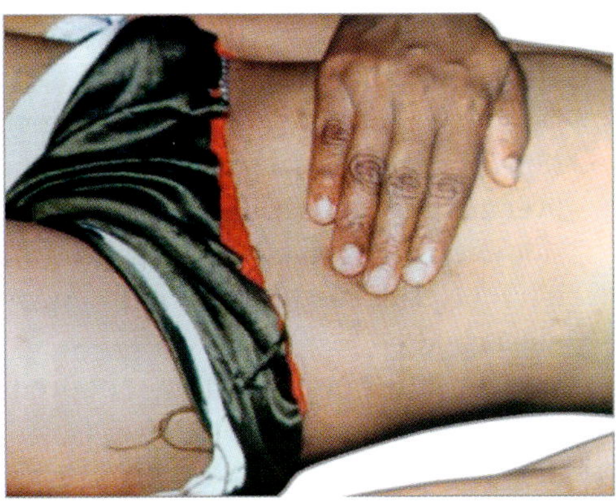

Fig. 20.25: Palpation of the abdomen, begin from L iliac fossa, use finger cushions with hand molded over.

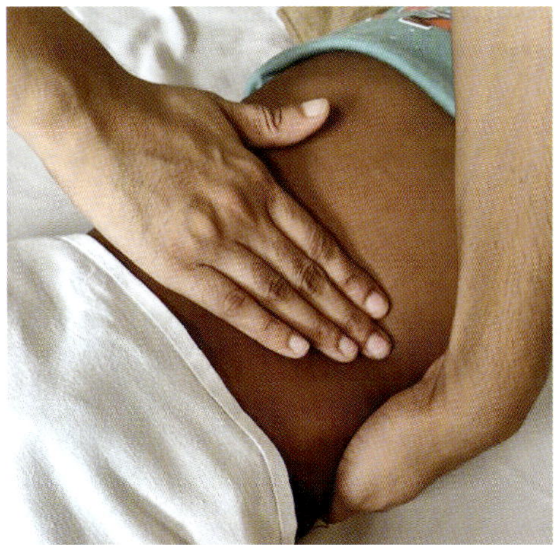

Fig. 20.26: Bimanual palpation of the (left) kidney. *Courtesy:* Dr Divya. D, JR (Peds), Govt Med College, Kottayam, Kerala

twice enlarged to become palpable. Spleen tip (<2 cm) may be normally palpable in newborns and young infants. In massive splenomegaly, the contour of the spleen can be visualized per abdomen **(Fig. 20.17B)**. Stand on the (right) side of the patient and palpate from the right iliac fossa towards the left hypochondrium, i.e., in the direction of enlargement of spleen. To palpate the minimally enlarged spleen, with the left hand press the posterolateral lowermost aspect of the rib cage medially and downward. Introduce the right hand beneath the left costal margin at the same time and palpate deeply. If the spleen is not palpated, gently turn the patient half towards the right side and repeat the examination **(Fig. 20.27)**. In irritable young children, the spleen can be palpated by holding the child in prone position over the mother's shoulder; the examiner should stand on the back of the child and gently palpate the spleen. The spleen is dull on percussion and moves downwards with each inspiration. An enlarged spleen can be differentiated from (left) kidney by the presence of splenic notch; absent bimanual palpability, inability to feel the upper border (cannot get above the mass), and absence of the band of colonic resonance (present anterior to enlarged left kidney). Based on the size, splenomegaly is graded as mild (<3 cm below costal margin), moderate (>3 cm up to the umbilicus), and gross (beyond the umbilicus).

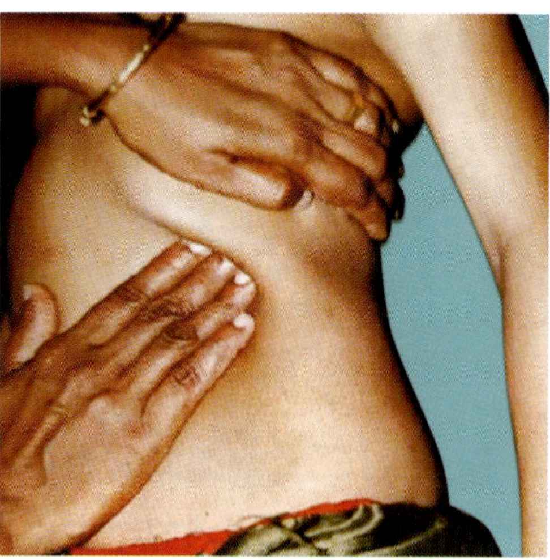

Fig. 20.27: Palpation of spleen.

Causes of splenomegaly are congenital (cysts, hamartomas, hemangiomas, lymphangiomas, polysplenia, etc.), infections (bacterial, viral, and protozoal), inflammatory diseases [systemic lupus erythematosus (SLE) and juvenile idiopathic arthritis (JIA)], hemolytic anemias, splenic cysts, polysplenia, neoplasms, storage diseases, and PHT.

- *The right kidney* is palpated by the horizontally placed right hand anteriorly over the right lumbar region. Place the left hand posteriorly in the right loin and push forward.
- *Liver:* The examiner should sit beside the patient so as to apply hands parallel to the abdomen. One method of palpation is by *both hands* placed side by side on the right hypochondrium lateral to the rectus muscle with the fingers pointing towards the ribs **(Fig. 20.28)**. Move the hands downward or upward till the liver margin is felt as a sharp regular border, which rides beneath the fingers. Now trace the liver margin from the lateral to the medial side toward the epigastrium to palpate the left lobe. This method is better done in older children.

  The alternate (widely adapted) method of palpation of the liver is with the radial border of the right index finger directed parallel to the right subcostal margin **(Fig. 20.29)**. For this, start from the RLQ and move the hand gently

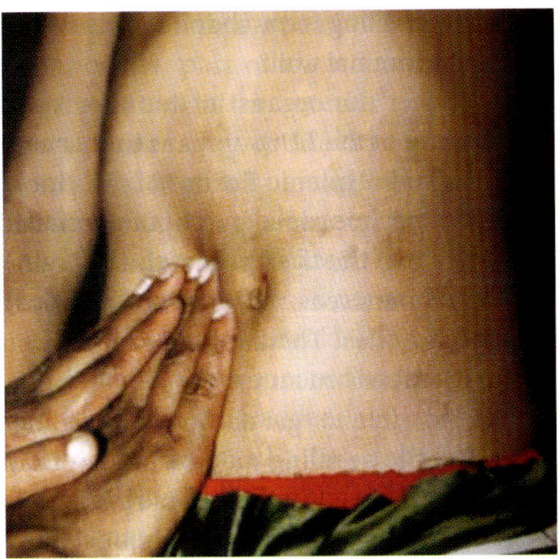

Fig. 20.28: Palpation of liver-ideal method.

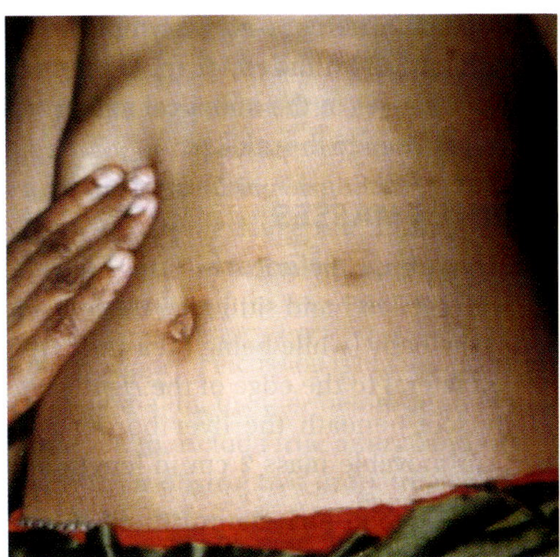

Fig. 20.29: Palpation of the liver—alternate method.

upwards, keeping the radial border of the index finger parallel to the costal margin, while the child is taking breaths. Once the border is felt, follow it to the epigastrium.

Assess the liver border whether regular or irregular. Feel the consistency (should be soft) and surface (smooth). The liver is normally felt up to 2 cm below the costal margin in the right midclavicular line. If >2 cm, it may be due to true hepatomegaly or pushed-down liver, which can be differentiated by measuring the liver span (see percussion). The liver is abnormal if enlarged or small, has abnormal consistency (firm or hard), nodular surface, irregular margin, or if there is isolated left lobe enlargement.

- *Gallbladder* is palpated in the same way as the liver. The distended gallbladder is palpated as a globular swelling just lateral to the right rectus abdominis near the tip of the ninth costal cartilage. *Murphy's sign* is pathognomonic of acute cholecystitis and is elicited in older children by asking the child to breathe deeply while palpating for the gallbladder. At the height of inspiration, the breath is arrested with a gasp (due to pain) as the inflamed gallbladder touches the palpating hand. Acute cholecystitis with or without calculi or choledochal cysts are not uncommon in children.
- *Urinary bladder* is not normally palpable in children. It is felt as a smooth, firm, oval shaped swelling "arising out of the pelvis" (since the lower margin cannot be made out). Persistent bladder distention may occur in the posterior urethral valve, spinal cord lesions, polyneuropathy, bladder diverticulum, urethral strictures, constipation, voiding dysfunction, and voluntary retention. The possibility of pregnant uterus (firmer, mobile side-to-side) mimicking distended urinary bladder has to be considered in adolescent girls. Ovarian cyst (usually placed to right/left) is another possibility in girls.
- *Aorta and paraaortic lymph nodes* are difficult to palpate in children unless enlarged. The aorta is palpated with the tips of extended fingers in the midline of the epigastrium. Aneurysm of the abdominal aorta is palpated as a pulsatile

thrill due to the movement of the fluid can be appreciated by the hand, held flat in the lumbar region when a large amount of ascitic fluid under tension is present.

Puddle sign helps to diagnose minimal ascitic fluid by placing the child in knee elbow position so that the small quantity ascitic fluid collects around the umbilicus. Percussion of the mid abdomen around the umbilicus elicits dullness, which was resonant in supine position. Common causes of abdominal distention are ascites, large ovarian cysts, and intestinal obstruction. The clinical diagnostic signs of ascites are dullness in the flanks and shifting dullness (revealed by percussion) and fluid thrill. In large ovarian cysts, the flanks will be resonant. In intestinal obstruction, the abdomen will be resonant throughout **(Figs. 20.30A to C)**.

Auscultation of the abdomen helps to detect bowel sounds and their nature, arterial sounds (bruits), venus hum, succussion splash, and peritoneal friction rubs. To detect bowel sounds, sit near the patient, and place the diaphragm of the stethoscope on the abdomen on the right side of the umbilicus for at least 5 minutes. The bowel sounds are loud and gurgling and persist in fasting also because of the swallowed air and secreted fluid. They are absent in paralytic ileus (silent abdomen). An increase in intensity and frequency occurs in colicky abdominal pain and intestinal obstruction.

Bruits are harsh high-pitched arterial sounds. Most of them are nonpathological. Compression, stenosis, aneurysmal dilatation of arteries, increased flow to vascular tumors (hemangioendotheliomas), and hepatoma are rare diseases with bruits. To detect aortic bruit, place the diaphragm of the stethoscope on the abdominal wall over the aorta (above and to the left of the umbilicus). Other areas to auscultate for bruits are over the *iliac arteries in the iliac fossae*, in the *epigastrium* to detect stenosis of the celiac axis or superior mesenteric artery, over the *liver area* in hepatoma and on *either side of midline* over mid abdomen for renal artery stenosis.

Venous sounds: Venous hum is low pitched continuous sound, heard over the liver, spleen, and periumbilical regions, indicating increased blood flow through the portal systemic venous shunt.

Succussion splash (SS) is the splashing noise heard on shaking the abdomen, by the naked ear or on auscultation resembling the sound made by a hot water bag partially filled with water and air. To elicit SS, the patient

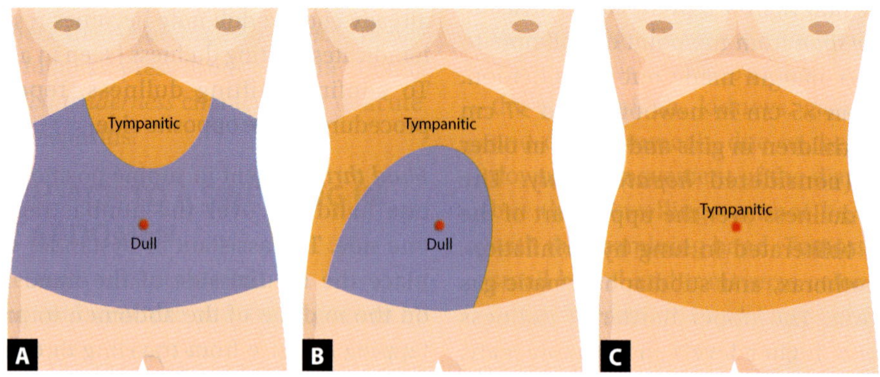

Figs. 20.30A to C: Differences in percussion notes in three diseases with abdominal distension. (A) Gross ascites; (B) Large ovarian cyst; and (C) Intestinal obstruction.

in supine position is rolled from side to side to agitate the fluid inside the abdomen. The sound is perceived through the stethoscope placed over the epigastrium. It can be normally heard up to three hours after a meal. Pathological conditions for SS are pyloric stenosis, intestinal obstruction, and paralytic ileus.

Peritoneal friction rubs are produced by the upper abdominal viscera rubbing the peritoneal surfaces as they move normally during respiration. They are dry, soft, scraping sounds heard in peritonitis. Friction rubs heard over the liver biopsy area indicate bleeding at the surface of the liver after the procedure. Over the splenic and hepatic areas such friction sounds indicate perisplenitis and perihepatitis (in sickle cell anemia, liver abscess, and leukemic infiltrates). The sounds are perceived through the stethoscope placed over the surface of these organs.

THE GROINS

Examine for inguinal hernias or any mass. Palpate for femoral pulses (Ref. Ch. 7 for details).

- *External genitalia, perineum, anus* (Ref. Ch. 7)
- *Rectal examination* is an essential but often forgotten/ignored procedure in GIT examination. After explaining the procedure gently, the child is made to lie in the left lateral position. The right thigh and right knee are flexed. Look at the perianal area for excoriations, ulcers, skin tags (not of significance), fissures, and fistula.
- Well lubricated, gloved little finger is used in newborns and infants and the index finger in an older child. Place the pulp of the finger flat on the anus and press firmly and slowly in a slightly backward direction. Initial resistance is followed by relaxation of the anal sphincter. Discontinue the examination if there is severe pain. Rotate the finger to 360°. The common conditions diagnosed in children are polyps, intussusception, intestinal obstruction, Hirschsprung's disease, and the hard fecal mass in habitual constipation. The examining finger should be observed for blood, mucus, and fecal matter.

The format of stating final diagnosis should be the clinical diagnosis first followed by the functional impairment and lastly the probable etiology.

CLINICAL CASE SCENARIO

Deksha, 6 yr old, girl, is brought to the OPD with yellowish discoloration of eyes for 2 w duration. She was on ayurvedic medicine on these days without any relief. She had progressive pallor and lethargy for the past 3 m for which no consultation was done. No history of fever, loss of appetite, vomiting, or high-colored urine. Her mother had abdominal surgery at 12 yr of age for repeated episodes of fever, abdominal pain, vomiting, and jaundice and the symptoms subsided after surgery. On examination she is jaundiced, anemic, afebrile, pulse rate 96/min, BP 110/72 mm Hg, no signs of dehydration, weight is 17 kg, height 112 cm, spleen 6 cm below the costal margin; liver palpable 2 cm below the costal margin, soft and smooth, liver span 7 cm, nontender. There are no signs of liver failure.

- *Clinical diagnosis:* Splenomegaly with jaundice and anemia, with family history suggestive of hemolytic anemia and gallbladder stones (mother) relieved by abdominal surgery.
- *Functional impairment*: Anemia leading to lethargy and jaundice.
- *Probable etiology*: Inherited hemolytic anemia.

- Loss of consciousness, paralysis, syncope, clumsiness, blurring or loss of vision, deafness, inability to speak/abnormal speech (negative features resulting from loss of function).
- Complaints related to other organs/systems due to brain disorder—vomiting in raised intracranial pressure (RICP), urinary retention in spinal cord lesions.
- Children with developmental delay (due to perinatal and postnatal insults, genetic, or chromosomal disorders) and developmental deviation should be detected at the outset itself from history.

Symptom Analysis

Each symptom has to be analyzed as given below:

Seizures are transient episodes of neurological signs and/or symptoms due to abnormal neuronal activity. A seizure episode is best diagnosed from the history given by an eyewitness. Enquire the time of onset, type (tonic-clonic, myoclonic, loss of posture), duration, evolution, body parts involved (focal or generalized), sensorium (alert/lost), post ictal paralysis/drowsiness, involuntary micturition and/or defecation, injuries sustained, the precipitating factors (trauma, fever, underlying diseases), past history of seizures, developmental delay and family history of febrile seizures and epilepsies. Beyond the neonatal period, the most common cause of convulsions in young children is *febrile seizure*. Clarify the details of febrile fits from the history so as to categorize the episode as simple/complex febrile seizure or febrile status epilepticus and the risk factors for the recurrence of febrile seizure. **Table 21.1** gives age-wise common causes of seizures in children.

Headache in neurologic diseases is produced by the stretching of pain-sensitive intracranial blood vessels (supplied mainly by the three divisions of the trigeminal nerve), meningeal irritation, or RICP. Ask the details of headache—severity, location, duration, frequency, activity restriction, photophobia, phonophobia (intolerance to sound), school absenteeism, and the need and response to drugs.

In *RICP*, headache is intense and progressively increasing. Typically, the child wakes up in the night, has projectile vomiting

TABLE 21.1: Common causes of seizures according to age group.

Neonates	*Infants*	*Children*
HIE	Febrile seizures	Encephalitis
ICH	Meningitis	Meningitis
Metabolic	Encephalitis	Epilepsy
Hypoglycemia	Trauma	Metabolic
Hypocalcemia	Drugs and poisons	ICH
Congenital anomalies of brain	Epilepsy	ICSOL
Meningitis	ICSOL	
Drug withdrawal		
Benign familial seizures		
Pyridoxine dependency		

(HIE: hypoxic ischemic encephalopathy; ICH: intracranial hemorrhage; ICSOL: intracranial space occupying lesion)

followed by transient relief in the early stages. Associated signs like blurring of vision, ataxia, multiple cranial nerve palsy and limb weakness, bulging anterior fontanel and/or papilledema will help to localize clinically the level of lesion in the brain.

Migraine headache is recurrent with moderate-to-severe intensity, focal and throbbing in nature, can have aura, nausea, vomiting, photophobia, and phonophobia.

Other causes of headache should be identified which are nonspecific fever, sinusitis, meningitis, encephalitis, visual defects, hypertension, and psychological problems.

Vomiting is also an important symptom in conditions with RICP and hence mostly occurs along with headache.

Loss of consciousness [LOC (Ref. Ch. 9)] can occur in diseases of the brain or in any systemic illness or disorders with metabolic impairment.

Paralysis indicates loss or impairment of motor function due to neural lesions (more common) and/or muscular damage which can be of varying grades. Time of onset, progression (rapid/slow), associated symptoms as fever, pain over the muscles, erythema, rashes or peeling of skin should be enquired. It is not unusual to come across children brought with myasthenic like paralysis after krait bite (history may not be present because krait bite is painless) and revealing progressive paralysis.

Syncope is sudden transient LOC with inability to maintain postural tone. It can mimic seizures especially if there are past episodes. The most common cause is vasovagal episode characterized by hypotension and bradycardia. Circumstantial factors like poor sleep, reduced fluid intake, illness, drug intake, injection received, severe pain, sight of blood, standing for a long time especially in a congested area or school assembly should be enquired. The child will be *fully aware of the episode of feeling uneasy* followed by diaphoresis and lightheadedness prior to the LOC (Ref. Ch. 17 for cardiac causes of syncope).

Enquire the onset, nature of clinical presentation, duration, evolution, associated symptoms, response to treatment, and adherence to treatment in all other symptoms. After a detailed history, the student should be able to reach a reasonable clinical hypothesis based on the following points:

- Onset and duration of the symptoms (*acute* within 24 hours, *subacute* within a few days, and *chronic* within a few weeks)
- Topographic distribution (parts of the body affected, sequence of involvement and possible anatomical structures affected in the nervous system)
- Evolution (*rapidly* deteriorating, *stepwise* or *gradually* progressing, static, partially or gradually improving, relapsing or remitting, resolving or having residual disability)
- Possible etiologies (congenital, traumatic, infectious, inflammatory, vascular, demyelinating, degenerative, neoplastic, metabolic, toxic, and deficiency states).

Neurological Examination (Ref. Ch. 14, 15 for Newborn Evaluation)

Additional tools needed for evaluation are updated development kit (Ref. Ch. 12), pediatric knee hammer, bright torch with rubber adapter, common toys to assess stereognosis, wisp of cotton, wooden tongue depressor, spatula, tuning forks (128 Hz for vibration sense, 256 Hz for Rinne test), snellen letter and picture charts, orange peel/coffee powder, ophthalmoscope, measuring divider (for two point discrimination) salt, sugar, vinegar, and quinine solutions (divider and solutions to examine older children only).

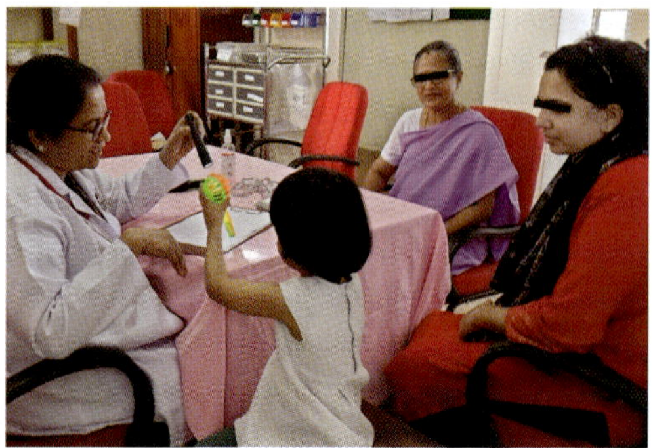

Fig. 21.1: Observing the child for neurological and developmental problems.

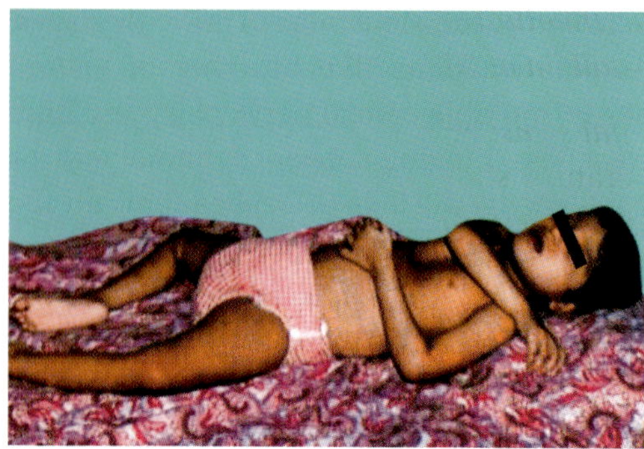

Fig. 21.2: Flaccid posture-pithed frog appearance.

To develop rapport with the child, utilize the history taking time to be interesting and gentle. Observe and assess the current developmental status during this period. Before touching the child, observe the sensorium, social interaction, personal cleanliness, attachment with parents, whether dull, hyperactive or irritable. The observation should be as if it is conversation with the parents. Check the posture of the patient, paucity of movements, and handedness by offering an attractive toy **(Fig. 21.1)**, and obvious cranial nerve deficits. Look for involuntary movements (at rest and while active) and gait. The examination should be in a nonthreatening setting (Ref. Ch. 12) and enjoyable to the child as a game. If a hearing assessment is to be considered from history, attention should be directed initially to that portion so as to get full cooperation.

SENSORIUM (REF. CH. 9)

Evaluate the unconscious child as in Chapter 9. *Posture* may be flaccid-pithed frog appearance **(Fig. 21.2)**, decorticate (flexion of upper limbs and extension of lower limbs—indicating lesion higher up in the brainstem or basal nuclei) or decerebrate [hyperextension of upper and lower limbs, pronation of upper limbs and plantar flexion of feet—due to lesion at the level of superior colliculus **(Fig. 9.3)**]. Cortical thumb and persistent hand fisting **(Fig. 21.3)** above 3 m age indicate early signs of spastic cerebral palsy.

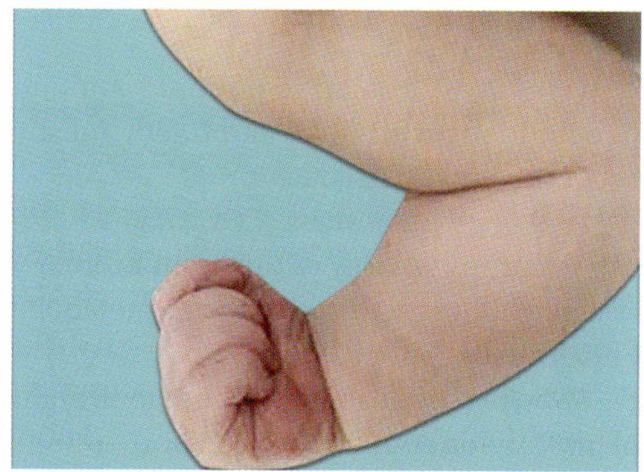

Fig. 21.3: Persistent fisting with cortical thumb in a 9-month-old baby.

Paucity of movements—detect by lack of spontaneous activity or in response to stimuli by gentle scratching of the distal part (with your finger nail), after informing the parent and getting consent.

Handedness is established after 2 yr of age and is assessed by observing the child, handling play materials or from spontaneous movements. Early handedness indicates weakness of the opposite hand.

Involuntary movements and gait (see details in motor function)

Vital signs: Pulse, BP, respiration, and temperature should be evaluated in relation to the neurological problem. Bradycardia, apnea, and hypertension indicate *Cushing triad* in the advanced stage of RICP. Observe abnormal breathing patterns (Ref. **Figs. 19.2A to D**). In a child with depressed sensorium, they reveal severe brainstem dysfunction due to structural brain disease, poisoning or a metabolic crisis (*e.g.*, diabetic ketoacidosis) all requiring urgent intervention. Fever indicates intracranial infections which may be meningitis, encephalitis, brain abscess, malaria and cerebral venous thrombophlebitis or other systemic infections.

Head: It is ideal to examine the head in the beginning (Ref. **Ch. 7, 11**) but measurement should be the last to maintain the child's cooperation. Assess the size, shape, fontanels, sutures, swellings, and evidence of injury. Suspect battered child if multiple injuries are seen. *Battle sign* is oval shaped bruising of the skin behind the pinna, a sign of basal or temporal bone fracture indicating serious head injury (Ref. **Fig. 9.2**). Percussion of the skull helps to detect RICP by the cracked pot or *Macewen's sign*. To elicit the sign, hold the patient's head on your nondominant hand (without support on the cot), and with the back of the index finger of the dominant hand, percuss the patient's parietal bone **(Fig. 21.4)**. RICP and subsequent sutural separation are revealed by the elicited sound, simulating to that produced by the percussion of a cracked pot. The test is irrelevant if fontanels are open. Common causes of RICP are meningitis, hydrocephalus, subdural effusion, ICH, and tumors. Auscultation of the skull may reveal bruits over the anterior fontanel, temporal regions, and the orbits. These can be normal up to 4 yr of age and during fever. Such bruits may indicate arteriovenous malformations of the middle cerebral artery or vein of Galen.

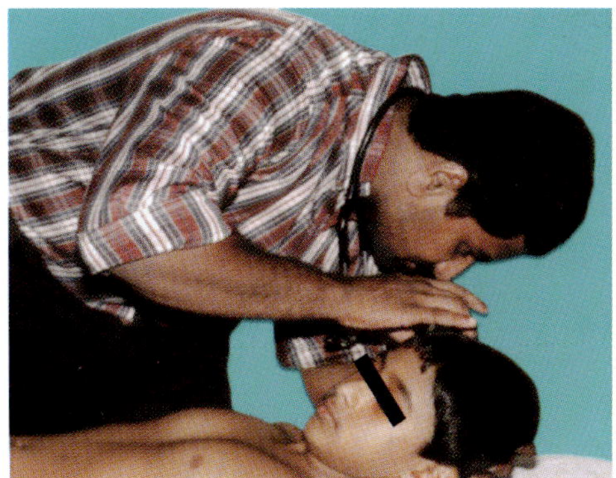

Fig. 21.4: Eliciting the Macewen's sign.

Transillumination of the skull (indicated in all infants below 1 yr of age) is useful to detect fluid collection within the cranium. The test is done in a dark room applying a bright torch with black applicator, over the frontal, parietal, and occipital areas on both sides. Illumination if it exceeds 2 cm in the frontal and 1 cm in the occipital areas respectively, suspect intracranial fluid collection. The entire skull may glow in large hydrocephalus, hydranencephaly, and porencephalic cyst if the thickness of the cerebral cortex is <1 cm. Positive test in the frontoparietal region is seen in subdural effusion, and in the suboccipital region in Dandy-Walker malformation. Transillumination is impaired in caput succedaneum, cephalohematoma, scalp edema, and thick black hair.

Special points in general examination (Ref. Ch. 7): Look for coarse facial features and dysmorphism, major/minor congenital malformations, neurocutaneous markers **(Figs. 10.1, 10.8, 10.23, 10.24, 15.8, and 21.5A and B)**, and other skin/eye/hair changes. They help to diagnose genetic

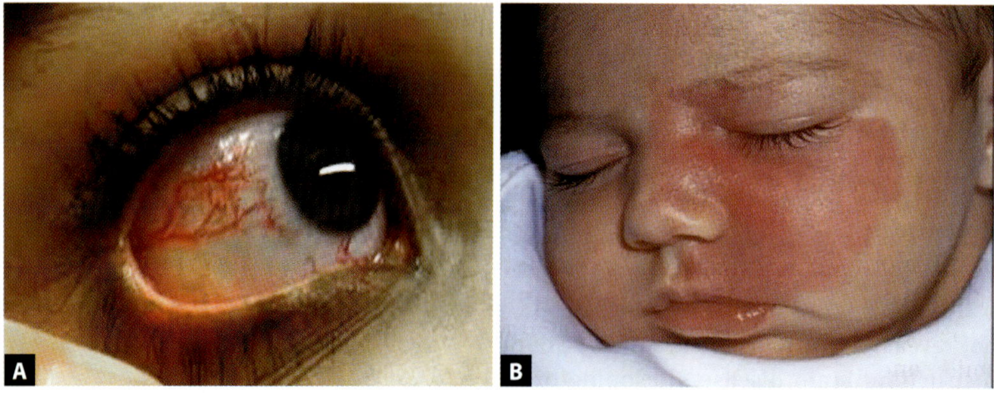

Figs. 21.5A and B: (A) Ocular telangiectasia; (B) Facial hemangioma.

syndromes and chromosomal disorders. Search for BCG scar, bed sores, and knuckle pigmentation (pathognomonic sign of vitamin B12 deficiency).

Anthropometry (Ref. Ch. 11) should be completed initially to detect failure to thrive, obesity, or short stature which may suggest important etiological factors.

SYSTEMATIC EVALUATION OF THE NERVOUS SYSTEM

Systematic evaluation of the nervous system can be proceeded in the stable child under the following headlines:

- *Higher mental functions (HMF)*
- *Cranial nerves*
- *Motor functions*
- *Sensory system*
- *Signs of meningeal irritation*
- *Soft neurological signs*
- *Tests for autonomic functions*

Higher Mental Functions

Age-wise modification is required in test procedure.

Infants and toddlers: Observe the basic biologic functions (feeding, sleeping), interaction with people (mother recognition by 1 m age, social smile by 3 m, and stranger resentment by 8 m age). Note the reaction to the surroundings (attracted by wall pictures and toys) and playfulness.

Children (2–5 yr age)—assess the response to praising the child ("you are so cute", "this frock is very attractive") and age appropriate questions (name, age, pointing to body parts, asking who gave the toy). For the older child (5–10 yr), address, name of the school, drawing a picture, and counting the numbers are advised. Above 10 yr of age, formal HMFs testing as in adults can be done. To assess the comprehension and attention span of the child, ask to count digits forwards and backwards. HMFs include *orientation* (time, space, and person), memory, intelligence, emotional state, and speech of the patient.

Orientation: Ask the following questions to the older child—name, year, month, date, day, time, the place the child is currently staying, and names of parents. Younger children reveal irritability in the unfamiliar environment and will cling to the parent which is equivalent to the person and the surroundings.

Memory includes registration, retention, and recollection of events. Loss of memory can be of immediate, recent, or past items.

To test immediate memory, ask the patient to repeat forwards and backwards a series of digits (*digit repetition test*) as 6, 3, 8, 0 and backwards in the same sequence. At the age of 6 yr, a child is able to repeat five digits forwards and three digits backwards. To test *recent memory,* ask about the food item taken in the morning. To test *past memory,* ask about a *past memorable event.*

For young infants, mother regard, social smile, and stranger resentment and above 2 yr age recognizing the close relatives and speech reveal memory.

Intelligence: An idea can be obtained from the report of scholastic performance and the ability to solve age-appropriate arithmetic problems in the older child. Detailed IQ testing is advised if needed. For the younger babies, fine motor, social and language milestones attained from assessing development are equivalent to the intelligence level.

Emotional state: Assess whether the patient appears cheerful, depressed, cooperative, aggressive, anxious, irritable, impulsive, and interested in surroundings.

Speech is meaningful production of sound. Language is understanding and use of symbols. Speech centers are situated in the dominant cerebral hemisphere and are usually on the *left side* for in left-handed people. The areas of representation are the frontal (1 "Brocas area" for spoken and written speech) and the superior temporal gyrus (2 "Wernickes area" for comprehension) **(Fig. 21.6)**. For speech assessment, the examiner should have adequate knowledge of the language acquisition skills at various ages of the child (Ref. Ch. 6, 12) as revealed from history and by listening to the child. Older children can be formally tested by asking to show the eyes or teeth (cover your mouth while instructing the child to avoid lip reading) and to repeat letters like "Ka" "Ta" "Pa". These simple orders are for testing comprehension. Use of consonants "Ka" "Ta" "Pa" reveals the function of main components of articulation namely the palate, tongue, and lips respectively. Written speech is tested by writing answers to questions like "how old are you?"

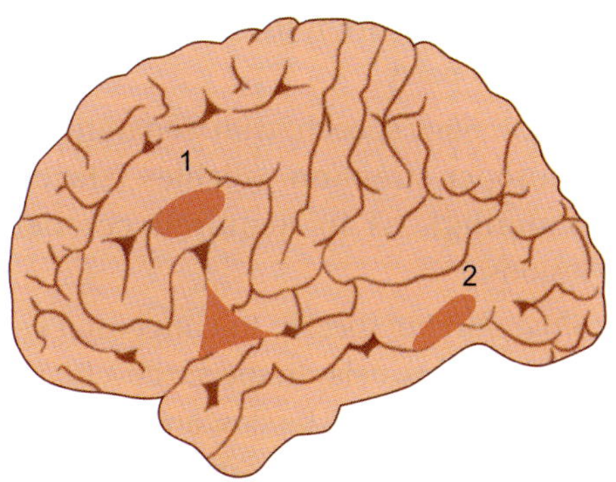

Fig. 21.6: Location of the speech centers *(1) motor and (2) auditory.*

Disorders of speech are *aphasia* (defective language) and *dysarthria* (defective articulation). Aphasia is *loss of acquired language* function and may be global (all functions lost), motor (expressive speech loss—Broca's aphasia), sensory (loss of comprehension—Wernicke's aphasia), and conduction aphasia (impairment of repetition). Aphasia indicates damage of the cortical speech centers seen in stroke, encephalitis, and meningitis. *Dyslexia* is speech disorder of developmental origin. *Mutism* is the complete absence of speech from birth. *Stammering or stuttering* is repetition of sounds, syllables or words, mostly emotional.

Common types of dysarthria are:

- *Spastic:* Slow, labored, hypernasal explosive rhythm, interfering with respiration. Seen in bilateral upper motor neuron (UMN) lesions producing pseudobulbar palsy, but not in hemiplegia. The most common situation in children is spastic cerebral palsy.

- *Ataxic:* Slow speech, wide separation and improper stress on syllables (staccato/scanning), as in acquired cerebellar lesions.
- *Slow slurring speech:* In congenital cerebellar lesions, delay in speech development occurs, speech will be slow and slurring but will not be grossly abnormal.
- *Dyskinetic:* Explosive, coming in rushes or slow monotonous. Seen in extrapyramidal lesions depending on the type and location of lesions.
- *Nasal speech:* Seen in palatal palsy and cleft palate with nasal twang
- *Dysphonia:* Is abnormality in speech volume—may be due to disorders of voice production in paralysis or dystonia of vocal cords and in respiratory muscle paralysis.

Cranial Nerves

The twelve cranial nerves can be categorized as sensory, motor, and mixed in type depending on their functions **(Table 21.2)**. The nuclei of 3rd to 12th cranial nerves are located in the brainstem; the motor nerve nuclei are placed more medially.

TABLE 21.2: Cranial nerves with their functions.

No.	Nerve	Function
1.	Olfactory	Sensory
2.	Optic	Sensory
3.	Oculomotor	Motor
4.	Trochlear	Motor
5.	Trigeminal	Mixed
6.	Abducens	Motor
7.	Facial	Mixed
8.	Vestibulocochlear	Sensory
9.	Glossopharyngeal	Mixed
10.	Vagus	Mixed
11.	Accessory	Motor
12.	Hypoglossal	Motor

First (Olfactory) Nerve

Function: Perception (olfactory pathway) and identification (olfactory cortex) of smell.

Anatomy: The central processes of the bipolar sensory cells of the olfactory nerve in the nasal epithelium pass through the cribriform plate of the ethmoid bone. They reach the olfactory bulb on the inferior surface of the frontal lobe where cells of the secondary olfactory neurons lie. Nerve fibers from here project through the olfactory tract to the *olfactory area of the cerebral cortex—parts of the temporal and frontal lobes.*

Test objects and clinical testing: Use familiar materials like orange peel (young children), coffee powder, soap, tooth paste, and asafoetida (older age group). Avoid pungent substances which stimulate the 5th nerve. Before testing, ensure that the nasal passages are patent by observing the movement of a cotton wisp brought in front of each nostril. Test each nostril separately with the other nostril and eyes closed. Formal testing is possible above the age of 5 yr. In infants and retarded children, note the behavioral response which need not be diagnostic.

Smell can be appreciated as early as the *32nd week* of gestational age so that *healthy newborns are able to perceive their mother's smell and breastmilk*. Abnormalities are anosmia (loss of smell), parosmia (perverted smell), hyperosmia (increased sensitivity), and hyposmia (reduced ability). The most common cause of *anosmia* is upper respiratory infection, especially *coronavirus* infection. See **Box 21.1** for causes of anosmia.

BOX 21.1: Causes of anosmia.

- Upper respiratory infections
- Allergy
- Intranasal drugs
- Head trauma leading to ethmoid fracture
- Pyogenic meningitis
- Toxins (acrylates, methacrylates, cadmium)
- Hydrocephalus
- Frontal lobe tumors
- Congenital (Kallmann syndrome)

Second (Optic) Nerve

Note: Complete evaluation of the eyes and orbit should be done before neurologic examination of 2, 3, 4, and 6 cranial nerves since affection of many structures of the orbit can mimic diseases of these nerves.

Parent's complaints regarding defective vision—in babies <3 m are absent visual fixation and following of an object and not looking at mother's face. Roving movements of eyes, sluggish/absent pupillary reaction, squint and nystagmus are the other features to suspect visual defects. *Even if there are no complaints, visual assessment is a must for all babies.*

Functions: (1) Vision and (2) afferent pupillary function in the initial part of the nerve.

Components of examination are acuity of vision, field of vision, color vision, and fundus examination. Test materials are a torch, bright colored (red, orange, yellow, green, blue) toys, (balls, pellets, dolls, pin), Snellen letter chart, Snellen picture book and/or wall pictures and ophthalmoscope. Baby may be in the mothers lap or over the examination table up to 3 yr age.

Anatomy: The fibers of this sensory nerve arise from the inner retina and reach the optic disk to enter the optic nerve. The nerve then passes through the optic canal to the optic chiasm from where the optic tracts arise. The fibers from the inner or nasal half of each retina, representing the temporal visual field, decussate. Those from the outer or temporal half, representing the nasal visual field, remain on the same side. Thus each optic tract consists of fibers from the temporal half of retina on the same side and nasal half of retina on the opposite side, which represent the visual field on the opposite side. They pass to the lateral geniculate body of the same side. Prior to the decussation, fibers destined for pupillary function decussate toward the midbrain Edinger–Westphal nucleus so that any fibers distal to this will not involve the pupillary reflexes. From the lateral geniculate body, the optic radiation originates and passes through the posterior limb of the internal capsule and projects to the occipital cortex around the calcarine fissure (visual cortex).

Visual acuity: Method of testing depends on the age and cooperation of the child and the clinician's choice. One should master the most comfortable and reliable method for the test. Each eye should be evaluated separately. A plastic occluder is the ideal one to cover the baby's nontesting eye, or the parent should be instructed to cover the eye gently, with the palm.

0–5 m: Ask the history for visual fixation on mothers face. Observe blinking, fixation, and tracking of a lighted torch or bright toy held 20 cm in front of the baby.

6–18 m: Test near vision by the visual fixation to small pellets and pincer grasp which develops at 9 m age. For distant vision, observe fixation of vision to rolling balls.

1½–3 yr: Near vision as above. Distant vision by picture book or wall pictures [Snellen picture chart **(Fig. 21.7A)** at a distance of 15–20 feet is advisable].

3–5 yr: Child can be on the mothers lap or sit independently. Test near and distant vision by letter matching test—*tumbling E test,* in which the child indicates the direction the letter *E* is facing—or use picture book/wall pictures **(Fig. 21.7B)**.

6 yr and above: By this age, the child is able to read letters. A formal vision test can be done with an adequately lit Snellen letter chart **(Fig. 21.7C)**. The child should sit/stand 6 meters away facing the chart. Gently instruct to read the lines. If unable to complete the lines, the child is allowed to come nearer to the chart till able to read. Vision can be stated as the value of *d/D* (*d*—distance where the patient stands from the chart; *D*—ideal distance of 6 meters). Suspect visual defect and consider ophthalmologist's evaluation.

Finger counting is an easy screening method to detect defective vision. Seat the child at *1 meter* distance facing the doctor. Test each eye separately. Show your fingers in changing numbers and clarify whether the numbers are correctly counted. The child can be made to sit nearer to the examiner and repeat the process if the counting is wrong. The test can be stated as finger counting at "—" meter distance. If the child fails in finger counting, examine for *hand movements* (HM) perception by waving your hand in front of the patient's eye and then observe for blinking. If HM perception fails, test for *perception of light* (PL) by showing a bright light beam over the eye. If no response, vision is stated as "no PL". **Box 21.2** reveals causes of defective vision.

Visual acuity age wise is—newborns 20/150, 3 yr 20/40, 4 yr 20/30, and by 6 yr 20/20.

Color vision: Test whether the child is able to appreciate the three primary colors (red, green, and blue) by showing colored toys. Child at 3 yr is able to name 1 color and at 5 yr, 4 colors. Blindness for red and green colors is seen occasionally only. Being X-linked, only boys are affected and become obvious by 6 yr of age. The acuity of vision is not affected. Objective assessment for color vision is by the Ishihara chart **(Fig. 21.7D)**.

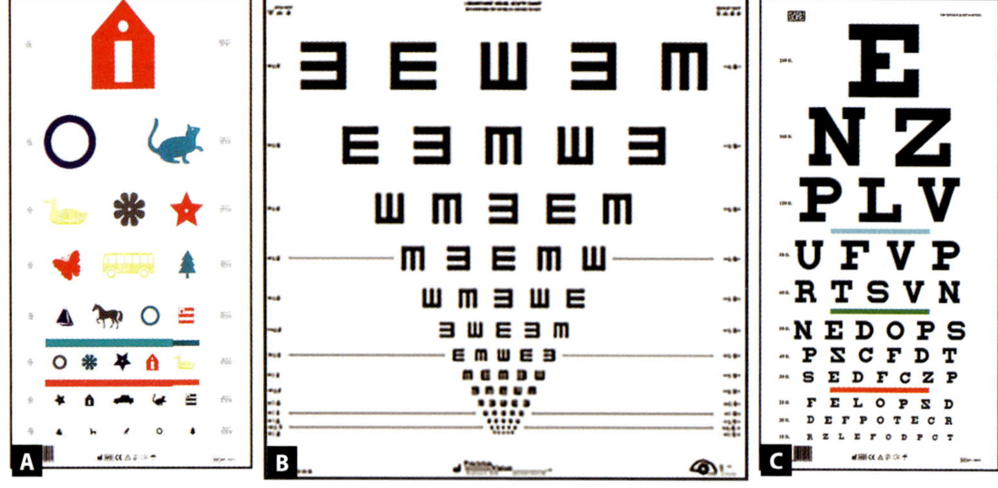

Figs. 21.7A to C: (A) Snellen picture chart; (B) "Tumbling E" test chart; (C) Snellen letter chart.

BOX 21.2: Causes of defective vision in children.

- Refractive errors
- Vitamin A deficiency
- Cerebral palsy
- Cataract
- Trauma to the eye
- Corneal opacities
- Toxins
- Raised ICP
- Chorioretinitis
- Neoplasms of optic nerve
- Demyelination
- Vascular problems of retina
- Optic atrophy
- Psychogenic

(ICP: intracranial pressure)

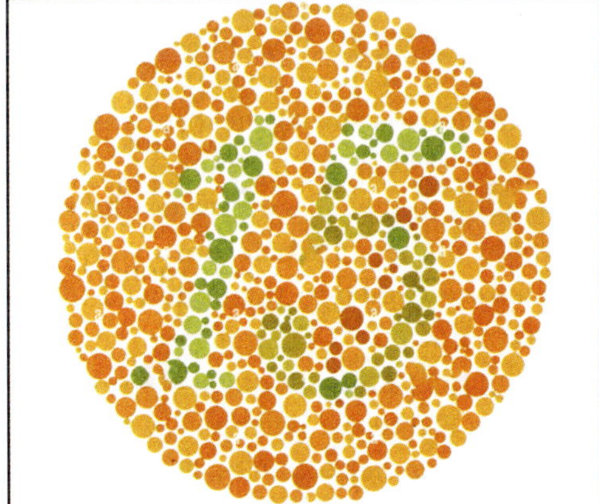

Fig. 21.7D: Ishihara chart for color vision test.

Visual fields: Infants and young children are tested with both eyes uncovered to maintain cooperation. Menace reflex is blinking of the eyes when the examiner's hand is suddenly brought towards the eye; may be unreliable as the air current by the hand can act as a stimulus. For infants >3 m age, move a light or red ball into the visual field from behind forwards and observe the response, as the test material enters the visual field *(Ref. Ch. 12)*.

Visual induced refixation: Mother is directed to attract the infant's attention from front; the examiner flashes light in various fields of vision; if vision is normal, the infant turns and looks at light.

Confrontation tests are applicable to children of 3–4 yr of age and above. The eyes can be tested together or separately. Examiner sits 1 meter away, facing the patient whose right eye is tested with the examiner's left eye and vice versa. The other eye is kept covered by the corresponding hands of the examiner and the patient. The patient is asked to fixate on the examiner's eyes. Different numbers of examiner's fingers/colorful toys/a red pen are presented in different quadrants of the visual field from the extreme periphery. The child is asked to mimic the number of fingers in each field or the name of the toy as soon as it is seen. This test detects central scotoma, bitemporal hemianopia, and homonymous hemianopia. The common visual field defects are unilateral nasal field loss and bitemporal hemianopia; trauma, tumors, cysts, aneurysms, hydrocephalus, and demyelination involving the optic chiasma are the common causes for defective vision. In cortical blindness caused by bilateral occipital lesions, pupillary response is maintained (very commonly seen in Cerebral Palsy) as opposed to lesions in other parts of the visual pathway.

Example 2: Boy, 3 yr old, with h/o difficult labor and delay in first cry, developmental delay (sits only), cannot recognize parents but identifies their speech and has meaningful speech. His vision reveals perception of HM only, pupillary reflexes are normal bilaterally.

Impression: Obviously the child has cerebral palsy (in which visual defects are common). Since the pupillary reflexes are preserved, it is cortical blindness.

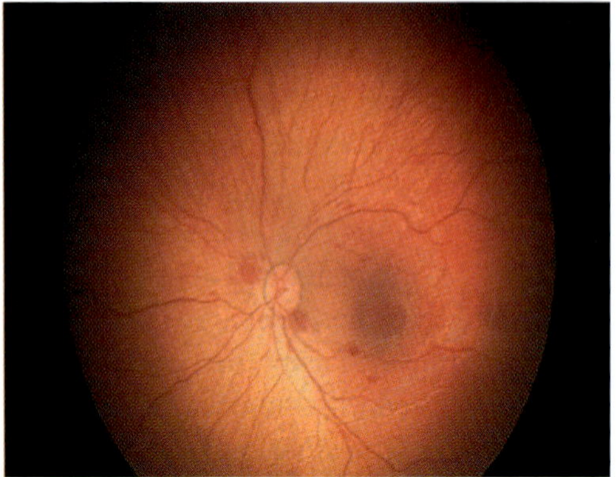

Fig. 21.7E: B/L fundus hemorrhage in nonaccidental trauma in a newborn.
Courtesy: Scruggs BA, Eyerounds.org The University of Iowa.

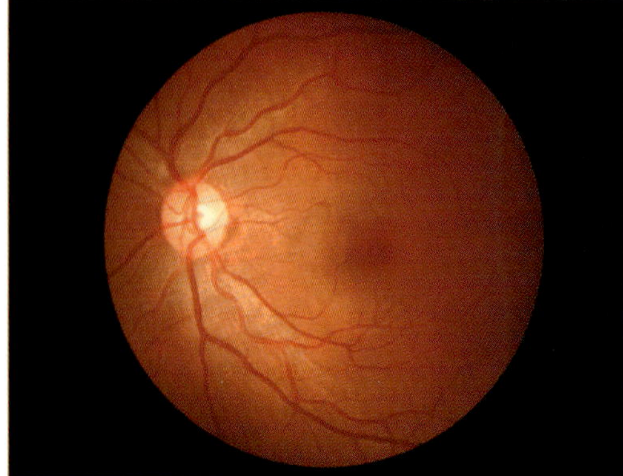

Fig. 21.7F: Fundus in retinitis pigmentosa.
Courtesy: Mandal A; news-medical.net/health/What is-Retinitis-Pigmentosa.aspx

Fundus examination: Sedation and mydriasis with short duration drugs (2.5% phenylephrine or 0.5–1% tropicamide) are needed in noncooperative children. Evaluate the optic disk for optic atrophy, papilledema (swelling of the optic disk due to raised ICP), and papillitis (localized swelling of optic disk due to inflammation). Common types of optic atrophy in children are primary (small pale disk with sharp margins) and secondary (gray disk with irregular margins following papilledema). Other points to be evaluated are retinal hemorrhages, macular cherry red spot, retinitis pigmentosa, chorioretinitis, lipemia retinalis, hypertensive retinopathy, phakomatosis, and choroidal tubercles **(Figs. 21.7E and F)**.

The visual evoked response, an electrophysiological method of evaluating the response to light, and preferential looking tests are others to be assessed by skilled persons in special situations.

Third (Oculomotor), Fourth (Trochlear), Sixth (Abducent) Nerves

Functions: Eye movements and pupillary reactions.

Anatomy: These nerves arise from brainstem nuclei close to the aqueduct of Sylvius extending between the superior colliculi and the floor of the 4th ventricle. The 3rd nerve nucleus is the farthest forward. The rostral nerve cells supply parasympathetic innervation to the ciliary muscles (Edinger–Westphal nucleus). Nuclei for extraocular muscles are caudal to this followed by the 4th nerve nucleus. The 6th nerve nucleus is at the floor of the 4th ventricle at the level of pons. The 3rd nerve emerges on the inner aspect of cerebral peduncles, and enters the lateral wall of the cavernous sinus. The fourth nerve, the only cranial nerve that decussates, emerges from the roof of the 4th ventricle and supplies the superior oblique. The 6th nerve emerges between pons and medulla, has the longest intracranial course and supplies the lateral rectus muscle. All three nerves finally enter the orbit through the superior orbital fissure along with the ophthalmic branch of the trigeminal nerve. All the other extraocular muscles, the sphincter pupillae, and the levator palpebrae superioris are supplied by 3rd nerve. **Figure 21.8** shows the actions of external ocular muscles.

The eye movements are adduction (horizontal medial), abduction (horizontal lateral), elevation (vertical upward), and depression (vertical downward). Rotary movements are also possible. The *common symptoms* of paralysis of these three nerves are diplopia, ptosis, squint, and head tilt **(Figs. 21.9 and 21.10)**.

Testing: Fix the patient's head while being examined. In infants and young children, observe the eye movements when a colored object tied to a string is moved in various directions of the visual field. Child above the age of 4 yr is asked to look at a red pen as it is moved in the direction of action of extraocular muscles. In noncooperative and unconscious patients, the doll's eye reflex is elicited. Clinical signs of 3, 4, 6 nerve palsy are given in **Table 21.3**.

Evaluation of pupils: Pupillary functions are mediated by the autonomic nervous system. Parasympathetic stimulation produces pupillary constriction and sympathetic fibers induce pupillary dilatation.

Cervical sympathetic originates from the ciliospinal center (lower cervical and upper thoracic regions of the spinal cord). It emerges through the first thoracic roots and supplies the eyeball and levator palpebrae superioris through the ophthalmic division of 5th nerve. Features of paralysis of sympathetic fibers *(Horner's syndrome)* are enophthalmos, ptosis and miosis with absence of mydriasis,

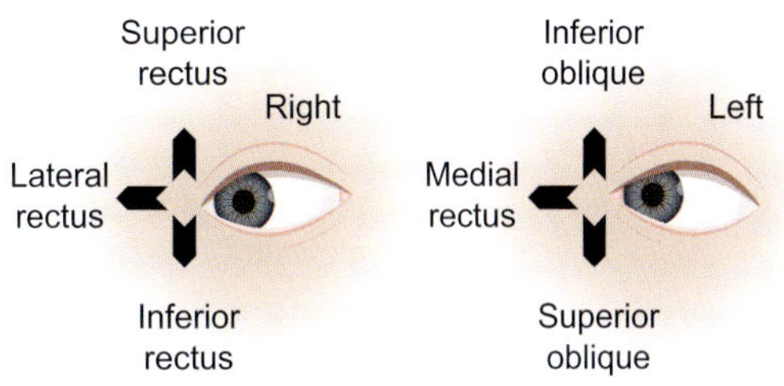

Fig. 21.8: Actions of external ocular muscles.

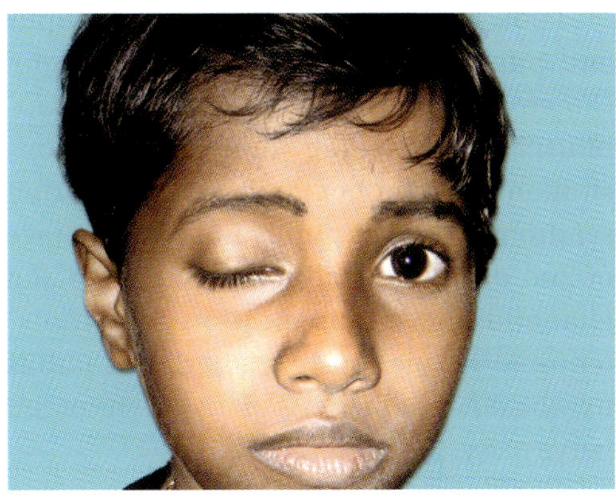

Fig. 21.9: Ptosis® eye.

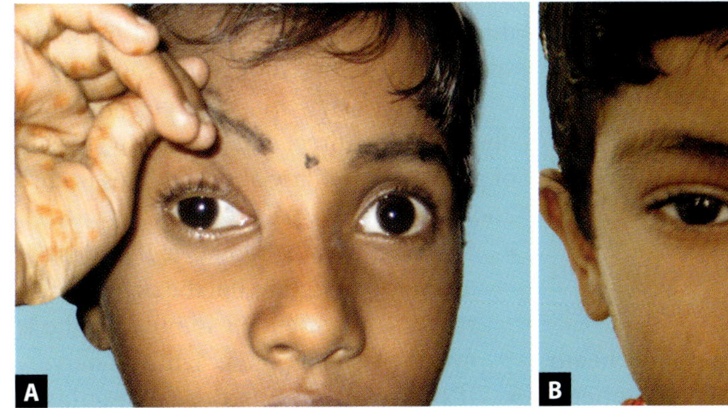

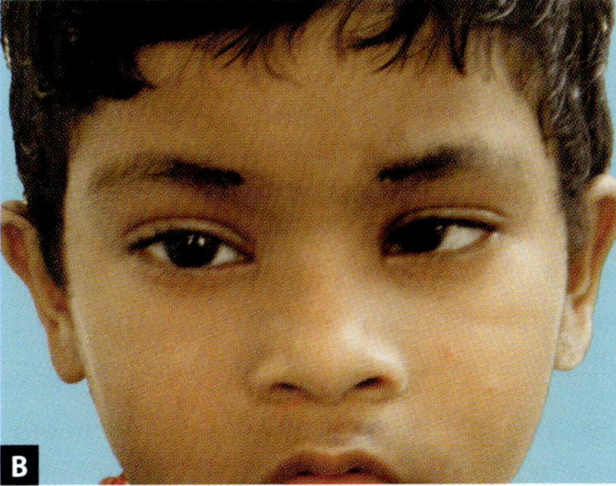

Figs. 21.10A and B: (A) Right lateral squint; (B) (L) Medial squint with abnormal light reflex.

TABLE 21.3: Clinical signs of III, IV, VI nerve palsy.

	III	*IV*	*VI*
Pupils • Size • Reaction	 Dilated Nonreacting (direct, consensual, accommodation)	 Normal Normal	 Normal Normal
Squint	Downward lateral	Outward rotation of eyeball on downward gaze	Convergent
Eye movements	Impaired adduction and elevation	As above	Impaired abduction
Eyelids	Ptosis	Normal	Normal

ciliospinal reflex, and sweating over the same side of head and neck.

Look for the size and shape of pupils and pupillary reflexes in moderate light. Constricted pupils are seen in organophosphate poisoning, morphine administration, pontine hemorrhage, and Horner syndrome. Dilated pupils indicate damage of 2nd or 3rd cranial nerves, atropine and guanethidine administration and transtentorial herniation. Irregularity of pupils may be due to adhesions of iris to lens or 3rd nerve palsy.

Pupillary reflexes include direct reaction to light, consensual reaction, accommodation convergence, and ciliospinal reflex.

Anatomy of pupillary reaction pathway: Afferent fibers pass through the optic nerve and tract and reach the superior colliculi; then cross the aqueduct of Sylvius, in front and behind, to the 3rd nerve nucleus. The efferent fibers from the 3rd nerve nucleus pass to the branch to the inferior oblique muscle, reach the ciliary ganglion and through the short ciliary nerves supply the constrictor pupillae.

Test: Bring a moderately bright light beam directed to the pupil from the periphery. Sudden constriction followed by dilation, some oscillations, and regaining of the normal size occur (direct reaction). The patient should be attracted to look into the distance to prevent accommodation reflex. When one eye is stimulated, the pupil of the other eye also constricts *(consensual reaction)* and dilates when the light is removed (the unilluminated eye should be shaded).

Accommodation-convergence reaction: Hold up a red pen close to the patient's nose. Ask the patient to look away (a wall picture) and then quickly look at the pen. As the eyes converge, pupils constrict. The reflex is impaired in 3rd nerve lesions.

Ciliospinal reflex: When the skin of the neck is pinched, dilatation of pupils is seen, due to the reflex excitation of the cervical sympathetic fibers (route value *C8 T1*).

Differentiate the involved nerve by observing the direct and consensual reaction of pupils as pupillary abnormalities occur in 2nd and 3rd nerve palsy only.

- Show light on the right eye: If both pupils are not constricting, but the right pupillary reaction is present on stimulating the left eye, the lesion is in the right 2nd nerve.
- If the right pupil is not contracting on stimulation, but consensual reaction is

present on the left eye, the lesion is on the right 3rd nerve.

Relative afferent pupillary defect (RAPD) may be observed in unilateral optic neuritis. The direct light reflex is stronger than the consensual reflex in the eye with normal visual function whereas the consensual reflex will be stronger in the affected eye and as a result the pupils dilate when the light is moved from the unaffected to the affected eye.

Gaze palsy: The supranuclear centers for eye movement control are in the frontal and occipital lobes. The fibers from these regions descend to the nerve nuclei in the brainstem. Damage to the cerebral cortex, midbrain, and pons results in paralysis of movements of both eyes in one direction (conjugate gaze palsy) without paralysis of individual ocular muscles (due to the loss of higher control). Thus, the patient may be unable to look to either side (conjugate lateral gaze palsy) in lesions of cerebral cortex and pons. Conjugate upward or vertical gaze palsy is seen in lesions of midbrain, inferior thalamic region, or around the 3rd nerve nucleus. In lesions causing damage to the cerebral cortex as in hemiplegia, the eyes are turned toward the side of the lesion, i.e., the patient "looks toward the lesion". An irritative lesion in the same region (e.g., epilepsy) causes deviation of both eyes toward the healthy side (patient "looks away from the lesion"). The direction of conjugate lateral gaze palsy is reversed in pontine lesion, i.e., the patient looks away from the damaged lesion and toward the irritating lesion. Impaired downward gaze may rarely occur with brainstem lesions at a lower level.

Examination for gaze palsy (Dolls eye reflex): Stand at the head end of the child, hold the head with both hands on either sides and briskly turn the head to right and then to left, observing the eye movements simultaneously. If the cortical centers are normal, the eyeballs move toward the opposite side of head rotation. If the eyeballs are not visible, gently pull the upper eyelids with the thumbs to visualize the movement. Extension and flexion of the neck will reveal upward and downward gaze palsies. This test is contraindicated in cervical spine disorders.

Squint or strabismus **(Figs. 21.10A and B)** is misalignment causing deviation of eyes which the patient cannot overcome. It can be nonparalytic (concomitant) or paralytic (in which there is paralysis of one or more extraocular muscles). In the former, range of eye movements is normal, patient has defective vision and onset is usually below 3 yr of age. In paralytic strabismus, range of eye movements is impaired in the direction of the physiological action of muscles affected, vision is not impaired and it can occur at any age. If the weakness is minimal or the unaffected muscles mask it, the defective movement will not be obvious. The tests for squint assessment are:

- *Assessment of visual acuity*—see description in cranial nerve 2.
- *Hirschberg corneal reflex test is the most rapid and easily performed diagnostic test for squint,* particularly in noncooperative children and those with poor ocular fixation. A light source is projected into the cornea of both eyes simultaneously, as the child looks directly at the light. In the normal situation, light reflex falls slightly nasal to the center of both pupils. The light reflex will be asymmetrical in the squint eye **(Fig. 21.10B)**.
- *Cover-uncover test* is applied to detect squint if the child is cooperative. Child is asked to look at a distant object (6 meters away). Cover one eye and watch

BOX 21.3: Causes of external ophthalmoplegia.

- Raised ICP (meningitis, encephalitis, hemorrhage, hydrocephalus, trauma)*
- Tumors—Pontine glioma
- Vascular—cavernous sinus thrombosis, ophthalmoplegic migraine
- Demyelinating disorders
- Myasthenia gravis
- Ocular myopathy

Note: *6th nerve paralysis occurs early due to its long course as false localizing sign.

the movement of the uncovered eye. If it deviates, it indicates strabismus of the uncovered eye. Repeat the test on the other eye.

Opsoclonus refers to the chaotic movements of both eyes. The common causes are viral encephalitis and demyelination and rarely neuroblastoma. It is due to cerebellar lesions. In *skew deviation* (seen in lesions of labyrinth and cerebellum), one eye is directed upwards while the other eye goes downwards.

External ophthalmoplegia is paralysis of all extraocular muscles with ptosis and normal pupillary reflex. See **Box 21.3** for the causes.

Internal ophthalmoplegia is revealed by completely dilated pupil not reacting to light or accommodation seen in diseases affecting the 3rd nerve nucleus and ciliary ganglion—always exclude drug (atropine)-induced mydriasis.

Nystagmus is the disturbance in ocular movements characterized by rhythmic to and fro oscillatory movements of one or both eyes in any or all directions of gaze, while looking voluntarily. Direction of nystagmus is toward the fast component. Causes of pathological nystagmus are visual defects, drug induced (anticonvulsants and tranquilizers), brainstem lesions (tumors and demyelination), and cerebellar and vestibular problems. The movements are horizontal, vertical, or pendular depending on cerebellar, brainstem, and visual pathway involvement respectively. Rotary and mixed types also occur.

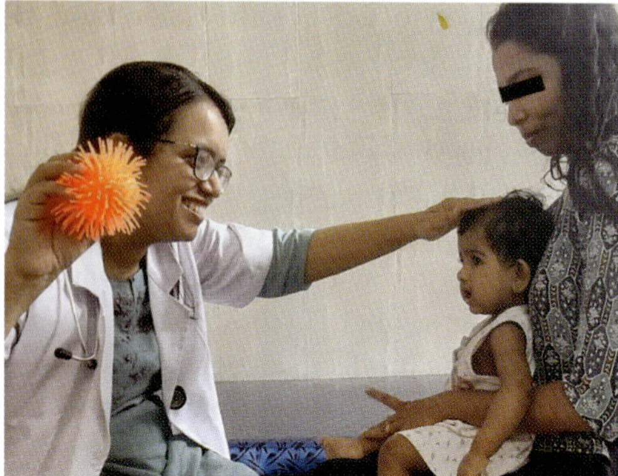

Fig. 21.11: Testing for nystagmus in young infant.
Courtesy: Dr Chinnu Chandran (SR in Pediatrics), Government Medical College, Kottayam, Kerala.

Detection of nystagmus: The methods are as for visual fixation and following for eye movements. Place young babies on mother's lap; eyes should be in level with the examiner. *The examiner should fix the child's head* prior to testing. Observe for nystagmus (type and direction of fast component) while the patient is looking directly at the light or a red toy **(Fig. 21.11)**. Move the test object about 30° medially, laterally, upwards, and downwards and observe the movements.

Optokinetic nystagmus is end gaze nystagmus revealing few beats of nystagmus on lateral gaze and is benign.

Ocular bobbing is downward jerks of eyes followed by a slow drift back to the primary position seen in *pontine lesions*.

Syndromes involving paralysis of 3rd, 4th, and 6th cranial nerves—*see midbrain lesions*.

Fifth Cranial (Trigeminal) Nerve

This is the largest cranial nerve.

Functions: Sensory to the face (excluding the angle of mandible) and head up to the vertex (includes intracranial structures—meninges of anterior and middle cranial fossae and cerebral vasculature). Sensory to the eyeballs, lacrimal glands, nasal mucosa and septum, nasopharynx, whole of the mouth up to pharynx, gums and teeth, anterior two-thirds of tongue, temporomandibular joint, tympanic membrane, lower lip and chin. **Figure 21.12** reveals the sensory areas supplied according to the divisions of the nerve. The sensations perceived are touch, pain, temperature, vibration, and proprioception. Motor to the muscles of mastication (masseter, temporalis, and lateral pterygoid).

Anatomy: The nerve arises from the pons and divides into three branches—ophthalmic, maxillary (both purely sensory), and mandibular (sensory and motor). The sensory impulses are carried by the first order fibers to the neuronal cells in the Gasserian ganglion. The sensory roots for light touch from there terminate in the nucleus in the pons. Pain and temperature afferents go down via the descending tract of trigeminal, which extends from lateral medulla to C2 segment of spinal cord. This can cause *dissociated sensory loss in the trigeminal area* (nonperception of pin prick in the area while light touch is preserved in lesions involving the medulla). Distal to the Gasserian ganglion the nerve splits into its divisions. The ophthalmic division (along with the maxillary branch) passes through the cavernous sinus. The former comes out through the superior orbital fissure (refer the course of 3, 4, and 6 cranial nerves). The maxillary and mandibular branches come out through the foramen rotundum and the foramen ovale respectively.

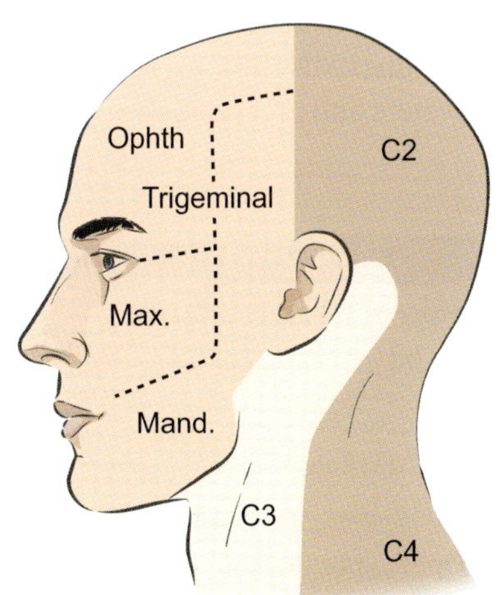

Fig. 21.12: Sensory supply of the trigeminal nerve.

The motor fibers arise from a small nucleus lying internal to the chief sensory nucleus in the pons, come out from the cerebellopontine angle, pass through the Gasserian ganglion, and join the mandibular division.

Clinical features: Isolated involvement of the 5th cranial nerve is rare in children. Deviation of the lower jaw, difficulty in chewing and swallowing are the main complaints. Loss of sensation over the face, mucous membranes of mouth (older children may complain of a broken cup feeling while drinking fluid), and nasopharynx are less common complaints. Rarely, trophic ulcers of cornea, nose, and mouth may be reported (due to diminished buccal, nasal, and lacrimal secretions).

Testing—motor part: Look for wasting of the temporalis muscle (seen as hollowing at the temporal region), flattening of the affected side of face and deviation of the jaw as the infant opens the mouth or cries. Deviation is toward the paralyzed side, being pushed over by the healthy lateral pterygoid muscle (scrutinize the deviation from the position of the incisors). For the older child, ask the patient to clench the teeth, and feel the temporal and masseter muscles which stand out prominently on this act. The pterygoids are tested by asking and showing the jaw moving side to side and also against resistance, with the mouth open. Isolated muscle involvement is seen in congenital myopathies and muscular dystrophies.

Sensory part: Touch at least three medial and three lateral points on each side of face (should represent all three divisions of the nerve) with a cotton wisp and ask the child how it feels and whether similar (child should not see the procedure). Temperature can be tested (see the sensory system) with cold and hot water test tubes. Sense of position and movement are tested by passively moving the pinna (with the patient's eyes closed) and asking to point the direction of the pinna.

Nasal tickle test is advised especially in infants, noncooperative or drowsy patients. Touch the child's anterior nares with a cotton wisp and observe the child's reaction. If the sensory part is intact, the child will grimace and will try to avoid this unpleasant stimulus with hands or moving the head.

Corneal reflex: Twist a *moist wisp of cotton* into fine hair. Fix the head of the child by holding at the forehead with one hand, ask the patient to look to the opposite side. Steady your testing hand by gently resting the little finger on the patient's cheek. Gently touch the lateral edge of the cornea with the moist cotton thread. Normal response is closure of both eyes (afferent 5th nerve, efferent 7th nerve). The reflex is absent on the same side in 5th as well as 7th nerve paralysis. *Do not use dry cotton since it may injure the cornea.*

Jaw jerk: Afferent and efferent are carried by 5th nerve. Keep the patient's mouth half open. The examiner's left index finger is placed across the chin and tapped gently with the right middle finger or percussion hammer. The response is sudden closure of the mouth. Jaw jerk is exaggerated in bilateral supranuclear lesions (associated with pseudobulbar palsy) and absent in nuclear and peripheral nerve lesions.

Common causes of 5th nerve palsy are brainstem glioma, cerebellopontine angle lesion, cavernous sinus thrombosis, malignancies, and demyelination. In spastic quadriplegic cerebral palsy, jaw jerk is exaggerated. Localize the 5th nerve lesion analyzing the divisions involved, other cranial nerves affected and associated findings as revealed in **Table 21.4**.

In bilateral UMN 5th nerve paralysis along with features of pseudobulbar palsy, emotional lability is usual. In bilateral lower motor neuron (LMN) lesions, jaw hangs loose and masseters and pterygoids are wasted and weak.

TABLE 21.4: Localization of 5th cranial nerve lesions.

Level of lesion	*Associated paralysis*	*Parts of 5th nerve affected*
Pons	Long tracts	Motor part complete sensory part ±
Cerebellopontine angle	Cranial nerves 7, 8	"
Floor of middle cranial fossa	Cranial nerves 3, 4, 6	All 3 divisions
Cavernous sinus	Cranial nerves 3, 4, 6	Ophthalmic and maxillary divisions
Superior orbital fissure	Cranial nerves 3, 4, 6	Ophthalmic division
Apex of petrous temporal bone	Cranial nerves 6, 7	All divisions

Seventh (Facial) Nerve

Functions: (1) Motor supply to all facial muscles except levator palpebrae superioris; (2) Taste (gustatory) sensation to the anterior two-thirds of tongue; (3) Secretory (parasympathetic) to salivary, lacrimal, and mucosal glands; (4) Sensory to the tympanic membrane, external auditory meatus, and tragus of the ear.

Anatomy **(Fig. 21.13A)**: The motor nucleus is in the caudal pons (ventrolateral to the 6th nerve nucleus). It receives supranuclear input from both cerebral hemispheres. The closely placed sensory and parasympathetic nuclei receive fibers from the geniculate ganglion. The fibers of the motor nucleus wind round the 6th nerve nucleus and emerge from the anterior surface of the brain between pons and medulla along with the sensory root, medial to the 8th nerve. It has a lengthy course, passing through the posterior cranial fossa along with 8th nerve, enter the internal acoustic meatus, traverses through the facial canal and internal ear, and expands to form the sensory geniculate ganglion **(Fig. 21.13B)**. From here, the nerve traverses backwards, gives a branch to the stapedius, and is joined by the chordae tympani, which contains taste fibers from the anterior two-thirds of tongue. The taste fibers pass through the geniculate ganglion to the sensory nucleus. The nerve emerges at the stylomastoid foramen, passes to the face through the parotid gland, and divides into branches to supply all the facial muscles including the platysma except levator palpebrae superioris.

Symptoms: Deviation of the angle of mouth and improper closure of the affected eye are the main complaints. Poor vigor in sucking, epiphora, and drooling can also be present.

Testing—motor part: Face becomes expressionless in 7th nerve paralysis.

Infants and young children: Observe the child while crying. Mouth deviates to the healthy side; there is inability to close the eye and flattening of nasolabial fold on the affected side. Impaired wrinkling of the forehead and drooling of fluid from the weak side of mouth are less prominent findings. Condition has to be differentiated from hypoplasia of DAO muscle *(Ref. Ch. 15)*.

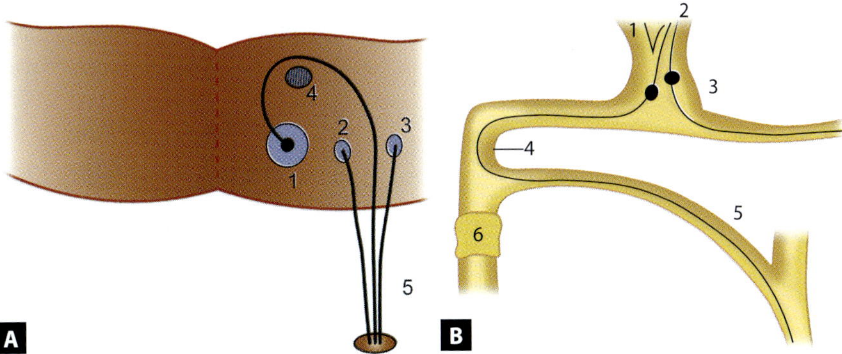

Figs. 21.13A and B: (A) Facial nerve nucleus and its connections: *(1) Main motor nucleus of 7th nerve; (2) Superior salivatory and lacrimal nuclei; (3) Sensory nucleus of 7th nerve; (4) 6th nerve nucleus; (5) Internal auditory meatus;* (B) Course of the facial nerve: *(1) Motor root; (2) Sensory root; (3) Geniculate ganglion; (4) Nerve to stapedius; (5) Chordae tympani; (6) Stylomastoid foramen.*

Older children: Formal testing is possible. Examiner should sit opposite the child. *Fix the patient's head while being examined.*

- Ask the patient to look upwards without tilting the head. For younger child, fix the head and bring a toy above the forehead to attract attention. The wrinkles on the forehead appear less prominent on the affected side.
- Ask the patient to shut the eyes tightly. Affected eye is not closed. On attempted closure, *Bell's phenomenon* (the normally present rolling up of eyeballs) becomes evident [*Bell's sign* **(Fig. 21.14A)**]. Try to open the closed eyes on both sides simultaneously by separating the eyelids with the index and thumb of each hand. The affected eye is easily opened.
- Ask the patient to say "eee" and show the teeth. The angle of the mouth deviates to the healthy side. The nasolabial fold on the affected side is flattened **(Fig. 21.14B)**.
- Ask the patient to whistle. It is not possible in facial nerve paralysis.
- Ask the patient to fill the oral cavity with air as in attempted blowing. Examiner should feel the tone and power of facial muscles on both sides by pressing with index and middle fingers simultaneously. The affected side yields easily and air escapes **(Table 21.5)**.

Sensory part: Test materials—Saline, glucose, vinegar, and quinine

Testing is possible in older children. Salt, sweet, sour, and bitter tastes should be tested in the order respectively. The patient is asked to put out the tongue and keep it protruding till the test is completed. Apply the test material on the middle of the anterior two-thirds of tongue on one side and ask "is it salt?" "is it sweet?", *etc.* The patient is directed to shake the head when the correct taste is mentioned. The mouth should be thoroughly rinsed after testing with each material. The sensation will be perceived in <10 seconds. In infants, taste sensation can be made out by facial expression when bitter solution is applied. The test may be done by using a weak galvanic current, which will provide a metallic taste.

Localization of the lesion: Facial nerve is affected very commonly in children.

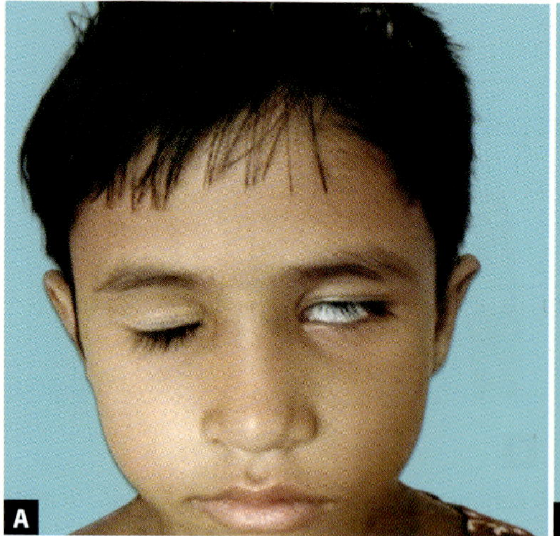

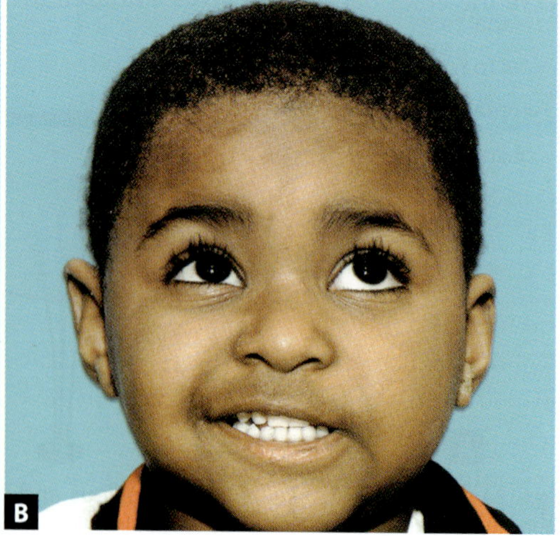

Figs. 21.14A and B: (A) Bell's sign (L); (B) Child with LMN facial palsy (L). See the flattened nasolabial fold. (LMN: lower motor neuron).

TABLE 21.5: Differentiating clinical features between UMN and LMN facial palsy.

Clinical feature	***UMN***	***LMN***
Affection of upper part of face	Spared (due to bilateral innervation)	Present
Spontaneous blinking	Present	Absent
Bell's phenomenon	Not seen	Seen
Lacrimation	Present	Present except for the lesion in geniculate ganglion
Affection of lower part of face	Present	Present
Atrophy of facial muscles	Absent	Present
Taste sensation over anterior two-third of tongue	Preserved	Lost when the lesion is between brainstem and origin of chordae tympani
Hyperacusis*	Absent	Present when the lesion is between brain stem and nerve to stapedius
Emotional movements	Preserved	Lost
EMG and nerve conduction	Normal	Abnormal

(EMG: electromyography; LMN: lower motor neuron; UMN: upper motor neuron)
Note: *Difficult to elicit in children

TABLE 21.6: Localization of LMN facial palsy.

Level of lesion	***Muscle paralysis***	***Taste***	***Hyperacusis****	***Lacrimation***
Motor nucleus	Present	Normal	Present	Normal
Pons (distal to motor nucleus)	Present	Normal	Present	Normal
Geniculate ganglion	Present	Affected	Present	Absent
Proximal to nerve to stapedius	Present	Affected	Present	Normal
Distal to nerve to stapedius	Present	Affected	Absent	Normal
Stylomastoid foramen	Present	Normal	Absent	Normal
Facial nerve branches	Partial paralysis	Normal	Absent	Normal

(LMN: lower motor neuron)
Note: **Difficult to elicit in children*

The manifestations differ depending on the level of lesion. **Table 21.6** reveals the salient clinical points in the localization of LMN facial palsy.

Table 21.7 reveals the common causes of different types of facial palsy. *Bilateral facial palsy may pass unnoticed unless not carefully looked for.*

Eighth (Vestibulocochlear) Nerve

It has two nerves with different functions in a single trunk.

Functions: (1) Maintenance of equilibrium, coordination and orientation (vestibular component); (2) sound perception (cochlear component).

TABLE 21.7: Common causes of facial palsy in children.

Unilateral UMN	***Unilateral LMN***	***Bilateral LMN***
Meningitis	Bell's palsy	Guillain–Barre' syndrome
Encephalitis	Otitis media	Brainstem glioma
Brain abscess	Guillain Barre' syndrome	Leukemic infiltrates
Stroke	Poliomyelitis	Post-diphtheritic paralysis
Brain tumors	Arachnoiditis Aneurysms CP angle tumor Secondary deposits Hansen disease	Hansen disease Systemic hypertension Syringobulbia

(LMN: lower motor neuron; UMN: upper motor neuron)

Anatomy: The fibers for the *vestibular part* arise from the vestibular ganglion in the internal acoustic meatus and reach the nuclear complex at the floor of 4th ventricle between pons and medulla. Different fibers pass uncrossed to the cerebellum, spinal cord, nuclei of 3, 4, 6 cranial nerves and to the cerebral cortex at the vestibular area in postcentral gyrus. The receptors of the *cochlear nerve* are in the organ of Corti and the cochlear ganglion. The auditory fibers arise from the ganglion and enter the pons lateral to 7th nerve and terminate in the nuclei in pons. Secondary fibers after partial decussation terminate in the inferior colliculus and medial geniculate bodies. Tertiary fibers from here pass through the posterior limb of the internal capsule to reach the auditory cortex located at the temporal lobe. Because of the decussation at various levels, unilateral hearing defect is uncommon and hence *unilateral hearing loss always indicates auditory nerve affection and not lesions in its pathway.*

Symptoms of auditory dysfunction: Most mothers and grandparents will be able to notice poor response to the sounds by the baby before 3 m age and will be reporting. Delayed acquisition of speech, absent babbling, abnormal speech, and temper tantrums are the symptoms in infants and toddlers. Older children with recent hearing loss or becoming hard of hearing will be able to complain about the problem. *It is mandatory to enquire about hearing ability in all ill babies as well as those coming for well baby checkup.* Ask for or observe the baby's response on telephone ringing, banging of door, calling the baby by name and sound of a motorcycle.

Testing for hearing is needed in all children with speech delay. Examine the external ear for wax impaction, integrity of the tympanic membrane and evidence of middle ear effusion; do the appropriate treatment and see the response before hearing evaluation.

Hearing ((*Ref. Ch. 12* for hearing screening): Audiometry can be done from 3 yr of age onwards and tuning fork tests in older children. Universal hearing assessment by 2 w after birth with otoacoustic emissions (OAE) is a must for early detection of hearing defect and to proceed for the corrective steps. *Brainstem auditory evoked response (BAER) is mandatory for any child suspected of hearing defect.* Hearing impairment in an older child can be due to auditory nerve disease or middle ear infection. This can be differentiated by tuning fork test for each ear as described below:

- *Rinne's test:* Activate the tuning fork (256 Hz) and hold it against the external auditory meatus and ask whether the sound is heard. Repeat the test by placing the handle of the tuning fork on the mastoid process and ask the child to compare both sounds. Normally directly heard sound (air conduction) is better than bone conduction. In middle ear disease, bone conduction is better than air conduction and in nerve deafness both are diminished or lost.
- *Weber test:* Activate the tuning fork and place the handle at the center of the patient's forehead at the anterior scalp line. Normally the sound is equally appreciated in both ears. In middle ear disease, the patient hears the sound better in the affected ear. In nerve deafness, sound is heard only in the normal ear.

Hearing loss in children may be partial (hard of hearing) or complete (deafness), can be conductive or sensorineural. **Boxes 21.4 and 21.5** reveal the common causes of conductive and sensorineural hearing loss respectively.

Disturbances of vestibular function are vertigo and nystagmus. *Vertigo* is the feeling of external objects moving round the patient. It is mostly due to ear disease and rarely due to benign paroxysmal vertigo. Older children complain of a feeling of spinning. Complaints in younger ones are the infant becoming clumsy or getting frequent falls. *Nystagmus with fast component directed away from the affected* nerve is typical of vestibular nerve dysfunction.

Fukuda stepping test: Ask the patient to stand with eyes closed and arms outstretched. The limbs tend to drift toward the affected side. On marching in place, the patient slowly pivots toward the affected side.

Romberg test: Ask the patient to stand erect with both feet close together, eyes open and arms outstretched on the sides. The patient falls toward the abnormal ear side.

Tandem gait test: Ask the patient to walk with feet one behind the other. The patient falls toward the side of the affected ear.

BOX 21.4: Common causes of conductive hearing loss in children.

Congenital
- Ear anomalies
- Fibrous dysplasia
- Osteogenesis imperfecta
- Osteopetrosis
- Osteosclerosis

Acquired
- Otitis media with effusion
- Trauma (skull, tympanic membrane)
- Histiocytosis
- Parotid tumors
- Rhabdomyosarcoma

BOX 21.5: Common causes of sensorineural hearing loss in children.

Genetic:
- Isolated (AR, AD, XLR)
- Syndromic (Waardenburg, Pendred, Alport)
- Chromosomal anomalies (Trisomies, Turner syndrome)
- Craniofacial anomalies
- Mitochondrial diseases

Acquired:
- Wax impaction
- Otitis media
- Foreign body ear
- TORCH infections
- Meningitis
- Mumps
- Drug induced (gentamicin)
- Toxic (bilirubin encephalopathy)
- Demyelination
- Tumors (acoustic neuroma)
- Postsurgical

(AR: autosomal recessive; AD: autosomal dominant; XLR: X-linked recessive)

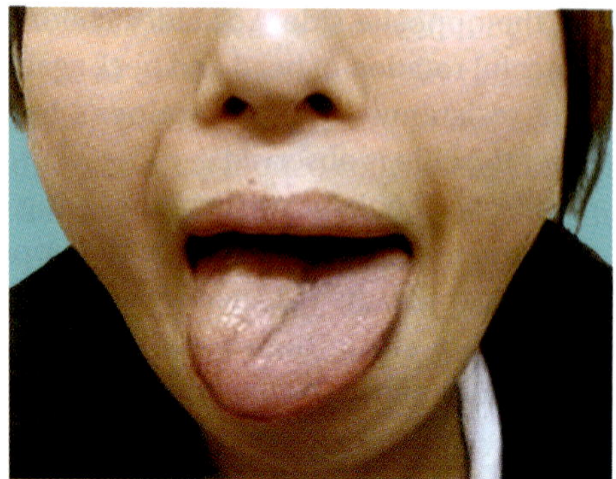

Fig. 21.16: LMN palsy (R) hypoglossal nerve.

from side to side and push the cheek with the tongue from inside. Assess the strength by pressing the cheek over the tongue with a finger during such movement.

In UMN lesions, tongue is spastic, thin, and pointed without atrophy or fasciculation. The leading cause of LMN palsy in infants is Werdnig-Hoffmann disease. Other causes are poliomyelitis, trauma, cerebrovascular accidents (CVA), and anomalies and tumors in the region of foramen magnum **(Fig. 21.16)**.

Bulbar and pseudobulbar palsy: Bulbar palsy is due to the damage of mainly 9th, 10th, 11th, and 12th cranial nerves or their nuclei in the medullary region resulting in flaccid paralysis of the muscles supplied by them. The symptoms are pooling of secretions in the throat, sialorrhea, dysphagia, dysarthria, nasal regurgitation of liquids, absent cough reflex, frequent aspiration and nasal twang of voice. The lower jaw hangs loosely. The jaw jerk and gag reflex are lost. Respiratory and cardiac irregularities and fluctuations in blood pressure may occur due to vasomotor and respiratory center involvement. The common causes are Guillain-Barre syndrome, encephalitis, meningitis, demyelinating diseases, poliomyelitis, and brainstem glioma. In pseudo- or suprabulbar palsy, due to the affection of UMNs, jaw is stiff, mouth is difficult to open fully, sialorrhea is present, jaw jerk is brisk and there may be jaw clonus. The tongue is small and stiff, the movements are difficult, chewing and feeding become difficult. The gag and the cough reflexes are preserved and aspiration, though present, is not as frequent as in bulbar palsy. The most common cause is spastic cerebral palsy following perinatal asphyxia. Other causes are late hypoxic insults, encephalitis, CVA, and infantile Gaucher disease.

Motor System

Anatomy and Physiology

For practical purposes, the motor system is divided into (1) upper (UMN) and (2) lower motor neuron units (LMN). UMN (pyramidal system) fibers arise from the pyramidal cells in 5th layer of motor cortex, pass through the corona radiata, anterior two-thirds of the posterior limb of internal capsule, cerebral peduncles, pons and decussate in the lower part of medulla and finally end up in the motor neurons in the brainstem and spinal cord. The pyramidal system is concerned with initiation of voluntary and skilled motor acts. *LMN units* include the motor neuron cells in the brainstem and spinal cord, nerve roots, cranial and peripheral nerves, myoneural junction and muscles. Function is muscular movements.

The major centers influencing the motor system are the extrapyramidal system and cerebellum. The extrapyramidal system consists of basal ganglia (caudate nucleus, putamen, globus pallidus), subthalamic nuclei, substantia nigra, and other structures in the brainstem. The connections to the LMN are indirect through various pathways arising in the brainstem. The function is regulation of muscle tone and posture. The cerebellum influences LMN through its connections. The function is regulation of rate, rhythm and force of muscular contractions on the ipsilateral side. The midline vermis is involved in maintenance of equilibrium and control of gait.

Assessment parameters are (1) muscle bulk, (2) tone, (3) power or strength, (4) locomotion and motility, (5) involuntary movements, (6) coordination of movements, and (7) reflexes.

Motor parts of cranial nerves are mentioned in the concerned section. Subsequent order of examination is upper limbs, trunk, and lower limbs.

Muscle bulk: Assess by inspection, palpation, and measurements of suspected parts and then compare with the opposite side. When bulk is reduced (wasting, atrophy), muscles are smaller, flabby, and softer. As fibrosis sets in they become harder, inelastic, and short (contractures). Severe and early wasting is seen in LMN lesions. Moderate wasting occurs in long-standing UMN lesions. Wasting is a feature of PEM, disuse and chronic illnesses. Pseudohypertrophy is muscle tissue replaced by fat and connective tissue giving a bulky appearance with reduced strength and occurs in Duchenne muscular dystrophy.

Muscle tone is an unconscious, continuous partial contraction of the muscle creating resistance to passive movements of a joint. It can be *phasic* (rapid contraction to high intensity stretch as in deep tendon reflexes) or *postural* (prolonged contraction of antigravity muscles in response to low intensity stretch of gravity). *Assess by*:

Inspection reveals "frog leg posture" in hypotonia characterized by partial flexion, complete abduction, and external rotation at hip joints **(Fig. 21.2)**. In hypertonia, the lower limbs are extended at hips and knees, plantar flexed and feet laterally rotated.

Palpation: Flabby in hypotonia and firm in hypertonia.

Passive movements of joints: The degree of resistance offered is assessed. The velocity of passive movement should be steadily increased to detect the increasing tone, as it is velocity dependent.

Dropping the limb: Elevate the limb to a height of 1 foot and suddenly release it to bed. The examiner should get hold of the testing limb with the other hand to prevent injury. Flaccid limb falls limply and hypertonic limb falls slowly.

Posture against gravity: Limb is placed in a posture against gravity and the patient is asked to maintain that posture, e.g., for the lower limb, keep the hip and knee flexed with foot on bed. As the examiner releases support, the hypotonic limb falls down sideways.

Shaking the limb: Hold the wrist and shake the distal part. Hypotonic hands are easily shaken and go into flexion limply.

In newborns and infants traction response, ventral suspension, angles of joints, vertical suspension at axillae are observed (Ref. Ch. 12, 15).

Deformities secondary to hypo- or hypertonia should be noted; cerebral palsy, arthrogryposis multiplex, dislocation of hip, and spinal muscular atrophy are some examples.

Abnormalities in tone are hypo- and hypertonia. Hypotonia can occur in acute cerebral lesions, cerebellar, spinal cord, and lower motor unit diseases. Cerebral, cerebellar, and UMN spinal cord lesions are characterized by normal or brisk deep tendon reflexes (DTR). The main differentiating clinical sign is *absent or sluggish DTR in LMN* lesions.

Hypertonia following UMN lesion is *spasticity* and extrapyramidal system is *rigidity.*

TABLE 21.9: Muscle power testing around joints.

Muscles	***Method of testing***
Neck	Ask the patient to flex, extend, and rotate the head in both directions with and without resistance; offer resistance over the occiput for extension and over chin for the other movements. Infants reveal head lag or head drop laterally and forwards on pulling to sit.
Upper limbs	
Shoulder	Ask the patient to abduct and elevate the arm with and without resistance, offer resistance at mid arm. Young children—offer toys above the shoulder level; infants—vertical suspension reveals shoulder weakness *Adductors:* Test both sides together—ask the child to abduct both arms with flexed elbows, apply resistance at midarm, ask the child to press downward *Flexors:* Ask the child to bring the arm flexed at elbow across the chest, offer resistance at midarm *Extension:* Ask the child to bring the arm flexed at elbow backwards, offer resistance at midarm
Elbow	Flexion—ask the patient to flex the forearm against resistance (at mid forearm) in full supination. Extension—ask the patient to extend the forearm against resistance at the same area. For young children and infants, offer toys. Observe spontaneous activity or the reaction to scratching at the distal part of the limb
Wrist	Ask the patient to make a fist and flex and extend the fist against resistance. This test is difficult in young children in whom observe for wrist drop and claw hand
Hand	Ask the patient to grasp your index and middle fingers simultaneously on both sides. In young children, assess the force of holding a pencil. In infants, assess the grasp reflex
Trunk muscles	
Intercostals	Observe the inspiratory movements. Lower intercostals are pulled in during each respiratory cycle in intercostal paralysis. Splint the diaphragm (compress the abdomen from both sides with your hands below the costal margin). Dyspnea increases if intercostals are paralyzed
Diaphragm	Observe paradoxical respiratory movements (abdomen is pulled in during inspiration if diaphragm is paralyzed). Splint the chest by compressing from both sides and observe for increasing dyspnea
Erector spinae	Ask the patient to raise his head, neck, and trunk in the prone position. Normally muscles stand out prominently. Infants and young children—observe the movements in prone position
Abdominal muscles	
Upper part	In supine position, ask the patient to raise his head and chest with the arms held behind the occiput. In weakness of the upper part, the umbilicus is pulled downwards
Lower part	In supine position, ask the patient to raise his extended lower limbs without any support. The umbilicus is drawn upwards in weakness (Beevor's sign—pulling of umbilicus to opposite side of paralysis of lower abdominal muscles)

Contd...

Contd...

Muscles	*Method of testing*
Lower limbs:	
Hip flexors	In supine position with the limb in extension, ask the patient to raise the leg off the bed against resistance offered at mid-thigh
Hip extensors	In prone position with the limb extended, ask the patient to raise the thigh against resistance offered at mid-thigh
Knee flexors	In prone position with the limb extended, ask the patient to flex the leg against resistance offered at mid-calf
Knee extensors	In supine position, ask the patient to extend the flexed knee against resistance offered at mid shin
Hip adductors and abductors	In supine position with the limb extended, ask the patient to adduct and abduct the thigh against resistance offered at mid-thigh
Hip rotators	In supine position with limbs extended, ask the patient to rotate the limb externally and internally against resistance offered at leg
Ankle—dorsiflexors, plantar flexors, supinator, pronator	Ask the patient to do dorsiflexion, plantar flexion, supination, and pronation of foot against resistance

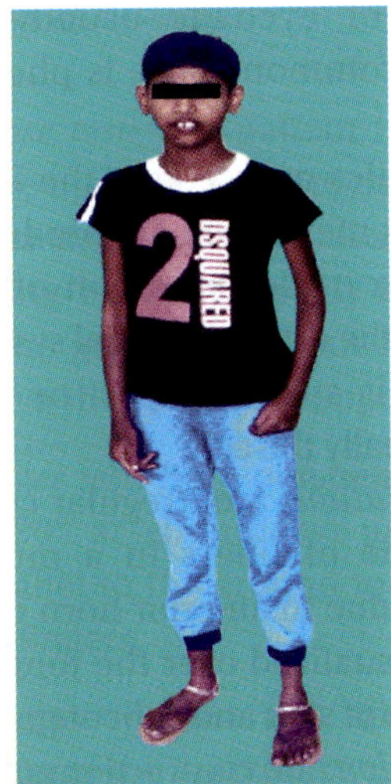

Fig. 21.20: Girl with spastic CP-(L) hemiplegia.

muscular dystrophy due to bilateral weakness of the gluteus medius muscle which normally tilts the pelvis upwards. Can also occur in bilateral hip damage as in bilateral DDH.

- *High steppage gait:* The patient lifts the leg too high due to foot dorsiflexion weakness—typical of peripheral neuropathy.
- *Hysterical gait* is a bizarre gait not resembling any pattern.

Involuntary movements are many. They can be the sole manifestation of the disease or associated sign/symptom, aiding in the diagnosis or the severity of that illness.

Chorea: Irregular, nonrepetitive semi-purposive mostly proximal movements associated with emotional instability. It is classically seen in Sydenham chorea, other causes being acute encephalitis (all types), Wilson disease, drugs, choreoathetoid CP, and metabolic disorders. The movements can be augmented by the following methods:

- *Extension of limbs:* Ask the patient to sit still with all limbs extended and tongue protruded. Choreic movements become evident in limbs and tongue after a few

Pendular knee jerk: The patient is seated with both legs hanging loosely. Elicit the knee jerk. The limbs swing unusually freely (more than 3 swings) in cerebellar lesions.

Note: Weak muscles can mimic ataxia.

Titubation is involuntary nodding movements of the head while sitting.

Truncal ataxia: The patient sways or even falls when made to sit; *gait ataxia*—see gait.

Titubation and truncal and gait ataxias indicate lesions of cerebellar midline structures and vermis. Limb ataxia indicates cerebellar hemisphere involvement.

Reflexes

Reflex is an involuntary response to a stimulus. They are of three types—(1) superficial, (2) deep, (3) organic. **Table 21.10** details the superficial reflexes (Refer: Cranial nerves 5, 9, 10 for corneal and gag reflexes).

Superficial reflexes will be abolished in conditions which cause damage to any part of the reflex arc. In infants (<1 yr), plantar reflex is normally extensor. More medial scratching produces plantar grasp response.

Deep tendon reflexes (DTRs) are elicited by putting the muscle into stretch and its tendon is sharply struck. The patellar hammer should be withdrawn immediately. The muscle suddenly contracts. **Table 21.11** reveals the details of common DTR. Grading is done as absent 0, reduced +, normal ++, brisk +++, exaggerated ++++/with clonus. See **Fig. 21.22** for the diagrammatic representation of reflexes.

Clonus is repetitive rhythmic contractions of a muscle evoked by a stretch stimulus and indicates severe degree of hyperreflexia.

TABLE 21.10: Superficial spinal reflexes.

Reflex	*Spinal level*	*Method*	*Response*
Abdominal **(Fig. 21.23)**	T6 to T12	Use a key or wooden stick. Stroke the abdominal wall below costal margins and iliac fossae, starting at the level of umbilicus from lateral to medial aspect	Contraction of abdominal muscles
Cremasteric	L1, L2	Stroke the skin at the upper and inner aspect of thighs	Drawing up of the testes
Anal	S3, S4	Stroke the skin around anus	Contraction of anal sphincter
Plantar **(Fig. 21.24)**	L5, S1	Stroke the outer edge of sole of foot from heel to little toe Press heavily along the inner border of tibia (Oppenheim's sign) Pinch the tendoachilles (Gordon's reflex) Stroke the outer edge of the dorsum of foot below the lateral malleolus (Chaddock sign) Rossolimo sign: Tap the ball of the big toe at the sole proximally—no response in normal people	• Flexor response normally—all toes are flexed and drawn together. Babinski's extensor plantar response occurs in lesions of the corticospinal tract characterized by dorsiflexion of the great toe, followed by spreading out and extension of other toes, dorsiflexion of the ankle and flexion of the hip and knee. Flexor and extensor spasms occur in bilateral upper motor neuron lesions at a higher level • Flexion of all toes in pyramidal tract lesion above the spinal cord

TABLE 21.11: Deep tendon reflexes.

Root value	***Name of DTR***	***Method***	***Response***
5th cranial nerve	Jaw jerk	Read cranial nerve 5	
C5, C6	Biceps jerk	Flex the elbow to 90° and place the forearm in a semipronated position. Place the examiners' left thumb over the patient's biceps tendon. Strike over the thumb with the hammer	Contraction of biceps Flexion of elbow
C5, C6	Radial supinator	Patients arm in the same position as the biceps jerk, strike on the styloid process of radius with a hammer	Supination of the forearm. Lesions of C5, C6 cause loss of supinator reflex but brisk flexion of fingers occurs (inversion of the reflex due to hyperexcitability of anterior horn cells below C5, C6)
C6, C7	Triceps	The Patient's elbow is flexed to 90° with the wrist placed across the patient's chest. Strike the triceps tendon above the olecranon	Contraction of triceps Extension of elbow
L2, L3, L4 **(Fig. 21.25)**	Knee jerk	(i) Patient supine, flex the knee at 120–150° which rests on the examiner's left palm or knuckle. Tap on the patellar tendon midway between origin and insertion. (ii) Patient sitting up legs dangling freely over the edge of bed. Strike the patellar tendon*	Brief extension of knee
S1, S2	Ankle jerk	Keep the lower limb everted on the bed with slight flexion at the knee. With the left hand of the examiner placed under the sole dorsiflex the foot to 90° so that the tendoachilles is stretched. Strike gently on the posterior surface of tendoachilles with the hammer	Contraction of calf muscles. Plantar flexion of foot appreciated by hand under the sole

Note: If difficulty in eliciting the reflex, try reinforcement by asking the patient to clench the teeth/by distracting attention.

*Infants allowed to breastfeed with the body on mother's lap and legs resting on mother's thigh. Strike the patellar tendon.

(DTR: deep tendon reflex)

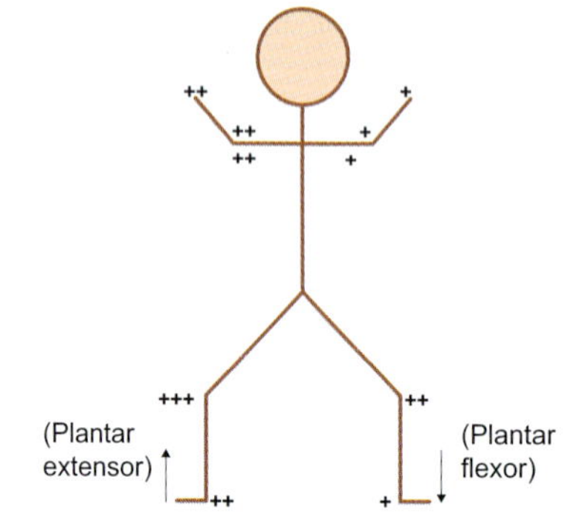

Fig. 21.22: Diagrammatic representation of reflexes.

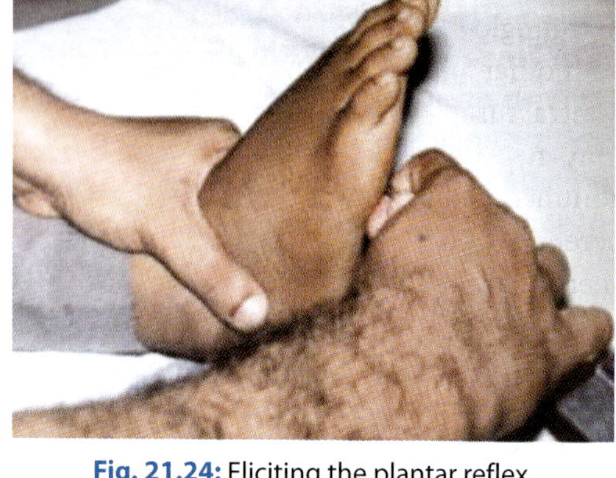
Fig. 21.24: Eliciting the plantar reflex.

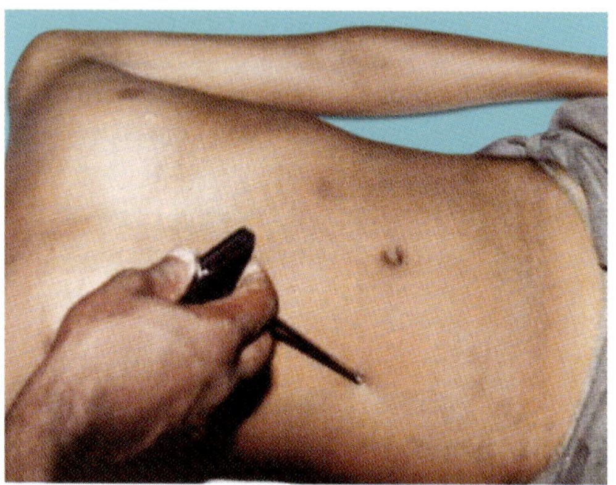
Fig. 21.23: Eliciting the abdominal reflex.

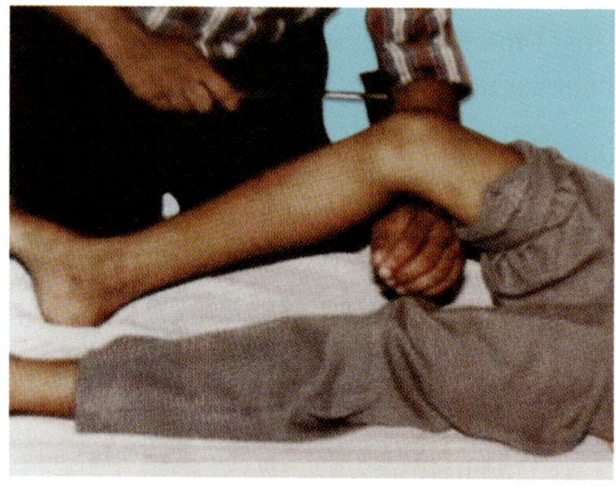
Fig. 21.25: Eliciting the knee jerk.

To elicit *ankle clonus*, standing on the patient's side, flex the patient's knee slightly and support the popliteal fossa with your less dominant hand. Suddenly dorsiflex the forefoot with the dominant hand from the plantar aspect and continue to apply the pressure. Sustained clonic contractions occur in calf muscles. Contractions *>10* in infants and *3* in older children are abnormal.

Patellar clonus: Keep the limb in extended position, push the patella from above toward the foot and maintain the pressure. A series of clonic contractions of quadriceps occur.

Palmomental reflex: Scratch or tap the thenar eminence of hand. Normally there is no response. In frontal lobe lesions, the orbicularis mentalis muscle contracts on the same side.

Hoffmann sign in the upper limb is equivalent to Babinski's reflex. Grasp the terminal phalanx of the patient's middle finger (arm extended with palm facing down) with your thumb and index. With the other index finger sharply flick the terminal phalanx. Adduction of thumb and flexion of fingers on the same hand is the positive sign suggesting pyramidal lesion above C7.

Abnormalities in DTR: The reflexes are diminished or absent in LMN lesions and muscle affections. They are exaggerated in UMN lesions, tetanus, and thyrotoxicosis and also in anxiety. Hence, these are considered pathological if asymmetrical or associated with other UMN signs. In UMN lesions with contractures and in neuronal shock, DTR may not be exaggerated. In myxedema, contraction and relaxation are prolonged. In cerebellar disease, pendular nature may be seen. Hung up knee jerk occurs in chorea.

Organic reflexes mediate respiration, deglutition, micturition, and defecation. They are ascertained from history. Anal sphincter can be assessed by anal reflex and tone of the sphincter.

Primitive reflexes (neonatal reflexes): Most important are Moro reflex, grasp, and glabellar tap.

Glabellar tap reflex: Tap repeatedly over the nasion with your finger. Normally the eyes close for 3–4 taps followed by conditioning. In bilateral UMN lesions, eye closure persists till tapping is stopped.

Urinary bladder: Higher centers of micturition are in frontal (inhibitory) areas and pons (facilitatory). Lesions in the frontal cortex produce "frontal lobe incontinence" characterized by urgency, frequency, and inappropriate voiding of urine. The sympathetic supply is from T11 to L2 (inhibitory) which determines the bladder capacity and urine storage. The parasympathetic and somatic innervation (both motor and sensory) are from S2 to S4 segments. Damage of the spinal cord between pons and sacral centers produces *atonic bladder* (distended bladder with overflow) in the early spinal shock phase. The typical UMN or *automatic reflex bladder* (reflex contraction to low volumes as in infants) is established after some weeks. Lesions of the sacral segments produce LMN or *autonomous bladder* (continuous dribbling). The common causes for bladder dysfunction are congenital [spinal anomalies, myelomeningocele (**Fig. 15.16**)], spinal injuries, infections (arachnoiditis and myelitis), demyelination and neoplasm (primary and secondary).

Bowel disorders: Innervation for bowel control is similar to the urinary bladder. Parasympathetic innervation is responsible for bowel emptying. Local nerve plexuses mainly control defecation. Sympathetic fibers cause relaxation of sigmoid and rectum with increased sphincter tone. Lesion above the sacral spinal cord causes increased sphincter tone and fecal retention. Segmental lesion of the sacral spinal cord leads to paralysis of sphincter ani (anus is patulous with absent anal reflex) leading to fecal incontinence. The most common neurological condition is myelomeningocele (Ref. **Fig. 15.6**) in which the level of lesion can be diagnosed by the anal sphincter tone.

Sensory System

Anatomy and Physiology

Sensations are- (1) cutaneous (touch, pain, and thermal sensation), (2) deep (pressure sensation, muscle, tendon, joint and bone sensation and vibration sense), and (3) cortical (tactile localization, two-point discrimination, sensory inattention, and stereognosis). Pain and temperature sensations ascend in the lateral spinothalamic tract and crude touch in the anterior spinothalamic tract. Posterior column fibers carry the sense of position, movement, stereognosis (size and shape of objects), vibration, and fine touch. Along with cranial nerve sensory fibers, they rely on thalamus. From there, they are carried by the thalamocortical fibers passing through the posterior one-third of the posterior limb of the internal capsule to the sensory cortex in the posterior central gyrus of the parietal lobe. The system has intimate connections to the cerebellum through spinocerebellar

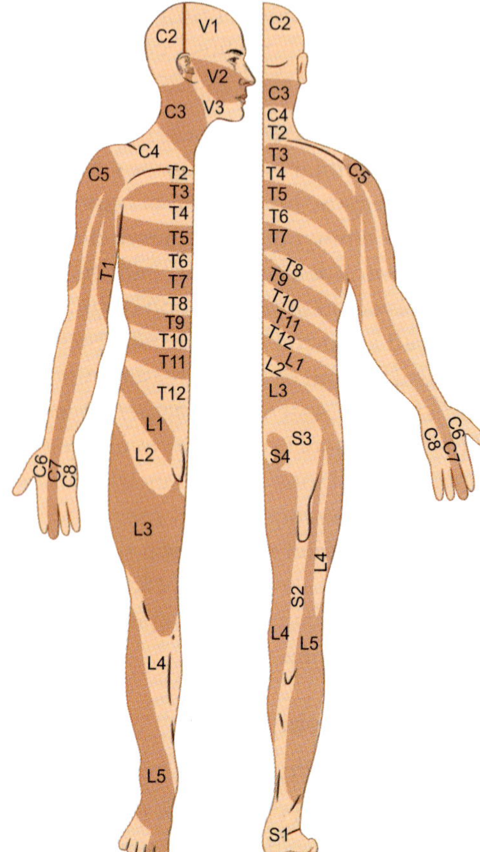

Fig. 21.26: Cutaneous sensory distribution.

tracts. **Figure 21.26** reveals the cutaneous areas supplied by sensory roots.

Testing: In children under 3 yr and patients who are noncooperative, only pain sense can be tested by observing facial expression or withdrawal of limb. There are six parameters—touch, pain, temperature, vibration, stereognosis, and position sense. The latter two are less important in children.

Testing should be done when the patient is alert, be quick, do from the abnormal to normal area and the process should not be visible to the child.

Touch (tactile sensibility): It includes light touch and pressure, tactile localization, and discrimination. *Light touch*—gently touch the skin with a wisp of cotton (tissue paper/soft brush). Tell the patient to say "yes" when touch is felt. Compare with the opposite side. Infants usually perceive the sensation and reveal it by irritation, looking at the examiner or crying.

Deep (pressure) touch: Repeat the process with a finger or a blunt object as the touch stimulus.

Cortical sensory impairments as deficits in tactile localization, two-point discrimination, stereognosis, and sensory inattention need be tested only if the primary sensations are intact. After each touch, the patient is asked to point to the exact site. Tactile localization is lost in cortical damage.

Two-point discrimination: A pair of blunt dividers are applied to the skin surface and gradually brought closer until the patient is unable to distinguish between the two points. Point discrimination varies with the area tested (2 mm over tip of index fingers to 1 cm on the pulp of toes). This ability is lost in parietal cortical, posterior column or peripheral nerve lesions.

Stereognosis (recognition of size, shape, weight, and form): Place common objects like a spoon, key, or pencil in patient's one hand and ask to identify the object. Repeat the test on the opposite side.

Sensory inattention: Mirror points on both sides of the body are simultaneously touched. If the touch on one side is not appreciated, the lesion is in the opposite parietal lobe. There is no actual loss of sensation on the abnormal side when tested separately.

Abnormalities in touch are anesthesia (loss of touch), hypoalgesia (partial loss), hyperesthesia (painful touch), and mislocalization.

Pain sensation: Use a sterilized or disposable domestic pin and prick the skin from affected to normal area. Compare with the opposite side. Abnormalities are analgesia (absence of pain sensation), hypoalgesia (partial loss of pain), hyperalgesia (exaggerated pain), and paresthesia or tingling sensation felt by the patient spontaneously or in response to light cutaneous stimuli.

Pressure pain: Squeeze a distal muscle or *Achilles tendon*. It is a poorly localized pain.

Temperature: Apply two test tubes with hot (*44°C*) and cold (*30°C*) water alternately to the skin. Patient responds by saying warm or cold. As a bedside test, the cold metallic sensation of the touch of a key can be used.

Vibration sense: The handle of a vibrating tuning fork of 128 Hz per second is applied over the skin of bony prominence—medial malleolus of tibia or olecranon process of ulna. Normally a person feels vibrations till he/she reports that vibrations are no longer felt. The examiner should then keep the fork on his own bone to verify whether the vibrations still continue. Vibration sense is lost in peripheral neuropathies and posterior column disorders.

Position sense and sense of passive movement: The patient in relaxed supine position, the toe or phalanx is moved up and down. The patient is directed to report the joint movements as "moving" and the direction as "up" or "down". *10°* movement can be appreciated normally at all joints.

Joint sense is tested in larger joints as the ability to appreciate the position of a limb. Distract the patient's attention by looking away. The examiner puts the patient's one limb in a particular position and directs the patient to keep the other limb in the same position.

Signs of Meningeal Irritation

Neck rigidity: Keep the patient in supine position without a pillow behind the head. With the nondominant hand hold the patient's head and gently flex the neck as if trying to touch the anterior chest wall with chin, which is normally possible **(Fig. 21.27)**.

In meningeal irritation, the procedure produces pain and resistance to neck flexion due to the spasm of extensor muscles of the neck and the child's chin cannot touch the anterior chest wall. Extreme neck rigidity produces head retraction. In struggling children to differentiate voluntary resistance from true neck stiffness, place the recumbent patient's shoulders at the edge of the table, support the weight of the occiput only in your hand and flex the neck anteriorly. In doubtful cases, repeat the test in the sitting posture with lower limbs extended. The most common cause of neck stiffness in children is infections of brain and coverings (meningitis, encephalitis, and brain abscess). Others are subarachnoid hemorrhage, raised ICP, brain and spinal cord tumors, drugs (phenothiazine), and infantile Gaucher disease. Congenital anomalies and infections of cervical spine and neck, tetanus, retropharyngeal and lateral pharyngeal

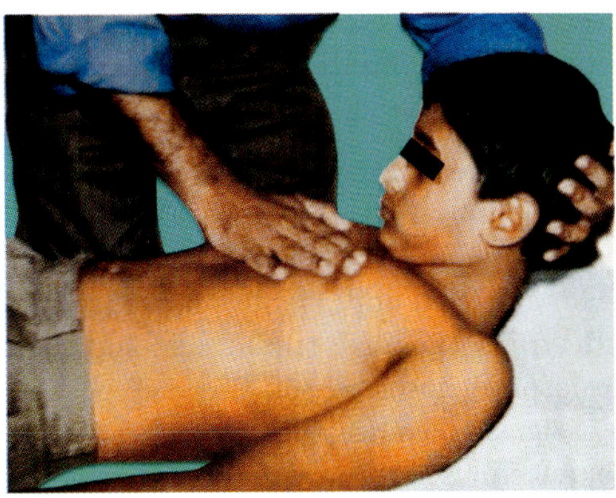

Fig. 21.27: Testing for neck stiffness.

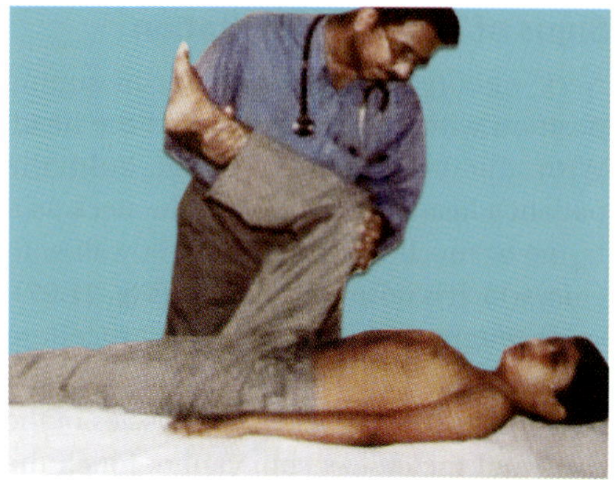

Fig. 21.28: Eliciting the Kernig sign.

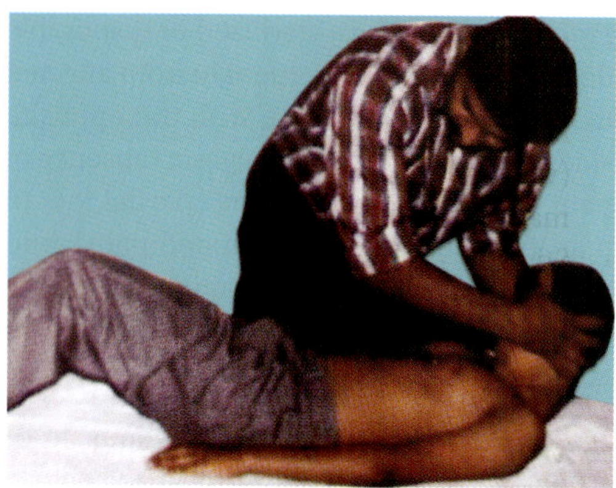

Fig. 21.29: Eliciting Brudzinski sign.

abscess are other causes. In spastic cerebral palsy, neck stiffness may be present.

Kernig sign (described by Vladimir Kernig, Russian physician, in 19th century): Standing on the right side of the supine patient, flex the patient's hip to 90° and extend the knee passively. More than 135° knee extension should be possible. Positive Kernig sign is indicated by pain and limitation of extension to more than 90° at knee due to hamstring spasm **(Fig. 21.28)**. Kernig originally described this sign in the sitting posture of the patient.

Brudzinski sign: (1) On eliciting neck rigidity, involuntary flexion of hips and knees occurs—*neck sign* **(Fig. 21.29)**; (2) eliciting Kernig sign produces involuntary flexion of opposite knee. Brudzinski neck sign is more reliable than Kernig sign.

Tripod sign: Ask the patient to sit erect with lower limbs fully extended. The child is unable to sit erect and supports the trunk with extended upper limbs on bed, behind the trunk. Positive tripod sign indicates paraspinal muscle spasm.

Signs of meningeal irritation are produced by reflex muscle spasm due to the stretching of the spinal nerve roots with inflamed meninges. In infants since the intervertebral foramina are larger, this effect is not pronounced and these signs may not be evident in meningitis.

Examination of spine: Look for congenital deformities, defects, dimple, tuft of hair, swelling, tenderness, gibbus deformity, and pressure sores.

Other points to be remembered are examination of carotids, palpation of peripheral nerves, and observation for trophic ulcers, soft neurologic signs, and autonomic functions.

Soft Neurologic Signs

Soft neurologic signs are deviant performance on a motor or sensory test, abnormal beyond a particular age. Some of them are:

- Minimal choreoathetoid movements persisting beyond 8 yr of age.
- *Synkinetic (mirror) movements:* One side of the body mimics exactly an act performed by the other side. Ask the child to oppose the thumb and index repeatedly on one side. The other side does the same action. Persistence beyond 8 yr is abnormal.
- Associated unnecessary movements—while the patient does one act, other parts of the body make unnecessary movements like head movements, chewing, foot tapping, *etc.*

- Dysdiadochokinesia
- Finger agnosia is inability to name the fingers. Hold some fingers of the child (without the patient seeing). Ask how many are held.
- Stimulus extinction is inability to perceive a stimulus when simultaneously two are presented. The child (eyes closed) is touched on face and hand at the same time and is asked to point the areas. If only the facial stimulus is perceived, it is "rostral dominance". Persistence of stimulus extinction beyond 7 yr is abnormal.
- Lateral dominance—hand dominance should be established before 4 yr and eye dominance by 2 yr of age respectively. Delay in establishing clear dominance and mixed dominance are abnormal.
- Left right discrimination is the ability to name left and right and should be attained by 6 yr.

The persistence of two or more soft neurologic signs herald neurological dysfunctions like cerebral palsy, attention deficit disorder, learning disability, autism, etc.

Tests for Autonomic Dysfunction

The autonomic nervous system has sympathetic and parasympathetic divisions. It is concerned with cardiovascular, gastrointestinal, respiratory and temperature regulation, bowel and bladder control and sexual reflexes. Features of autonomic disorders are pupillary dysfunctions, postural hypotension, resting tachycardia, incontinence of urine, poor urine stream, impotence, constipation, fecal incontinence, gastro intestinal dysmotility, impaired sweating, snoring, and sleep apnea. Resting tachycardia is made out by the *Valsalva test*—the patient blows into a sphygmomanometer maintaining 40 mm of Hg pressure for 15 seconds. The ratio of the highest pulse rate in the preliminary test period to the lowest pulse rate during the test is >1.5 in normal subjects and <1.1 in patients with autonomic dysfunction.

ANALYSIS OF THE LESIONS OF NERVOUS SYSTEM

The following points for the neurologic lesion are to be analyzed at the completion of evaluation:

Is there a neurologic problem? Is it trivial or grave? Is it acute, subacute, or long standing? Is it recovering, progressing, remitting and relapsing or static? Which part of the nervous system is affected, e.g., UMN/LMN/combined/others? Where is the lesion? Can all the features be explained with a single lesion? What may be the pathological nature of the lesion? What is the probable etiology?

Salient Features of Lesions at Different Areas of the Brain

Lower motor neurons: Severe and early wasting, hypotonia and weakness, absent superficial and deep reflexes. Distribution of weakness depends on the site of lesion (motor neuron, nerve root, or peripheral nerve). Fibrillations and fasciculations may be observed.

Pyramidal lesions: Muscle wasting (mild to moderate) due to disuse in chronic patients. Spasticity and weakness of *cortical nature* (shoulder abduction, finger movements, hip flexion, and ankle dorsiflexion more affected) will be present. Abnormal gait (hemiplegic, scissoring), absent superficial reflexes, extensor plantar response, and exaggerated deep tendon reflexes are other features. *Babinski's rising up sign* is useful to distinguish spastic and hysterical paralysis. The patient in supine posture with extended legs is asked to rise up without the support of hands. In spastic paralysis, affected limb rises first which is not seen in hysterical paralysis.

Extrapyramidal involvement: The features are abnormal postures and various involuntary movements and rigidity.

Cerebellar lesions: Hypotonia, intention tremor, dysmetria, nystagmus, titubation, truncal ataxia, and pendular knee jerk are the diagnostic features. Wasting and weakness are insignificant.

Localization of Lesions in Nervous System Diseases

The salient features are:

Cerebral cortex: Altered sensorium of varying degrees, convulsions, contralateral paralysis (usually monoplegia, hemiplegia—not dense), cortical sensory loss, and aphasia

Frontal lobe: Weakness, disinhibition, incontinence, and appearance of grasp reflex

Temporal lobe: Complex hallucinations, dysphasia, and psychomotor seizures

Parietal lobe: Cortical sensory loss, dysphasia, and visual field defects

Occipital lobe lesions: Visual hallucinations and field defects

Subcortical: The differentiating features from cortical lesion are absence of convulsions and altered sensorium.

Internal capsule: Contralateral dense hemiplegia, sensory involvement if the posterior one-third of the posterior limb of the internal capsule is also affected, may also have homonymous hemianopia.

Thalamus: Contralateral sensory loss or hyperalgesia

Midbrain—upper level: Weber syndrome: Ipsilateral 3rd nerve palsy with contralateral hemiplegia. *Midbrain—lower level: Benedikt syndrome*: Ipsilateral 3rd nerve palsy with contralateral hypertonia, tremor, and ataxia due to involvement of red nucleus.

Pons: Millard-Gubler syndrome: Ipsilateral 6th and 7th nerve nuclear palsy with contralateral hemiplegia

Foville's syndrome: Ipsilateral 6th and 7th nerve palsy with contralateral hemiparesis

Medulla: Jackson syndrome: Ipsilateral 12th nerve palsy with contralateral hemiplegia. Varying combinations of vertigo, ataxia, nystagmus, ipsilateral facial anesthesia and intention tremor and contralateral loss of position and vibration sense may be present.

Wallenberg syndrome (lateral medullary syndrome): Ipsilateral loss of facial pain and temperature with preservation of light touch and corneal reflex. It is due to infarction of lateral medulla secondary to vertebral or posterior inferior cerebellar arterial occlusion.

Spinal Cord Lesions

Physiologically the spinal cord is made up of a series of superimposed segments with a pair of nerve roots arising from each segment. To locate the spinal segment, add 1 for cervical vertebrae, 2 for thoracic 1–6, and 3 for thoracic 7–9. 10th thoracic arch overlies lumbar 1st and 2nd, 11th thoracic over lumbar 3rd and 4th and first lumbar arch over sacral and coccygeal segments.

The common symptoms are back pain, gait disturbance, sphincter disturbances, and weakness depending upon the level of lesion. The type of myelopathy can be compressive or non-compressive.

Compressive Myelopathies

Extramedullary: Asymmetric weakness, root pain, complete sensory loss, late bladder involvement, trophic changes.

Intramedullary: Symmetrical weakness, early bladder involvement, trophic changes, descending pattern of sensory loss, LMN paralysis at the level of lesion.

Localization: In acute lesions of the spinal cord in the initial spinal shock stage (variable period from few days to few weeks), there is flaccid paralysis. Typical localizing signs appear after some days and will be present in slowly evolving lesions. See **Table 21.12** for the salient features of spinal cord lesions depending on the level of lesion. The causes of compressive myelopathy are trauma, tumors, caries spine, abscess, and hemorrhage. Noncompressive myelopathies are produced by demyelination, degeneration, toxic and nutritional factors. Combined picture of UMN, LMN, and root involvement is seen in spinal arachnoiditis.

Brown-Sequard syndrome is transection of the spinal cord revealing pyramidal weakness on the same side with spinothalamic sensory loss on the opposite side.

Anterior horn cell disease is characterized by gross wasting, flaccid weakness, loss of DTR, and preservation of sensations. Fasciculations may be observed, e.g., spinal muscular atrophy.

Radiculopathy (spinal root disease) reveals root pain, paresthesia, sensory dulling, and LMN weakness of mainly proximal muscles, e.g., Guillain-Barre syndrome.

Peripheral nerve disease is characterized by distal symmetrical LMN weakness and distal sensory loss or paresthesia (glove and stocking anesthesia).

TABLE 21.12: Localization of spinal cord lesions.

Segment	*Clinical features*	*Reflexes involved*
C3, C4	Spastic tetraplegia (upper limb more affected), diaphragm paralysis	
C5	Spastic tetraplegia	Loss of biceps jerk
C7	Spastic paraplegia	Loss of triceps jerk
C8 T1	Spastic paraplegia. Paralysis of flexion of hand and wrist	Upper limb DTR normal
T6	Spastic paraplegia. Intercostal paralysis	Loss of upper abdominal reflex
T9–T10	Spastic paraplegia	Upper abdominal reflex present. Loss of lower abdominal reflex
T12–L1	Spastic paraplegia	Abdominal reflexes present Loss of cremasteric reflex
L2, L3,	Spastic paraplegia	Loss of knee jerks
L4		Ankle jerks brisk
S1, S2	Paraplegia with flexion at hips and extension at knees, ankle dorsiflexion **(Fig. 15.16)**	Knee jerk normal Absent ankle jerk and plantar response
S3, S4	No paraplegia, retention of urine and feces	Loss of anal reflex Normal DTR

(DTR: deep tendon reflex)

Neuromuscular junction disease features are symmetrical predominantly proximal muscle weakness with diurnal variation and fatigability on exertion. Ptosis is characteristic. No change in muscle tone, DTR, and sensory capacity, e.g., myasthenia gravis.

Muscle diseases have symmetrical proximal muscle weakness. No sensory loss. Muscle wasting and loss of DTR are late, e.g., myopathies.

SUGGESTED READING

1. Brett EM. Pediatric Neurology, 1st edition. London: Churchill Livingstone; 1983.
2. Farmer TW. Paediatric Neurology, 3rd edition. Philadelphia: Harper & Row.; 1983.
3. Kliegman RM. The Nervous System. Nelson Textbook of Pediatrics, 21st edition. Amsterdam: Elsevier; 2019.
4. Menkes JH. Textbook of Child Neurology, 5th edition. Philadelphia: Lippincott Williams and Wilkins; 1995.
5. Paul VK, Bagga A. Ghai Essential Pediatrics, 10th edition. New Delhi: CBS Publications and Distributors Pvt Ltd.; 2024.
6. Richard SS. Clinical Neuroanatomy for Medical Students, 3rd edition. Philadelphia: Lippincott Williams and Wilkins; 1992.
7. Rodney WH, Walker NS, Glynn M, Drake WM. Hutchison's Clinical Methods, 24th edition. Amsterdam: Elsevier; 2018.
8. Russel ND. The Neurological Examination, 2nd edition. London: Pitman Medical Publishign Co. Ltd.; 1959.
9. Shikin K, Noda K, IkusalesM. Transient idiopathic isolated hypoglossal nerve palsy. J Gen Int Med. 2013;28:593.
10. Sondhi V, Patnaik SK. Unilateral palatal palsy. Indian Pediatr. 2011;48:237-8.
11. Spillane JA. Bickerstaff's Neurological Examination in Clinical Practice, 6th edition. Hoboken, New Jersey: Wiley-Blackwell; 1996.
12. Swaiman KF, Stephen A. Paediatric Neurology: Principles and Practice, 3rd edition. Maryland Heights: Mosby; 1999.

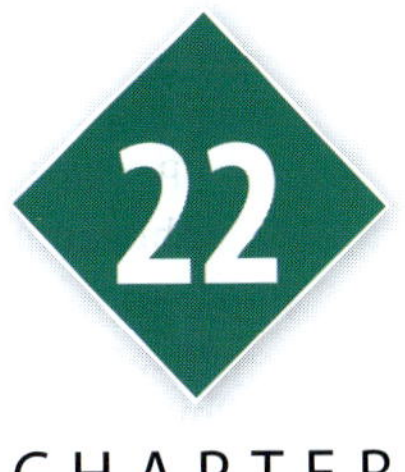

CHAPTER

Neurological and Neuromuscular Investigations in Children

Vaishakh Anand, KP Vinayan

Chapter Outline

- Introduction
- Cerebrospinal Fluid Studies
- Electroencephalogram
- Nerve Conduction Study
- Electromyography
- Evoked Potentials
- Polysomnography
- Neuroimaging
- Genetic Investigations

INTRODUCTION

Advanced investigations are increasingly established in neurology because of the complexity of the diseases encountered, the need for their early diagnosis to provide timely treatment to reduce death and disability, as well as for genetic counseling. These include cerebrospinal fluid (CSF) studies, electrophysiological methods to assess the functional integrity of the central and peripheral nervous systems, neuroimaging procedures to detect structural problems, and genetic processing. These investigations have helped neurologists to avoid many invasive and painful procedures.

As most children require sedation for procedures, parents/caretakers should be counseled about the diagnosis, need for the investigation as well as sedation and the problems following the investigation procedures (Ref. Ch. 3). If the child is of understandable age, a briefing of the procedure in a simple, nonthreatening way (using a dummy demonstration if available) need be given. Allowing the parent to be with the child in possible situations will be consoling. These will provide much cooperation from the patient and the parent. Written informed consent from the caretaker is a must before any procedure.

CEREBROSPINAL FLUID STUDIES

Lumbar puncture (LP) established for more than a century is a simple bedside procedure for CSF collection. The indications are diagnostic (meningitis, encephalitis, subarachnoid hemorrhage, Guillain-Barré syndrome, demyelinating and degenerative disorders, collagen vascular diseases, idiopathic intracranial hypertension, and metastatic leukemia) and therapeutic [intrathecal drug administration in leukemias and to relieve raised intracranial pressure (RICP)] purposes. The contraindications are Glasgow coma scale (GCS) <8, RICP with neurologic deficit, infections over the puncture site and bleeding tendency (LP can be done after correction of bleeding).

Procedure

Stabilize the patient prior to LP, if sick (adequate hydration; airway, breathing and circulation support). Place the child on a wooden couch in the left lateral decubitus

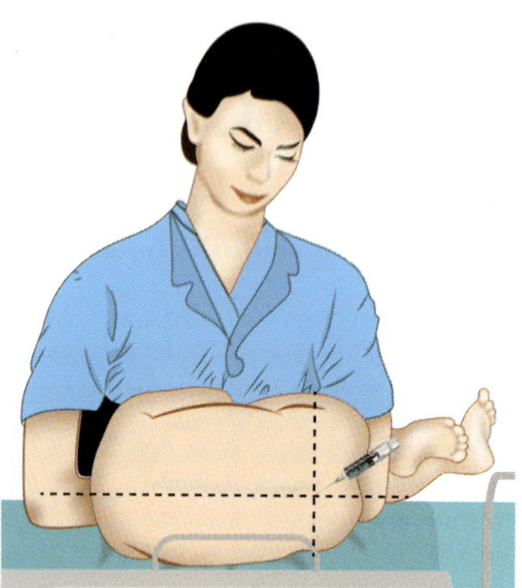

Fig. 22.1: Preparing the child for LP. (LP: lumbar puncture)

position (can be sitting also). A competent assistant should hold the child to bring the spine near the edge of the couch. Keeping the child's hands between the knees flex the knees toward the chest. The assistant should hold the child with one hand at the buttocks so as to bend the back. With the other hand, flex the neck of the child to the chest (the airway should not be compromised). The performer should scrub the hands and wear sterile gloves. Locate the space between the 3rd and 4th lumbar (L3-L4 space) vertebrae (L3 is at the junction of the line from the highest point of the iliac crests passing through the vertebral column) **(Fig. 22.1)**.

Clean the area with povidone iodine followed by alcohol from the located puncture site toward the periphery up to 10 cm, sponging in widening circles. Drape the area with a sterile towel; infiltrate 1% lignocaine into the skin and soft tissues for local anesthesia (topical application of EMLA 30 min prior to LP is the noninvasive local anesthesia advised). Select the LP needle with stylet (22G for young and 20G for older child). Insert the needle at the middle of the intervertebral space at 90°, aiming toward the umbilicus and advance it with uniform force. Sudden decrease in resistance indicates the puncture of dura. The stylet can be withdrawn now and the CSF will come out as clear drops. Document the pressure and color of the CSF. Collect four samples of 0.5–1 mL CSF in four separate sterile containers, one each for culture, biochemistry, preservation for later analysis, and the last sample for cell count. The specimen should reach the concerned laboratories within 30 min. Withdraw the needle quickly after reinserting the stylet. Press over the puncture site for 30 sec and seal the area with sterile dressing. Keep the child in prone position for 2 hr to avoid post-LP headache. Rare complications encountered are post-LP headache, low back pain, iatrogenic infections, and brainstem herniation in symptomatic RICP.

ELECTROENCEPHALOGRAM

Electroencephalogram (EEG) measures the electrical activity from the cerebral cortex by recording the amplified potential differences between electrodes placed on the scalp (scalp EEG), or cortex (subdural electrodes), or within the brain (depth electrodes). These field potentials are generated by the excitatory and inhibitory postsynaptic potentials at the dendrites of pyramidal cells in the cortex and are recorded extracellularly, but do not record single neuronal activity, glial cell activity, or subcortical structures. Standard 10-20 system is used to place electrodes on the scalp along the line connecting nasion with inion in the sagittal plane and the line connecting preauricular points in the coronal plane. Though EEG is inevitable in the management of epilepsy, a normal EEG does not rule out epilepsy. A standard EEG recording should include a minimum of 20 min.

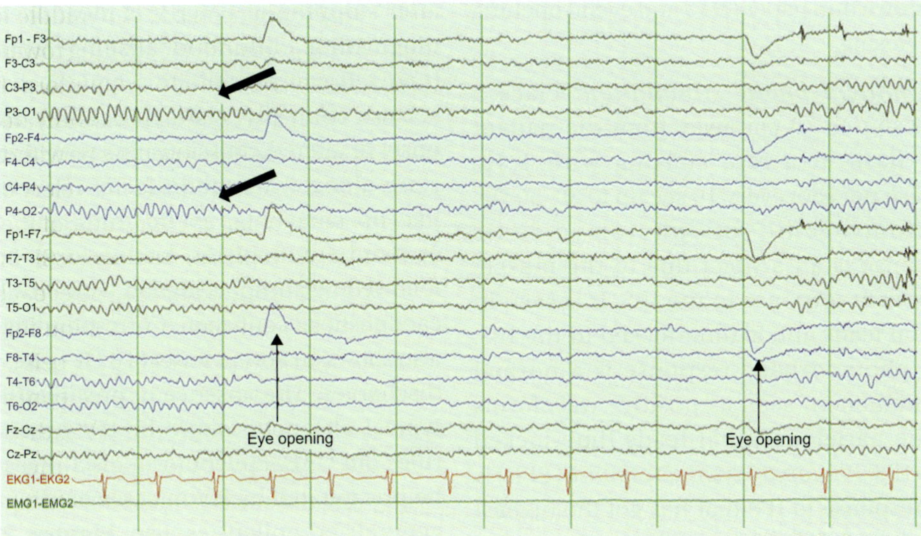

Fig. 22.2A: Normal awake EEG of a 12 yr old boy showing posterior alpha rhythm of 9 Hz (block arrows). Alpha attenuation and accentuation with eye opening and closing is seen. (EEG: electroencephalogram)

Indications for EEG are: (1) first unprovoked seizure, (2) seizure like movements, (3) to evaluate the risk of recurrence after withdrawal of treatment in a well-controlled epilepsy, (4) in status epilepticus management during general anesthesia, (5) suspected nonconvulsive status epilepticus (NCSE), (6) syncope without definite cardiac or vascular cause, (7) unexplained encephalopathy, cognitive and behavior decline, and (8) suspected brain death. **Figure 22.2A** reveals a normal EEG.

Video-EEG is simultaneous recording of the video of the patient along with the EEG. It differentiates a paroxysmal nonepileptic event (PNEE) from true seizures and ictal localization of seizures delineating the epileptogenic zone in the presurgical evaluation for epilepsy surgery.

Montages

The orderly arrangement of different electrodes on the scalp is known as a montage, classified as bipolar or referential. In a *bipolar montage (BM)*, the potential difference between adjacent electrodes is amplified to form a channel depicted by a line in EEG (e.g., : Fp1-F3). In *referential montage*, the potential difference between a particular electrode and a common referential electrode is used. The reference electrodes commonly are the ipsilateral ear (e.g., : Fp1-A1), contralateral ear (e.g., : Fp1-A2), cz electrode (e.g., : Fp1-Cz), and common average reference (e.g.: Fp1-Avg). *BM* detects focal epileptiform activity by locating the leads showing reversal of polarity. As per the sequence of the connection of electrodes, the montages can be longitudinal, transverse, or circular.

Activation Procedures

Activation procedures are employed during routine EEG recording to increase the diagnostic yield—as intermittent photic stimulation *(IPS)*, sleep deprivation, hyperventilation by asking the patient to blow on a thin paper *(HV)* and eyelid opening and closing.

Intermittent photic stimulation: Place a light source 30 cm away from the patient and flash at a rate starting with 1 Hz (1 flash per sec) every 10 sec up to 30–50 Hz. Photomyogenic or photomyoclonic response is an artifact due to the muscle activity in response to the IPS. It is seen in frontal leads and is time-locked to the IPS. The photic driving response is a normal phenomenon, seen as positive waveforms in the parietooccipital leads time-locked with IPS. *Photoparoxysmal response* (PPR) is the response to IPS that has got the highest correlation with clinical epilepsy. It consists of generalized or posterior predominant spike-wave or polyspike discharges which may outlast the stimulus. The discharge does not start with the first flash of light and the frequency of the discharge is not time-locked to the IPS. Identification of PPR during EEG recording is an indication for stopping IPS since prolonged stimulation may precipitate a clinical seizure. PPR is most commonly associated with progressive myoclonic epilepsy *(PME)* followed by generalized epilepsies such as juvenile myoclonic epilepsy *(JME),* juvenile absence epilepsy *(JAE),* and idiopathic generalized epilepsy *(IGE).*

Hyperventilation (HV): The patient is asked to breathe regularly and deep at a rate of 20–30/min for 3–4 min. The most dramatic EEG changes following HV are seen in children between 8 and 12 yr; become less prominent with advancing age. Diffuse slowing occurs initially followed by high amplitude delta activity known as hyperventilation-induced high amplitude rhythmic slowing (HIHARS) which may persist up to 1 min after stopping of HV. HV is most useful in diagnosing childhood absence epilepsy (CAE). It can precipitate a typical absence seizure clinically, characterized by abrupt onset of altered consciousness with a vacant stare along with subtle facial movements like lip smacking, eyelid fluttering, and/or hand automatisms, lasting for 4–20 sec followed by abrupt cessation with no significant postictal confusion. Corresponding EEG also shows an abrupt onset of 3 Hz spike-wave discharges. The absence of precipitation of typical absence seizure by HV practically rules out CAE. Epileptiform discharges may be precipitated by HV in cases of idiopathic generalized epilepsies also. **Figures 22.2B to D** reveal EEG in various types of seizure disorders.

NORMAL SLEEP

Sleep activity in children may be composed of high-voltage waves with a spiky appearance, mistakenly giving the impression of epileptiform activity to inexperienced eyes. Vertex waves start appearing during stage 1 NREM. They are frontocentrally located and are diphasic with an initial negative wave (revealed as upward deflection) followed by a positive wave which starts appearing by 3–5 m of age. Sleep spindles consist of spindle-like waves with a frequency of 10–12 Hz. They define stage 2 sleep and are not consistently present before the age of 2–3 m. K-complexes are also seen during stage 2 sleep, are large triphasic waves with fast, slow, and fast components and are consistently seen after the age of 18 m.

Ontogeny of sleep: Preterm EEG reveals discontinuity (brief high amplitude slow waves interspersed with longer discontinuous periods of low voltage activity)

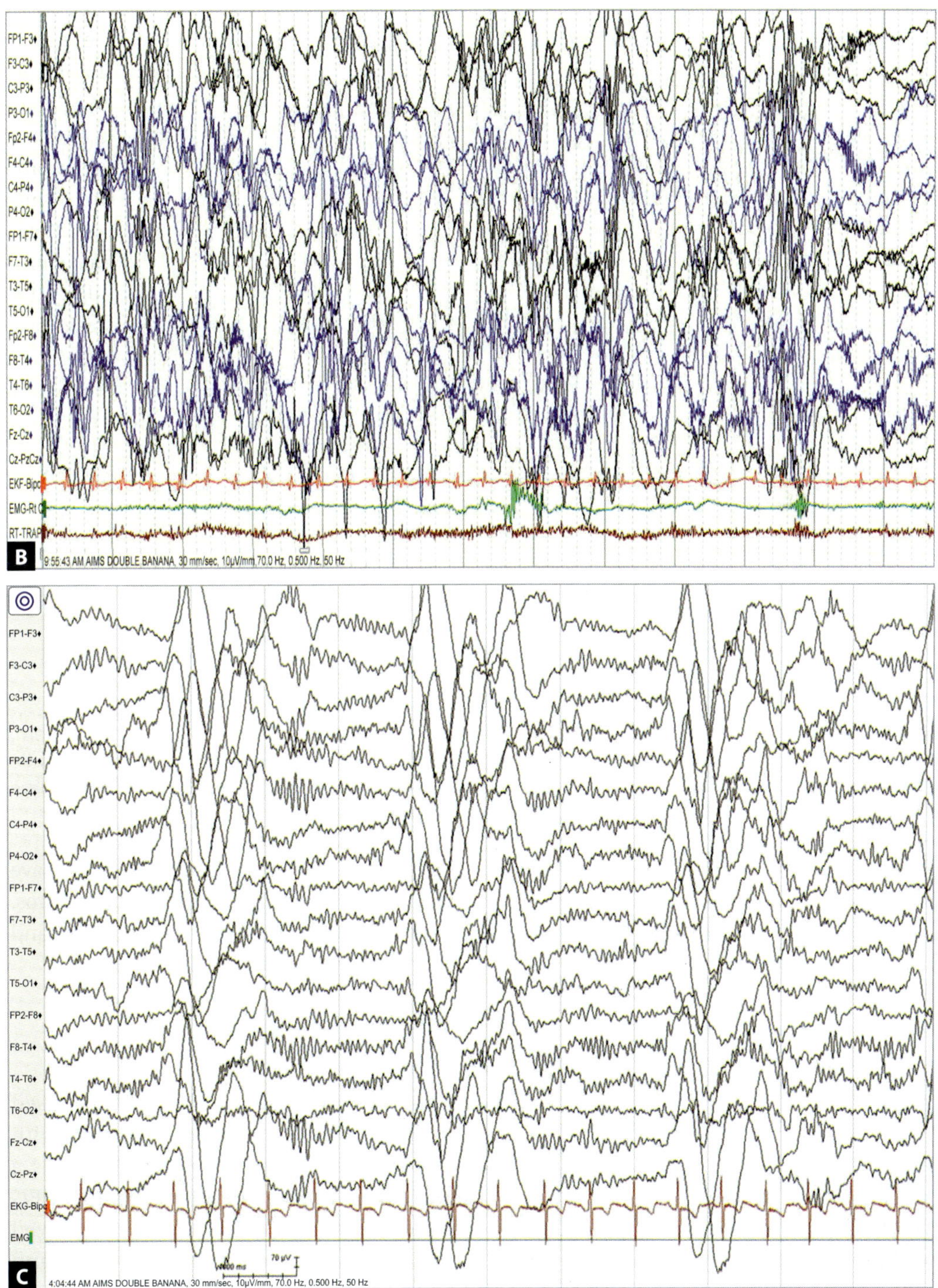

Figs. 22.2B and C

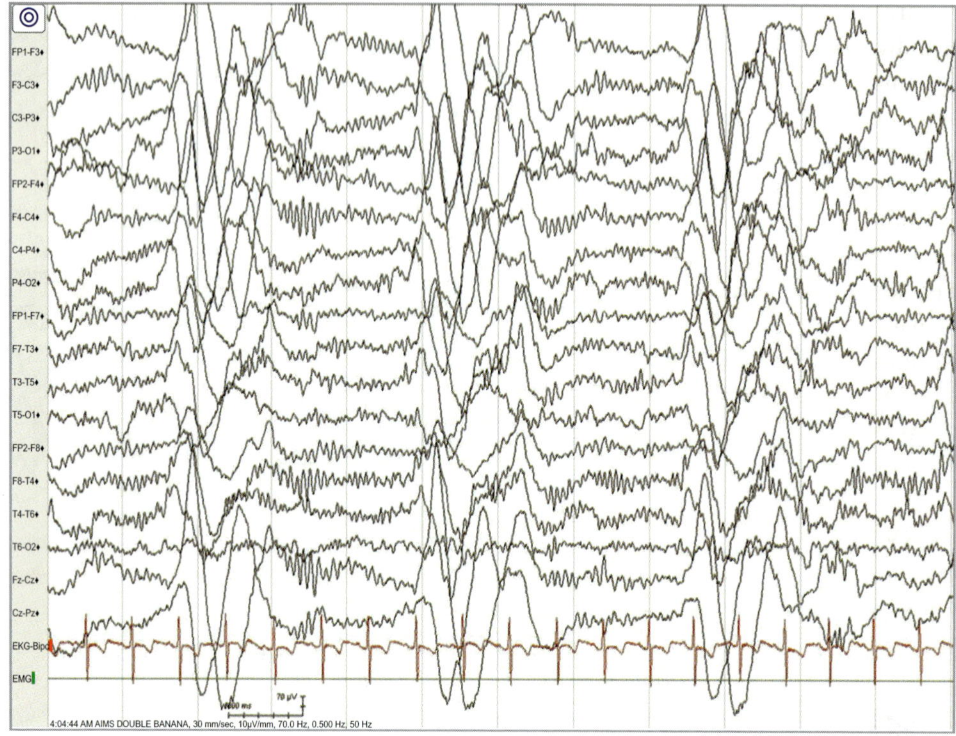

Fig. 22.2D

Figs. 22.2B to D: (B) EEG of a 6 m old baby with infantile spasms showing hypsarrhythmia pattern; (C) EEG of an 8 yr old girl with subacute sclerosing panencephalitis (SSPE) showing periodic large amplitude slow wave discharges; (D) EEG of a 7 yr old girl showing abrupt onset of generalized 3-Hz spike and wave discharges during a typical absence seizure. (EEG: electroencephalogram)

which decreases as the brain matures and becomes continuous by the age of 2 m. The first EEG pattern to differentiate between sleep and awake state is Tracé discontinu (TD), between 30 and 34 wk of gestational age. From a wakeful state, transition to active sleep followed by quiet sleep occurs. Mature adult sequence of wakefulness-quiet sleep-active sleep occurs by the age of 3 m.

Abnormal Patterns

The EEG patterns, consistently associated with seizure disorders, are referred to as epileptiform. A sharp wave is surface negative with a duration between 70 and 200 ms. A spike is sharper with a lesser duration (20–70 ms). A slow wave may follow a spike or sharp wave and have a duration between 200 and 1000 ms. **Figures 22.2A to D** reveal normal awake and few characteristic abnormal EEG patterns.

Amplitude-integrated Electroencephalogram

Amplitude-integrated EEG (aEEG) is used in NICUs where a conventional EEG with multiple leads may not be feasible. It is a simplified version of conventional EEG and correlates well with it. aEEG is derived from raw EEG which is filtered (<2 Hz and >15 Hz filtered), rectified, smoothened, time-compressed (6 cm/hr), and plotted semilogarithmically. Three aspects of aEEG are utilized clinically—background, electrophysiological maturity, and behavioral states including sleep and seizures. The upper margin of the aEEG bandwidth is the peak-to-peak amplitude of the EEG bursts and the lower margin is the peak-to-peak amplitude of the interburst EEG period. Normal term neonates have a voltage of >10 μV for the upper margin and >5 μV for the lower margin. A seizure is represented by elevation of both upper and lower margins and thereby a narrow bandwidth. The band width in sleep is broad due to the lowering of the lower margin.

NERVE CONDUCTION STUDY

Nerve conduction study (NCS) is stimulating peripherally accessible nerves with small amounts of currents and recording the velocity and amplitude of action potentials with electrodes placed over distal muscles. Poor patient cooperation and age-dependent normative data make NCS difficult in pediatrics. The study aids in the diagnosis and characterization of peripheral neuropathy, radiculopathy, and neuromuscular junction disorders **(Fig. 22.3)**.

Indications are to differentiate: (1) primary nerve disease from muscle disease, (2) axonal neuropathy from demyelinating neuropathy, (3) polyneuropathy from mononeuropathy multiplex, (4) to diagnose sensory, motor, and mixed peripheral neuropathy, and (5) to determine the site of injury in traumatic neuropathy.

For motor responses, place the stimulator first distally over the nerve and then proximally. The active recording electrode is placed over the belly of the muscle being

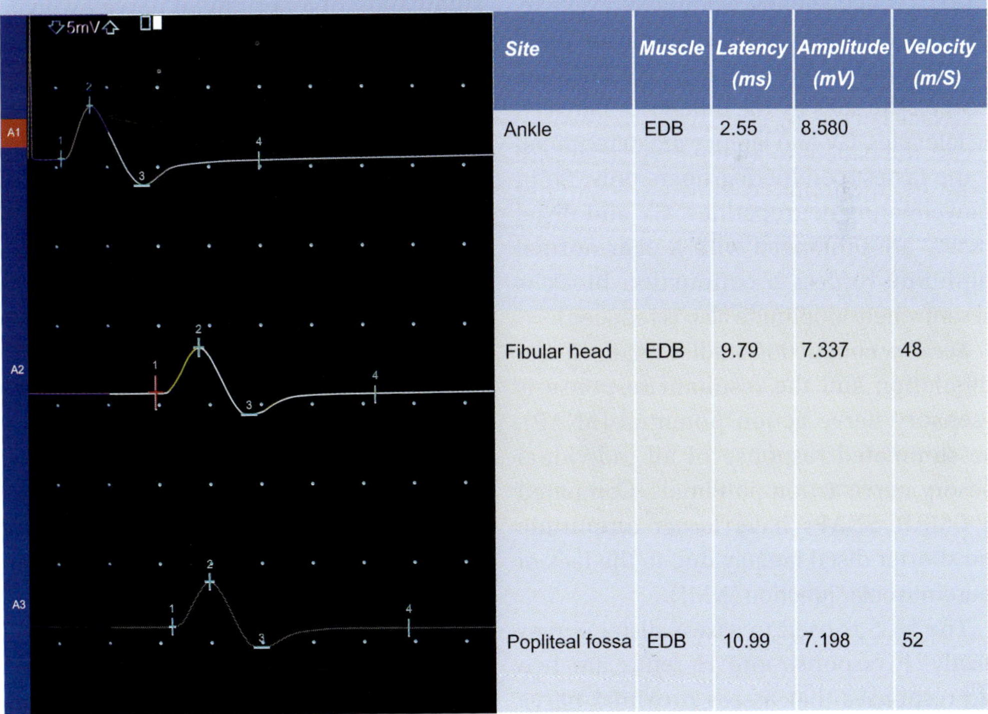

Site	Muscle	Latency (ms)	Amplitude (mV)	Velocity (m/S)
Ankle	EDB	2.55	8.580	
Fibular head	EDB	9.79	7.337	48
Popliteal fossa	EDB	10.99	7.198	52

Fig. 22.3: Normal nerve conduction study in the peroneal nerve of a 12 yr old boy. (EDB: extensor digitorum brevis)

recorded and the reference electrode distally over the tendon. The recorded potential is the compound muscle action potential (CMAP), representing the summated APs of all muscle fibers. CMAP is a biphasic potential with an initial negative phase followed by a positive phase (i.e., upward first and then downward). The amplitude of the CMAP is measured from baseline to negative peak and is contributed by all muscle fibers. Low CMAP amplitude indicates axonal loss, characteristic of axonal neuropathy. Other causes of low amplitude CMAP are a conduction block typical of an acquired demyelinating neuropathy, e.g., acute inflammatory demyelinating polyneuropathy (AIDP), chronic inflammatory demyelinating polyneuropathy (CIDP), presynaptic congenital myasthenic syndromes, and severe myopathies. The time lag from stimulus to the initial deflection of CMAP is called latency. Conduction velocity (CV) is calculated by stimulating proximal and distal sites and dividing the distance between the sites by the difference between the latencies. CV and latency are determined by the fastest conducting fibers only. So in demyelinating neuropathies, CV and distal latency are prolonged with a near-normal amplitude (unless a conduction block is present where amplitude also is reduced).

Sensory conduction studies require lesser stimulation and the resultant response is a sensory nerve action potential (SNAP), the summated response of all individual sensory nerve action potentials. Compared to CMAP, SNAPs have lesser amplitude and shorter distal latency due to the lack of neuromuscular junction (NMJ).

The NCS is used to assess distal nerves mostly. F response and H reflex are two late responses that assess proximal nerve conduction. During nerve stimulation, conduction occurs in both directions, distally and proximally. While the distal conduction traverses crossing NMJ and stimulates the muscle, some amount of conduction occurs antidromically toward anterior horn cells in the spinal cord. This leads to the backfiring of a few anterior horn cells (AHC) which again travels orthodromically toward the muscle and creates a small CMAP after the CMAP created by the direct stimulation and is called F-response. This represents only 1–5% of the nerve fibers but assesses the proximal parts including the motor radical. In early GBS where only radicals are involved or suspected cases of motor radiculopathy, F-waves are either absent or F-estimate is prolonged. H-reflex is the electrical correlate of ankle reflex and is abnormal in S1 radiculopathy.

Repeated Nerve Stimulation Test

Repeated nerve stimulation test (RNST) is stimulation of a peripheral nerve by giving back-to-back stimulation at low frequency (3 Hz), high frequency (50 Hz), after prolonged exercise, after short exercise, with cooling, warming, etc. and the decrement or increment in the amplitude of each CMAP is compared with the first CMAP. RNST when performed at 3 Hz, the initial response is a decrease in amplitude till 3rd or 4th stimuli (never >10% of the amplitude of the first CMAP) followed by gradual increase. In myasthenia gravis, a postsynaptic neuromuscular junction abnormality, the decrement will be >10%. While doing RNST, proper technical factors should be observed. Improper immobilization, not giving supramaximal stimuli and temperature variations may produce spurious results.

ELECTROMYOGRAPHY

Electromyography (EMG) involves inserting an EMG needle into a muscle (any skeletal muscle can be tested) and assessing the electrical activity during the insertion, at rest, and after activation. The time of injury, severity, and the extent of renervation in nerve injuries can be assessed. EMG assesses spontaneous activity at rest and motor unit action potentials (MUAP) during action.

Normal muscle is silent at rest; muscle pathologies produce different types of spontaneous activities. Fibrillation potentials are the most common, revealing active denervation and spontaneous depolarization of single muscle fibers, appear 2–6 wk after the nerve injury, depending on the severity of the injury and the distance of the muscle from the site of injury. It may occur in inflammatory myositis and NMJ disorders also. They are identified by the regularity and the characteristic "rain on tin roof" sound in the loudspeaker. Positive sharp waves are also commonly associated with fibrillation potentials and have the same clinical significance. Myotonic discharges are spontaneous discharges from single muscle fibers with a characteristic waxing and waning amplitude leading to a peculiar "revving engine" sound. They are associated with myotonic dystrophy, Schwartz-Jampel syndrome, myotonia congenita, and paramyotonia congenita. Fasciculation potentials are markers of AHC injury. In contrast to fibrillation potentials which arise from muscle fibers, fasciculation potentials originate from the motor unit and have the morphology of normal MUAP produced during voluntary muscle activation. They differ from normal MUAP by their low frequency (usually less than 2–3 Hz) and irregularity whereas voluntary contractions start with a frequency of 4–5 Hz.

Analysis of MUAP is done by asking the patient to contract the muscle voluntarily. An MUAP represents a single motor unit which is defined as a motor neuron with its axon, its NMJ, and all the muscle fibers supplied by it. Normal MUAP duration is 5–15 ms. MUAP duration prolongs with an increase in the number of muscle fibers and with age; prolonged duration suggests renervation following chronic denervation. The number of phases of MUAP is a measure of synchrony with which fibers within a motor unit contract. Normally 2–4 phases are present in the MUAP. Polyphasic MUAPs indicate renervation following long-standing denervation. The normal amplitude of MUAP ranges from 100 μV to 2 mV. In contrast to the duration of MUAP which is a collective of all fibers of that motor unit, amplitude reflects only the fibers which are closest to the EMG needle.

During voluntary muscle contraction, the force of contraction can be increased by increasing the firing frequency of the motor unit from 4–5 Hz to a maximum of 30–50 Hz called activation, a centrally mediated process and recruiting other motor units (peripheral nerve process). Normally both processes participate in an orderly manner (5:1) to increase the force gradually. Interference pattern in EMG at maximal muscle contraction will be showing multiple MUAPs which overlap and cannot be identified singly. Incomplete interference patterns may be due to poor activation by central nervous system (CNS) lesion or due to poor recruitment because of a nerve lesion. Incomplete interference due to neuropathic lesions are characterized by MUAPs showing polyphasia, high amplitude, and prolonged duration. Myopathic lesions are characterized by early recruitment with small amplitude MUAPs.

EVOKED POTENTIALS

Evoked potentials (EPs) are electrographic responses to various sensory stimuli; three EPs are routinely performed—visual evoked potential (VEP), brainstem auditory evoked potential (BAEP), and somatosensory evoked potential (SSEP).

Visual Evoked Potential

Visual evoked potential assesses the functional integrity of the visual pathway from the retina to the occipital cortex. It helps to diagnose prechiasmatic lesions which are difficult to visualize by neuroimaging. Pattern reversal VEP (PRVEP) using a checkerboard as a visual stimulus is the most common method requiring much patient cooperation. In children, flash VEP (FVEP) is done using strobe light or LED goggles. The most important waveform identified in PRVEP is a positive polarity wave at approximately 100 ms latency called P100. Parameters assessed are the latency, amplitude, morphology, and topography of P100, latency being the most useful. A unilaterally prolonged latency indicates a prechiasmatic lesion on that side like optic neuritis. In FVEP, a prominent positive peak occurs between 50 and 100 ms, termed as P1. Since the latency and amplitude of P1 vary widely between patients, FVEP is interpreted only as P1 response present or absent. P1 response in FVEP and P100 in PRVEP are demonstrable by 6–8 m of age.

Brainstem Auditory Evoked Potentials

Brainstem auditory evoked potential consists of waveforms arising from the auditory nerve and brainstem within 10 ms of acoustic stimulation. Five waveforms are commonly assessed for clinical purposes with their generators provided in **Table 22.1**. Out of this, wave I, III, and V are obligate waveforms which mean that their absence indicates an audiological or neurological abnormality. Wave V is the most significant and persistent wave and occurs about 5.5 ms after the stimulation. Absolute latencies of waves I, II, III, and interpeak latency (IPL) of waves I-III, III-V, and I-V are assessed **(Fig. 22.4)**. Prolongation of the absolute latency of wave indicates an abnormal peripheral auditory pathway up to the distal auditory nerve. Wave I-III IPL measures the lower brainstem pathway from the distal auditory nerve and cochlear nuclei in the rostral medulla till the superior olivary complex in the pons. Wave III-V IPL measures the upper brainstem pathway from the superior olivary complex to the inferior colliculus in the midbrain.

TABLE 22.1: Origin of BAEP waveforms.

Waveform	*Localization*
I	Distal auditory nerve
II	Dorsal and ventral cochlear nucleus
III	Superior olivary complex
IV	Lateral lemniscus
V	Inferior colliculus

(BAEP: brainstem auditory evoked potential)

Brainstem auditory evoked potential is preferably done in sleep/mild sedation and can be used to evaluate brainstem function and hearing evaluation in young children; can be used as a screening tool for hearing in neonates. Waves I, III, and V are demonstrable in normal term neonates but with half the amplitude of adult values which is achieved by 2 yr of age. Other indications for BAEP in childhood are to assess hearing loss after meningitis, in demyelinating disorders like multiple sclerosis (MS) and neuromyelitis optica spectrum disorder (NMOSD); in dysmyelinating leukodystrophies like Krabbe disease, metachromatic leukodystrophy (MLD), and adrenoleukodystrophy (ALD); different types of coma and brain death.

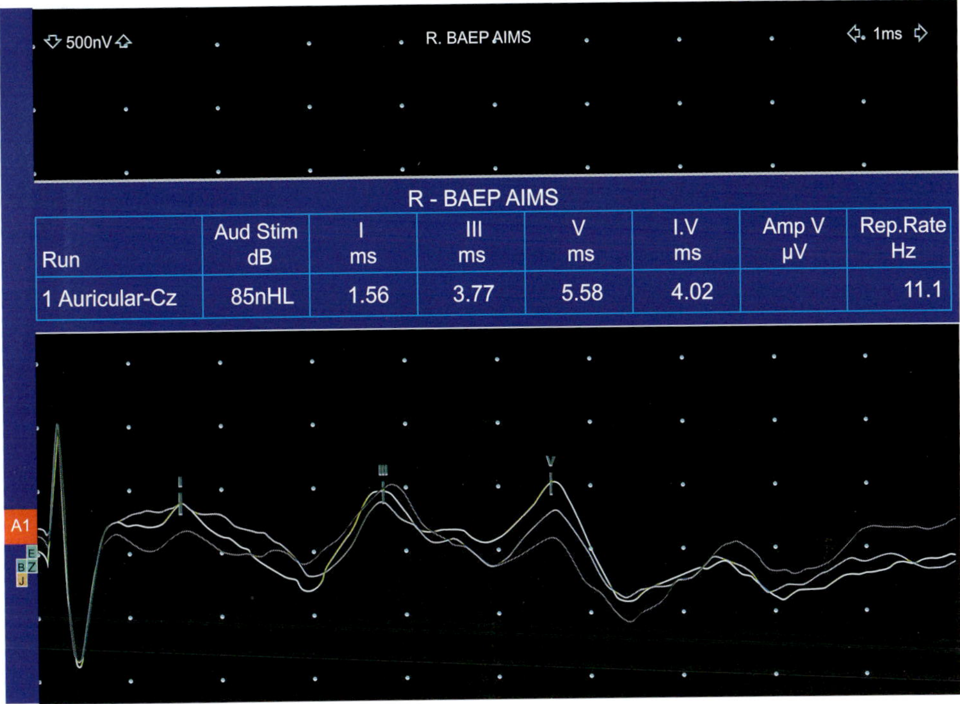

Fig. 22.4: Normal BAEP in a 14 yr old girl. (BAEP: brainstem auditory evoked potential)

Somatosensory Evoked Potential

Somatosensory evoked potential is obtained by electrical stimulation of peripheral nerves. The electrically induced sensory impulse travels from the peripheral nerve to the brachial plexus, dorsal column, spinal cord, brainstem, and somatosensory cortex and is useful to assess the dorsal column function. Different waveforms are recorded from various points of this ascending pathway. The median and ulnar nerves of upper limbs and tibial nerve of lower limbs are the sites used routinely for SSEP. Various waveforms are named according to the polarity and latency after stimulation, e.g., N30 is a negative potential occurring 30 ms after median nerve stimulation and is generated from the somatosensory cortex. The presence of various waveforms, their absolute latencies, and inter-peak latency (IPL) are assessed for abnormalities. The test is useful to determine the outcome of hypoxic-ischemic encephalopathy, in which an absent N20 waveform denotes poor prognosis. Other clinical indications are demyelinating disorders, dysmyelinating disorders like Krabbe disease, MLD, ALD, and Pelizaeus-Merzbacher disease (PMD).

POLYSOMNOGRAPHY

Overnight polysomnography (PSG) is the gold standard investigation for diagnosing sleep disorders such as parasomnias, sleep-related breathing disorders, narcolepsy, and excessive daytime sleepiness. It is a multiparametric study assessing various biophysiological changes occurring during sleep. The parameters monitored and recorded include sleep stages using EEG, tone assessment with chin and leg EMG, eye movements by electro-oculogram (EOG), ECG waveform, snoring, continuous airflow via thermistor and nasal pressure transducer, chest and abdominal effort, oxygen saturation, body position through a position sensor, and video monitoring.

Indications

- *Suspected obstructive sleep apnea (OSA):* OSA is diagnosed by the cessation of airflow in the nasal thermistor/nasal pressure transducer for at least 10 sec in the presence of breathing efforts detected by the chest and abdominal belts. Central apnea is the presence of airflow cessation in the absence of breathing efforts. A mixed apnea begins as central apnea and toward the end has some breathing efforts.
- *Narcolepsy* is diagnosed in the presence of daily periods of excessive and irrepressible need to sleep along with episodes of cataplexy, PSG criteria, and low levels of CSF hypocretin. PSG criteria are sleep latency of <8 min in MSLT (multiple sleep latency test: 5 naps are recorded for 20 min, each every 2 hr and mean sleep latency, i.e., mean time from lights out to NREM1 stage is calculated) and >2 SOREMPs (sleep-onset REM periods: time from sleep onset to REM stage <15 min).
- *Others:* Excessive daytime sleepiness, insomnia, parasomnias and sleep-related hypermotor epilepsy (SHE)/nocturnal frontal lobe epilepsy (NFLE).

NEUROIMAGING

Skull Radiography (Ref. Ch. 26)

- *Neurosonogram (NSG):* This is the most frequently utilized neuroimaging technique in the pre- and perinatal periods. Inability to assess the posterior fossa structures and cerebral convexities as well as observer dependency are the shortcomings.
- *Computed tomography (CT):* Easy availability, lower cost, and quick acquisition are the merits, the disadvantage is radiation hazard. Air, fat (myelin), and liquid (CSF) attenuate the CT radiation very less which appear as hypodense dark areas. Bone, calcification, and fresh bleeds appear as hyperdense or bright images. Indications are acute cerebral hemorrhage, traumatic brain injury, temporal bone evaluation, detection of calcifications, and craniosynostosis. Contrast-enhanced CT (CECT) helps to diagnose suspected infectious, vascular, or neoplastic etiologies. ALARA ("as low as reasonably achievable") principle is used in children to limit the radiation exposure.
- *Magnetic resonance imaging (MRI)* provides multiplanar imaging of the brain with good resolution without radiation hazard. Radiofrequency pulses are sent to the patient lying in a magnetic field to create images. As per the differences in time to echo (TE) and time for relaxation (TR), two types of images are generated. T1-weighted image (T1W) with a short TE and short TR and T2-weighted image (T2W) with a long TE and long TR are obtained. After myelination is completed by 2 yr of age, white matter appears hyperintense (white) and gray matter as gray in T1W. The pathological changes appear hypointense (dark) or isointense in T1W, except fat, subacute hemorrhage, melanin, and contrast material (all appear hyperintense or bright) in T1W. Structural malformations and focal cortical dysplasia (FCD) are readily visualized in T1W. Postcontrast T1W shows enhancement

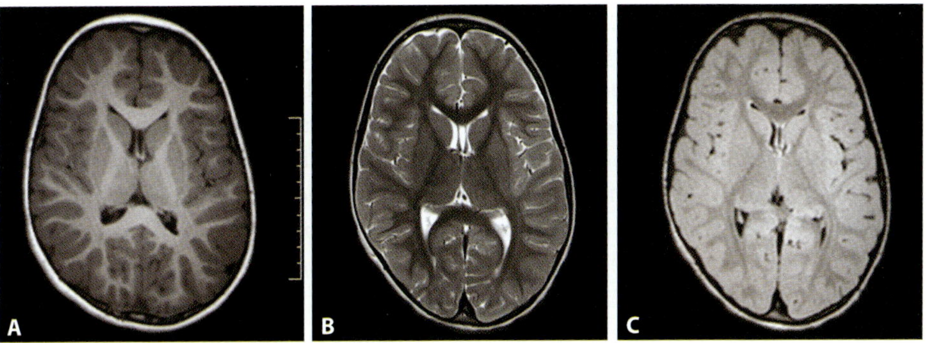

Figs. 22.5A to C: Normal MRI of a 3 yr old boy. (A) Axial T1-weighted image; (B) Axial T2-weighted image; (C) Axial T2 FLAIR image.

in infections, demyelination, and tumors because of the breach in the blood–brain barrier. In T2W images, after 2 yr of age, white matter appears dark and gray matter as gray. Most pathologies like demyelination, dysmyelination, edema, infarct, and bleed appear hyperintense on T2W. Since CSF also is hyperintense on T2W, periventricular pathologies may be difficult to visualize. Fluid-attenuated inversion recovery (T2 FLAIR) sequences suppress the CSF signals so that CSF also appears dark making the detection of hyperintensities in other areas more easy **(Figs. 22.5A to C)**.

Gradient-recalled echo (GRE) sequence detects paramagnetic substances such as iron and calcium and is useful in bleeding and calcifications. Susceptibility-weighted imaging (SWI) also detects iron and calcium as areas of hypointensities (called blooming) but delineates microbleeds more efficiently than GRE sequences and is useful in diffuse axonal injury (DAI) in traumatic brain injury. Diffusion-weighted imaging (DWI) measures the diffusion of water through tissues. In cases of infarcts, HIE, abscesses, acute demyelination and highly cellular tumors, the restriction of diffusion of water molecules due to intracellular cytotoxic edema reveals hyperintense lesions. DWI is superior in suspected stroke, where acute infarct is visible as an area of diffusion restriction within an hr of insult and before the changes appear in conventional T1W and T2W images.

- *Magnetic resonance angiography (MRA)* is used to assess the cerebral blood vessels. It can be done using flow-dependent techniques (e.g., TOF—time of flight) or phase contrast (PC). MR arteriography is used in stroke, arteriovenous malformations, aneurysms, and Moyamoya disease. MR venography is done in suspected cases of cerebral sinus venous thrombosis (CSVT) or cortical venous thrombosis.
- *Proton magnetic resonance spectroscopy (proton MRS/1H-MRS)* detects and quantifies certain brain metabolites. N-acetylaspartate (NAA) is a neuronal marker and is detected as a peak at 2.0 ppm. Its level is increased in Canavan disease due to the deficiency of aspartoacylase which promotes the breakdown of NAA. Creatine (Cr) is a marker of brain energy metabolism and its peak is detected at 3.0 ppm. The absence of Cr peak is characteristic of

cerebral creatine deficiency. The response to creatine supplementation can be assessed by demonstrating the restoration of Cr-peak. Choline (Ch), a marker of cell membrane disruption, is detected at 3.2 ppm and is high in increased cell turnover like tumors, leukodystrophies, and demyelination. Lactate is detected as an inverted doublet peak at 1.3 ppm indicating anaerobic metabolism or mitochondrial dysfunction. MRS can differentiate tumor recurrence from postradiation necrosis since the latter shows low NAA, Cr, and Ch peaks.

- *Functional MRI (fMRI)* is used to study regional brain activity in response to sensory, motor, or cognitive stimulation. The assumption is that while a task is performed, the corresponding cortical area is stimulated which leads to an increase in glucose metabolism and blood flow locally. This produces a small change in the local MRI signal and is called the BOLD (blood oxygenation level dependent) effect. In pediatrics, fMRI is used mainly for cortical mapping before epilepsy surgery or tumor removal.

  Absolute contraindications for MRI include metallic and electronic implantations like cardiac pacemakers, cochlear implants, metallic stents, aneurysm clips, and orthopedic implants.
- *Positron emission tomography (PET)* is a functional imaging modality that uses positron emitting radioisotopes labeled biomolecules. The most commonly used compound in PET is fluorodeoxyglucose (FDG-PET) which can map glucose metabolism in the brain. The images obtained are fused with corresponding CT (PET-CT) or MRI (PET-MRI) so that the anatomical areas with increased or decreased metabolism are clear. FDG-PET is commonly used in focal seizures when MRI images do not find any obvious focal lesion and in brain tumors to differentiate between residual tumor and tumor recurrence after radiation necrosis.
- *Single-photon emission computed tomography (SPECT)* is most commonly used in epilepsy surgery workup. It is based on the observation that in the epileptogenic zone, there is hyperperfusion during a seizure whereas the blood flow and metabolism are low interictally. The radioisotope should be injected within sec of seizure onset for proper ictal SPECT images. The interictal images then are digitally subtracted from ictal images and then coregistered on MRI using software support. This provides a three-dimensional anatomical localization of the epileptogenic zone.

GENETIC INVESTIGATIONS

Karyotyping detects aneuploidies (numerical abnormalities—trisomy and monosomy), aberrant chromosomes, ring chromosomes, balanced translocations, large deletions, and duplications of more than 5 Mb size.

Gene Sequencing

The human genome possesses around 20,000 genes out of which >80% are expressed in the brain. Though costly, molecular diagnostic facilities are widely available now. Genetic diagnosis helps in prompt and apt therapy and preconception counseling of epilepsy, intellectual disability, movement disorders, neurodegenerative disorders, and inborn errors of metabolism (IEMs).

Sanger sequencing: DNA sequencing analysis is mostly done by the Sanger method, used in cases of a clear phenotype of a single gene disorder with a known gene. It detects the variations in the sequence of that particular gene like a single nucleotide change or small insertions and deletions (indels) and helps in validating the results of NGS (next-generation sequencing). The inability to detect copy number variations (large deletions or duplications) is the disadvantage.

Next-generation sequencing (NGS): It utilizes high-throughput technology by which simultaneous sequencing of thousands to millions of DNA molecules is performed. It is useful in cases where the phenotype does not indicate any particular disorder strongly and a structural genomic variation (variations involving DNA segments more than 50 base pairs) is not suspected. NGS can sequence any predefined genomic region of interest. It is called whole-exome sequencing (WES) when the exons of all the known ~20,000 genes are tested. Specific targeted panels are available currently where a particular set of genes associated with a phenotypic category are tested as in epilepsy panel, muscular dystrophy panel, etc. The testing if restricted to the genes known to be associated with disease states only (~6,000 genes), it is called clinical exome sequencing (CES).

The variants detected are then filtered for significance through various filters and the final variants are reported as one of the five categories as per ACMG 2015 guidelines [pathological, likely pathological, variant of uncertain clinical significance (VUS/VOUS), likely benign and benign]. NGS also cannot detect copy number variations (CNVs) and alterations in introns which may be pathogenic occasionally.

Multiplex ligation probe amplification (MLPA): It analyzes deletion or duplication at the exon level in disorders with exon or gene deletions (Duchenne muscular dystrophy, spinal muscular atrophy) or duplications (Charcot–Marie–Tooth neuropathy 1A). MLPA also detects microdeletion syndromes (Williams syndrome, Cri-du-Chat syndrome, Wolf–Hirschhorn syndrome); but is not suitable to detect unknown point mutations and balanced translocations.

Comparative genomic hybridization (CGH)/ chromosomal microarray (CMA): CNVs are DNA segments larger than 1 kb which repeat at variable copy number. CGH basically compares the genome of the subject to the reference genome for CNVs. It has greater resolution than the conventional karyotype. It is applied in intellectual disability (ID) or dysmorphism of unknown cause, autism spectrum disorders (ASD), major congenital anomalies not explained by any well-described syndromes, and recurrent abortions. It cannot detect balanced translocations, polyploids, and low-level mosaicism.

Fluorescence in situ hybridization (FISH): It detects specific chromosomal regions or chromosomes through hybridization of fluorescently labeled DNA probes to the target DNA sequence. Detects chromosomal aberrations too small to be detected by karyotyping and too large to be detected by DNA sequencing methods. It is useful in diagnosing microdeletion syndromes for which FISH probes are available and in the identification of marker chromosomes.

Others: Southern blot technique is used to detect trinucleotide repeat disorders [Friedrich's ataxia (GAA), fragile X syndrome (CGG), Huntington's disease (CAG), and myotonic dystrophy (CTG)]. Methylation studies are utilized in suspected parental imprinting disorders like Angelman syndrome and Prader–Willi syndrome.

SUGGESTED READING

1. Brakovich AJ, Raybaud C. Pediatric Neuroimaging, 5th edition. Philadelphia: Wolters Kluwer; 2011.
2. Ebersole JS. Current Practice of Clinical Electroencephalography, 4th edition. Philadelphia: Lippincott Williams and Wilkins; 2014.
3. Preston DC, Shapiro BE. Electromyography and Neuromuscular Disorders, 3rd edition. Philadelphia: Saunders; 2013.
4. Radhakrishnan K, Murthy JMK, Rathore C. EEG in Clinical Practice, 1st edition. Manipal: Manipal Universal Press; 2018.
5. Schomer DL, da Silva FL. Niedermeyer's Electroencephalography, 6th edition. Philadelphia: Lippincott Williams & Wilkins; 2012.
6. Swaiman KF, Ashwal S, Ferriero DM, Schor NF, Finkel RS, Gropman AL, et al. Swaiman's Pediatric Neurology, 6th edition. Amsterdam: Elsevier; 2017.

23

CHAPTER

Confirmation of Death

Davidson Devasia, KP Vinayan

Chapter Outline

(Read Chapter 3 also)

INTRODUCTION

Death is defined as the end of life, an irreversible cessation of all vital functions, indicated by the permanent stoppage of the heart, respiration, and brain activity. Brain death (BD) occurs when an insult to the brain causes a neuropathologic vicious cycle of brain edema, raised intracranial pressure (RICP), and a decrease in cerebral blood flow (CBF), compromising blood supply to the brain leading to ischemia, a situation that resembles "total brain infarction." Research about brain death involves adults mostly and the main concept of this situation in the pediatric age group is extrapolated, producing inherent weaknesses in its assessment and diagnosis. Brain in children is a developing one, continuing throughout childhood, myelination is mostly completed by 2 yr. Resilience to certain forms of injuries producing cerebral edema and the subsequent increase in cerebral volume could be found in neonates and infants, due to open fontanels and the capacity of the sutures to separate in response to the increase in intracranial pressure. Hence, for the interpretation and confirmation of brain death in children, these factors should be considered.

HISTORICAL FACTORS

In 1968, an ad hoc committee of the Harvard Medical School published the first definition of brain death. The first specific guidelines on brain death in children were published in 1987 by the American Academy of Pediatrics (AAP). An update was followed in 2011 in which specific criteria were put forward for the newborn (37 w gestation to 30 days of life), which was a little different from one proposed for infants and older children from 31 days of life to 18 yr. There are certain differences in the concepts of brain death across the countries. In the USA, Australia, and New Zealand, a whole brain death definition is accepted where the entire brain function should be absent electrocerebral silence and absent brainstem reflexes. On the contrary, in the UK, India, and Canada a brainstem-based definition of death is in place and the term "death by neurological criteria (DNC)" is adopted where the strong driving point is absent brainstem reflexes. Regardless of the differences in terminology, brain death has to be considered in a person with acute irreversible coma along with absent brainstem reflexes and apnea. In short, brain death is a clinical diagnosis.

CAUSES OF BRAIN DEATH

- Severe traumatic brain injury
- Severe infection
- Tumors
- Cerebrovascular accidents
- Acute global anoxic/ischemic injury following severe respiratory failure, drowning, shock, or cardiac arrest.
- Acute toxic neuronal injury—metabolic diseases or cellular hypoxia-cyanide poisoning.

Where the cause of the coma is not identifiable, the physician should specify the cause of the coma as "other."

NEED FOR BRAIN DEATH POLICY

Certification of "Death"

Certification of "death" should be done with utmost care. If a patient reveals signs of life after having been certified dead by a doctor, it indicates gross negligence from the concerned doctor and the health care system and will lead to serious medicolegal consequences in the professional life of the doctor. Hence doctors should strictly adhere to the standard protocol in certifying death to avoid such an error. Most critically ill patients may be on life-supporting measures, such as mechanical ventilation, vasopressors, and parenteral fluids so that at a time when brain death is already established, the heart may be beating in a few cases.

When the doctor is called to assess a patient in the terminal stage of illness suspecting death, a systematic approach for confirmation of death and correct documentation of the findings should be done. Obtain a brief history from a reliable bystander (if seeing the patient for the first time) or review the patient's details from the hospital record as well as from a close relative of the patient, if he/she was seen earlier. Ascertain the probable cause of coma as not treatable or reversible. Evaluate the patient for coma, apnea, and cardiac compromise. Provide intense cardiopulmonary resuscitation for 30 min while the vitals are being monitored. The absence of heartbeats and spontaneous respiration for 30 min are adequate criteria for clinical death. If the patient is on a ventilator, spontaneous respiratory efforts must be watched by periodically switching off the ventilator [maintain partial pressure of carbon dioxide ($PaCO_2$) = 60 mm Hg or >20 mm Hg >above normal baseline value before switching off the ventilator]. Cardiac asystole is to be depicted by electrocardiogram (ECG) tracing which should be attached to the patient's hospital case record. The parameters for brain death are coma, apnea, and absence of brainstem reflexes which are detailed in "Clinical Parameters of Brain Death" further.

In this era, the requirements to define brain death are legally necessary because of the rapid advances and acceptance in organ transplantation between living donors. The major milestone in this regard was the first heart transplant by Dr Christian Barnard in 1967 from a brain-dead person. The priority of the medical system is to save lives rather than to obtain organs and hence the public must feel confident that they would become organ donors only after all reasonable attempts to save their lives have failed. Robust guidelines for diagnosing brain death will help to confirm the situation and to decide on the discontinuation of medical support in brain-dead patients.

Guidelines

In 2011, a multidisciplinary committee was formed by the Society of Critical Care Medicine (SCCM) and the AAP to update the 1987 Task Force Recommendations for the diagnosis of brain death in children. According to the guidelines, brain death is a clinical diagnosis based on the absence of neurologic function with a known diagnosis that has resulted in irreversible coma. *Coma, absent brainstem reflexes,* and *apnea* are the parameters to diagnose brain death.

Prerequisites

The known reversible causes of coma should be excluded. The evolution of brain damage to brain death ideally be depicted with computed tomography (CT) or magnetic resonance imaging (MRI). Since neuroimaging may not show any significant findings in the early stage of the disease, serial examinations may be needed occasionally. All the major potentially influencing factors must be corrected in advance and all the following preconditions must be met:

- *Cardiovascular stability:* Mean or arterial systolic pressure should be normal for age with inotropic and vasomotor support if needed. Direct arterial pressure measurement is recommended if possible, for monitoring, blood gas analysis, and $PaCO_2$ evaluation, especially for apnea testing.
- *Normothermia:* Hypothermia is a depressant to central nervous system activity and may lead to a false diagnosis of brain death. Metabolism and clearance of medications are retarded, which can interfere with examination. As therapeutic hypothermia is increasingly used after neurological injury, neurological examination should be delayed until after rewarming at least 72 hr before the examinations. The patient's core body temperature should be >35°C (95°F) before the first examination and be maintained throughout the observation period.
- *Homeostasis:* The most common metabolic disturbance during brain death is hypernatremia due to diabetes insipidus which should be ideally corrected with the administration of antidiuretic hormone or desmopressin. Hyperglycemia is common and monitoring of blood glucose and insulin therapy is indicated. As per recent guidelines, correction of hypernatremia is not mandatory if other preconditions are met.

  Hyponatremia, hypoglycemia, hypothyroidism, severe pH disturbances, severe hepatic or renal dysfunction, or inborn errors of metabolism are some of the causes of potentially reversible coma in children.
- *Neuromuscular blocking agents (NMBAs):* Adequate clearance of NMBA is a must before proceeding with confirmation of brain death. If residual NMBA action is doubted, a peripheral nerve stimulator to evoke a sustained "train of four" muscle twitch (good neuromuscular activity with 4/4 responses in "train of four" testing) needs to be tried.
- *Drug intoxications:* Intoxications with barbiturates, opioids, sedatives, anesthetic agents, antiepileptics, and alcohol require adequate clearance (based on the age of the child, presence of organ dysfunction, the total amount of medication administered, the elimination half-life of the drug and any active metabolites) before confirming brain death. Lab tests should be done to confirm

if residual drug effect is suspected. Since there is evidence that subtherapeutic and therapeutic barbiturate levels (phenobarbital at 15–40 ug/mL) did not interfere with the reliability of diagnosis of brain death, it is advisable to be at the low to midtherapeutic range before the examination. Consider unusual causes such as neurotoxins (snake venom—Krait bite, usually painless, during sleep in the night) and exposure to carbamates and organophosphates, if the etiology for coma is not established.

Other potential causes to be excluded are locked-in syndrome, Guillain–Barré syndrome, brain stem encephalitis, and high spinal cord injury before the confirmation of brain death.

Examination

- *Age definition (age is counted after birth)*: For newborns 37 w gestation to 30 days of life; infants and children—31 days of life to 18 yr.
- *Timing of first examination:* Timing of the examination from the neurological insult as in cases of cardiac arrest with successful resuscitation or other severe neurological insult is 24 hr for patients aged from 37 w of gestation to 30 days of life and 12 hr for patients aged 31 days of life to 18 yr.

It is reasonable to defer neurologic examination to determine brain death for longer than 24 hr if dictated by the clinical judgment of the treating physician. Neonates who probably suffered from hypoxic/ischemic insult during the neonatal period and had been put in therapeutic hypothermia deserve a longer observation time before the first examination. Immediately following cardiopulmonary resuscitation or other severe acute brain injuries, assessment of neurological function may be unreliable and hence brain death assessment should be deferred for at least 24–48 hr or longer if there is variability in findings. The first clinical examination may be performed once the etiology of coma is determined, and the condition of the patient is established as irreversible with the confounders corrected.

Clinical Parameters of Brain Death

Irreversible coma: Irreversible coma is the absence of higher neurological functions—complete loss of consciousness, vocalization, volitional activity, profound state of non-response, flaccid tone without any spontaneous or induced movements.

- *Tests:* Apply noxious stimuli in the cranial nerve distribution (deep supraorbital and/or condyle mandibular pressure—fifth cranial nerve) and all four limbs (deep bed nail pressure), and trunk (sternal rub) and observe the response. Responsiveness to central (in the territory of cranial nerves) and peripheral (outside the territory of cranial nerves) noxious stimuli must be absent. Complete absence of movement equates to a Glasgow Coma Scale (GCS) score of 3. Decerebrate or decorticate posturing, true extensor or flexor motor responses to painful stimuli, and seizures are not compatible with the diagnosis of brain death.

Suspect spinal reflexes in patients with motor responses, in a somatic distribution, after stimulation in the peripheral nerve territories and not after a stimulus in the cranial nerve distribution. They present a wide range of movements that are reflexive, appear to be spontaneous and purposeful, and raise suspicion about the diagnosis of brain death. The most common reflexes are plantar response, myoclonus, triple flexion and pronator extension, and undulating toe reflex. Seen mostly in patients who are hemodynamically stable after medical intervention. Caregivers should be informed about these reflexes.

Brainstem Reflexes

All brainstem reflexes should be absent, confirmed by physical examination, as per the parameters detailed below:

- *Pupillary reflex (afferent II, efferent III—midbrain):* Pupils must be >4 mm up to 9 mm with absent pupillary response to bright light in both eyes. Fixed midsize or fully dilated pupils are common. If uncertain, use a magnifying glass. Interpret with caution if pupil size is <4 mm—small constricted pupils may be due to drug intoxication; or *severe facial or ocular trauma and in those with preexisting pupillary abnormalities, this test is inconclusive,* and ancillary tests should be considered.
- *Corneal reflex (afferent V, efferent VII-pons):* Touch the cornea with a moist cotton swab wisp/a piece of gauze/paper/water squirts (take special care not to damage the cornea). Eyelid movements should be completely absent.
- *Absence of facial or bulbar musculature movement to noxious stimuli (afferent V, efferent VII):* Deep pressure on the condyles at the level of the temporomandibular joints and at the supraorbital ridges should not produce any grimacing or facial muscle movement.
- *Oculovestibular reflex (caloric reflex, afferent VIII, efferent III, VI—pons and midbrain):* Check for patency of the external auditory canal with otoscopy before examination. The eardrum should be visible, or it should be cleared before the test. Irrigate each ear with ice water (Ref. Ch. 21 for the caloric test) after the head is elevated to 30° to place the semicircular canals in a horizontal position. Each external auditory canal is irrigated (one ear at a time) with >10–50 mL of ice water. Movement of the eyes should be absent during 1 min of observation. Test both sides, with an interval of several min.
- *Oculocephalic reflex (Doll's eye reflex):* (Afferent VIII, efferent III, (VI—pons and midbrain)—this test is not considered mandatory in many guidelines such as AAP 2011 and ANZICS 2013 due to the facts that the findings may be equivocal and the risk of exacerbating possible cervical spinal trauma **(Fig. 23.1)**.
- *Gag reflex [afferent IX, efferents IX and X—medulla (Refer to Chapter 21)]:* Use a tongue depressor to stimulate the posterior pharynx, taking care not to dislodge the patient's endotracheal tube (ETT). In neonates and infants <3 m of age, sucking, and rooting reflexes are sought.
- *Cough reflex—tracheal reflex (afferent X—medulla):* Examine the cough response to tracheal suctioning. Insert the suction catheter into the trachea and advance it to the level of the carina followed by one or two suctioning processes. The efferent limbs for this reflex are the phrenic nerve and the thoracic and abdominal musculature. Hence, it cannot be assessed in patients with high cervical cord injury.

Apnea Test

Apnea testing is conducted, only if all the above reflexes are absent because high

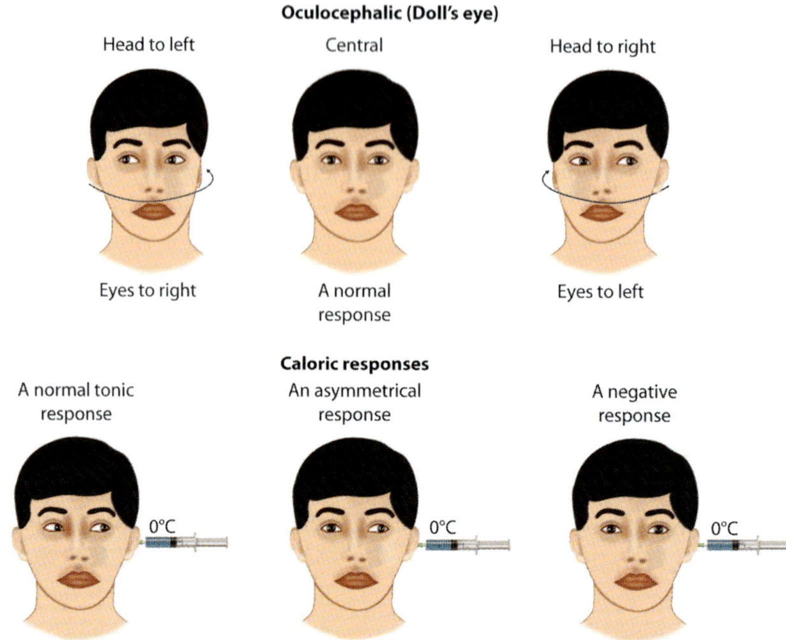

Fig. 23.1: Oculocephalic and oculovestibular reflexes.

$PaCO_2$ in an apnea test should not confound the testing of the other cranial nerves. Apnea testing is the cornerstone for the diagnosis of brain death in all age groups and is conducted similarly.

The rationale behind the apnea test is that in a patient on ventilator, an intense stimulus, such as hypercapnia and respiratory acidosis, is needed to stimulate respiratory drive centers in the medulla to start respiratory efforts. During this procedure, concomitant hypoxia should be avoided by administering 100% O_2. According to AAP 2011 guidelines, if no respiratory effort is observed from the initiation of the apnea test to the time the measured $PaCO_2$ is ≥60 and ≥20 mm Hg above the baseline, the apnea test is consistent with brain death. Patients with chronic respiratory disease and chronic hypercapnia may need a higher respiratory stimulus, and in this case, the limit of ≥20 mm Hg above baseline is advised. CO_2 rises approximately 4 mm Hg/min of apnea. The rate may be lower in the setting of brain death due to the loss of brain metabolism. At this rate, it will take at least 5 min of apnea for the pCO_2 to rise by 20 mm Hg; often it requires 7–9 min. Hence draw blood gas at 5–6 min of apnea and continue the apnea observation while awaiting the results. Stop the testing if hypoxia or hypotension or hypothermia develops during the procedure. Maintenance of homeostasis is a must during the procedure.

Before initiating the test, preoxygenation using 100% oxygen, aiming at nitrogen removal and oxygen enrichment should be applied for at least 10 min. Apneic oxygenation is attempted during the test with the oxygen-diffusion technique—with tracheal insufflation of oxygen at a rate suitable for the age of the child. Mandatory intermittent mechanical ventilation is discontinued once the patient is well oxygenated and the normal $PaCO_2$ around 35–40 mm Hg is achieved. The patient could also be changed to a T-piece attached to the ETT, or a self-inflating bag such as a Mapleson circuit connected to the ETT or continuous positive airway pressure (CPAP) in cases of hypoxemia. Heartbeats, blood pressure, and oxygen saturation should be continuously monitored while observing carefully for spontaneous respiratory effort (any respiratory muscle activity that results in abdominal or chest excursions or activity of accessory respiratory muscles) throughout the entire procedure.

If the patient is well-oxygenated [peripheral oxygen saturation (SpO_2) >85%] and hemodynamically stable, keep apnea duration to 10 min and then draw arterial blood gas (ABG) for analysis. The longer the apnea time, the more the possibility for a positive apnea test. AAP 2011 guidelines suggest serial follow-up ABG to monitor the rise in $PaCO_2$ while the patient remains disconnected from mechanical ventilation. If oxygen saturation falls below 85% or hemodynamic instability limits completion of apnea testing, draw ABG at this time, discontinue the test, and return the patient to the ventilator with full support. If a $PaCO_2$ level of ≥60 and ≥20 mm Hg above the baseline has not been achieved at that time, another attempt to test for apnea may be performed at a later time or an ancillary study may be pursued to assist with the determination of brain death.

During the examination, the patient's chest and abdomen should be exposed to detect any chest wall movement or respiratory effort. Any respiratory effort is inconsistent with brain death and the apnea test should be aborted.

Brain death should be confirmed by two examinations by two different physicians; each physician after a complete neurological examination should conduct the apnea test. The examinations should be separated by an observation period. For term neonates (from 37 w of gestation up to 30 days old), the observation period recommended is 24 hr; for infants >30 days old to children 18 yr old, a 12 hr period is advised. Some recent guidelines in adults recommend shorter intervals (6 hr). The first examination is to establish that the patient has met neurological criteria for brain death. The second examination is to confirm brain death.

ANCILLARY STUDIES

The 2011 AAP guidelines recommend that ancillary studies [electroencephalogram (EEG) and radionuclide CBF] are not required to establish brain death and are not substitutes for neurologic examination. The term "ancillary study" is preferred to "confirmatory study" since these tests assist the clinician in making the clinical diagnosis of brain death. These studies are not common in places where the direct numerical control (DNC) concept is accepted but are more common where the whole concept of brain death, including the death of the brain and brainstem, is acknowledged. Under current consensus guidelines, ancillary testing is not required to make a diagnosis of brain death, unless the neurological examination and apnea test cannot be completed. They are used to decrease the observation period especially when the clinical examination is doubtful. There is no specific recommendation about the second clinical examination with an apnea test to be performed after the ancillary study to make confirmation of death for children of all ages.

If ancillary testing supports the diagnosis of brain death, then a second clinical examination and apnea test should be performed, but repeat ancillary testing is not necessary. If the ancillary test is equivocal, then a 24 hr waiting period is recommended before retesting. Imaging studies such as CT or MRI scans are not considered ancillary studies to make a determination of brain death. The ancillary tests are EEG, four-vessel cerebral angiography that determines CBF, and radionuclide CBF. Both EEG and CBF have similar confirmatory values.

The "Gold standard," four-vessel cerebral angiography requires moving the patient to an angiography suite. Useful in high-dose barbiturate therapy, is difficult to perform in smaller infants and children and is less sensitive in newborns.

Ancillary studies that are not yet completely validated in children are transcranial Doppler, CT angiography, CT perfusion with spin labeling, nasopharyngeal somatosensory evoked potential studies, MRI + magnetic resonance angiography, and perfusion MRI.

The time of death is the time of the second examination, including apnea and/or ancillary test completion. When a patient meets all criteria for brain death, they are legally dead. Once it is diagnosed, always *communicate as "dead"* and not "brain dead" to avoid confusion for the relatives.

Kerala guidelines for brain death (not age specific) updated on 19 January, 2020 insist on examination by 4 doctors, 2 examinations with a minimum 6-hr interval between 1st and 2nd examination, and following the above guidelines with an emphasis on *death by neurological criteria.*

CONTRAINDICATIONS

Circumstances under which clinical neurological examination and/or apnea test cannot be performed are ocular trauma, severe maxillofacial injuries, basal skull fractures running through the external ear canal, or eardrum rupture. Cervical spinal trauma with possible involvement of the phrenic nerve limits the spontaneous breathing ability during apnea testing. Apnea testing cannot be performed in cases of severe hypoxia as in acute respiratory distress syndrome (ARDS) patients even under CPAP conditions and/or in patients with severe hemodynamic instability.

SPECIAL CONSIDERATIONS

- *37 w (corrected gestational age) up to 1 m:* Unfortunately, the accepted medical standards that apply for adults such as EEG and CBF measurements, are not reliable in newborns because of the open fontanel and lack of increase in intracranial pressures. Hence in newborns, consider "brainstem death" rather than brain death in the evaluation of coma.

  Infants with anencephaly frequently have physical abnormalities, including ocular and otic congenital defects that prevent a complete neurological clinical examination. Since these patients lack normally formed cerebrum, ancillary tests such as EEG and CBF are unable to be obtained and hence these infants cannot be declared brain dead.

  Assessment of pupillary reactivity and ocular motility may be difficult in a compromised infant on ventilator support and requires both oculocephalic (Doll's eye) and oculovestibular (caloric) reflexes to be examined. Assessing caloric response may be difficult in newborns owing to their small external ear canal. Corneal reflex is easy to examine in neonates and its presence indicates intact brain-stem function but is the least reliable test. Assessment of auditory function is difficult in a comatose infant; if necessary, a brainstem auditory evoked response test should be obtained. Assessment of the lower cranial nerves is limited to assessment of the gag reflex only.

Apnea testing can be successfully performed in all infants >32 w gestational age. Few ineffectual respiratory efforts should not be considered reversible brain defects. Carbon dioxide accumulates slowly in brain-dead infants owing to a lack of production of CO_2 by the brain. Generally, this test should take 5–15 min to reach the CO_2 threshold of 60 mm Hg. Compressive brain-stem lesions may mimic brain-stem death, which could be seen in newborns with posterior fossa subdural hematomas, Dandy–Walker syndrome, Arnold–Chiari malformation, and brain tumors.

- *EEG:* Therapeutic levels of phenobarbital (15–40 mg/mL) do not affect the EEG. If the EEG shows electrocerebral silence, repetition of EEG is not necessary.
- *CBF studies:* The open fontanels in the newborns will not reveal RICP after acute injury as in older children and the perfusion pressure may not decrease despite low mean arterial pressure. Thus, CBF may be present in brain-dead newborns, making this test somewhat unreliable.
- Doppler CBF measures the progression of velocity changes in brain-dead neonates and children. These changes include the loss of diastolic blood flow, the appearance of retrograde diastolic blood flow, a decrease in systolic blood flow in the anterior cerebral artery with unchanged flow in the common carotid artery, and finally no flow in all the cerebral vessels. Digital subtraction angiography is another technique used to measure blood flow. Limited data exist to use these methods in children to determine brain death. Assessment of brain metabolic activity using spectroscopy has also been described in brain-dead neonates.

POINTS TO REMEMBER

- Neurodiagnostic tests, such as EEG and radionuclide scanning measuring CBF, reconfirmed clinically determined brain death in only one-half to one-third of the patients.
- Electrocerebral silence confirms brain death if clinical findings remain unchanged in the absence of barbiturates, hypothermia, or cerebral malformations during a 24 hr period.
- Absence of radionuclide uptake associated with initial electrocerebral silence can be correlated with brain death.
- Term infants clinically brain dead for two days and preterm infants brain dead for three days did not survive despite EEG or CBF status.
- Phenobarbital levels >25 mg/mL may suppress electroencephalographic activity in these infants.
- The above facts suggest that the determination of brain death in the newborn can be made solely by using clinical criteria. Supplemental diagnostic studies are of potential value to shorten the period of observation.

SUGGESTED READING

1. Government of Kerala, Health and Family Welfare Department. (2020). Guidelines for Brain Death Certification, G.O(Ms) No.7/2020/ H and FWD. [Online] Available from https://nhrc.nic.in/sites/default/files/AR_2021-2022_EN.pdf [Last accessed September, 2024].
2. Martin SD, Porter MB. Performing the Brain Death Examination and the Declaration of Pediatric Brain Death. J Pediatr Intensive Care. 2017;6(4):229-33.
3. Nakagawa TA, Ashwal S, Mathur M, Mysore M, Kolinski L, Retford L, et al. Clinical report—Guidelines for the determination of brain death in infants and children: An update of the 1987 task force recommendations. Pediatrics. 2011;128(3):e720-40.
4. Sekar KC. Brain death in the newborn. J Perinatol. 2007;27:S59-62.
5. Volakli EA, Mantzafleri P, Kalamitsou S, Violaki A, Chochliouro E, Svirkos M, et al. Brain death in children. [Online] Available from https://doi.org/10.5772/intechopen.68468 [Last accessed September, 2024].

24

CHAPTER

Endocrine System

M Vijayakumar, Lalitha Kailas

Chapter Outline

- Introduction
- Endocrine History
- Endocrine Symptoms
- General Examination

INTRODUCTION

Please read Chapters 6, 7, 8, 9, 11, and 12 before you proceed.

Endocrine disorders in children are often complex in nature, difficult to diagnose clinically alone, requiring costly investigations for confirmation. Lack or delay in appropriate treatment can end up in untimely death or chronic disability in these patients. Timely diagnosis is possible at present by improved laboratory tests thus enabling prompt and correct treatment a reality.

Most endocrine disorders originate from the newborn period itself. Affected babies may die if not diagnosed correctly and treated in time. Many of these diseases are genetically transmitted so that subsequent generations also get affected. Hence, it is mandatory for all pediatricians to have correct knowledge regarding these disorders to diagnose and treat, detect, and manage promptly the complications as and when encountered and also to counsel the families properly.

The endocrine system comprises the classic endocrine glands which include the hypothalamus, pituitary, thyroid, parathyroids, adrenals, pancreatic islet cells, and gonads (ovaries and testes). The glands synthesize and secrete hormones directly into the blood or lymph which produce specific effects on different organs or systems in the body. Most endocrine diseases do not present with pain or visible/palpable abnormalities of the affected glands except for the thyroid and the testes. Unlike other body systems, actions of these glands are not at all restricted to one organ or system at any time, so that the manifestations occur on different body parts on different occasions even for the same person. Systematic patient approach will enable the doctor to target a particular gland aberration and proceed for diagnostic confirmation.

ENDOCRINE HISTORY

Elicit the history in detail carefully, since many patients with endocrine disorders narrate lengthy history with irrelevant points. Chief complaints in temporal sequence, their duration and severity, treatment taken (including alternate systems), type, duration, route of administration of drugs, response to the treatment given, reasons for stopping any drug, course of the illness, details of investigations done, diet changes made, inpatient treatment received, past illness, details of surgeries done, restriction of schooling done with the reasons for that, parental consanguinity, details of endocrine disorders in parents, siblings and among close blood relatives, present status of their illness and the details of treatment taken by the affected persons, all should be documented.

ENDOCRINE SYMPTOMS

The symptoms can present as acute life-threatening emergencies or with classical features of the suspected hormonal disorder or less often with subtle and vague complaints necessitating detailed workup to confirm the endocrine etiology.

Acute Life-threatening Endocrine Emergencies

Acute life-threatening endocrine emergencies usually encountered are vomiting, respiratory distress, seizures, lethargy, altered sensorium, coma, shock, dehydration, dyselectrolytemia, menorrhagia, severe anemia, neonatal jaundice, high fever with cardiac irregularities, and failure to thrive (FTT) with dehydration.

Vomiting

Repeated episodes of vomiting may indicate diabetic ketoacidosis *(DKA)* or acute adrenocortical insufficiency (AACI) of which DKA is the leading one. Clinical features of dehydration **(Table 7.5, Fig. 7.7)**, dyselectrolytemia, shock, deep breathing and varying grades of coma are usual. Abdominal pain and vomiting are common in older children with DKA due to ketogenesis. Exclude other causes of abdominal pain (Ref. Ch. 20) clinically and by relevant investigations.

Almost 40% of type 1 diabetes mellitus *(T1DM)* children present as DKA at their first hospital visit. DKA is less common in type 2 diabetes mellitus *(T2DM)*. Factors precipitating DKA are high blood sugar with low body insulin causing impaired glucose metabolism and defective energy liberation. Body adapts to lipid breakdown as the alternate mechanism for energy source, leading to the accumulation of ketone bodies as end metabolite which provokes abdominal pain and vomiting.

Key points

In a sick child with vomiting, dehydration, and abdominal pain, consider the possibility of DKA always. DKA should be an important differential diagnosis or added illness in all children who are critically ill, unconscious, severely dehydrated and in those with organ failure.

Table 24.1 and the footnote reveal the salient clinical features of common endocrine emergencies and their diagnostic criteria.

TABLE 24.1: Clinical presentation of common endocrine emergencies.

Clinical presentation	*Possible endocrine emergency*
Vomiting, dehydration, deep breathing, and coma	Diabetic ketoacidosis (DKA)
[1]*NN* seizures + tetany	Pseudohypoparathyroidism (PHP)
[1]*NN* seizures + severe hypoglycemia	Multiple pituitary hormone deficiency (MPHD)
[1]*NN* hyperbilirubinemia	Hypopituitarism (HP), congenital hypothyroidism (CHT)
Repeated vomiting, dehydration, shock	Acute adrenocortical insufficiency (AACI)
Vomiting, dehydration, weight loss ± ambiguous genitalia	Congenital adrenal hyperplasia (CAH)
Bleeding PV ± anemia	Abnormal uterine bleeding (AUB)

Contd...

Contd...

Clinical presentation	*Possible endocrine emergency*
Hyperthermia, delirium, tachycardia in a hyperthyroid child	Thyroid storm (TS)
Excessive hunger, tiredness, tremors, sweating, tachycardia, irritability, drowsiness, coma, and convulsions	Hypoglycemia (HG)
Irritability, irregular fever, unaccountable dehydration, [6]*FTT*	Diabetes insipidus (DI)

[1]Neonatal, [2]Growth hormone, [3]Thyroid-stimulating hormone, [4]Adrenocorticotropic hormone, [5]Hydroxyprogesterone, [6]Failure to thrive

- *DKA*—affects T1DM group. Usual features—repeated vomiting with abdominal pain (due to ketoacids), increasing dehydration, Kussmaul breathing, fruity odor in breath, dry mucosa and altered sensorium deteriorating to coma. H/O polyuria, polydipsia, weakness and weight loss (due to hyperglycemia) may be present. Laboratory criteria for DKA: (1) Nonfasting blood glucose ≥*200 mg/dL*, urine sugar >3+; (2) metabolic acidosis—venous blood pH <7.3; (3) Ketosis—blood ketones ≥3 mmol/L, serum bicarbonate <15 mmol/L, urine ketones >2+. Nonketotic hyperosmolar coma in T2DM presents as depressed sensorium deteriorating to deep coma and seizures. High blood sugar (blood glucose *>800 mg/dL*), hyperosmolarity (serum osmolarity ≥350 mOsm/kg) and absent ketoacidosis are the differentiating diagnostic parameters from DKA.
- *PHP:* Clinical—short stature with round face, limb anomalies and the metacarpal sign **(Fig. 7.38)**. Lab findings—persistently low S. Ca with high/normal S. parathyroid hormone blood level.
- *MPHD:* Newborns—apnea, cyanosis, resistant hypoglycemia often with seizures and progressive neonatal jaundice (conjugated and unconjugated), progressing to neonatal hepatitis; older children have prominent frontal bones, small saddle shaped nose, crowded teeth, short neck, linear growth failure of >2SD below sex adjusted MPH, reduced skeletal age and decreased [2]*GH <10 ng/mL* with IGF1, GH-dependent IGFBP3 matched values for skeletal age. Additional investigations for hypothyroidism, hypocortisolism, hypogonadism and precocious puberty are mandatory.
- *HP:* Hyperbilirubinemia can be the sole manifestation of hypopituitarism. Low serum [2]*GH* is diagnostic. Micropenis, if present, is a diagnostic clue for HP.
- *CHT:* Big head with wide AF and PF, excessive sleepiness, poor feeding, hoarse cry, constipation, cold dry skin, prolonged neonatal jaundice, macroglossia, and umbilical hernia **(Appendix 1, Fig. 24.5)** are features of hypothyroid newborn. Raised serum [3]*TSH* levels along with low levels of T_4 *(total and free) and T3* are diagnostic.
- *AACI (Addisonian crisis):* Recurrent vomiting, weight loss, orthostatic hypotension (may present in frank shock), and H/O salt craving are usual. Hyperpigmentation of sun exposed body parts occurs in secondary adrenal cortical insufficiency due to melanocyte stimulation; diagnostic laboratory criteria are hypoglycemia, hyponatremia, ketosis, low serum cortisol, and high [4]ACTH.
- *CAH:* With 11 beta and 17 alpha hydroxylase deficiencies hypertension can manifest. Girls often have ambiguous genitalia **(Fig. 7.41)**. Early postnatal virilization can occur in both sex groups. Diagnostic laboratory criteria are high levels of serum [4]*ACTH* and [5]*17OHP*, low serum cortisol, hyponatremia, hyperkalemia, and hypoglycemia.
- *AUB:* Abnormal uterine bleeding is menstrual bleeding lasting >7 days/cycle or infrequent bleeding within 20 days of menstrual cycle, passing clots larger than1 inch size, frequent number of pads changed hourly (any one criterion is diagnostic). Exclude other causes of uterine bleeding (inherited bleeding disorders, uterine vascular malformations, uterine anomalies with USG abdomen and coagulation studies).
- *TS:* Acute life-threatening complication of hyperthyroidism—presents with high fever, tachycardia progressing to atrial fibrillation, rapid progression to cardiac failure, delirium, coma and death if not treated.
- *HG:* Hypoglycemia is whole blood glucose <*55* mg/dL in newborns and plasma glucose *<60 mg/dL* in older children; fatal complication in children with diabetes mellitus, HP, AACI, and CAH.
- *DI:* Features are irritability, [6]*FTT* and unaccountable dehydration. Diagnostic laboratory criteria—serum osmolality >300 mOsm/kg along with urine osmolality <270 mOsm/kg with normal renal function.

Diabetes mellitus (DM) is an endocrine disorder of impaired glucose metabolism due to low levels of body insulin in T1DM and peripheral insulin resistance in T2DM leading to hyperglycemia and its complications. T1DM is an autoimmune disorder ending in pancreatic beta cell destruction, severe insulin deficiency, and hyperglycemia requiring exogenous insulin for survival. Hyperglycemia produces hyperosmolarity, polyuria, ketosis (due to lipid breakdown for energy), and weight loss. The clinical presentation may range from asymptomatic hyperglycemia to life-threatening DKA. **Footnote of Table 24.1** details the diagnostic features of DKA. **Table 24.2** shows the severity grading of DKA in children.

Type 2 diabetes mellitus affects adults mainly and adolescents less frequently. Family history of T2DM and gestational diabetes in blood relatives are helpful diagnostic clues. Polyuria, polydipsia, recent weight loss, and nocturia are the symptoms, may be asymptomatic detected incidentally.

Acute adrenocortical insufficiency (AACI) is a potentially fatal endocrine emergency due to acute dysfunction of the adrenal cortex resulting in reduced synthesis of glucocorticoids (cortisol), mineralocorticoids (aldosterone), and sex hormones. Clinical severity depends on the extent and rapidity of adrenal cortex damage, blood levels of the concerned hormones and the fluid and electrolyte status of the host prior to the episode.

Acute adrenocortical insufficiency in newborns: Suspect in traumatic birth if the baby develops dehydration, shock, poor feeding, and nonbilious vomiting. Other causes of adrenal bleeding such as severe sepsis, coagulopathies, and blunt abdominal injury (battered baby, accidents) are to be excluded. Presence of ambiguous genitalia indicates CAH as the etiology.

Acute adrenocortical insufficiency in infants manifests as unexplained dehydration, shock, poor feeding, nonbilious vomiting, weight loss or poor weight gain, failure to thrive and poor activity. Causes are as stated as for the newborns except traumatic birth.

Older children present with recurrent vomiting, orthostatic hypotension or shock and lethargy. Abdominal pain due to ketoacidosis, asthenia, and progressive darkening of complexion are important diagnostic clues in history; leading questions may be required. The causes are autoimmune adrenalitis, blunt abdominal trauma [accidental/intentional (battered child)], hemorrhagic fevers (dengue illness, meningococcemia, Ebola fever, and rickettsial diseases), inherited coagulopathies, tuberculosis, adrenal gland malignancy, and drug intake (rifampicin and etomidate). In chronic adrenocortical insufficiency,

TABLE 24.2: Severity grading of DKA in children.

Parameter	Mild	Moderate	Severe
Symptoms	Vague	Drowsy, but arousable	Deepening coma
Signs	Fatigue	Some dehydration	Severe dehydration
Venous pH	>7.25–7.35	>7.15–7.25	<7.15
Care area	ER	HDU	PICU

(DKA: diabetic ketoacidosis; ER: emergency room; HDU: high dependency unit; PICU: pediatric ICU)

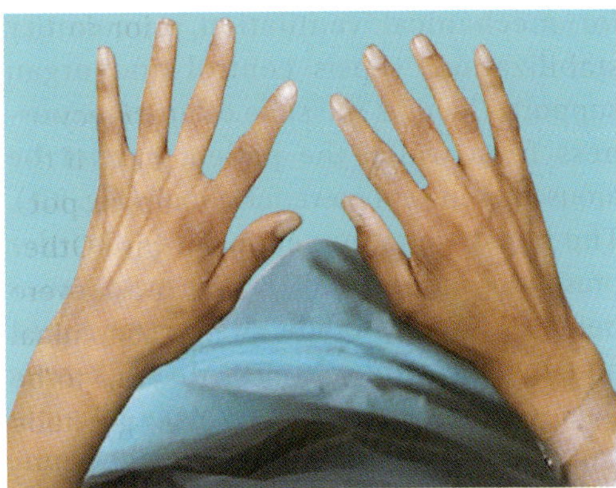

Fig. 24.1: Hyperpigmentation of knuckles in Addison's disease.

hyperpigmentation of the sun-exposed body parts is an important feature **(Fig. 24.1)**. Read **Footnote of Table 24.1** for the diagnostic criteria of AACI and CAH.

Breathing Difficulty (Ref. Ch. 19)

Breathing difficulty in endocrine disorders is often due to severe systemic acidosis. Deep and rapid "Kussmaul breathing" is the pattern seen in DKA **(Fig. 19.2C)**. Other causes of respiratory distress such as acute asthma, pneumonia, empyema, pneumo-/hemothorax, pleural effusion, cardiac failure, myocarditis, pericarditis, renal failure, inborn errors of metabolism, and salicylism should be excluded. In young children with severe respiratory distress without any clinical signs of respiratory illness, the possibility of DKA should be excluded.

Key points

In all DKA patients with breathing difficulty, other causes of respiratory distress like acute asthma, pneumonia, empyema, pneumo-/hemothorax, pleural effusion, cardiac failure, myocarditis, pericarditis, renal failure, inborn errors of metabolism and salicylism should be excluded.

The differentiating points between T1DM and T2DM are given in **Table 24.3**.

TABLE 24.3: Differentiating features of T1DM and T2DM.

Features	***T1DM***	***T2DM***
Onset	Rapid	Slow
Age of onset	6 m to 18 yr	Usually at puberty, rare <10 yr
Obesity	No role	Predisposes
Acanthosis nigricans	Rare	Present in 85% cases
Family history	10%	Strong
Ketoacidosis	25%	5–20%
Need for insulin	Universal	May require for initial control

(T1DM: type 1 diabetes mellitus; T2DM: type 2 diabetes mellitus)

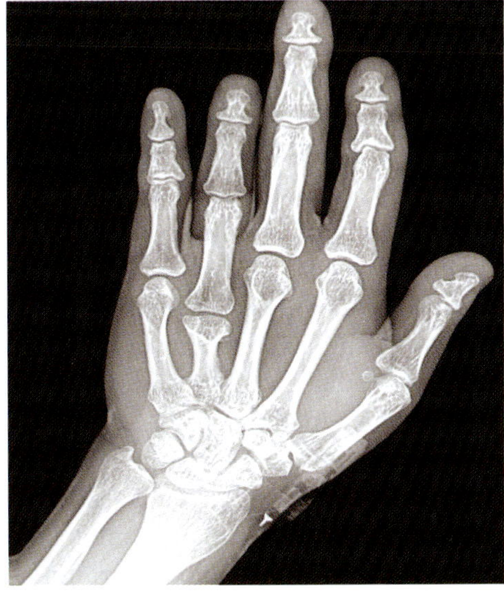

Fig. 24.2: Short 4th metacarpal bone in pseudohypoparathyroidism.

Seizures

Intractable seizures with tetany is typical of *pseudohypoparathyroidism (PHP)* from neonatal period onwards. Short stature, rounded face, skeletal deformities like shortening of 4th metacarpal bone **(Fig. 24.2)** causing brachydactyly and the metacarpal sign **(Fig. 7.38)** are the obvious clinical findings in pseudohypoparathyroidism.

In neonates with recurrent seizures and hypoglycemia, consider the possibility of *multiple pituitary hormone deficiency (MPHD)*. Micropenis (Ref. Ch. 7) is a diagnostic clue in neonates for HP and MPHD which can be clinically confirmed by measuring the stretched penile length (SPL). SPL value <–2.5 SD is diagnostic of micropenis. **Footnote of Table 24.1** details the confirmatory tests for MPHD.

Key points

Stretched penile length to detect micropenis is an important diagnostic clue for hypopituitarism in newborns.

Lethargy, Altered Sensorium, Delirium, and Coma (Ref. Ch. 9)

Altered sensorium is a change in mentation to different levels of reduced alertness ranging from drowsiness to varying grades of coma. *Delirium* is confused mental status with slurred speech and disordered thoughts. In endocrine disorders, such problems are often due to fluid and electrolyte imbalance and hypoglycemia and carry grave prognosis unless treated in time. AACI, DKA, HG, and less frequently CAH are the endocrine disorders presenting with altered sensorium. In all situations with impaired mentation, cerebral pathologies such as traumatic injury, infection, inflammation, intracranial bleeding, venous thrombosis, tumors, brain edema and cerebral abscess and systemic diseases like severe sepsis, poisoning and metabolic disorders should be excluded. Grading of coma can be by AVPU, GCS, or FOUR score (Ref. Ch. 9). AVPU score ≤P or GCS score ≤8 indicates critical illness (Ref. Ch. 9) and forewarns the need for mechanical ventilation, circulatory stabilization, sepsis control and organ support. *Coma* is the state of unconsciousness from which the patient cannot be aroused even with powerful stimuli **(Fig. 9.1)**. The most common endocrine disorder presenting in coma is T1DM, the main causes being DKA, dehydration, dyselectrolytemia, and hypoglycemia. In T2DM, nonketotic hyperosmolar coma due to hyperglycemia can occur less commonly. Hypoglycemic coma may manifest in both types. Superadded CNS infections, cerebrovascular accidents, trauma, tumors, metabolic disorders, and poisoning are the other problems presenting with coma to be excluded.

Key points

Urgent blood sugar estimation is a must in all diabetic children presenting in coma to detect hypoglycemia so that emergency intravenous glucose can be given to save the life.

Shock

Children with AACI, DKA, and CAH may present in shock following repeated vomiting and severe dehydration. Rapid deterioration to hypovolemia, unresponsiveness and coma can occur. High index of suspicion is a must to detect shock in time. Low pulse pressure (Ref. Ch. 17) if detected early heralds shock.

Dehydration and Dyselectrolytemia

Dehydration and dyselectrolytemia present as an emergency in children with AACI, DKA, CAH, and diabetes insipidus (DI). Severity of dehydration is unaccountable to the quantity of fluid loss by vomiting, loose stools, aspirates/drainage and reduced fluid intake as perceived from the history. In patients with DI, history of excess thirst with fluid intake and signs of dehydration (Ref. Ch. 7) are helpful for diagnosis.

Hyponatremia, hyperkalemia, hypoglycemia, and acidosis are the other common problems encountered in dyselectrolytemia. See **Footnote of Table 24.1** for the diagnostic criteria of CAH.

Severe Menorrhagia and Anemia

Menorrhagia (pads requiring hourly, passing clots of >1 inch size, bleeding exceeding >7 days/cycle or infrequent bleeding within 20 days of menstrual cycle—one or more criteria) can lead to severe anemia (*Hb <8 g/dL*). Assess clinically the severity (Ref. Ch. 7, **Footnote of Table 24.1**) and complications of anemia and also for signs of any other disease leading to severe anemia. Though the cause is immaturity of hypothalamic-pituitary-gonadal axis with anovulatory cycles in most patients, detailed evaluation for underlying coagulation defects, uterine anomalies, infections, impacted foreign bodies, sexual assault, etc. should be excluded.

Key points

Teenage girls with severe anemia should be enquired about their menstrual flow details and evaluated to assess the complications of anemia and other causes of anemia.

Neonatal Jaundice

Prolonged jaundice (both conjugated and unconjugated) is an occasional neonatal problem in congenital hypopituitarism. Unconjugated hyperbilirubinemia is common in congenital hypothyroidism. Diagnosis is by excluding other causes of neonatal jaundice and confirming the endocrine etiology by low serum levels of the hormones. **Footnote of Table 24.1** reveals the hormonal abnormalities in congenital hypothyroidism. Deficiencies of glucocorticoids, mineralocorticoids, and thyroxine can coexist in hypopituitarism. Assess the visual fixation of the baby (normally intact at birth) and examine for nystagmus. Absent visual fixation along with the presence of nystagmus at birth indicates *septo-optic dysplasia*.

Key points

In babies with hyperbilirubinemia due to hypopituitarism, absent visual fixation with presence of nystagmus indicates septo-optic dysplasia.

Fever with Tachycardia

Fever with tachycardia can indicate thyroid storm or thyroid crisis in infants with hyperthyroidism. Tachycardia unaccountable to the degree of fever may lead to atrial fibrillation, heart failure, and death. Trauma, infections, radioactive iodine treatment, or surgery in the hyperthyroid host are the precipitating factors. Hyperpyrexia, agitation, delirium, seizures, and coma can occur.

Key points

The possibility of fatal thyroid storm should be considered in hyperthyroid children presenting with fever and tachycardia.

Hypoglycemia

Hypoglycemia (HG) is encountered in T1DM, T2DM, AACI, HP, and CAH. See **Table 24.1** and the footnote along with the table for the clinical signs and diagnostic parameters of HG.

Classical Symptoms

Most endocrine disorders present with classical symptoms so that history and physical examination are almost diagnostic in them. Disorders of growth and nutrition, pubertal problems, anomalies of genital organs, developmental delay and physical affections of endocrine glands come in this group.

Refer Chapters 6, 7, 8, 9, 11, and 12 for the definition, terminologies, and diagnostic criteria of disorders of growth and nutrition, puberty, anomalies of genital organs and developmental delay.

Disorders of Growth and Nutrition

Disorders of growth and nutrition are short stature (growth retardation), tall stature (overgrowth syndrome), obesity, wasting, failure to thrive (FTT), and PEM.

Short stature (SS) (Ref. Ch. 11): Short stature in children is usually perceived by parents, grandparents, relatives, school teachers, or the staff in school health programs. In the routine clinical check-up of children, stature assessment is given importance always to detect short stature. Endocrine disorders with SS are hypothyroidism, hypopituitarism, Cushing's syndrome, and pseudohypoparathyroidism **(Fig. 24.3)**. Read **Footnote of Table 24.1** for the diagnostic features of *congenital hypothyroidism*. Family history of thyroid disease (autoimmune thyroiditis in mother), hypothyroidism, and goiter are common in babies with hypothyroidism. *Acquired hypothyroidism* predominantly affects older children and adolescents, presents as recent weight gain, declining school performance, cold intolerance, constipation, tiredness, hair loss, pubertal delay (rarely precocious puberty can occur), restlessness, nervousness, emotional instability and heat intolerance.

In *congenital hypopituitarism*, the salient diagnostic clues in history are neonatal apnea and severe hypoglycemia with intractable seizures; older children have SS and characteristic facial features **(Footnote of Table 24.1 MPHD)**.

Cushing syndrome babies present with excessive weight gain and chubby appearance **(Fig. 24.4)**. Older children have increased weight gain and linear growth retardation.

Children with *pseudohypoparathyroidism* have recurrent seizures with tetany and growth retardation. *Bone age (BA)* estimation is an important investigation to detect the cause of short stature in endocrine disorders, other major pathological conditions with growth failure and during therapy for any

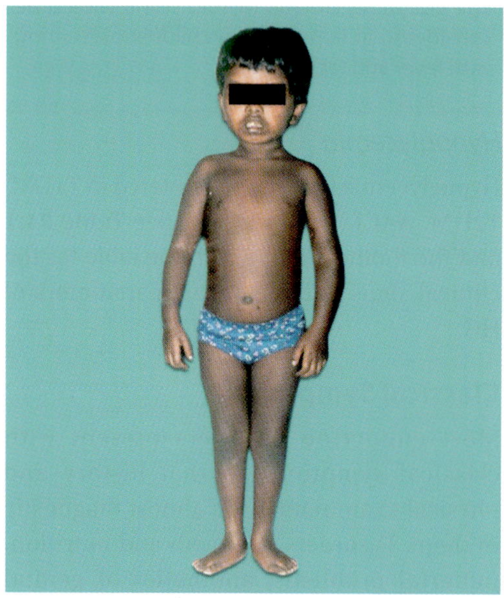

Fig. 24.3: Girl, 6 yr old with SS and intellectual subnormality due to hypothyroidism.

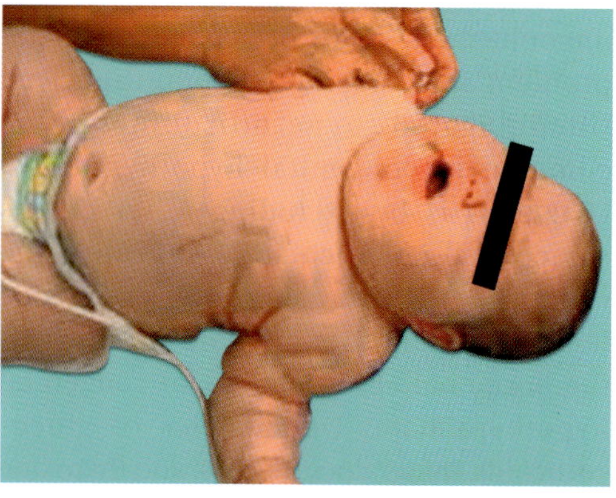

Fig. 24.4: Baby with Cushing's syndrome.

form of growth failure. In normal children, an orderly and predictable sequence of maturation of epiphyseal centers of growing bones occurs, the degree of maturity correlating with the biological age of the child. BA is the age in years that correlates well with sexual maturity and reveals the child's growth potential. Children with delayed BA have adequate growth potential if rectifiable, e.g., GH therapy in GH deficiency. Skiagram of the left hand (AP view) is the selected site for BA evaluation. The film should include the lower ends of ulna and radius, carpal bones and all digits up to the distal phalanges. Compare the maturation status of various epiphyses in the skiagram of the hand with age and sex matched standards such as Greulich and Pyles atlas or Tanner and Whitehouse chart. Software-based bone age assessment methods (BoneXpert) are available at present. **Table 24.4** shows the bone age of the normal child and different disorders of growth retardation. Significant retardation of bone age >2 yr age is a marker of pathological cause of SS over normal variants like constitutional delay in growth and puberty (CDGP) commonly referred as *"the late bloomers".*

TABLE 24.4: Bone age interpretation in growth retardation.

Diagnosis	*Parameters*
Normal growth	BA = CA = HA
FSS	BA = CA > HA
CDGP	BA = HA < CA
Endocrine diseases*	BA <HA < CA
Precocious puberty	BA = HA > CA

*Hypothyroidism, hypopituitarism, and Cushing syndrome

(BA: bone age; CA: chronologic age; CDGP: constitutional delay in growth and puberty; FSS: familial short stature; HA: height age)

Tall stature (TS) (Ref. Ch. 11): Tall stature is less common and is a rare complaint especially in boys. Rapid increase in growth in the pubertal period is perceived as pubertal growth spurt more so in boys. The main differential diagnosis is constitutional tall stature in which the parents and siblings are all tall and the patient's height exceeds the MPH. Endocrine causes of TS are fetal overgrowth in maternal diabetes, pituitary gigantism, estrogen receptor syndrome, McCune-Albright syndrome with excess GH secretion, the initial acceleration phase of precocious puberty and hyperthyroidism. TS is most often detected on routine growth assessment or incidentally during clinical examination of the child for some other illness.

Obesity (Ref. Ch. 11): It is increased body weight due to generalized accumulation of fat. Endocrine causes of obesity are hypothalamic disorders (hamartoma, trauma, tumors, cranial irradiation, TB, pyogenic meningitis, and demyelination), adrenocortical adenomas (Cushing syndrome), hypopituitarism, ACTH-secreting pituitary adenomas (Cushing disease), hypothyroidism, pseudohypoparathyroidism, hyperinsulinism, and ovarian disorders (PCOS). The commonest cause is iatrogenic obesity after prolonged corticosteroid therapy **(Fig. 11.15)** in nephrotic syndrome, malignancies, rheumatologic, inflammatory, and immune disorders. The main differentiation is from simple obesity in which height of the child exceeds the MPH, compared to the endocrine disordered obese child whose height is below the MPH. Clinical clues to suspect endocrine obesity are irregular menses, hirsutism, acne (PCOS), polyuria, polydipsia, acanthosis nigricans, constipation, developmental

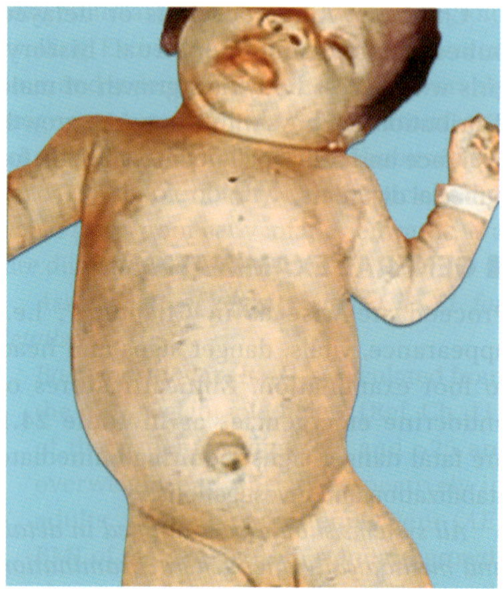

Fig. 24.6A: Infant with hypothyroidism—has puffy face, big tongue, distended abdomen, umbilical hernia and short lower segment.

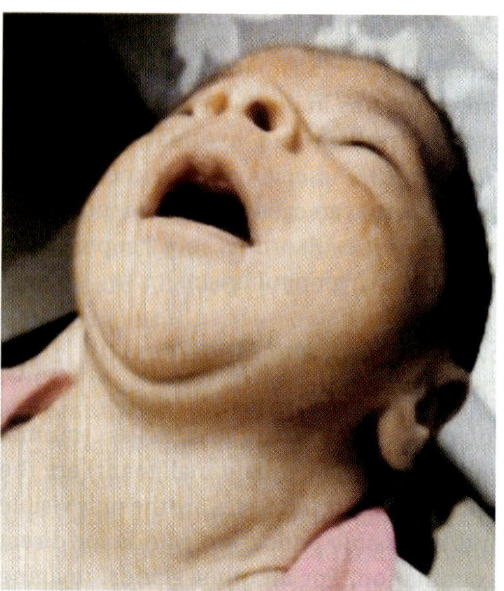

Fig. 24.6B: Rare picture of a hypothyroid infant with goiter.

apart from the features given in **Footnote of Table 24.1** for newborns. **Fig. 24.6A** is the picture of an infant with congenital hypothyroidism with macroglossia and umbilical hernia. Goiter (thyroid swelling) is more common in older children with acquired hypothyroidism. **Fig. 24.6B** shows the rare picture of a newborn with goiter.

Children with *growth hormone (GH) deficiency* have immature facies, protuberant eyes, midline cleft lip, single central incisor, truncal obesity, linear growth failure, and high-pitched voice **(Fig. 24.7)**.

In *septo-optic dysplasia*, characteristic visual field defects will be present. See **Footnote of Table 24.1** for the additional clinical features of hypopituitarism.

Cushing syndrome is the endocrine disorder caused by high blood levels of cortisol or other glucocorticoids. The most common cause is iatrogenic as in nephrotic syndrome and lymphoproliferative disorders on prolonged glucocorticoid therapy. Endocrine diseases with excess endogenous cortisol production are very rare **(Box 24.1)**. Infants (<1 yr) present with obesity, linear

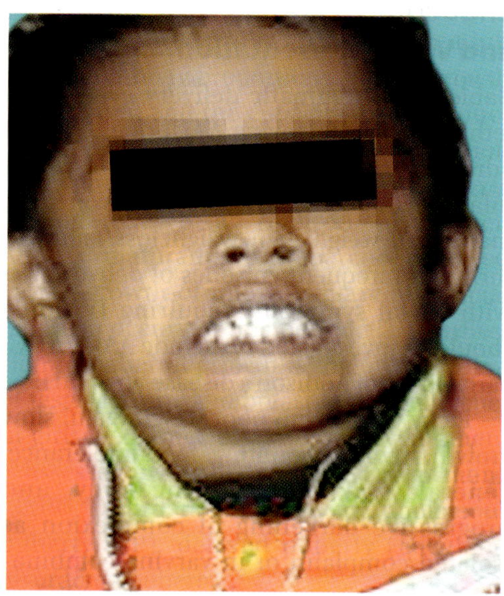

Fig. 24.7: Child with hypopituitarism and solitary median maxillary central incisor.

BOX 24.1: Causes of hypercortisolism (Cushing syndrome).

- *Iatrogenic:* Prolonged glucocorticoid therapy, exogenous corticotropin
- Bilateral adrenal hyperplasia, adrenocortical tumors (Adenoma)
- Hypersecretion of corticotropin (Cushing disease)
- *Ectopic ACTH secretion:*
  - Islet cell carcinoma pancreas
  - Neuroblastoma
  - Wilms tumor
  - Thymic carcinoma
- *ACTH independent syndromes:*
  - Primary pigmented nodular adrenocortical disease (PPNAD)
  - Carney complex
  - McCune-Albright syndrome

(ACTH: adrenocorticotropic hormone)

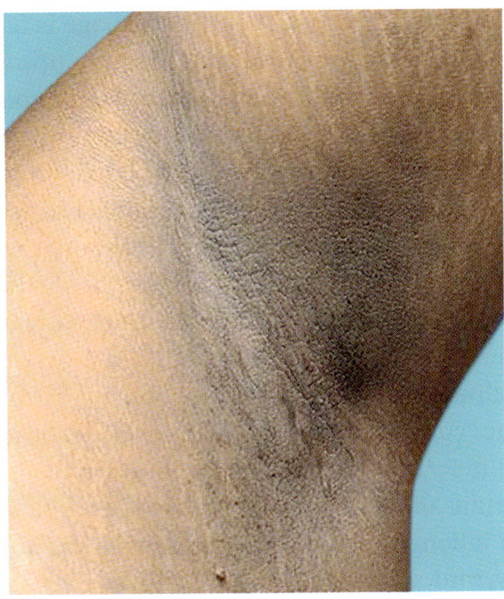

Fig. 24.8: Striae and hyperpigmentation over axilla in a child with Cushing syndrome.

growth retardation (length <3rd percentile), moon face [rounded face, prominent cheeks, and flushed appearance **(Fig. 24.4)**], and hypertension. Children reveal superficial striae (over hip, thigh, and abdomen), hirsutism, acne, central obesity, buffalo hump, muscle wasting, fatigue, abnormal masculinization (hirsutism over face and chest and deepening of voice in boys and clitoromegaly in girls) and axillary and pubic hair growth **(Fig. 24.8)**. Hyperglycemia and osteoporosis occur especially in iatrogenic patients. Hypertension and excess androgen effects are variable depending on the extent of hypersecretion of androgen and mineralocorticoids.

Hyperthyroidism or Grave's disease patients have eye pain, reveal proptosis with lid lag, chemosis, redness of conjunctiva, and warm moist skin. Exophthalmos is rare.

Examination of the thyroid gland: This butterfly-shaped gland (weight 10–20 g) is placed in front and sides of the trachea, between the cricoid cartilage and suprasternal notch, corresponding to the space between C_5-T_1 vertebrae. Sternocleidomastoid muscles on the sides form the lateral boundaries of the space. The patient may stand or sit on a stool (or on mother's lap), comfortably in a well-lit room. (For adolescent girls during examination, a chaperone should be present.) The gland is examined better from the back of the patient. Keep the neck in neutral or slightly extended position. On extending the neck further, the overlying tissues will be stretched which makes the gland more prominent and the abnormalities are revealed better.

Inspection: Inspect the gland directly, then turn the patient's head to right and left to see the lobes. Flash of a torchlight from the sides gives a better view of the gland. Normal thyroid gland is visible only in lean patients after neck extension. Swellings, pulsations, and changes in contour are better seen when the gland is enlarged.

Palpation: Move the tip of the index finger from the mentalis downward through the midline of the neck. Thyroid cartilage is felt as a firm mass with a notch at the upper midline part of the neck. Below the thyroid cartilage is the cricothyroid membrane followed by the firm cricoid cartilage. Palpate the isthmus of the thyroid gland just below the cricoid cartilage. For palpating the lobes of the gland, move the fingers on both sides laterally along the trachea, just medial to the sternocleidomastoid muscles. Palpate with the pulp of fingers and assess the consistency, symmetry, tenderness, diffuse/nodular feel of the lobes and the details of the regional lymph nodes (tender in inflammation, hard in malignancy of the thyroid gland). The gland moves up and down on swallowing saliva or a sip of water. The consistency is firm with bosselated appearance in hypothyroidism and soft and fleshy feel in hyperthyroidism.

Demonstration of goiter in neonates: Place the baby in supine position on the bed. The examiner's left hand is placed under the back and shoulder blades of the baby. Infant's trunk is slowly raised from the bed with this hand. As the head falls backwards, goiter becomes evident. In older children, evaluate the size of thyroid using *"rule of thumb"*. Each lobe of the normal thyroid gland has approximately the size of the terminal phalanx of the child's thumb. *Auscultation* over the thyroid mass may reveal bruit. Continuous bruit suggests Grave's disease. Systolic bruit is mostly carotid in origin or less often part of the cardiac cycle. *Disorders of thyroid gland* are reduced and excessive hormone synthesis (hypo- and hyperthyroidism), thyroid dysgenesis, and goiter **(Fig. 24.6B)**. Primary hypothyroidism is decreased thyroxine secretion by the diseased thyroid gland. Central hypothyroidism due to pituitary disorders is secondary hypothyroidism and those due to hypothalamic disorders are tertiary hypothyroidism. **Box 24.2** reveals the causes of congenital hypothyroidism.

Ectopic thyroid presents as lingual thyroid **(Fig. 20.16)** or as a mass along the line of migration of thyroglossal duct to the diaphragm. Pressure effects of goiter as *dysphagia* (by lingual thyroid or esophageal compression), *dysphonia,* irritant cough, stridor, and choking due to laryngeal compression and *dyspnea* from tracheal compression are the usual symptoms. *Thyroid dysgenesis* often presents as hypothyroidism. *Goiter* is detected incidentally or on routine clinical examination. Thyroxine synthesis is reduced due to enzyme defects in thyroid dyshormonogenesis in which goiter often coexists. In *hypothalamic and pituitary disorders,* growth problems (obesity and short stature) and neurologic deficits with features of hypothyroidism will be present. Transient hypothyroidism occurs in preterms, sick newborns, and babies of mothers with autoimmune thyroiditis or those on thyroxine therapy. **Box 24.3** shows the diseases producing goiter in children.

Hashimoto's thyroiditis is autoimmune destruction of thyroid gland *(chronic lymphocytic thyroiditis)* and is the leading cause of acquired hypothyroidism in children >6 yr affecting girls mainly. Thyroid is uniformly enlarged, nontender, and usually euthyroid (can be hypothyroid or rarely

BOX 24.2: Causes of congenital hypothyroidism.

- *Thyroid dysgenesis:*
  - Ectopic thyroid
  - Athyreosis (absent thyroid)
- Thyroid dyshormonogenesis
- Thyroxine resistance
- Hypothalamic diseases
- Pituitary disorders
- Transient hypothyroidism

hyperthyroid). USG thyroid and T_4, TSH assay confirm the diagnosis. Thyroiditis is detected by increased levels of serum TPO-Abs (Thyroid peroxidase antibodies) and Tg-Abs (thyroglobulin antibodies). Thyroid scintigraphy and biopsy are rarely needed for diagnosis. WHO grading system to assess the goiter size initially and on follow-up is given in **Box 24.4**.

Iodine deficiency is worldwide; it is endemic in Himalayan areas in India. Endemic goiter and endemic cretinism are the manifestations. The latter presents as neurologic or myxedematous types. Intellectual disability, deaf mutism, gait disturbances, and pyramidal signs appear in both types. Normal growth and development along with goiter occur in the neurologic group whereas in the myxedematous patients growth and sexual development are delayed and myxedema is present without goiter. Low serum T_4 (total and free) and high TSH are diagnostic.

BOX 24.3: Causes of goiter in children.

- Autoimmune thyroiditis
- Iodine deficiency disorders
- Goitrogens
- Familial dyshormonogenesis
- Idiopathic simple goiter
- Inflammatory thyroiditis

BOX 24.4: WHO grading of goiter.

- *Grade 0:* No goiter is present (the thyroid impalpable and invisible)
- *Grade 1:* Neck thickening is present as a result of enlarged thyroid, palpable, however, not visible in normal position of neck; the thickened mass moves upward during swallowing. Grade 1 includes also nodular goiter if thyroid enlargement remains invisible
- *Grade 2:* Neck swelling, visible when the neck is in normal position, corresponding to enlarged thyroid found in palpation

Goitrogens are foods which compete with iodine against thyroid uptake leading to compensatory hypertrophy of the gland. The common ones are Cassava, linseed, sweet potato, cabbage, cauliflower, broccoli, turnips, soy and millets.

Idiopathic simple goiter affects adolescent girls and is often familial. Periodic evaluation is a must to exclude pathologic transformation.

Inflammatory thyroiditis follows bacterial or viral infections of the respiratory tract. Common pathogens are alpha hemolytic streptococci, *Staphylococcus aureus*, gram-negative bacteria, and anaerobes. Mycobacterial, fungal, and pneumocystis infections occur in immunocompromised children. Recurrent or mixed infections indicate underlying thyroglossal duct remnant or pyriform sinus fistula.

Nodular thyromegaly is due to benign or malignant tumors of the thyroid. It is rare in children and has the risk of malignancy up to 25%. Regional lymphadenopathy of hard consistency and rapid deterioration are common.

Skeletal anomalies should be scrutinized in all children with endocrine disorders. Limb anomalies are usual in pseudohypoparathyroidism which include brachydactyly, dorsal dimpling of the hand and feet due to short metacarpals [Archibald's metacarpal sign **(Fig. 7.38 and Fig. 24.2)**] and metatarsals. The index finger and second toe are longer than the middle finger and third toe, due to the sparing of the second metacarpal and metatarsal from shortening.

Sexual maturity rating (SMR): (Ref. Ch. 11 for SMR). Assess the SMR in all children to exclude precocious or delayed puberty. The first sign of puberty in boys is testicular enlargement by 9–14 yr and in girls breast bud development (thelarche) by 8–12 yr age. Pubic hair development closely follows thelarche in girls and testicular enlargement in boys.

Testicular volume is ideally measured by the Prader orchidometer (Dr Andrea Prader, Swiss endocrinologist, 1966). It consists of a string with groups of wooden beads of different colors arranged in increasing size **(Fig. 7.42)**. The beads are numbered as per the volume of testis in mL as 1, 2, 3, 4, 5, 6, 8, 10, 12, 15, 20, and 25. Compare the patient's testes with the beads. The testis which matches in size with the number written on the bead is selected as the one with that volume. Each testis should be assessed separately. Testicular volumes of 1, 2, and 3 mL are prepubertal size. *Volume ≥4 mL* indicates the onset of *true puberty*.

If an orchidometer is not available, testicular length can be measured in the longest diameter. Preadolescent testes are 1.5–2 cm. Adult testes are up to 3.5–5 cm. The left testis is slightly smaller than the right and remains lower in the scrotum compared to the right.

Pubertal disorders are *precocious puberty* [(PP) first sign of puberty appearing in boys <9 yr and in girls <8 yr], *delayed puberty* [(DP) failure of development of secondary sexual characters by 13 yr in girls and 14 yr in boys] and *disordered puberty* (puberty with chaotic functions of internal sex organs). PP can be gonadotropin dependent [primary/idiopathic/central (CPP)] due to premature activation of hypothalamic-pituitary-gonadal (HPG) axis or organic/secondary (SPP) in which the sex steroids are produced by gonads stimulated by the CNS disorders. In *peripheral precocious puberty (PPP)*, which is gonadotropin independent, sex steroids are produced from the gonads or other organs and the presentation can be isosexual or heterosexual in type.

Evaluation of the child with precocious puberty (Ref. ***Box 24.5****):* In *primary (central) PP*, the HPG axis set point is preponed, starting and completion of the pubertal process occurs at an earlier age. History will reveal increased growth velocity and younger age of attainment of puberty in parents and siblings. These patients reveal early growth spurt and advanced osseous maturation. Girls outnumber boys four times, pubertal process starts by 6–8 yr; the SMR stages of puberty and the duration of puberty simulate normal puberty. LH (assay done at mid puberty) and estradiol >50 pg/mL (assay done 20–24 hr after leuprolide stimulation) are confirmatory points for the diagnosis of CPP. Physiologic enlargement of pituitary from MRI scan of the brain and pelvic ultrasonography reporting normal pubertal changes of ovaries and uterus are supportive for the diagnosis of CPP.

In *secondary PP (isosexual)*, age of onset is often <4 yr, boys are affected more and the most common cause is hypothalamic hamartoma. Pubertal process is faster and the final pubertal stage may not be similar to normal puberty. Neuroendocrine manifestations [gelastic seizures, diabetes insipidus, hyperthermia, adipsia (lack of thirst), obesity/cachexia, and unusual laughing and crying] or visual defects and proptosis may appear 1–2 yr prior to the radiological detection of such tumors. Imaging studies confirm the diagnosis. Growth hormone deficiency may coexist which may be unnoticed because of the growth spurt induced by gonadal steroids. *Peripheral PP* is the *least common* seen in less than one-fourth of all children with sexual precocity. These patients have increased estrogen or testosterone values with low gonadotropins and lack of pubertal response to gonadotropin-releasing hormone

BOX 24.5: Common causes of precocious puberty.

Central precocious puberty (CPP) in both sex groups:
- *Primary (idiopathic):* Familial (advancement in HPG axis set point)
- *Secondary (organic—CNS affections):*
  - *Tumors:* Hamartoma, germinoma, astrocytoma, adenoma, glioma
  - *Malformations:* Hydrocephalus, arachnoid cyst, myelomeningocele
  - *Infections:* Postmeningitis/encephalitis, abscess, neuro-TB
  - *Insults:* Head trauma, neurosurgery, perinatal asphyxia, cerebral palsy
  - Demyelination
  - *Iatrogenic:* Low dose cranial irradiation (18–24 Gy), chemotherapy
  - Miscellaneous

Peripheral precocious puberty (PPP):
- *Girls:*
  - Long-standing hypothyroidism
  - McCune–Albright syndrome
  - Benign follicular cysts
  - *Tumors:* Granulosa—theca cell tumors, arrhenoblastoma, teratoma
  - *Adrenal estrogen:* Feminizing adrenal neoplasia
  - *Exogenous estrogen:* Medications and phytoestrogens
- *Boys:*
  - *Adrenal source of androgen:*
  - Congenital adrenal hyperplasia (CAH)
  - *Adrenal tumors:* Virilizing adenoma, carcinoma
- *Testicular source of androgen:*
  - *Tumors:* Leydig cell tumor, adrenal rest tumor
  - *Apparent LH excess:* Testotoxicosis (FMPP)
  - *hCG-secreting tumors:* Germinoma, choriocarcinoma, hepatoblastoma
  - *Exogenous androgen exposure:* Testosterone creams, medications
- *Heterosexual precocity:*
  - *Virilization in girls:* CAH, virilizing ovarian/adrenal neoplasia, PCOD
  - *Feminization in boys:* Estrogen secreting adrenal tumor, exogenous estrogens
- *Variations in pubertal development:*
  - Premature thelarche
  - Premature adrenarche/pubarche
  - Premature isolated menarche
  - Adolescent gynecomastia in boys
  - Macroorchidism

(CNS: central nervous system; hCG: human chorionic gonadotropin; HPG: hypothalamic-pituitary-gonadal; LH: luteinizing hormone; PCOD: polycystic ovarian disease)

(GnRH) stimulation. History and physical examination with relevant investigations will unveil the diagnosis. See **Table 24.5** for the evaluation of a child with PP.

Premature thelarche is early onset of isolated breast development by 1–2 yr age (usual type) and is self-regressing. Rarely the enlarged breasts may remain as such till the onset of true puberty. Other features of puberty (linear growth acceleration, hormonal surge, uterus enlargement, external genitalia changes, and bone age acceleration) will be absent. It is due to the sensitization of the infant's breast tissue to

TABLE 24.5: Evaluation of a child with precocious puberty.

History	*Physical examination*
• Family H/O early puberty • H/O neurological illness, congenital adrenal hyperplasia (CAH) • H/O medications—steroids (O/T*)	Plot accurate height, weight, growth velocity: • *Girls-look for;* early estrogenic effects (staging of breasts, pink color of vaginal mucosa); androgenic effects: stage of pubic hair and clitoromegaly • *Boys—assess;* testicular volume, penile size, and pubic hair • Both groups—examine the skin for acne and cafe-au-lait spots proceed for detailed neurological examination as well as other systems

**Topical*

the ovarian estrogens following transient gonadotropin release or transient estrogen release from the follicular ovarian cysts. Patient follow-up will reveal normal pubertal development.

Premature adrenarche or pubarche is premature (<*8 yr* in girls, <*9 yr* in boys) development of pubic hair followed by axillary hair. It is more frequent in females. Excess growth acceleration, advanced bone age >2 SD from the mean age, cystic acne, adult type body odor due to premature production of adrenal androgens if detected in girls, nonclassic CAH due to 21-hydroxylase deficiency is to be excluded by ACTH stimulation test with 17-OHP estimation. Acanthosis nigricans indicates PCOS requiring investigation.

Premature isolated menarche is regular menstrual bleeding cycles without other pubertal changes and gets self-corrected after a short period. Transient rise in ovarian activity leading to isolated follicular cyst development and increase in estradiols with normal gonadotropins will be seen. Increased sensitivity of the endometrium to circulating estrogen levels too low to produce breast development is considered another possibility. Hypothyroidism, MAS, ovarian pathologies, sexual abuse, vaginal foreign body, or tumor, all should be excluded.

The most common cause of PP is CAH which should be suspected clinically as given below:

Female neonate: Can reveal varying degrees of virilization of genitalia from minimal clitoromegaly to complete fusion of the labia mimicking “male” genitalia without gonads, pigmentation of the areola and genital skin.

Male neonate: Symptoms range from mild (failure to thrive) to catastrophic (sudden infant death); vague complaints as poor feeding, lethargy, weight loss with failure to thrive; persistent vomiting, unaccountable dehydration and hemodynamic collapse with impending salt losing adrenal crisis.

Simple virilizing form of CAH: Female babies present with signs of virilization; males normal at birth, may present in early childhood with signs of precocious pseudo-puberty (sexual precocity, pubic hair development or growth acceleration due to premature androgen excess).

Delayed puberty (DP): The most common cause of DP is constitutional delay in growth and puberty (CDGP), more common in boys. Causes of DP can be disorders of hypothalamus or pituitary (hypogonadotropic hypogonadism) or primary gonadal failure (hyper gonadotropic hypogonadism). The causes of DP are given in **Box 24.6** and the evaluation of DP in **Table 24.6**.

Micropenis (Ref. Ch. 7) is stretched penile length (SPL) < –2.5 SD below the mean for the age or stage of sexual development. Mean penile length of a newborn is 3.5 cm. *SPL <1.9* cm in a newborn is micropenis and a child with *SPL <4 cm* must be evaluated. Technique of measuring the SPL is in Chapter 7. **Box 24.7** reveals the disorders with micropenis. **Table 24.7** gives the clinical clues for diseases with micropenis.

Disorders of sexual development (DSD) mainly manifest as ambiguous genitalia. They are 46 XX DSD, 46 XY DSD, or ovotesticular DSD. The common causes of ambiguous genitalia are CAH and gonadal dysgenesis. Dysmorphic features with life-threatening cardiac or renal defects indicate Campomelic

BOX 24.6: Causes of delayed puberty.

Physiological: Self-limited delayed puberty
Pathological:
- *Hypergonadotropic hypogonadism:*
  - *Male:* Klinefelter syndrome, congenital anorchia, testicular regression, mumps
  - *Female:* Turner syndrome, premature ovarian insufficiency
  - *Both:* Chemotherapy, radiotherapy, galactosemia, gonadal dysgenesis
- *Hypogonadotropic hypogonadism:*
  - Isolated hypogonadotropic hypogonadism
  - Protein–energy malnutrition syndrome
  - Combined pituitary hormone deficiency
  - Drug-induced (prolonged steroid therapy)
  - CNS tumors, infiltrative diseases
  - Kallmann syndrome
  - Chemotherapy and radiotherapy
  - Functional hypogonadotropic hypogonadism
  - Systemic illness (heart disease, IBD, celiac disease)
  - Hypothyroidism
  - Excessive physical activity

(CNS: central nervous system)

TABLE 24.6: Evaluation of children with delayed puberty.

History	*Physical examination*
• Family H/O of childhood growth pattern and age at pubertal onset; delayed menarche in mother and delayed adult height completion in father indicate CDGP • F/H of Turner/Klinefelter suggests chromosomal anomalies with pubertal delay • H/O chronic systemic illness (IBD, celiac disease, thyroid/cardiac/RS disorders, diabetes, mumps) • *Neurological symptoms:* Headache, visual disturbances (midline lesions), anosmia (Kallmann syndrome) • Nutritional history (undernutrition) • Medication history (prolonged steroid therapy) • H/O undescended testis, trauma/radiation to testes (gonadal damage) • H/O chemotherapy/radiotherapy (gonadal damage)	• Growth parameters, features of undernutrition/chromosomal anomalies/chronic illness • Pubertal assessment—SMR staging; genital anomalies for micropenis, absent testes; urethral anomalies • Features of chromosomal anomalies—Turner syndrome **(Figs. 24.9A and B)**, Klinefelter syndrome • Signs of hypothyroidism; thyroid anomalies • CNS examination in detail, fundus evaluation

(CDGP: constitutional delay in growth and puberty; CNS: central nervous system)

BOX 24.7: Disorders with micropenis.

- *Hypogonadotropic hypogonadism (hypothalamic and pituitary disorders):*
  - Isolated growth hormone deficiency
  - Multiple pituitary hormone deficiencies
  - Kallmann syndrome
  - Laurence–Moon–Biedl syndrome
  - Prader–Willi syndrome
- *Hypergonadotropic hypogonadism (testicular disorders):*
  - Anorchia (vanishing testis syndrome)
  - Chromosomal abnormalities (Klinefelter and poly-X syndromes)
  - Gonadal dysgenesis (incomplete form)
  - Testosterone steroidogenesis (incomplete form)
  - Androgen receptor defects (incomplete form)
  - 5-α reductase deficiency (incomplete form)
- *Developmental abnormalities:*
  - Penis agenesis (aphallia)

TABLE 24.7: Clinical clues for diseases with micropenis.

Clinical findings	***Disease***
Neonatal hypoglycemia, prolonged jaundice, midline facial defects, short stature	Hypopituitarism **(Fig. 24.7)**
Hyperpigmentation, hypoglycemia, weight loss, dehydration, shock, ambiguous genitalia	Congenital adrenal hypoplasia (CAH) **(Fig. 7.41)**
Failure to thrive	Genetic syndromes
Family history of unexplained sibling death/similar illness among blood relatives	Defects in steroidogenesis (e.g., CAH), androgen insensitivity syndrome

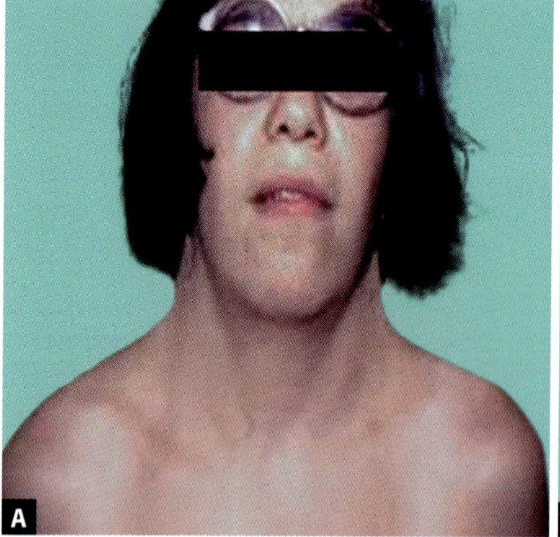

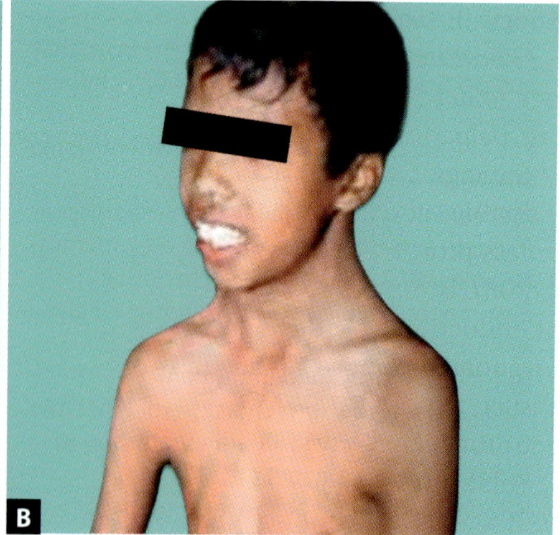

Figs. 24.9A and B: (A) Turner syndrome girl 12 yr with webbing of the neck, delayed puberty; (B) Boy with Noonan syndrome—note webbing of neck and shield chest.

BOX 24.8: Classification of disorders of sexual development.

46XY DSD (male pseudohermaphrodite):
- *Gonadal development disorders:* Ovotesticular DSD, complete or partial gonadal dysgenesis, testicular regression
- *Androgen synthesis abnormalities:* STAR, CYP11A1, 3B2HSD, POR, CYP17A1, 17B3HSD, SRD5A2
- *Androgen action problems:* Complete and partial androgen insensitivity
- *Others:* Persistent Müllerian duct syndrome (PMDS), severe hypospadias

46XX DSD (female pseudohermaphrodite):
- *Gonadal development disorders:* Ovotesticular DSD, testicular DSD, gonadal dysgenesis
- *Androgen excess:* CAH, placental aromatase deficiency, exogenous administration

Sex chromosomal DSD 46 XX DSD (female pseudohermaphrodite):
- *45X:* Turner syndrome and variants
- *47XXY:* Klinefelter syndrome and variants

(CAH: congenital adrenal hypoplasia; DSD: disorders of sexual development)

TABLE 24.8: Clinical clues for diseases with DSD.

Pointers	*Disorders*
Dysmorphic features	Chromosomal disorders
No palpable gonads	Gonadal dysgenesis/external virilization of a genetic female
Sick baby/hyperpigmentation of genitalia	Congenital adrenal hyperplasia
Asymmetry of genitalia	Mixed gonadal dysgenesis

(DSD: disorders of sexual development)

dwarfism, Denys-Drash syndrome, and Antley-Bixler syndrome.

Locating the gonads is the most important step to determine the child's sex in DSD. For this, palpate the gonads through the full length of the inguinal canal from above downward. Palpable gonads are usually the testes unless proven otherwise. Testicular volume *<12 mL* is *microorchidism* which can occur in endocrine disorders, genetic syndromes or gonadal damage as given in **Box 24.7**. Testicular volumes >20 mL before puberty or >30 mL after puberty indicate *macroorchidism*. Fragile X syndrome, idiopathic sexual precocity, FSH-secreting pituitary macroadenomas, testicular tumors or teratoma and aromatase deficiency are the causes of macroorchidism.

Assess the symmetry of external genital structures, severity of virilization, and the position of the urethra. Symmetrically virilized external genitalia with absent gonads is female with CAH. Asymmetrical external genitalia is mixed gonadal dysgenesis (45X/46XY). Symmetrical but incomplete genital development with palpable gonads suggest male with incomplete sexual differentiation. **Box 24.8** reveals the classification of DSD and **Table 24.8** gives the clinical clues for diseases with DSD.

SUGGESTED READING

1. Amanizadeh M. Higher prevalence of permanent congenital hypothyroidism in the Southwest of Iran mostly caused by

dyshormonogenesis: a five-year follow-up study. Arch Endocriol Metab. 2018;62(6): 602-8.

2. Desai PM, Menon PSN, Bhatia V. Pediatric Endocrine Disorders, 3rd edition. Hyderabad: Universities Press (India) Private Ltd.; 2014.
3. Dutta D, Jain R, Kumar M. Solitary median maxillary central incisor, a clinical predictor of hypoplastic anterior pituitary, ectopic neuro-hypophysis and growth hormone deficiency. J Ped Endocr Metabol. 2013;26(9-10):1-2.
4. Khadilkar A, Ekbote V, Chiplonkar S, Khadilkar V, Kajale N, Kulkarni S, et al. Waist Circumference Percentiles in 2-18 Year Old Indian Children. J Pediatr. 2014;164:1358-62.
5. Kliegman RM. Nelson Textbook of Pediatrics, 21st edition, International Edition. Amsterdam: Elsevier; 2019.
6. Paul VK, Bagga A. Ghai Essential Pediatrics, 10th edition. New Delhi: CBS Publishers and Distributors Pvt Ltd.; 2023.
7. Sarna A, Porwal A, Acharya R, Ashraf S, Ramesh S, Khan N, et al. Waist circumference, waist-to-height ratio and BMI percentiles in children aged 5 to 19 years in India: A population-based study. Obes Sci Pract. 2021;7(4):392-404.
8. Singh M. Pediatric Clinical Methods, 6th edition. New Delhi: CBS Publishers and Distributors Pvt Ltd.; 2020.
9. WHO. (2008). Waist Circumference and Waist-Hip Ratio: Report of a WHO Expert Consultation. [online] Available from https://www.who.int/publications/i/item/9789241501491. [Last accessed September, 2024]

25

CHAPTER

Musculoskeletal System

S Letha, Suresh S Vadakedom, Suma Balan

Chapter Outline

INTRODUCTION

(Read Chapters 6, 7, 11, 12, and 21 before you proceed)

Musculoskeletal disorders (MSDs) are becoming increasingly common in pediatrics. They are characterized by chronic/recurrent pain, long-standing disability, loss of school days, poor academic achievement, progressive deformities, physical compromise in jobs and growth defects leading to tremendous economic loss for the family as well as to the nation. Though majority are benign in nature, progression to chronic and crippling situations can occur in a good number of patients mostly because of delay in treatment or improper/irregular treatment; malignancies or potentially life-threatening complications are increasingly recognized. Early and correct diagnosis by systematic clinical assessment and proper investigations and appropriate treatment can ameliorate the morbidity and bring down the mortality of these disorders.

CLINICAL APPROACH

History and physical examination are the main steps in diagnosis of MSD. The causes can be congenital (mostly affecting children) and acquired. Clinical diagnosis in congenital MSD is easy due to the obvious external anomalies from birth (e.g., *clubfoot*—***Fig. 12.6***), genetic disorders (*achondroplasia*—***Fig. 11.13***) or part of syndromic manifestation (Marfan syndrome). An important exception is developmental dysplasia of hip (DDH), which unless specifically examined will not be detected in time and finally ends up with obvious deformity and disability. In acquired diseases, infants are unable to report the symptoms or locate the site affected (e.g., septic arthritis/osteomyelitis), the communications by older children or the accompanying adult may be vague and nonspecific—all leading to late or wrong diagnosis. Timely diagnosis of MSD is crucial, since early appropriate treatment reduces death and disability.

The objectives of clinical approach to MSD should be—(1) to make a correct diagnosis at the earliest, (2) to assess the severity and outcome of the illness, and (3) to plan the immediate and long-term management.

Symptom analysis and physical examination are the important steps for correct diagnosis.

SYMPTOM ANALYSIS

Pain, limping, fever, paucity of movements, inability to bear weight, swelling, weakness, stiffness of limbs, deformity, erythema, and motor delay are the common symptoms. Skin lesions may be the initial presentation in systemic lupus erythematosus (SLE), Kawasaki disease (KD), and dermatomyositis. The possibility of MSD should be considered in children presenting with acute life-threatening situations like shock (KD), cardiac failure (Rheumatic carditis), and seizures, hypertension, and renal failure (SLE).

Pain is the leading symptom in MSD, the intensity ranging from mild to severe (can be quantified by pain rating scale from the facial expression as shown in **Figure 7.20**). Most children are unable to localize pain. Ask the child or parent to point to the exact area affected with one fingertip. Make an attempt to differentiate between joint pain and musculoskeletal pain. Note the *S*ite, *O*nset, *C*haracter, *R*adiation, *A*ssociated factors, *T*iming, *E*xacerbating and relieving factors and *S*everity (SOCRATES). Analyze when and how the problem started, relation to trauma (common in boys), fever (rheumatic fever, osteomyelitis, septic arthritis, and pyomyositis) and whether the symptoms are confined to bone, muscles, or soft tissues. High fever, joint pain (constant, increased by movement), swelling, local heat, and limitation of joint movement suggest septic arthritis. Past history of bleeding episodes or recurrent painful joint swelling in a boy denotes hemophilia **(Fig. 25.1)**.

Features if suggestive of arthritis, look for the distribution and the number and type of joints involved. Morning stiffness associated with arthritis is seen with inflammatory disorders. *Monoarthritis* is the presentation in trauma, septic arthritis, hemarthrosis, and gout **(Fig. 25.2)**. Polyarthritis usually indicates inflammatory or systemic disorders like infections, SLE, juvenile idiopathic arthritis (JIA), rheumatic fever (RF), or malignancies. *Symmetrical* involvement of multiple joints can occur in polyarticular JIA, SLE, and polyarteritis nodosa (PAN). *Asymmetrical* involvement is seen in ERA-JIA (enthesitis-related arthritis JIA) and psoriatic JIA. In *flitting* pain, joint inflammation begins in one joint and then serially involves other joints, usually affecting one at a time for about 1–3 days. It is typical of acute RF but is occasionally seen in gonococcal and meningococcal arthritis, acute leukemia, and inflammatory bowel disease. In *enthesitis* (inflammation of fascia and areas of tendon attachments to bones) seen in ERA-JIA and other rheumatoid diseases, pain is severe and increases with movement.

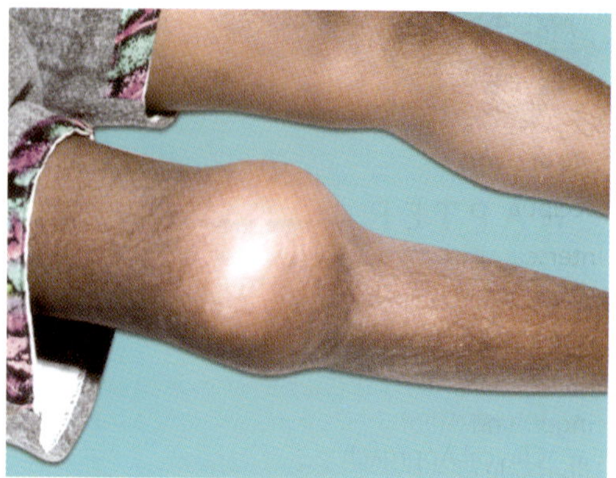

Fig. 25.1: Hemarthrosis R knee of boy with hemophilia.

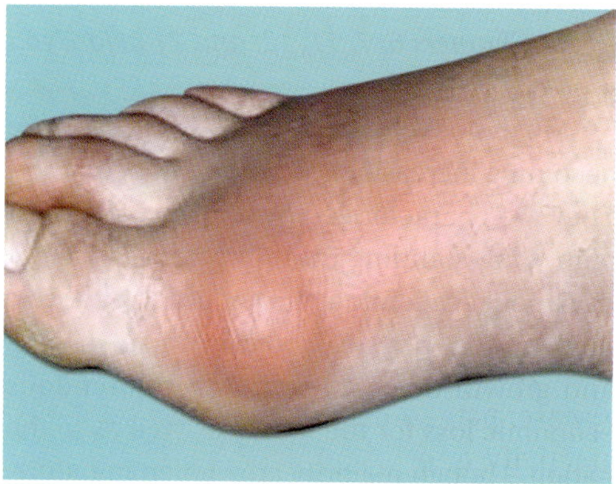

Fig. 25.2: Gouty arthritis of metatarsalphalangeal joint.

TABLE 25.1: Common patterns of referred and radicular musculoskeletal pain.

Site of pain perception	*Site of pathology*
Occiput	C1, 2
Interscapular region	C3, 4
Tip of shoulder, upper outer aspect of arm	C5
Interscapular region or radial fingers and thumb	C6, 7
Ulnar side of forearm, ring and little fingers	C8
Medial aspect of upper arm	T1
Chest	Thoracic spine
Buttocks, knees, legs	Lumbar spine
Lateral aspect of upper arm	Shoulder
Forearm	Elbow
Anterior thigh, knee	Hip
Thigh, hip	Knee

Pain on activity but getting relieved with rest is typical of mechanical joint disease; pain and stiffness after a period of inactivity and disappearing after up and active suggest degenerative joint disease. Early morning stiffness is characteristic of juvenile rheumatoid arthritis (JRA). Pain can sometimes be referred from adjacent structures, joints or nerve roots or radicular pain **(Table 25.1)**. Consider *referred pain* from the hip or thigh, when the child has knee pain without any evidence of localized disease at the knee. Morning stiffness (*synovial gel phenomenon*) and improvement of symptoms with activity suggest inflammatory arthritis, whereas improvement with rest suggests mechanical disorders.

Bone pain is deep, nonarticular and increases at night; may indicate occult trauma, osteomyelitis, fractures, and malignancies. Suspect primary osteoarticular malignancy in adolescents with localized bone pain. Other diseases presenting with bone pain are osteoid osteoma, chronic nonbacterial osteomyelitis, and chronic recurrent multifocal osteomyelitis. *Scurvy* due to vitamin C deficiency is a rare disease in children with bleeding tendency producing subperiosteal bleeding; this deficiency disease follows severe food restriction or food faddism **(Fig. 25.3)**.

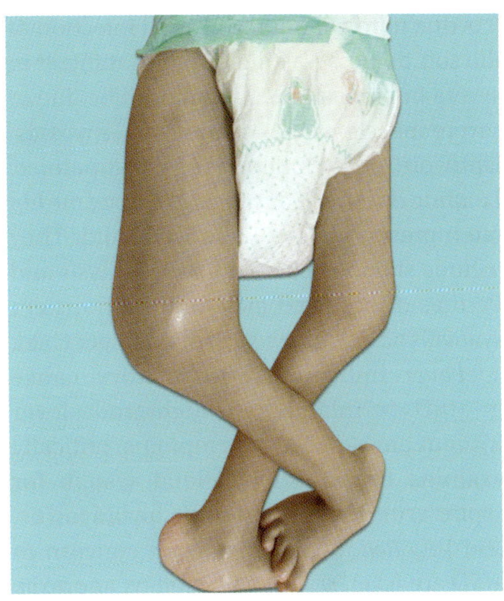

Fig. 25.3: Child with spastic CP revealing subperiosteal bleeding of right femur due to scurvy.

Muscle pain follows trauma or infection and can lead to localized weakness. Generalized muscle pain and tenderness occur in viral infections (echo, coxsackie, rubella, chikungunya, and dengue), leptospirosis (mainly affects pelvic girdle and calf muscles), and trichinosis (specifically involves masseters, intercostals, and diaphragm). Weakness of muscles due to neurological problems can be excluded, if superficial and deep reflexes of the area are preserved.

Limping is a complaint when the lower limb joints are affected minimally. Most often it is due to trivial trauma or mild infection of the soft tissues. Walking becomes difficult in severe inflammation. Limping can be due to severe muscle pain as seen in viral myositis, leptospirosis, or inflammatory myopathies. *Limping due to orthopedic problems of the hip* often presents acutely in a well child. They include slipped upper femoral epiphysis and Perthes disease and may follow a transient synovitis or *"irritable hip"* in the younger child.

Fever indicates inflammatory cause in MSD. In infants with high-grade fever without any associated symptoms, critically examine the musculoskeletal system for septic arthritis, osteomyelitis, pyomyositis, and JIA. *Red flags* that warrant concern *in MSD* are fever, malaise, irritability, anorexia, weight loss, or raised inflammatory markers.

Paucity of movements/inability to bear weight indicates severe MSD—former seen in infants and latter in older children. Unintentional trauma, battered child, severe local infections, hematoma, and malignancies are the common problems.

Swelling: The triad of arthritis is pain, swelling, and limitation of movements of the joint. In arthralgia, only pain is present. In a swollen joint, the normal hollows around the joint will be obliterated and the joint space will be increased as seen in **Fig. 25.1** revealing hemarthrosis of knee. Acute onset of swelling following injury can be due to contusion, fracture, or hemarthrosis, mostly in children involved in sports activities.

The *distribution of joint involvement* may suggest the underlying systemic diseases—the first metatarsophalangeal (MTP) joint is classically affected in gout [**(Fig. 25.2)** extremely rare in childhood]; the metacarpophalangeal (MCP) joints and proximal interphalangeal (PIP) joints in rheumatoid arthritis **(Fig. 25.4)**; and the distal interphalangeal (DIP) joints and the first carpometacarpal joint in osteoarthritis (unusual in children). Patients with inflammatory arthritis may have low-grade fever; high fever with chills usually suggests septic arthritis. Generalized edema or diffuse swelling may be noted in SLE, dermatomyositis, or other inflammatory conditions.

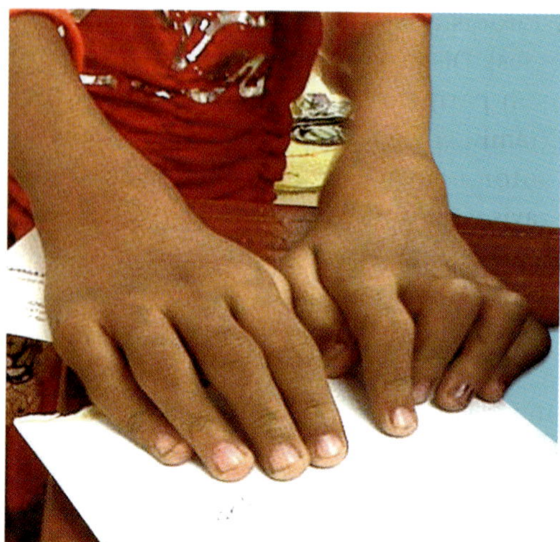

Fig. 25.4: Arthritis of PIP and wrist joints in JIA. (PIP: proximal interphalangeal; JIA: juvenile idiopathic arthritis)

Weakness denotes neurological or muscular problems. Weakness of neuro-muscular diseases should be differentiated from "pseudoparalysis" of painful conditions seen in osteomyelitis, septic arthritis, scurvy, and hematoma by eliciting deep tendon reflexes which will be normal in pseudoparalysis. Joint disorders cause limitation of movements often attributed as weakness. Weakness following trauma may also be due to peripheral nerve injury along with fracture or muscle injury. Predominantly proximal type of weakness suggests a primary muscle disease of inflammatory (polymyositis and dermatomyositis) or noninflammatory myopathy [thyrotoxicosis, drug induced (steroids and statins) or muscular dystrophies]. Distal weakness is often neurological as in peripheral neuropathy, vitamin B_{12}/thiamine deficiencies or hereditary sensory motor neuropathy. Suspect myasthenia gravis if the weakness worsens by evening or intermittent weakness follows activity.

Stiffness of joints or the reporting of reduced/uncomfortable range of movement is worst on awakening in the mornings and improves throughout the day in inflammatory arthritis. "Gelling" may occur after prolonged inactivity, such as sitting in a car or at a desk. It is important to establish what the patient means by stiffness. If stiffness predominates over pain, it can be due to soft tissue contracture or spasticity, the best example being cerebral diplegia. Inflammatory arthritis causes early morning stiffness that takes at least 30 min to wear off with activity. Noninflammatory mechanical arthritis causes stiffness after rest that eases rapidly on movement. Diseases of the soft tissues, rather than the joint itself, may cause stiffness. In polymyalgia rheumatica, stiffness commonly affects the shoulder and pelvic areas.

Deformities of limbs or spine are mostly congenial (isolated or syndromic) and can be progressive. Acute onset of deformity after trauma suggests fracture, joint dislocation, or hematoma. Most congenital MSDs are diagnosed by the pattern of multiple deformities and associated system/organ involvement. Arthrogryposis multiplex congenita, osteogenesis imperfecta, and mucopolysaccharidosis are some examples. Painless slow evolution of deformity occurs in neuromuscular disorders as contractures in cerebral palsy **(Fig. 25.5)**, myopathies, rheumatological diseases as in JIA **(Fig. 25.6)** and in DDH.

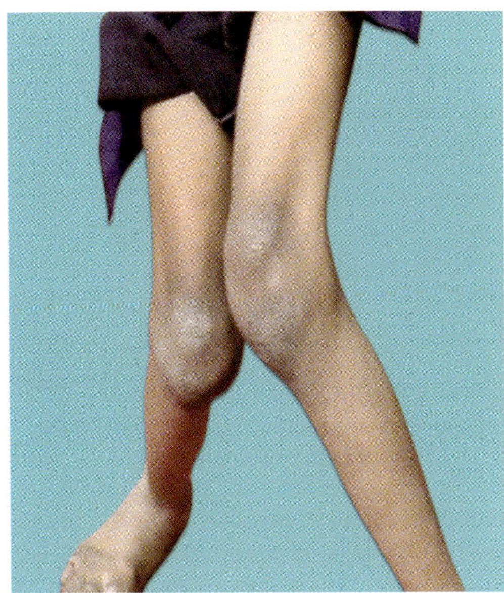

Fig. 25.5: Child with spastic CP. Note the hamstring and tendoachilles contractures (painless).

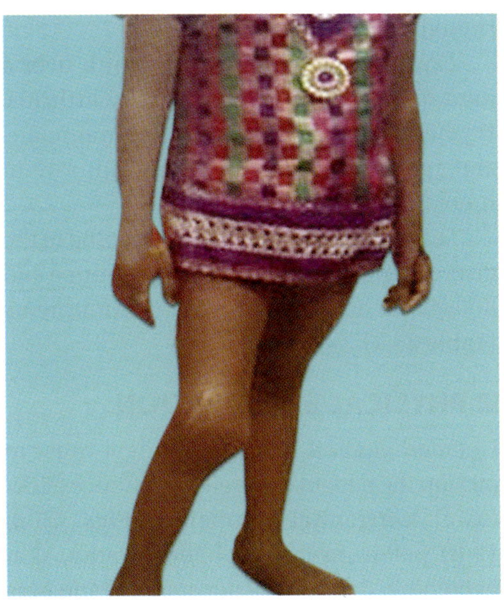

Fig. 25.6: JIA oligoarthritis R knee leading to fixed flexion deformity. (JIA: juvenile idiopathic arthritis)

Developmental delay: Isolated gross motor delay is mostly benign; exclude the possibility of DDH clinically and by investigations if any doubt. This is because if not corrected in time DDH may end up in gross limping

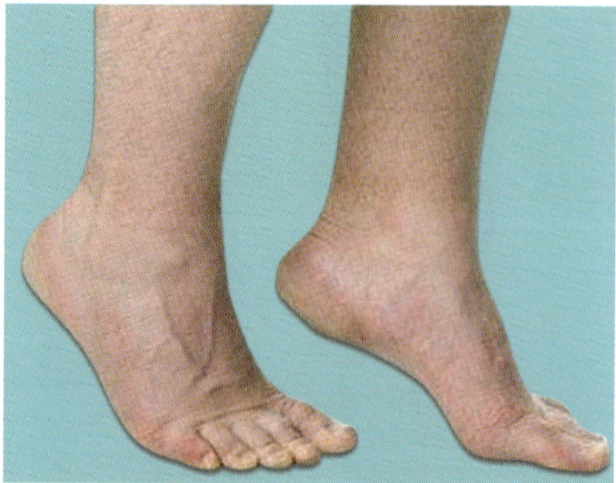

Fig. 25.7: Toe walking in a boy (10 yrs) with tendoachilles contracture.

TABLE 25.2: Grading of disability in MSD.

Grade	*Activity*
Class I	Complete ability to carry out all usual activities of daily living
Class II	Adequate normal activities despite handicap of discomfort or limited motion in one or more joints
Class III	Limitation of daily activities because of discomfort or limited motion in one or more joints
Class IV	Severe limitation to joint motion, incapacitated largely, bedridden, confined to wheelchair, little or no self-care

and physical disability. *Toe walking (equinus gait)* also causes isolated motor delay. Shortening of the tendoachilles **(Fig. 25.7)**, spastic diplegia, autism spectrum disorders, pseudohypertrophic muscular dystrophy, spinal dysraphism, and intraspinal tumors should be excluded.

Erythema (redness) and warmth over a joint occur in acute inflammatory arthritis. Erythema is common in infective, traumatic, and crystal induced conditions, but rare in JIA or SLE.

Disability is produced by worsening of the disorder; grade the severity by the routine and household activities or work commitments **(Table 25.2)**.

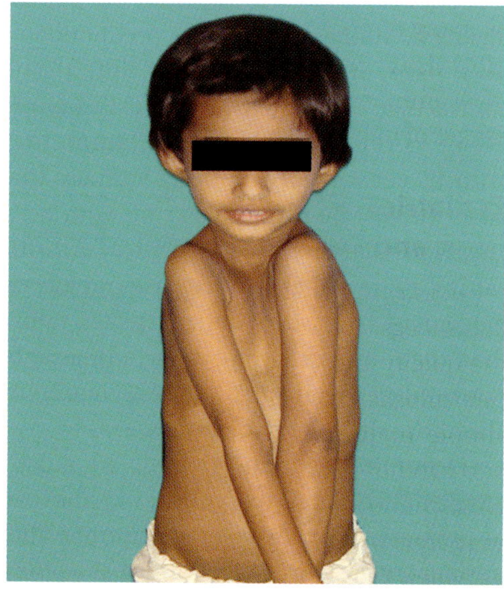

Fig. 25.8: Absent clavicles (B/L) (congenital).

PHYSICAL EXAMINATION

Detailed general examination is a must to pick up the patient's overall appearance (sick/toxic), congenital anomalies **(Figs. 25.8, 12.6)** pallor, rash, lymphadenopathy, skin tightening, deformities, ulcers and blue eyes typically seen in osteogenesis imperfecta **(Fig. 25.9)**.

Assess all aspects of growth and development to detect short stature, long stature, and developmental delay (Ref. Ch. 11, 12). Examination of the nervous system, cardiovascular system, and GIT is crucially important to pick up associated findings and secondary complications to confirm the final diagnosis.

Order of musculoskeletal system examination depends on the age, clinical condition, and the cooperation of the patient. If the child walks, runs, or struggles, preliminary observation of the gait, posture, and stance (manner of standing) is evident and separate testing is not needed. Practice examining

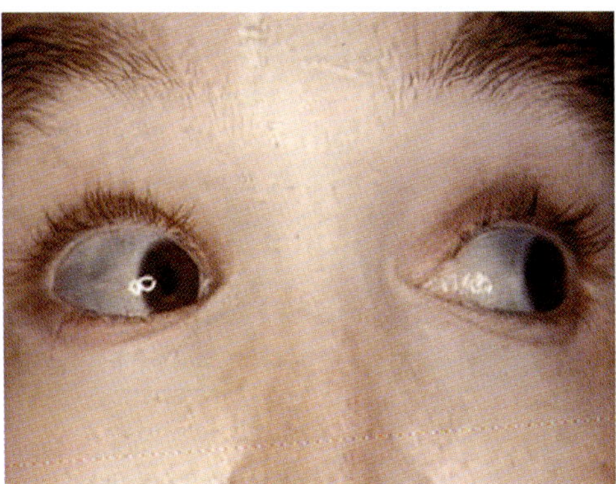

Fig. 25.9: Blue eyes in osteogenesis imperfecta.

as many joints as possible, in those without MSD also to become familiar with the method of examination, normal appearances and ranges of movement.

Pediatric Gait, Arms, Legs, and Spine

pGALS, i.e., the pediatric version of GALS (*G*ait, *A*rms, *L*egs, *S*pine—screening) has improved the quality and the confidence of doctors in musculoskeletal evaluation. It incorporates simple maneuvers acceptable to children and parents. pGALS starts with observing the child coming into the room, interaction with the parent or carer, and their interest in play or activities. The child should be barefoot and the limbs exposed to the knees, thighs, and arms completely. The torso can be exposed to assess the spine in due course.

Observe the child by standing on the *front, from behind and sides.* The upper limbs and neck are best examined with the child sitting on an examination couch facing the examiner. The child is then instructed to copy the various maneuvers as performed by the examiner. The child should then lie supine to allow the legs to be examined and then stand again for spine assessment. Throughout pGALS, the sequence of *"look, feel, move"* is followed, checking for verbal and nonverbal signs of discomfort. The examiner demonstrates the postures and the child is asked to follow so that the patient has the feel of a dance practice.

See **Table 25.3** for pediatric screening questions and the screening maneuvers for pGALS.

Gait (Ref. Ch. 21)

Gait is the position of the body while walking. Consider the age of the child while assessing. The toddler has a wide-based gait. The adult pattern of gait with narrow base and smooth reciprocal swing of upper limbs begins between 3–5 yr.

Pathologic gait: The child should walk with legs and feet fully exposed, without any footwear, first away from the examiner, turn around at a given point and then walk toward the examiner. Noncooperative children may be attracted by toys for facilitating the examination process or the parent can walk along with them. Abnormal gait may be due to:

- Pain—antalgic gait
- Structural deformities of bones and joints
- *Muscle weakness*:
  - Waddling gait
  - Quadriceps weakness
  - Foot drop gait
  - Abnormal limb control
  - Spasticity—hemiplegic gait and diplegic gait
  - Rigidity—parkinsonian gait
  - Ataxic—sensory ataxia, cerebellar ataxia

The gait differs according to the degree and location of weakness.

Waddling gait: Normally, when a person stands on one leg, the gluteus medius of the same side (the principal hip abductor), elevates the pelvis on the opposite side balancing the trunk

TABLE 25.3: The pGALS musculoskeletal screening examination.

The pGALS musculoskeletal screening examination

Screening questions:
Do you (or does your child) have any pain or stiffness in your (their) joints, muscles, or back?
Do you (or does your child) have any difficulty getting yourself (him/herself) dressed without any help?
Do you (or does your child) have any problem going up and down stairs?

Screening maneuvers	***Features assessed***	***Examples of abnormalities***
Observe the child standing (from front, back, and sides)	• Posture • Habitus	• Knock knees, bow legs, leg length discrepancy • Scoliosis, kyphosis
Observe the child walking and "Walk on your tip-toes/walk on your heels"	Feet and ankles	• Flat feet, antalgic gait • Inflammatory arthritis • Enthesitis (ERA) • Severe disease, tarsal coalition
"Hold your hands out straight in front of you"	Shoulders, elbows, wrists, hands	Inflammatory arthritis
"Turn your hands over and make a fist"	Wrists, elbows, small joints of hands	
"Pinch your index finger and thumb together"	Small joints index finger and thumb	
"Touch the tips of your fingers"	Small joints of fingers	
Squeeze the metacarpophalangeal joints (MCPs)	Metacarpophalangeal joints	
"Put your hands together palm to palms/put your hands together back to back"	Small joints of fingers, wrists	
"Reach up, 'touch the sky', and look at the ceiling"	Neck, shoulders, elbows, wrists	• Hypermobility • Inflammatory arthritis
"Put your hands behind your neck"	Shoulders, elbows	• Hypermobility • Inflammatory arthritis
Feel for effusion at the knee	Knee	Inflammatory arthritis
Active movement of knees and feel for crepitus	Knee	Anterior knee pain
Passive movement (full flexion, internal rotation of hip)	Hip	• Orthopedic causes (Perthes, Slipped Capital Femoral Epiphysis, hip dysplasia) • Inflammatory arthritis (enthesitis-related arthritis)
"Open wide and put three (*child's own*) fingers in your mouth"	Temporomandibular joints	Inflammatory arthritis

Contd...

Contd...

Screening maneuvers	*Features assessed*	*Examples of abnormalities*
"Try and touch your shoulder with your ear"	Neck	• Inflammatory arthritis • Torticollis
"Bend forwards and touch your toes?"	Thoracolumbar spine	• Spondylolysis, spondylolisthesis • Mechanical back pain • Inflammatory arthritis (ERA)
Helpful tips whilst performing the pGALS screening examination: • Get the child to copy you doing the maneuvers. • Look for verbal and nonverbal clues of discomfort. • Check for asymmetry (e.g., muscle bulk, joint swelling, range of movement). • Consider clinical patterns and associations (e.g., hypermobility and Marfanoid habitus, leg length discrepancy and scoliosis).		
(pGALS: pediatric gait, arms, legs, and spine)		

over the weight-bearing hip. If the gluteus medius is paralyzed on the side in which the patient stands, the opposite side of the pelvis drops so that the trunk also tilts to the opposite side. In bilateral gluteus medius weakness and in bilateral DDH, it produces waddling gait (simulated to the gait of a person walking on a country boat) or that of a duck—*wide based, body sways from side with each step, heels and toes brought down simultaneously.* Characteristically seen in pseudo-hypertrophic muscular dystrophy and bilateral DDH.

Calcaneus gait: The gastrocnemius and soleus muscles are responsible for the final forward propulsion in the push off portion of the stance phase of the gait. Paralysis of these muscles reveals lack of push off and tibia shifts posteriorly. The patient walks on heels with dorsiflexion of the foot—a common scenario of postpolio paralysis in olden days.

Drop foot (steppage, high stepping) gait: Paralysis of the foot dorsiflexors causes difficulty to hold the foot against gravity in dorsiflexion. The foot goes into plantar flexion (drops). To clear the toes, the patient externally rotates and raises the whole lower limb to a higher level flexing the knee and hip.

Weakness of the corresponding upper limb muscles causes drooping of the shoulders, winging of scapula, and wrist drop.

Structural deformities of bones and joints: If *one leg is short*, it may produce a limp but the length discrepancy may be well hidden by the tilt of the pelvis, revealing apparent scoliosis **(Fig. 25.10)**. Other means of compensation are to hold the foot and the ankle of the short limb in equinovarus posture and the knee and hip of the longer leg in flexion. When the hip is *ankylosed*, it can produce a pathological gait by greater movement of the pelvis on the lumbar spine. *Painful bones and joints* shorten the stance phase of gait and the patient will take quick short steps on the affected side with painful limp (*antalgic gait*). In congenital dislocation of the hip, the head of the femur does not have a fixed position in the acetabular cavity and rides high on the side of the pelvis. This impairs the action of the gluteus medius leading to a gluteus medius limp and *Trendelenburg gait*.

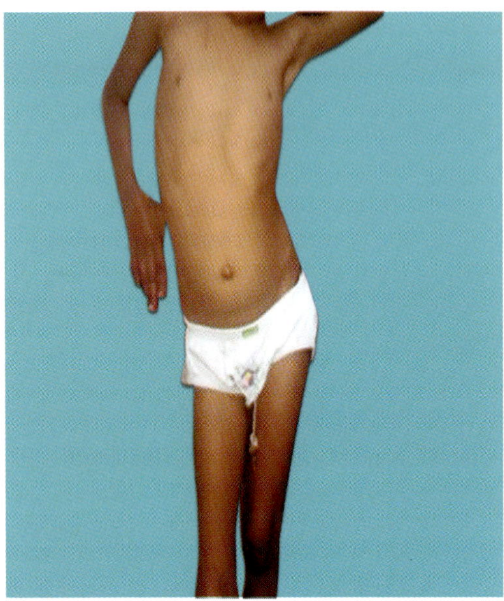

Fig. 25.10: Limb length discrepancy—apparent scoliosis by pelvic tilt.

Limb lengthening and limb length discrepancy can be a complication of long-standing untreated/poorly treated JIA due to unopposed synovial inflammation and increased blood flow to growing epiphyses.

Posture: Observe the natural standing posture and body outlines of the child from the back, front, and sides. Between 8 and 15 yr, regular screening for kyphosis and scoliosis is essential as detailed below:

- *From the back:* Uncloth except for shorts. Ask the patient to stand erect with feet together, arms hanging by the side, and occiput aligned over the inter gluteal cleft
- *Ask the child to bend 90°* forwards at the hips with knees straight and arms dangling from the shoulder, inspect parallel to the back from both ends
- *Examine from the side* while standing upright.

Kyphosis and scoliosis can be detected by this examination.

Limbs: Terms used in describing angular deformities indicate the position of the distal segment of the limb in relation to the proximal segments. Varus and valgus denote angulation toward and away from the midline of the body respectively, distal to the anatomic part named. Thus, cubitus valgus means the forearm is directed away from the midline distal to the elbow joint; cubitus varus is the forearm which is bent inward and toward the midline of the body. Coxa valga—the angle of the neck and shaft of femur is greater than normal; the distal segment is angulated away from the midline of the hip. Coxa vara is the reverse. Similar is the case with genu valgum and genu varus where the anatomic point is the knee.

Disparity in length: Lower limbs will reveal differences in the level of popliteal and gluteal creases, the pelvis and shoulders, when the child stands with both feet together, heels on ground and knees fully extended. Place the radial border of your index fingers on the uppermost part of each iliac crest and the thumb on the anterior superior iliac spines. Compare the height of the pelvis on both sides.

Place blocks of wood of various thickness under the short limb foot so as to make iliac crests and anterior superior iliac spines horizontal and measure the difference. The actual lower limb length can be measured from the underside of the anterior superior iliac spine to the lowest point of the medial malleolus or plantar surface of the heel, with both ankles in neutral position. If the anterior superior iliac spine is not easily palpable or distorted, the ischial tuberosity is taken as the proximal landmark. The apparent length, an index of the functional length of the lower limbs, is measured from the umbilicus to the lowest portion of the medial malleolus. An adduction deformity of the hip causes an apparent shortening on the side of involvement and abduction deformity produces an apparent lengthening on the same side.

Disproportion between thigh and leg length if observed, measure them separately. The medial knee joint line is the intermediate landmark, which is easily located by flexing the knee to 45°.

For assessing disparity between thigh lengths, two tests are helpful.

1. *Galeazzi test* or Allis sign (Ref. Fig. 15.18)
2. *Ellis test*: Turn the patient to the prone position with hips in full extension, knees flexed to 90°, ankles in neutral position and observe the level of sole of the heels. On the affected side, the sole will be at a lower level.

The total length of the upper limb is measured from the posterior tip of acromion to the end of the long finger with elbow, wrist, and fingers in neutral, zero degrees extended position. The upper arm is measured from the posterior tip of the acromion to the point of olecranon. The forearm is measured from the point of olecranon to the tip of the radial or ulnar styloid process.

The circumference of the calf is measured at the greatest diameter. The thighs are measured at specifically marked identical levels, several inches above the patella or below the anterior superior iliac spine. In the upper limb, the greatest circumference of the forearm and the mid upper arm circumference are measured.

Examination of joints: Proceed in the following steps—

- *Look (inspection)* the position of the joint at rest and its surface anatomy, contours, color, scar, size, muscle bulk, limb length, and whether swollen **(Figs. 25.1 and 25.2)**.
- *Feel (palpation)* for skin *warmth*, joint *swelling* (increase in joint size that alters the normal surface markings of the joint), and *tenderness*. Note the position, extent, and consistency of the swelling. If cystic, elicit fluctuation and try to reduce it into the joint. Intra-articular effusion, periarticular fluid, soft tissue changes (edema, joint capsule thickening and inflammation of muscle, ligament or subcutaneous or cutaneous tissues), or bone hypertrophy are the factors for joint swelling. Thickened synovium is felt as spongy and elastic. Though fluctuant its edge can be rolled under the finger unlike the edge of effusion.

Tenderness should be localized; determine whether it arises in the joint or neighboring structures. Joint margin tenderness or tenderness and inflammation at the site of the tendon insertion into bone or ligament, fascia, or joint capsule indicate *enthesitis*.

Feel for local *rise of temperature*. Feel the bony components starting at the articular end and gradually proceed toward the shaft. Muscle *wasting* is assessed by naked eye inspection, measurement, and the feel of the muscles.

Joint crepitus is detected by feeling the joint with one hand while moving it by the other hand. Differentiate from nonspecific clicking of the joints. Joint crepitus occurs in hematoma, gas gangrene, surgical emphysema, tenosynovitis, osteoarthritis, and Charcot's joint.

- *Range of motion:* Test for passive range of motion by the examiner and active range of motion by the patient noting pain or irritability, especially at the end range of joint motion.
- *Stability:* Assess joint stability, particularly for the ligaments of the knee (cruciate and collateral ligaments). Assess for pain

requires USG or MRI of the joint. Enthesitic points to be examined include the greater trochanter and anterior superior iliac spines.

Knees: Wasting of vastus medialis or gastrocnemius follows muscle atrophy due to reduced use or guarding of a painful joint. Subtle *loss of knee extension* is observed by applying relaxed passive extension of both knees, by lifting the patient's feet gently up off the table. *Mild swelling* obscuring the medial and lateral contours of the patella can be confirmed by palpating and inspecting for a *synovial fluid wave* or *bulge sign* (medial compression followed by lateral "re-expression" of the swelling) and by balloting the patella. *Joint margin tenderness* is maximal just medial to the lower patellar border. Key points for palpation of entheses are at the tibial tuberosity and the 2, 6, and 10 O'clock positions around the patella. Knee locking or giving way indicates a mechanical disorder requiring assessment of knee stability. To assess medial and lateral collateral ligament integrity, apply gentle valgus and varus pressure on the knee (held in 5° flexion) which will reveal abnormal abduction or adduction.

Bones: Pain confined to bones indicates trauma, infection, or rarely malignancy. Bone tenderness is revealed in fractures, infections, and bone destruction in malignancy. Look for swelling, deformity, tenderness, and crepitus. Change in shape can be congenital or due to metabolic problems as in rickets **(Figs. 25.14A and B)**.

Muscular system symptoms are pain, tenderness, and weakness (read Chapter 21 for neurological causes of muscle weakness).

Weakness is the most important muscle problem. Muscles appear flabby and limp and soft to touch. Generalized ligamentous relaxation with hypotonia can be present in many otherwise normal children. See **Box 25.1** for diseases with hypotonia. Detailed examination and relevant investigations should be done in such children especially with isolated gross motor delay before labeling it as benign.

Myalgia is most common complaint reported in leptospirosis, rocky mountain

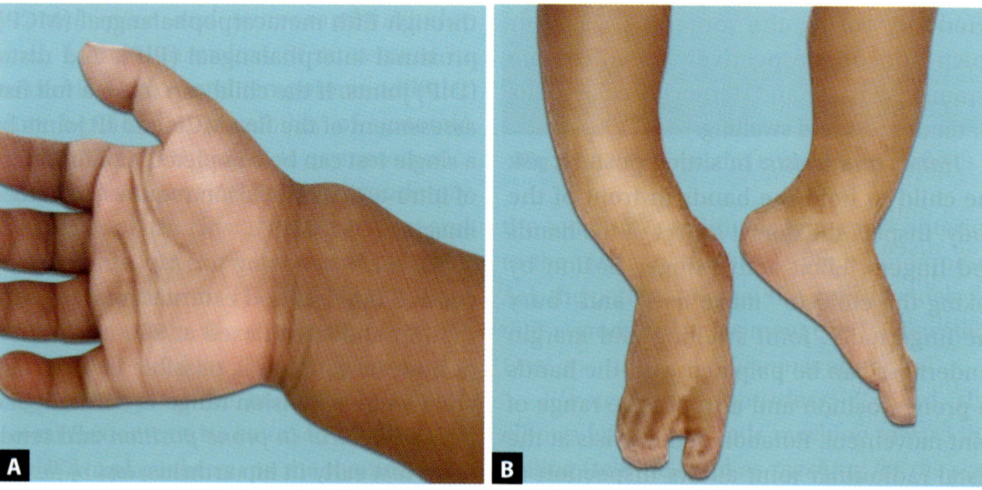

Figs. 25.14A and B: (A) Widening of lower ends of radius and ulna in rickets in an infant; (B) Bowing of legs in vitamin D deficiency rickets in a young child.

BOX 25.1: Diseases with hypotonia.

- Malnutrition
- Vitamin D deficiency
- Endocrine causes (hypoparathyroidism, hypothyroidism)
- Chromosomal anomalies (Down syndrome)
- Myopathies
- Storage disorders (Pompe, Tay-Sach's)
- Dyselectrolytemia (hypokalemia)
- Myotonic dystrophy
- Syndromes (Marfan, Prader–Willi, Zellweger)

spotted fever, bubonic plague, SLE, toxic shock syndrome, Guillain-Barre syndrome, poliomyelitis, and in many viral infections (dengue, chikungunya, influenza, corona, echo, and coxsackie).

Myotonia is slow relaxation of a muscle after contraction. Though not painful, wasting and weakness occur gradually. Slow relaxation of the muscle can be appreciated by asking the child to make a tight fist and then quickly open the hands. The clinical sign can be elicited by tapping a muscle belly with the reflex hammer. Local contraction and dimpling persist for about 30–60 sec. A sharp blow on the thenar eminence produces sustained adduction of the thumb.

Muscular dystrophy: Visible enlargement of the muscles with weakness **(Fig. 25.15)** is the characteristic feature. In the early stage of illness, the enlarged muscles are firm doughy or rubbery in consistency. As the disease progresses, muscular atrophy develops. Gait becomes waddling as the hip girdle muscles become weak and positive Gower's sign develops **(Fig. 21.16)**. Weakness of the shoulder muscles makes the child slip through the examiner's hands when being picked up by the axillae.

Myositis: Chronic myositis is common in connective tissue or collagen vascular diseases such as SLE, PAN, and occasionally rheumatoid arthritis. In dermatomyositis, there is involvement of skin also. Polymyositis is characterized by pain, tenderness, induration, and weakness of mainly proximal muscles from initially onward and is associated with swallowing problems.

Musculoskeletal pain: Limb pain is a common complaint in children. It may be due to benign conditions like growing pains, hypermobility syndrome, restless leg syndrome (nocturnal limb pain and insomnia due to anemia

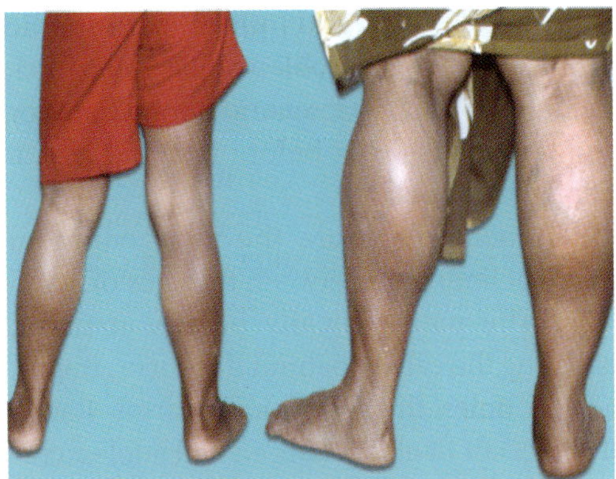

Fig. 25.15: Pseudohypertrophic muscular dystrophy—calf muscles of son and mother.

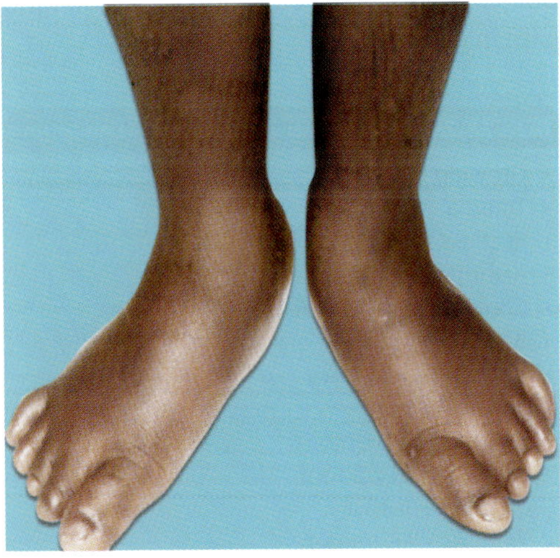

Fig. 25.16: Toeing out.

or genetic trait) and minor orthopedic problems. Serious problems like green stick fractures, primary or secondary malignancy should be ruled out before labeling it as a benign condition.

Growing pains are the most common cause of limb pain between the ages of 3 and 7 yr. The pain typically occurs at night, affecting the calves, behind the knees, thighs, and, at times, the arms and forearms. Rarely it can occur in older children and adolescents also. Nocturnal limb pain can also manifest due to muscle fatigue after vigorous physical activity or due to minor orthopedic problems. **Box 25.2** reveals the common causes of limb pain in children.

BOX 25.2: Common causes limb pain in children.

- Growing Pains
- Trauma
- Restless leg syndrome
- Arthritis
- Connective tissue diseases
- Bone tumors
- Vitamin D deficiency
- Perthes disease
- Hypermobile joints
- Hyperparathyroidism
- Sickle cell disease
- Tight Achilles tendon
- Leukemias
- Psychogenic

Normal musculoskeletal variants: Many minor musculoskeletal abnormalities in children get corrected during the period of growth. They include bowlegs, metatarsus varus, flat feet, toeing out **(Fig. 25.16)**, internal torsion of femur and tibia, toe walking, and knock knee (genu valgum). They should be considered normal after examination and necessary investigations.

SUGGESTED READING

1. Bayer M. Vitamin D-Deficiency Rickets-Where Do We Stand. Austin J Pediatr. 2014; 1(1):1001.
2. Foster HE, Jandial S. Examination of the musculoskeletal system in children—a simple approach. Paediatr Child Health. 2008;18(2):47-55.
3. Foster HE, Jandial S. pGALS – pediatric Gait Arms Legs and Spine: a simple examination of the musculoskeletal system. Pediatr Rheumatol Online J. 2013;11:44.
4. Graham T, Gianini EH. Juvenile Rheumatoid Arthritis Assessment. Indian J Pediatr. 1996; 63:283-91.
5. Green M. Pediatric Diagnosis, 5th edition. Philadelphia: WB Saunders Company; 1997. pp. 131-60.
6. Kaur S, Goraya JS. Images: Infantile scurvy. Indian Pediatr. 2017;54:699.
7. Kliegman RM. Nelson Textbook of Pediatrics, 21st edition. Amsterdam: Elsevier; 2019.

26

Pediatric Imaging: The Basics

CHAPTER

L Jayasree, R Vishnu

Chapter Outline

- Introduction
- Imaging Modalities
- Radiation Protection
- Contrast Studies
- Choice of Imaging Modality
- Imaging Different Body Areas

INTRODUCTION

Imaging is the health specialty that deals with the process of producing pictures of the inside of a patient's body for diagnosis. Sir Wilhelm Conrad Roentgen from Germany in 1895 accidentally detected "X" (meaning unknown) rays claimed as the first imaging modality. An upsurge in imaging started from the latter part of the 20th century, which has tremendously aided in the quick and astute diagnosis of diseases in all medical specialties facilitating apt and timely treatment.

"Infants and children are not miniature adults". This statement holds true in pediatric imaging also. Indications, procedures, and interpretation of the different pediatric imaging modalities are quite different from those in adults and correlation with clinical details is a must.

IMAGING MODALITIES

The imaging modalities are of two groups:

1. *With ionizing radiation:* These include X-ray imaging such as fixed X-ray units, portable X-ray and digital radiography (DR), computed tomography (CT), pediatric cath lab (PCL), C-arms (CA), and nuclear medicine imaging (NMI).
2. *Without ionizing radiation:* These are ultrasonography (USG) imaging and magnetic resonance imaging (MRI).

Imaging with Ionizing Radiation

X-rays and gamma rays are the ionizing radiations used for imaging, X-rays in radiological imaging and gamma rays in nuclear medicine imaging. These rays are high-energy radiation and can penetrate the tissues. They are photons or energy packets and on entering tissues get absorbed or scattered. These interactions of photons result in the removal of photons from the X-ray beam that reaches the X-ray film or image receptor which is stated as attenuation of the X-ray beam. The differential attenuation of X-rays by different tissues made of different elements and with different densities will result in variation in the amount of X-rays passing different regions of the patient and falling on the image receptor.

In earlier days, photographic films were used as image receptors. Now, it is replaced by photostimulable phosphor or flat panel detectors. In conventional radiography, the X-ray exposure results in the formation of metallic silver by reduction of silver halide (and enhanced during darkroom processing).

Metallic silver being opaque to light will appear dark when the film is viewed. The area of the film coming under lung will be dark since lung attenuates less X-rays; the more the radiations reach the film, more metallic silver is formed. This dark room processing is replaced nowadays by computed radiography (CR) system. The CR system uses a special detector (CR cassette) to receive X-rays using ordinary X-ray machines. The CR cassette is read in a CR reader to get a digital image. This digital image can be viewed on a computer or can be filmed.

Direct radiography or *digital radiography (DR)* uses a flat panel detector as an image receptor. The X-ray image can be directly viewed on a computer monitor without film processing. The advantage of portable X-ray and C-arm units is that they can be moved to the patient's station. The portable X-ray units are used for bedside imaging; C-arms are used in operation theaters to view real time (movie) X-ray images. Cath lab units are modified forms of X-ray or C-arm units with more degrees of freedom for the X-ray tube detector assembly. The digital subtraction angiography (DSA) uses image processing techniques to visualize the blood vessels during an interventional procedure.

The above mentioned techniques give only a two-dimensional image of a three dimensional patient, thus causing uncertainties in interpretation. In CT, patient information is acquired from multiple directions and a three-dimensional image is produced in the computer. CT has an advantage of identifying the type of tissues from their CT numbers. The CT numbers are generated from the attenuation value of tissues which are different for each tissue type as given in **Table 26.1**.

TABLE 26.1: Body tissues and their CT numbers.

Type of tissue	*CT number (HU)*
Fat	−300 to −100
Fluid	0 to +20
Blood	+50 to +80
Calcification	+100 to +300
Bone	+1,000 and above

(CT: computed tomography)

The data is collected in axial planes from which images can be reconstructed in any plane. This is called multiplanar reconstruction. Advanced reconstruction techniques such as volume rendering will enable the visualization of internal organs in three dimensions.

Nuclear medicine differs from other imaging techniques in the use of unsealed gamma emitting radioactive nuclide for the functional imaging of a patient by a gamma camera or PET. In gamma camera imaging, a radionuclide labeled to pharmaceutical agent (radiopharmaceutical, e.g.: Tc-99m to pertechnetate) is administered orally or intravenously. The pharmaceutical undergoing normal physiological processes will be taken up more by cells with more metabolic activity. More gamma radiation will be emitted from such metabolically active cells and the gamma camera records these areas as *hot spots* in the image.

Positron emission tomography (PET) is similar to gamma camera imaging except that the radionuclide is different (e.g.: Fluorodeoxyglucose) and that the image is three dimensional.

Imaging Modalities without Ionizing Radiation

Magnetic resonance imaging (MRI) uses radiofrequency waves to excite the hydrogen nucleus (proton H_1^1) inside the human tissues placed under a strong magnetic field. When the RF pulse is switched off, the protons will relax. The de-excitation or relaxation rates are

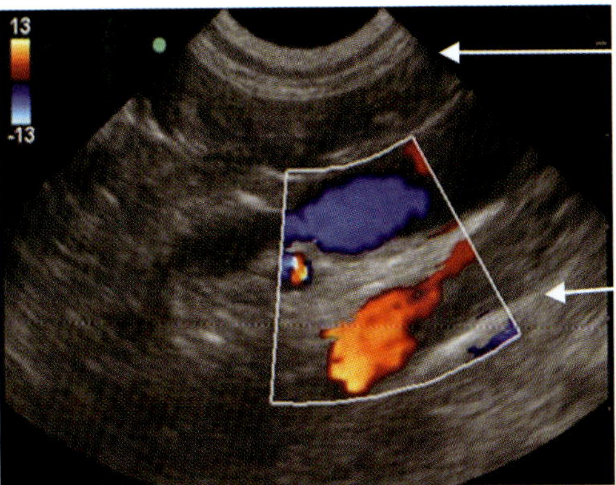

Fig. 26.1: Color Doppler imaging. The blue and red color represent blood flow in the two adjacent vessels, in the sampling box (3). Red indicates flow toward the transducer and the blue represents flow away from the transducer. Note that no color is seen outside the sampling box (2). Face of the transducer (1)

then monitored with the help of RF receiver coils and depending on the difference in the relaxation rates, a particular gray value is assigned for that tissue in the image.

Ultrasound imaging uses ultrasonic waves (sound waves of frequency *>20,000 Hz*). Sound waves are sent to the tissues with the help of a transducer (probe) placed on the surface of the body which travel through the tissues of different depths and get reflected by the tissues. These reflected waves are received by the same transducer to generate a gray scale *(2D)* image.

If the reflecting tissue is in movement (e.g.: moving blood in vessels), the direction and speed of flow can be observed *(color Doppler imaging)*. This information with proper color coding (*red* for motion toward the transducer and *blue* away from transducer) will give details of the flow **(Fig. 26.1)**.

RADIATION PROTECTION

Children are more susceptible to harmful effects of radiation due to the increased sensitivity of growing organs and longer life expectancy. CT (though an important diagnostic modality) has higher amount of radiation exposure compared to plain radiography. Repeated CT examinations impose higher radiation doses which can increase the risk of fatal cancer **(Table 26.2)**.

TABLE 26.2: Comparative radiation doses—CT Vs plain film.

Examination type	*CT effective dose (mSv)*	*Plain film effective dose (mSv)*
Chest	8.0	0.02
Head	2.0	0.07
Abdomen	10.0	1.0
Pelvis	10.0	0.7

Source: Task Group on Control of Radiation Dose in Computed Tomography. Managing patient dose in computed tomography. A report of the International Commission on Radiological Protection. Ann ICRP. 2000;30(4):7-45.

CONTRAST STUDIES

Contrast media are substances used for demonstration of internal organs like gastrointestinal tract and urinary system which are not normally visible on plain X-rays. The ideal contrast medium for gastrointestinal tract is barium sulfate suspension, given orally as barium swallow (esophagus), barium meal (stomach and duodenum), barium meal follow through (small bowel), and rectally for barium enema. Barium sulfate is water insoluble and cannot be given intravenously. Iodine containing water soluble contrast agents are used for intravenous urography *(IVU*—kidneys, ureters, and urinary bladder), micturating cystourethrography *(MCU)*, and contrast-enhanced CT (for structure and function of different solid organs and characterization of tumors). MRI uses derivatives of the heavy metal *gadolinium* as a contrast agent.

CHOICE OF IMAGING MODALITY

Ultrasound is the first priority (even for chest imaging in emergencies). The next choice is radiography with contrast medium, in selected cases. If the diagnosis is still not confirmed, MRI (no harmful radiation) or CT (has ionizing radiation) is the next choices. For emergency imaging as in polytrauma, acute abdomen, or respiratory distress, CT examination is the next immediate choice after ultrasound because of its availability and lower cost. MRI is the choice for brain and spine pathologies and for situations necessitating highest soft tissue details. Contrast administration (IV, per oral/per rectal) is needed for pathologic information in the latter two. PET-CT and PET-MRI are reserved for searching the secondaries and for the follow-up of malignancies.

Prerequisites for pediatric imaging studies are—(1) adequate immobilization (if needed sedation), (2) prevention of hypothermia, (3) reduction in radiation dose, and (4) judicious use of contrast media.

IMAGING DIFFERENT BODY AREAS

Chest

Plain radiograph is the investigation of choice in chest pathologies as it reveals the maximum natural contrast due to the air containing lungs surrounding the soft tissues of the mediastinum. Bones and soft tissues of the chest wall can be visualized both through the lucent lung fields and opaque mediastinum. *Abnormalities in chest radiograph* may be in lung parenchyma, airways, mediastinum, chest wall, or diaphragm. Interpretation of the radiographic patterns should be according to the age, clinical features, past history, previous imaging studies, and laboratory reports.

Systematic Approach

Note: All skiagrams should be evaluated through a viewer.

Step 1: Patient's basic data—should be verified always with the request form—name, age, side marker (may be on the right or left side); otherwise dextrocardia will be wrongly interpreted as normally placed heart **(Figs. 26.2A and B)** and misinterpretation of the side of lung disorders can also occur. Place the film on the viewer in such a way that the patient is facing the doctor (i.e., the left side of the film is opposing the right side of the doctor and vice versa).

Step 2: Assess the view: In neonates and young infants, supine anteroposterior (AP) view with arms elevated is preferred; upright sitting position as posteroanterior (PA) view is advised in older infants and children. **Table 26.3** gives the differentiating points between supine AP and erect PA chest views.

TABLE 26.3: Differentiating points between supine AP and erect PA views.

Parameters	*Erect PA*	*Supine AP*
Scapulae	Outside the lung fields	Inside the lung fields
Clavicle	Within the lung apex	Away from lung apex
Ribs	Posterior ribs well seen	Anterior ribs well seen
Heart shadow	Normal	Apparent cardiomegaly
Air in the fundus of stomach	Seen	Not seen

(AP: anteroposterior; PA: posteroanterior)

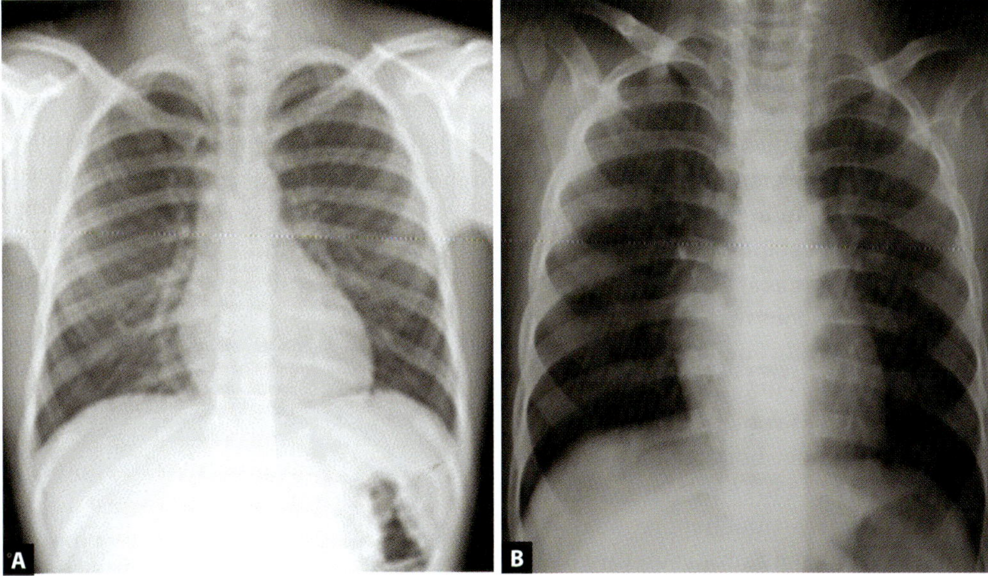

Figs. 26.2A and B: (A) Chest skiagram posteroanterior (PA) view; (B) Chest skiagram anteroposterior (AP) view.

Step 3: Check the position: In a correctly positioned (nonrotated) radiograph medial ends of clavicles are equidistant from the spinous processes **(Fig. 26.2A)**.

Step 4: Check the respiratory phase—should be inspiratory unless requested (as in partial occlusion of the airway by a foreign body). Anterior end of at least 5–7 ribs need be visualized above the diaphragm in inspiratory phase. In expiratory films, the ribs above the diaphragm will be less than 5 in number anteriorly and the lung fields reveal prominent bronchovascular markings.

Step 5: Assess the exposure: Penetration should be enough to see the vertebral bodies and light enough to see the peripheral vascular markings **(Fig. 26.2A)**.

Step 6: Reading the image: The headlines can be (1) soft tissue shadows, (2) bony cage, (3) mediastinum, (4) lung fields, (5) diaphragm, (6) subdiaphragmatic space, and (7) pleura.

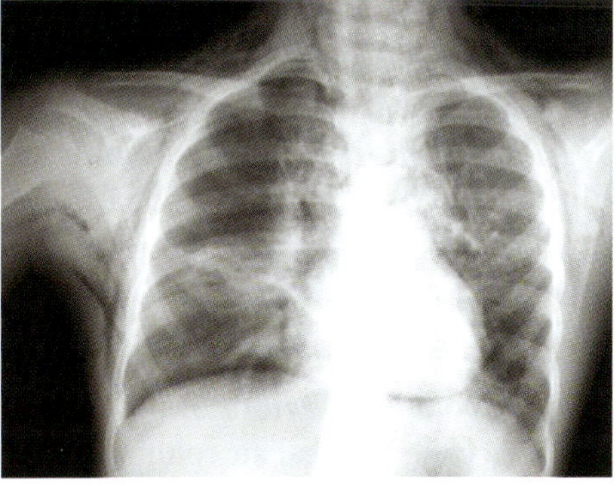

Fig. 26.3: Surgical emphysema in acute severe asthma revealing air collection at neck, (R) axilla, and mediastinum.

- *Soft tissue shadows:* Observe the skin, subcutaneous tissue, and muscles around the chest and neck for swellings, injuries, intercostal drainage tube placement, air in soft tissue, and mediastinum **(Fig. 26.3)** and calcification. Soft tissue air collection (surgical emphysema) is seen in acute severe asthma, chest trauma along with lung contusions, fracture ribs, after ICD insertion, and hemopneumothorax.

- *Bony cage:* Evaluate the ribs, thoracic vertebrae, clavicles, lower cervical spine, and visible parts of the humerus. Look for kyphosis and scoliosis. Count the vertebral bodies and ribs to see reduction or increase in numbers; check for anomalies or fractures. Alteration in numbers and structure of ribs and vertebrae occur in various syndromes and chromosomal anomalies. Bulbous expansion of anterior rib ends indicates *rachitic rosary* due to vitamin D deficiency. Isolated congenital absence of clavicles can occur. Fracture of clavicles in newborns follows difficult deliveries **(Fig. 26.4)**; in older children, it is usually accidental but may be due to child abuse. Multiple rib fractures at various phases of healing indicate nonaccidental trauma; exclude battered baby syndrome, endocrine/metabolic bone diseases or skeletal dysplasia. Funnel-shaped chest is seen in spinal muscular atrophy **(Fig. 26.5)**.
- *Mediastinum* is the central white area inside the thoracic cavity, which can be divided as superior and inferior regions for description purposes.

Superior mediastinum: The superior mediastinum has one-third width of the thoracic cavity. Trace the tracheal air column (central linear lucency) to the carina and proximal main bronchi. Suspect anterior mediastinal mass or lung atelectasis on the side of tracheal displacement **(Fig. 26.6)** and air or fluid collection/tumor infiltration on the opposite side if the air column is compressed or displaced.

Widening of the paratracheal stripe on either side with wavy margins suggests

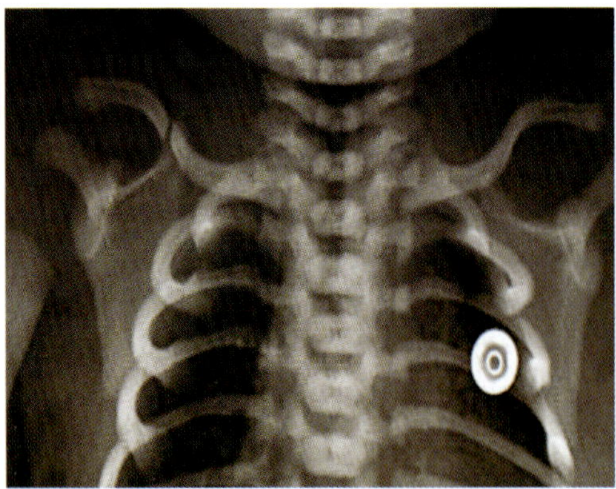

Fig. 26.4: Fracture (R) clavicle in a neonate on D1.

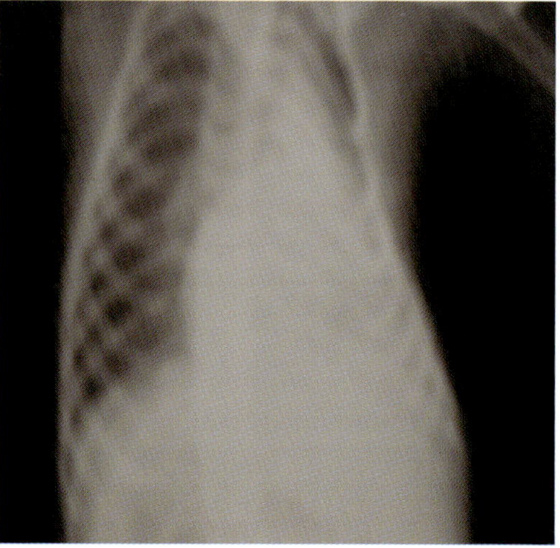

Fig. 26.5: Funnel-shaped chest in spinal muscular atrophy due to selective involvement of intercostal muscles and sparing of diaphragm.

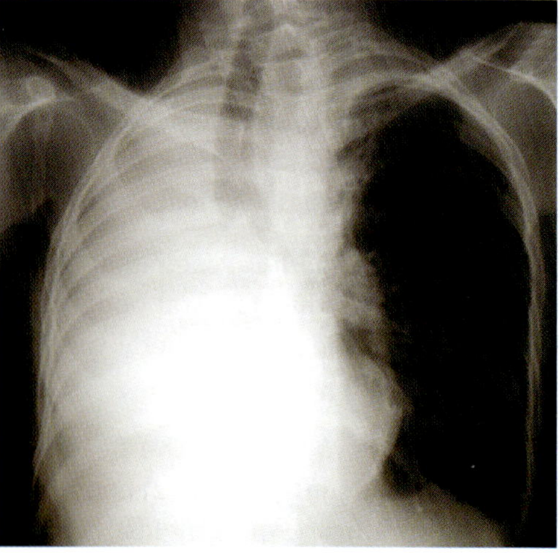

Fig. 26.6: Collapse R lung revealed by tracheal shift to (R).

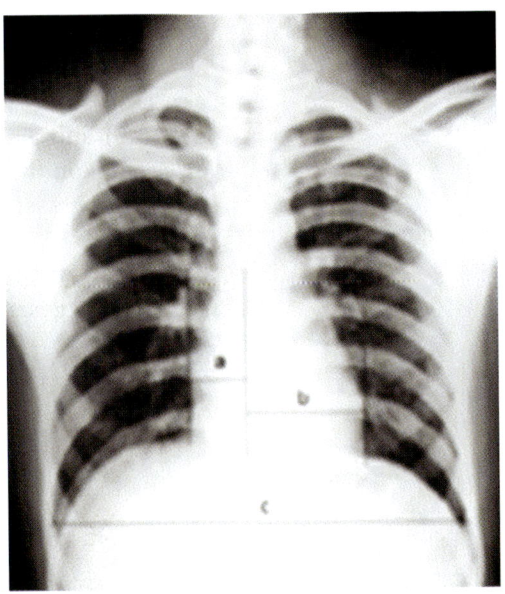

Fig. 26.7: Correct method of measuring transcardiac diameter [TCD (a + b)] and transthoracic diameter [TTD (c)]; CTR = TCD/TTD, i.e., (a + b)/c.

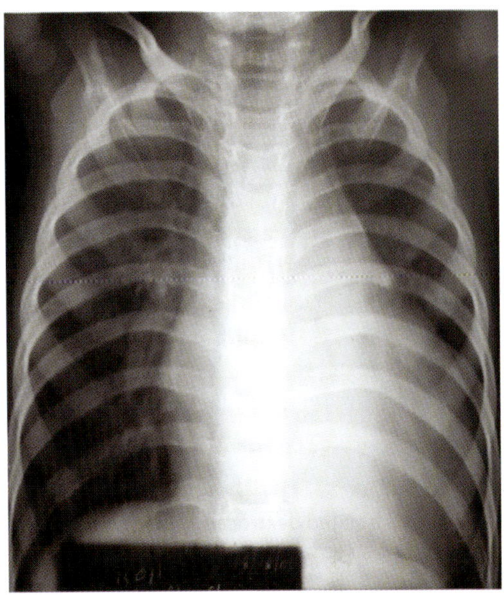

Fig. 26.8: Cardiomegaly in a child with large VSD and L→R shunt. (VSD: ventricular septal defect)

enlarged thymus (can be confirmed by USG). Mediastinal widening with lobulated contour is characteristic of enlarged lymph nodes. Check for any added opacities visible at the hila (mass/lymph nodes/cysts/aberrant blood vessels) or through the cardiac shadow (suggested by retrocardiac lung collapse). Posterior mediastinal mass like neurogenic tumors appears as paraspinal shadows with posterior rib destruction, intervertebral foramen widening, and may reveal calcification.

Inferior mediastinum: Assess the cardiothoracic ratio (CTR). With a transparent scale, measure the maximum cardiac width in the horizontal plane and the maximum thoracic cavity width at the highest point of the diaphragm and find out the ratio **(Fig. 26.7)**. CTR in children can be up to 60%; >60% is cardiomegaly **(Fig. 26.8)**. The common causes of cardiomegaly are cardiac failure, congenital heart diseases (CHD) with left to right shunt, pericardial effusion, cardiomyopathies and endocardial fibroelastosis. CTR <55% is microcardia, seen in Addison's disease and protein energy malnutrition (PEM). Normal cardiac apex is directed to the left (levocardia); dextrocardia is cardiac apex directed to the right **(Fig. 26.9)**. In isolated dextrocardia (in which the intestinal organs are normally aligned), probability for cardiac anomalies is more as compared with dextrocardia with situs inversus. Typical cardiac contours are seen in tetralogy of Fallot (TOF) as boot-shaped heart **(Fig. 26.10)** and in transposition of great arteries (TGA) revealing egg on a string sign **(Fig. 26.11)**. The diagnostic points of TOF in the chest skiagram are narrow cardiac pedicle, right ventricular apex, and pulmonary oligemia.

- *Lung fields:* For description of pathology, lung fields are divided into upper, mid, and lower zones which do not correspond to the anatomical lobes. The area

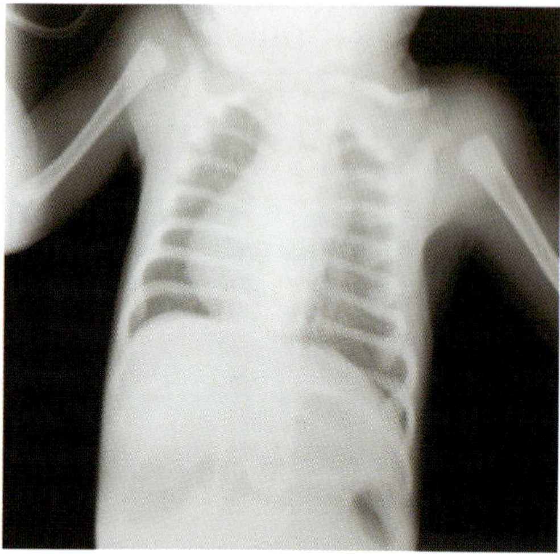

Fig. 26.9: Isolated dextrocardia, see fundal air shadow on left.

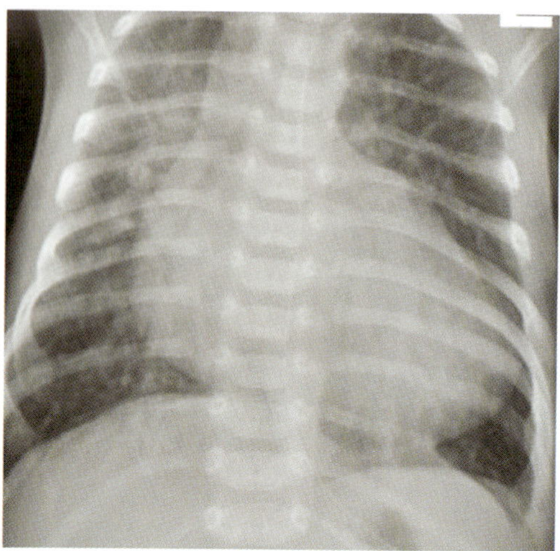

Fig. 26.11: TGA—egg on a string sign. (TGA: transposition of great arteries)
Courtesy: Radiopedia.com

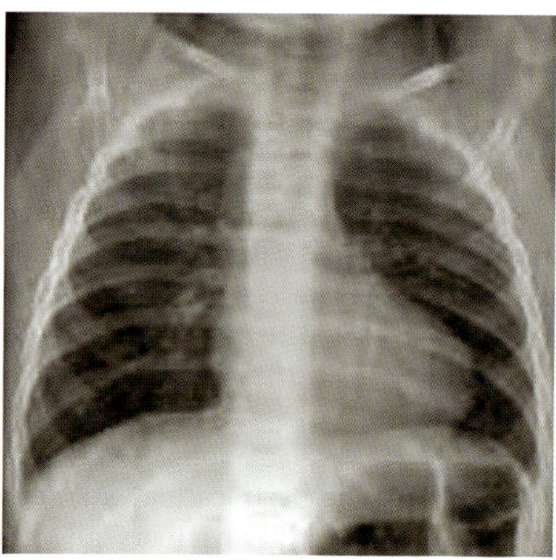

Fig. 26.10: TOF—boot-shaped heart. (TOF: tetralogy of Fallot)

between the lung apex and a horizontal line through the lower margin of the anterior end of the second rib makes the upper zone; the area between the first line and a horizontal line through the lower margin of the anterior end of the fourth rib makes the midzone. The lower zone is between the second line and the diaphragm. Parenchymal pathologies can produce lucent or dark (air collection) and opaque/white (collection of fluid, pus, cells, or blood) shadows. Exclude external bodies or artifacts causing opacities before considering pathological lesions.

Opacity in the lung fields: Assess the size, location, margins, presence of calcification or air within the opacity, signs of volume loss (displacement of fissures, hila, mediastinum, elevated diaphragm), whether associated with adjacent bone erosion, mediastinal lymph node enlargement, and pleural effusion. Multiple opacities can be due to multilobar consolidation, bronchopneumonia, or metastases. Causes of diffuse opacification of a hemithorax are massive effusion, pulmonary aplasia, multilobar consolidation and tumor infiltrates and should be interpreted with clinical details **(Fig. 26.12)**.

Lung lucencies: Dark shadows in chest skiagram are pneumothorax [air in the pleural cavity **(Fig. 26.13)**] pneumatoceles [thin-walled ring shadows or cavitary parenchymal

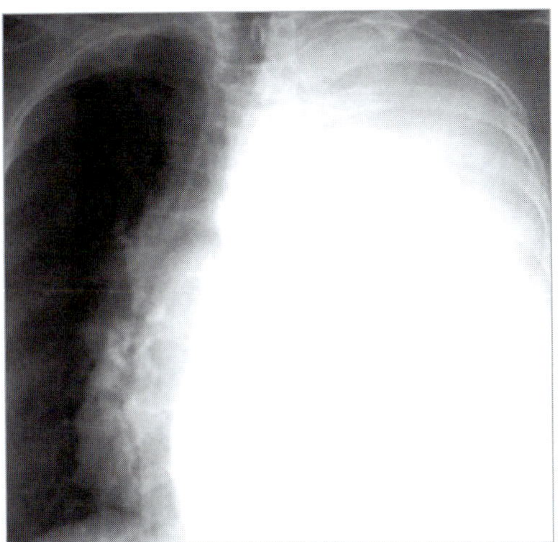

Fig. 26.12: Massive effusion L (increased chest volume and uniform opacity L), mediastinal shift to R.

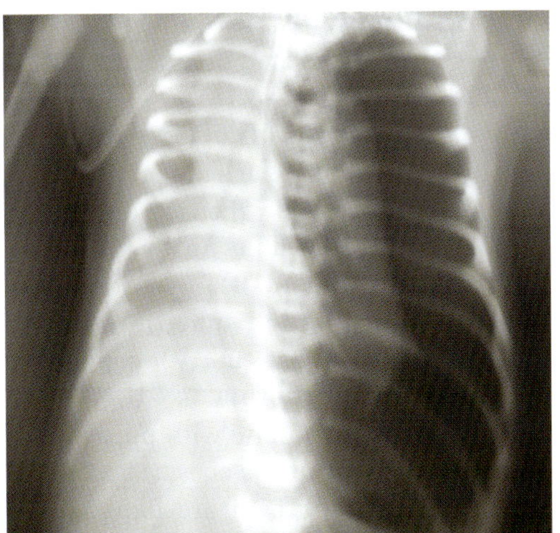

Fig. 26.13: Pneumothorax L [increased chest volume, dark air shadow, collapsed (L) lung], mediastinal shift to R.

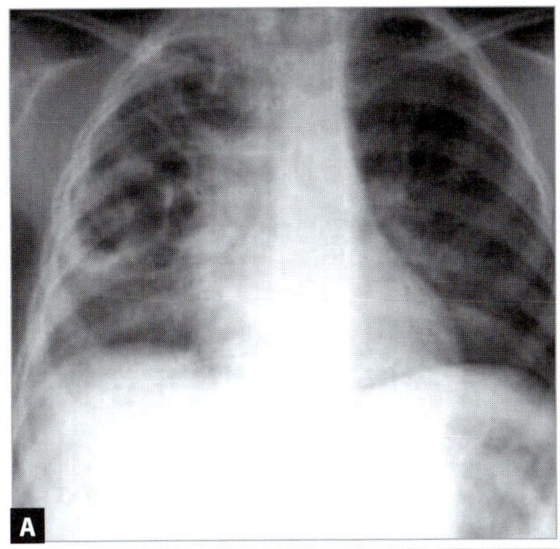

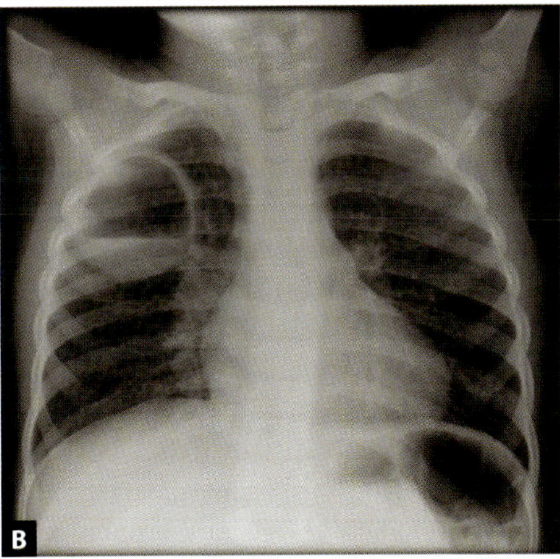

Figs. 26.14A and B: (A) Multiple pneumatoceles (thin walled air containing lung parenchyma) R upper and mid zones; (B) Lung abscess RMZ (thick walled with air fluid level).

lesions **(Figs. 26.14A and B)**], congenital lobar emphysema, air containing bowel loops in the chest [congenital diaphragmatic hernia **(Fig. 26.15)**], congenital cystic adenomatoid malformation and hyperinflated lung secondary to endobronchial foreign body obstruction. The differing features of lung abscess from pneumatocele are its thick wall and presence of air fluid level. The most common cause of unilateral hyperlucent hemithorax in a child is malpositioning (rotation to one side) during radiography.

Pulmonary vascularity: Trace the branches of the pulmonary arteries which are usually not visible in the peripheral third of the lung. If seen, it indicates increased pulmonary blood flow (this criterion has become controversial with the advent of digital radiography).

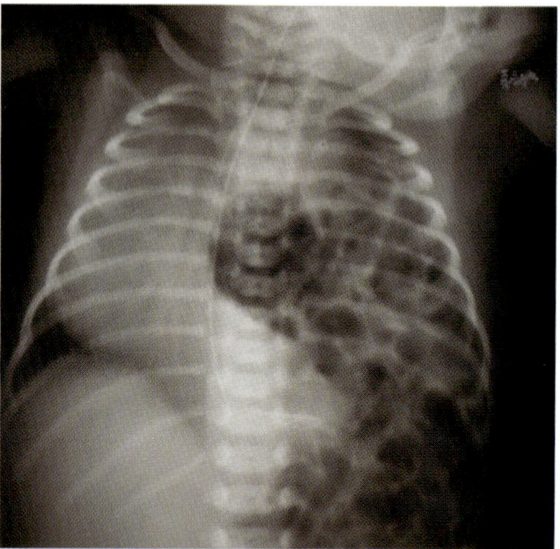

Fig. 26.15: Gas-filled diaphragmatic hernia (L): Mediastinal shift to (R)

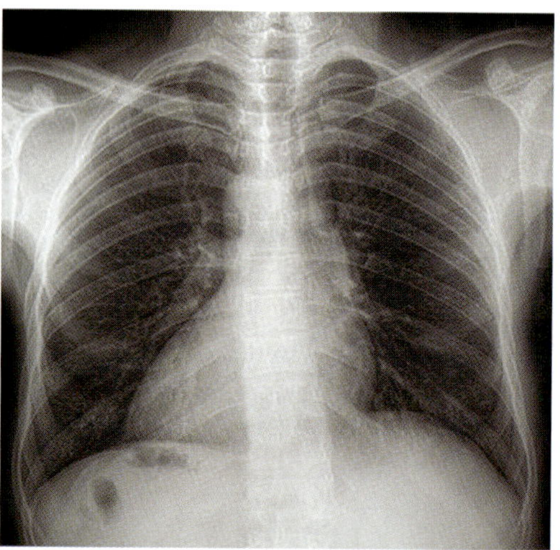

Fig. 26.16: Dextrocardia with situs inversus: Note the stomach bubble on R side.

In "plethora", the peripheral pulmonary arteries are nontapering and appear nodular. Nonvisualization of pulmonary vessels centrally indicates reduced pulmonary blood flow **(Fig. 26.9)**. Pulmonary arterial hypertension is indicated by "peripheral pruning of the pulmonary arteries" seen as dilatation of the proximal arteries and a sudden reduction in caliber distally. *Pulmonary hila* are the holes in the mediastinal pleura through which pulmonary vessels and bronchi pass through. Look at the position of the hilum and compare it with the opposite side. Normally the left hilum appears higher than the right. Displacement of hilum occurs in lobar and segmental collapse, i.e., right hilum is elevated in right upper lobe collapse or pulled down in right lower lobe collapse. The hilar shadows become enlarged due to vascular (dilated pulmonary arteries in left to right shunts) or added density by enlarged lymph nodes.

- *Assess the situs:* The atrial and visceral situs should be established by inspection of the bronchial anatomy, position of the stomach bubble, and side of the aortic arch. Normal cardiac apex is directed to left.

  In dextrocardia, it is directed to (R) which can be isolated or associated with situs inversus **(Fig. 26.16)**.
- *The diaphragm*: Right dome is normally at a higher level than the left; part of the left dome is obscured by the cardiac shadow but can be traceable up to the spine **(Figs. 26.14A and B)**. Eventration is abnormal elevation and thinning of the diaphragm **(Fig. 26.17)**; congenital diaphragmatic hernia is absence of diaphragmatic outline with presence of bowel loops inside the chest **(Fig. 26.15)**. Domes of diaphragm are flattened in emphysema **(Fig. 26.18)**. Basal consolidation in lower lobes obliterates the diaphragm producing "silhouette sign" **(Fig. 26.19)**. In an erect chest radiograph, search for free air under the diaphragm, especially in blunt trauma abdomen **(Fig. 26.20)**.
- *Costophrenic (CP) angles* are normally sharp at the lateral ends; fluid in the pleural cavity produces blunting of the angles **(Fig. 26.21)**.

  Pleural outlines are not visualized normally. In pleural effusion (accumulation

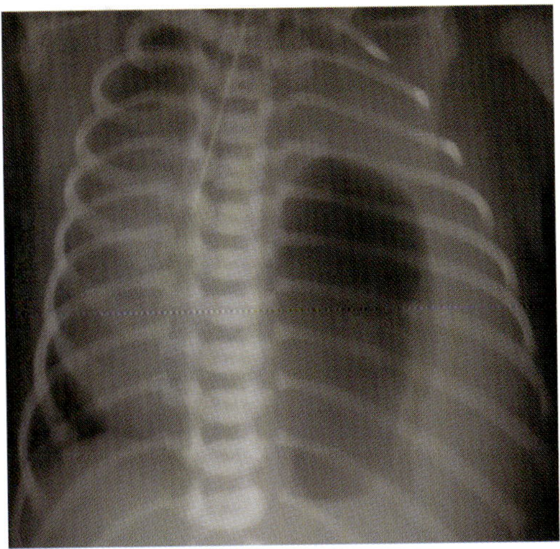

Fig. 26.17: Eventration (L) dome of diaphragm; stomach bubble on (L) thorax.

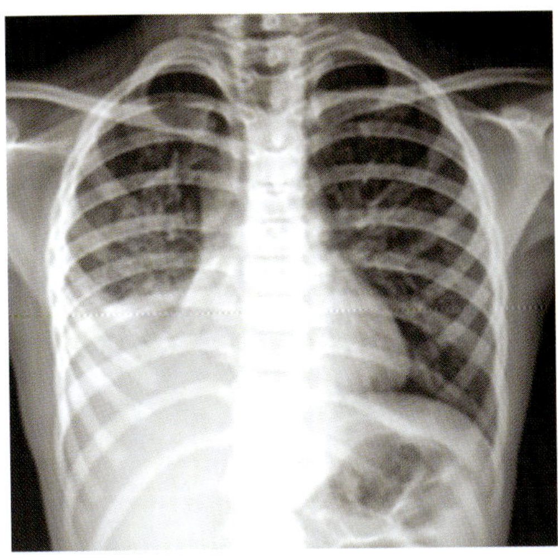

Fig. 26.19: Silhouette sign in R basal consolidation obliterating the R dome of diaphragm.

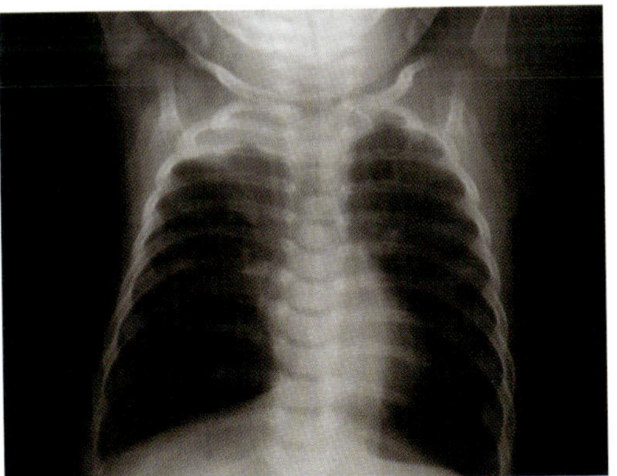

Fig. 26.18: RUZ collapse, with B/L hyper inflation and flattened domes of diaphragm.

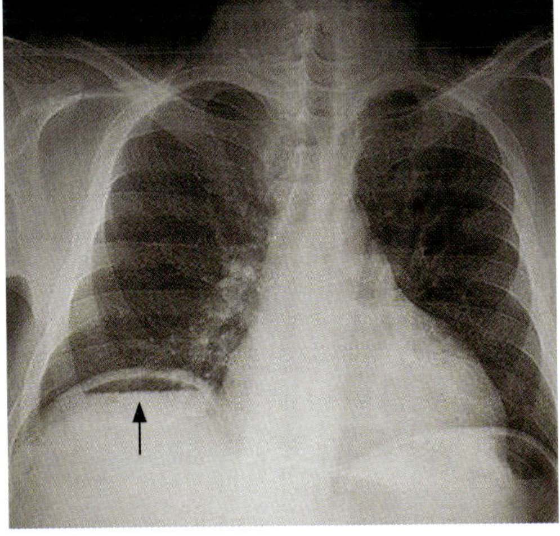

Fig. 26.20: Air under R dome of diaphragm following blunt injury abdomen.

of fluid between mediastinal and parietal layers), pleura appears white **(Fig. 26.12)**, in pneumothorax (air between two pleural layers), it is black **(Fig. 26.13)**; the most common pleural pathologies. Hydropneumothorax is accumulation of both air and fluid in the pleural cavity.

- *Lateral view of chest skiagram* is occasionally needed. The indications are to localize the lobar pathology **(Fig. 26.22; Sail shadow)**, to detect enlarged hilar lymph nodes, hyperinflated chest and to confirm thymic shadow. It is difficult to position young children correctly for lateral view; also radiation exposure is more than AP view. CT chest is superior in such situations to provide details in the third dimension with accuracy.

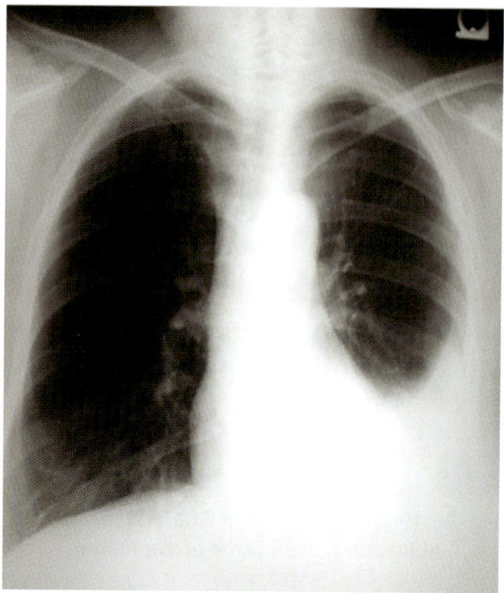

Fig. 26.21: Moderate pleural effusion (L) obliterating CP angle (L); normal CP angle (R).

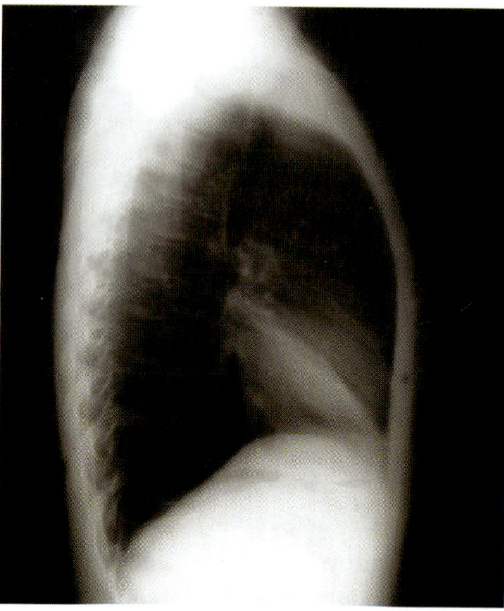

Fig. 26.22: (R) lateral view chest with middle lobe collapse (Sail shadow) and lung hyperinflation.

Ultrasound in chest imaging is gaining increasing importance for early detection of pleural and pericardial fluid collection and consolidation involving the lung margins **(Fig. 26.23)**. The limitation is the presence of air in the lungs preventing the penetration of sound waves. *Point of care ultrasound* (POC-US) is done in intensive care units to look for the onset of pulmonary edema and increasing pericardial and pleural effusions in ventilated patients.

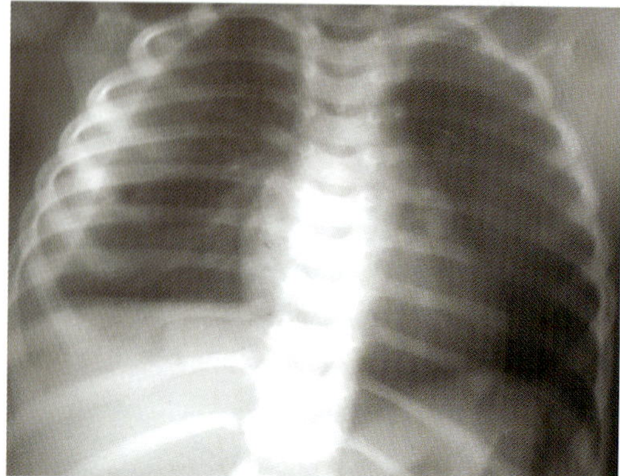

Fig. 26.23: Pneumonia with lamellar pleural effusion R.

Computed tomography chest: Axial sections of the chest are taken with the child supine on the CT table with hands raised above the head. The computer can reconstruct the axial images in coronal plane (chest skiagram AP view) and sagittal plane (lateral view). The images are displayed in two window settings—lung window to show lung and airway anatomy and pathology and the mediastinal window to show the anatomy and pathology of the soft tissues including heart and great vessels. Intravenous contrast is administered to differentiate masses from consolidation and mediastinal lymph nodes from vessels to demonstrate pleural enhancement in empyema and to delineate vascular anatomy and variations. Advanced reconstructions like virtual bronchoscopy can be useful in localization of intrabronchial foreign bodies.

See **Figures 26.24A to C**—chest skiagram and CT scan of a girl, 10 yr with recurrent respiratory infection for 2 yr.

Magnetic resonance imaging chest is rarely taken in pediatrics due to inadequate breath holding. Cardiac MRI is advised for congenital heart problems that need surgical correction.

Abdomen including Gastrointestinal Tract and Genitourinary Tract

Plain Skiagram Abdomen

It can be taken as supine anteroposterior (AP) or erect AP. Supine AP view demonstrates patterns of bowel involvement and helps in identifying involved segments of the bowel. **Figure 26.25** is the supine abdominal (plain) radiograph of a newborn with acute intestinal obstruction revealing grossly dilated air filled bowel loops distending the abdomen.

Gastrointestinal tract (GIT): Plain X-ray erect view detects bowel wall air (necrotizing enterocolitis), air fluid levels in intestinal obstruction **(Fig. 26.26)**, free peritoneal air [bowel perforation **(Fig. 26.20)**], impacted radiopaque foreign bodies **(Fig. 26.27)**, and as preliminary film of barium examinations. Neonatal surgical emergencies like intestinal atresia and meconium peritonitis can be strongly suspected from plain X-ray examinations (duodenal atresia, jejunal atresia, and peritoneal calcifications). A prone cross lateral view of the abdomen after placing a radiopaque marker in the expected anal orifice helps in identifying and classifying anorectal malformations in neonates [former invertogram **(Fig. 26.28)**].

Kidneys, ureters, and bladder (KUB): Plain film is routinely taken as a preliminary of IVU or MCU. It is beneficial in children with abdominal colic, chronic constipation, or hematuria to detect renal/ureteric/pancreatic calculi and impacted fecal matter. Ultrasound is superior in these situations.

Gastrointestinal contrast studies are advised in neonates and infants to confirm Hirschsprung disease **(Fig. 26.29A)**, midgut malrotation, idiopathic hypertrophic pyloric stenosis [IHPS **(Fig. 26.29B)**], to demonstrate gastroesophageal reflux disease in older children **(Fig. 26.29C)**, gastric bezoar and intussusception. Barium sulfate suspension is the preferred positive contrast agent for GIT. Water-soluble contrast mediums like diatrizoate sodium (urografin) or newer nonionic low osmolar contrast medium (iohexol) are used in suspected bowel perforation with leak into the peritoneal cavity where barium is contraindicated.

Intravenous urography and micturating cystourethrography are the two main special X-rays for the genitourinary tract (GUT). Present indications for IVU are limited as newer CT scans with excellent reconstructions (exactly simulate IVU film) with minimum radiation dose. MCU is ideal to detect vesicoureteric reflux [VUR **(Fig. 26.30)**], recurrent urinary tract infections (UTIs) in children, and for evaluating posterior urethral valve [PUV **(Fig. 26.31)**]. IVU has only a limited role for the follow-up of surgically corrected renal anomalies (pelviureteric junction obstruction and hydronephrosis) to avoid repeated CT studies **(Figs. 26.32A and B)**.

Ultrasonogram is the first investigation in a child with abdominal symptoms since it is cheap, easily available, repeatable without the hazards of ionizing radiation and is usually acceptable to those in distress. Solid viscera like liver, spleen, pancreas, and kidneys are easily assessed on USG. *Gallbladder (GB)* examination needs a period of fasting

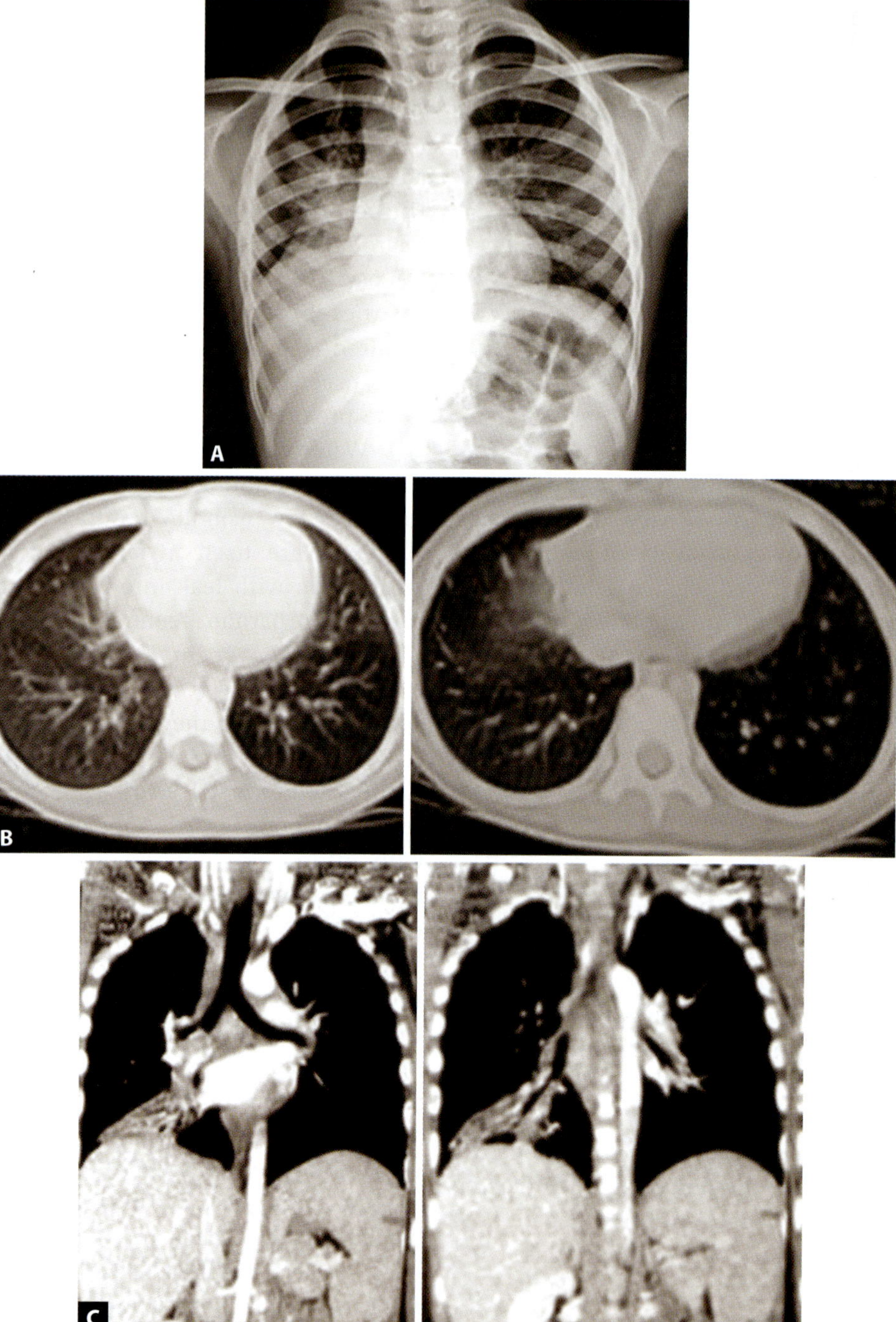

Figs. 26.24A and C: (A and B) R mid and lower zone opacities with straight lateral margin obliterating R dome of diaphragm with R hilum pulled down, R cardiac margin not obliterated; compensatory overinflation middle and upper lobes; (C) CT thorax axial sections and coronal reconstruction show resolving collapse consolidation R lower lobe.

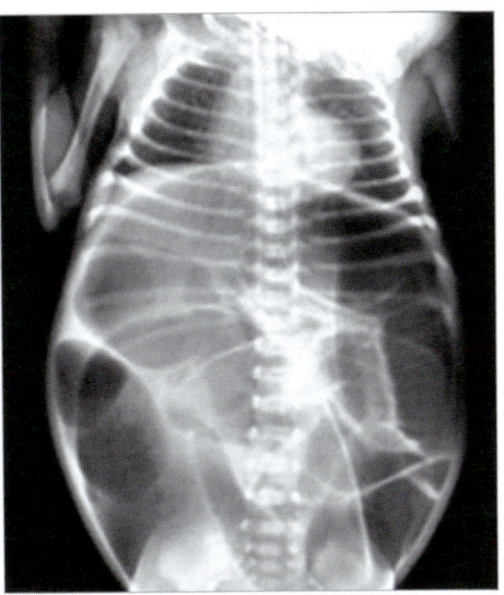

Fig. 26.25: Plain radiograph abdomen—supine AP, view of a newborn baby with intestinal obstruction—*see* distended bowel loops.

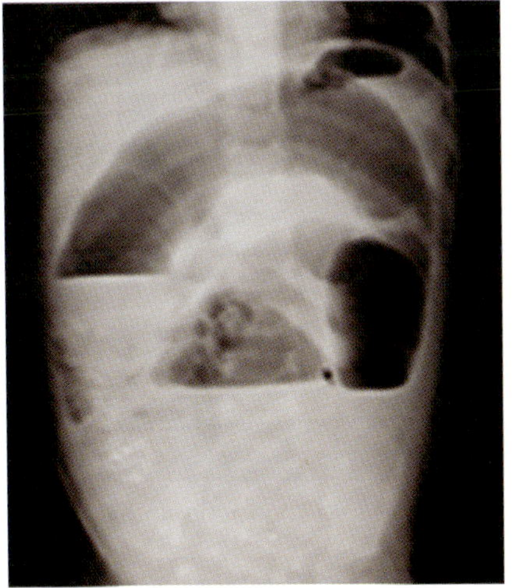

Fig. 26.26: Plain radiograph abdomen—erect view of a child with intestinal obstruction, see multiple air fluid levels.

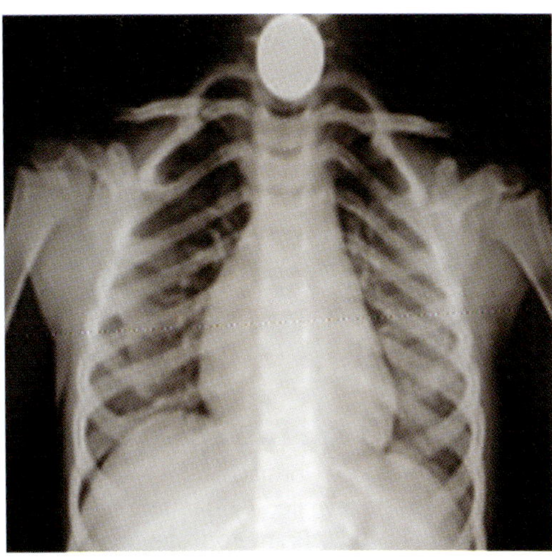

Fig. 26.27: Foreign body—metallic coin in the esophagus (coins in the esophagus are oriented in coronal plane); usual site of impaction at thoracic inlet.

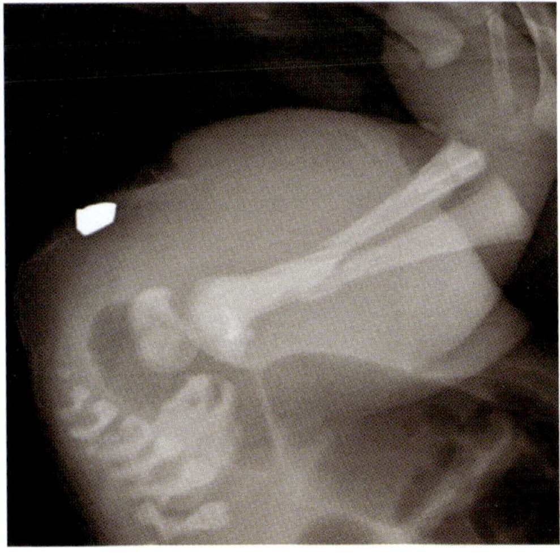

Fig. 26.28: Invertogram in diagnosing imperforate anus.

(2 hours, 4 hours, and 6 hours for newborn, infant, and older child respectively) before the examination, to get the GB distended with bile for easy visualization of its lumen and wall. Fasting also helps to eliminate bowel air which causes reflection of sound waves barring visualization of deeper structures. Intestinal loops can be assessed for distension, peristalsis, and evidence of obstruction like worm mass or intussusception. Ascites is identified as fluid accumulation in Morrison's pouch or pelvis.

Ultrasound of the pelvic organs, inguinal region, and scrotum is mandatory in all

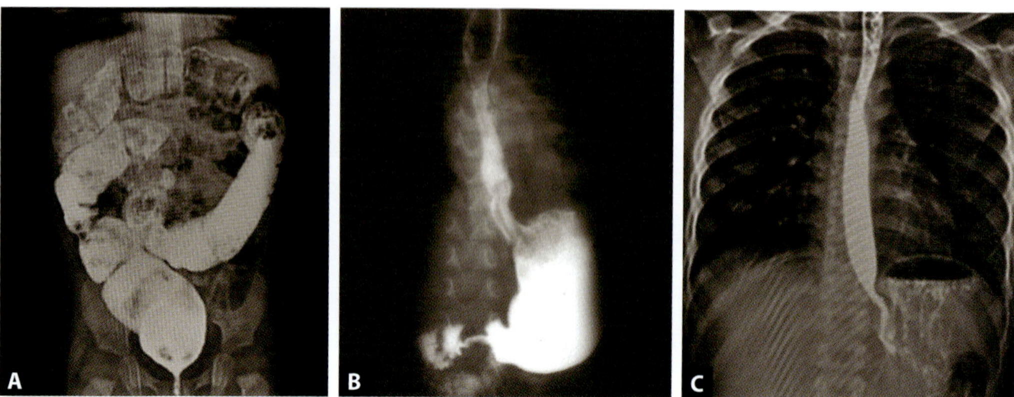

Figs. 26.29A to C: (A) Normal barium enema opacification up to hepatic flexure; (B) Idiopathic hypertrophic pyloric stenosis—revealed by barium meal studies; (C) Chest AP view—barium swallow opacifying the thoracic esophagus. (AP: anteroposterior).

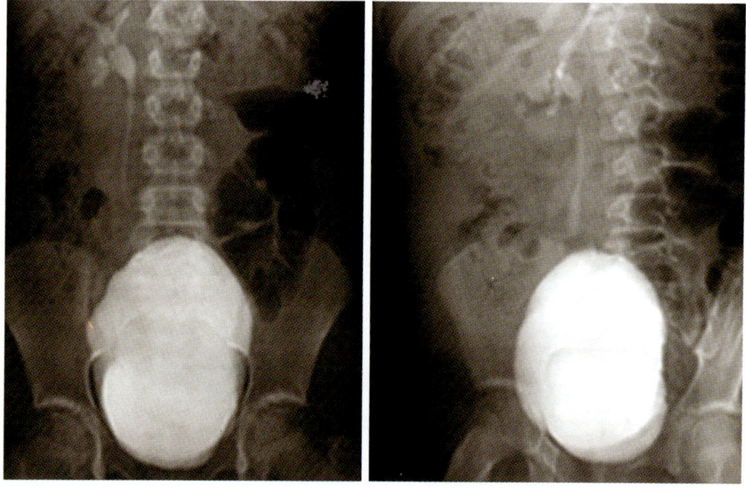

Fig. 26.30: MCU of a 10 yr old girl with B/L VUR-AP and oblique views show reflux into R ureter and pelvicalyceal system.

abdominal imaging. The female pelvis should be scanned both with full bladder and after urination, to detect a twisted ovarian cyst which can mimic a filled urinary bladder and cause acute abdomen. A positive ultrasound scan report of acute appendicitis or torsion testis obtained on the way to the theater adds to the confidence of the surgeon.

Color Doppler scanning is necessary to assess portal vein flow in cases of liver cirrhosis, superior mesenteric vein-superior mesenteric artery relationship in midgut rotation, preoperative assessment of vascularity and vascular invasion of malignant neoplasms and to evaluate children with malignant hypertension to detect renal vascular causes and vessel thrombosis. Substantiation by CT scanning or contrast studies is a must for USG findings, since apart from operator dependency, other

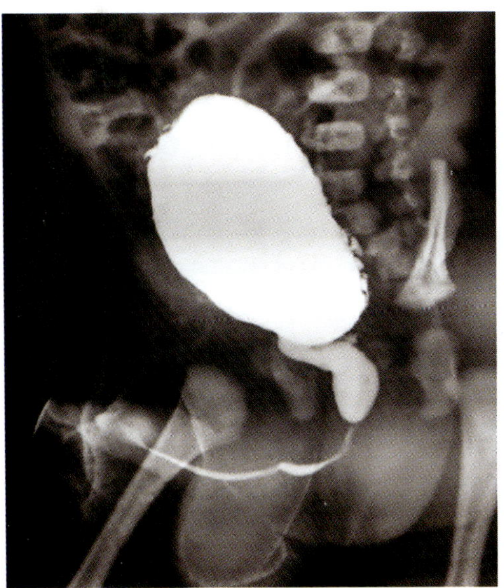

Fig. 26.31: MCU studies—baby boy revealing posterior urethral valve.
Courtesy: Dr Kundal AK, Pediatric surgeon indelhi.in/posterior-urethral-valve.

factors like presence of bowel air, adequacy of fasting, distension of urinary bladder, and the child's cooperation are also involved.

Computed tomography scanning of the abdomen is undertaken only after ultrasound and sometimes after contrast studies also, because of the risk of exposure to ionizing radiation. In young children, contrast-enhanced CT is undertaken, if plain CT alone is not answering the clinical queries. The type of CT contrast depends on the clinical indication. For babies with midgut rotation and Ladd's band obstruction or with suspected IHPS, CT with oral contrast administration (water-soluble contrast is ideal since barium can produce CT artifacts) is the choice study, whereas patients with liver mass or pancreatic tail injury (blunt trauma abdomen) need post-intravenous (IV) contrast CT. Older children with appendicular mass or suspected ovarian malignancy need CT scanning with oral, rectal, and IV contrast administration. CT enterography involves dedicated examination of the bowel after proper distension of the lumen by water or polyethylene glycol (PEGLEC) followed by CT scanning with IV contrast administration. Indications for CT enterography are inflammatory bowel disease (Crohn's disease or ulcerative colitis) or demonstration of polyps in the lumen (intestinal polyposis syndromes).

Preoperative staging or pretreatment planning of Wilms tumor, neuroblastoma, and lymphoma in children needs CT scanning as the baseline examination. CT scan of the abdomen is the ideal in pediatric trauma, especially when hemoperitoneum is noted on USG. CT scan with IV contrast administration can reliably rule out solid visceral injury.

Magnetic resonance imaging of the abdomen in pediatrics is considered in situations where IV contrast is dangerous as in neonates and in renal failure. MRI has superb resolution and advanced MRI techniques help in differentiating tissues without IV contrast administration (MR urogram). It can also delineate the intraspinal extension of neuroblastoma.

Radionuclide studies are important in assessing differential renal function in cases of bilateral hydronephrosis [dimercapto succinic acid (DMSA) scan **(Fig. 26.33)**].

Positron emission tomography (PET) scanning is used to search for metastases in a known malignancy.

Musculoskeletal System

The most common indication for imaging of the musculoskeletal system (MSK) in pediatrics is trauma, to confirm/rule out fractures and dislocations **(Fig. 26.34)**. Radiograph of the involved part can easily answer this. Osteomyelitis is not an uncommon condition in children; in young babies, the diagnosis may be easily missed

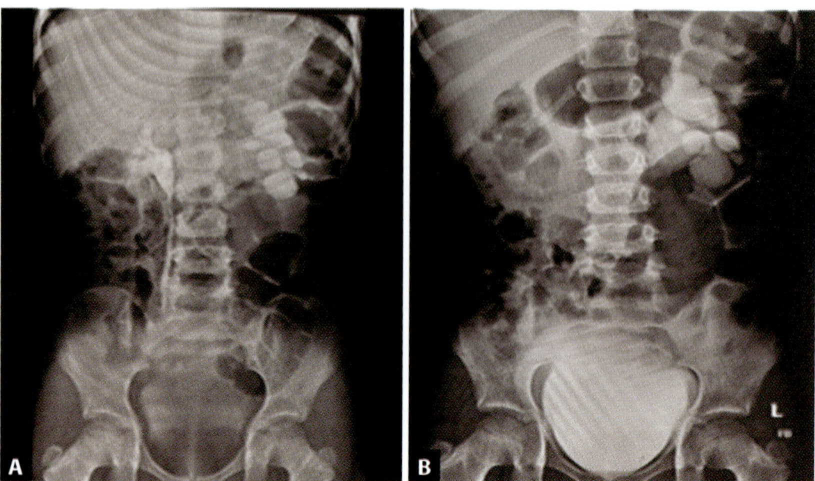

Figs. 26.32A and B: (A) IVU of boy 7 yr old—at 10 min shows dilated pelvicalyceal system (L), (R) side normal. See F/U after 45 min; (B) 45 min delayed film—further dilatation pelvicalyceal system without excretion into (L) ureter; (R) side normal. See F/U after 45 min (L) pelviureteric junction obstruction, normal (R) side.

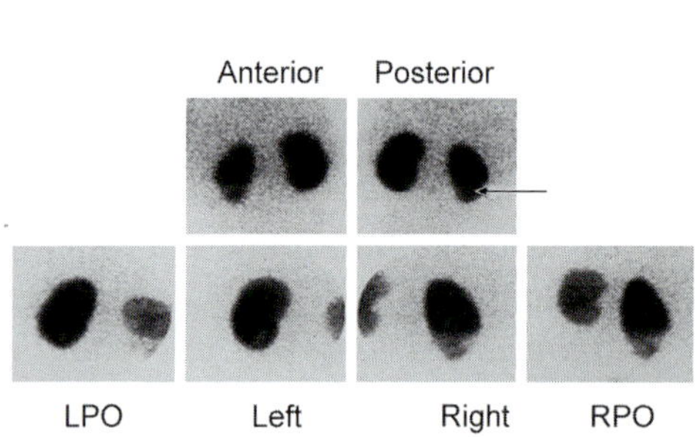

Fig. 26.33: DMSA cortical renal scintigraphy on a 5 m old baby with AN diagnosis of R hydronephrosis revealing reduced uptake in the nonfunctioning hydronephrotic lower moiety (black arrow). (DMSA: dimercapto succinic acid)

Source: Sandler MP. Turnaround: Time to Take a Look. J Nuclear Med. 2001;42(1):1-2.

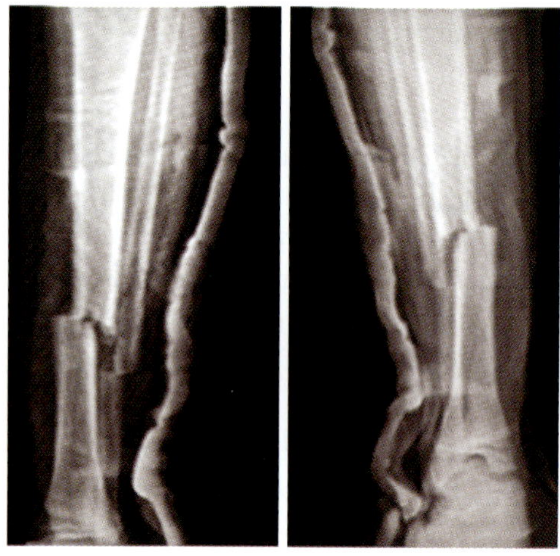

Fig. 26.34: Radiograph of leg of a child AP and lateral views revealing fracture fibula and tibia. (AP: anteroposterior)

clinically **(Fig. 26.35)**. Other indications are skeletal surveys for age determination, skeletal dysplasias, and endocrine/metabolic disorders to prove the diagnosis. Plain radiograph is the investigation of choice in focal bone pain and is almost diagnostic, second only to MRI with all its added advantages.

Ultrasound of MSK system is a very useful tool in newborn infants with suspected developmental dysplasia of the hip for initial diagnosis and treatment follow-up. USG can diagnose joint effusions, fluid collections or hematoma in soft tissues related to trauma and infections. Color Doppler

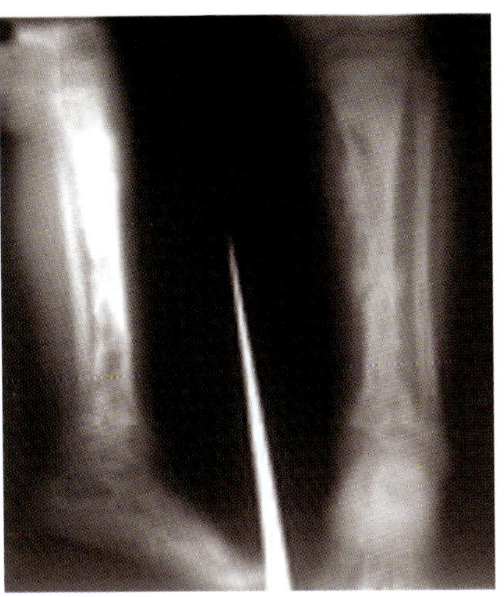

Fig. 26.35: Skiagram of (L) leg of a 23 m old child with osteomyelitis lower end of tibia.

Fig. 26.36: 3D reconstruction of normal human cochlea and semicircular canals. Reconstructed from high-resolution CT images of temporal bone in a boy 2 yr old, waiting for cochlear implantation.

imaging contributes to the assessment of neurovascular bundles in bone and soft tissue tumors and compression by fracture hematoma, especially the status of distal vessels.

Multidetector raw CT (MDCT) with its three-dimensional applications can demonstrate the minute details of fractures and dislocations and is essential in operative management **(Fig. 26.36)**. In infections, dysplasia, and tumors, the patient is directly taken up for MRI, after the initial evaluation by plain radiograph.

Role of bone scintigraphy is limited to demonstration of unsuspected metastases as in neuroblastoma and hematological malignancies.

Head and Neck, Brain, and Spine

Indications for radiographs of head, neck, and spine in the pediatric population are limited to local trauma or pain and swelling and as part of skeletal survey. *Skeletal survey* means a series of radiographs performed systematically to prove or disprove a specific clinical entity; e.g., suspected child abuse, skeletal dysplasias, rickets, juvenile rheumatoid arthritis, etc. It can involve the entire skeleton or the anatomic regions appropriate for the indication. *Ultrasonography of the neck* can identify lesions of thyroid, enlarged lymph nodes, salivary glands and branchial cyst and cystic hygroma. Complete diagnosis may not be possible in all cases by ultrasonography; CT or MRI may be required.

Neurosonogram (NSG) can diagnose hydrocephalus, germinal matrix bleed, hypoxic ischemic encephalopathy, anomalies such as corpus callosum dysgenesis and Dandy–Walker malformation, ventriculitis and white matter echogenicities. Follow-up by NSG can be done till the AF is open. USG of the spine can be done in the neonate with myelomeningocele to assess the level of termination of cord and to look for a lipoma and other masses in the spinal canal. *CT scan is not advised* for brain imaging, especially in the newborn period. A well-scrutinized NSG by an experienced sonologist along with clinical correlation can provide a working diagnosis in most of the neonatal problems.

MRI is the next choice for further workup as CT has the risk of ionizing radiation. Neonatal meningitis can be effectively managed by serial NSG, but MRI is superior for diagnosing complications like subdural effusion and vascular pathologies. After infancy, in emergencies such as head injury, suspected intracranial bleeding, or space-occupying lesions, the choice is CT scan because of better availability and low cost. In spinal injuries, CT is preferred, as bony details are better appreciated in CT than MRI in which fractures may be missed. Another advantage of CT over MRI is for the differentiation between blood and calcium. *The safest and most informative modality* in imaging of the pediatric brain, head and neck, and spine is MRI. It is the choice imaging modality in white matter diseases, inborn errors of metabolism, diagnosis of brain tumors (by advanced techniques), intractable infections, epilepsy imaging, and head and neck tumors. MRI is the only modality which depicts the status of spinal cord in conditions of trauma, tumors, and spinal dysraphism.

SUGGESTED READING

1. Arthur R. Interpretation of the pediatric chest X-ray. Curr Paediatr. 2003;13:438-47.
2. Burdi AR, Huelke DF, Snyder RG, Lowrey GH. Infants and children in the adult world of automobile safety design: Pediatric and Anatomical considerations for Design of child restraints. J Biomech. 1969;2(3):267-80.
3. Caffey J, Silverman FN, Kuhn JP. Caffey's Pediatric X-ray Diagnosis: An Integrated Imaging Approach, 9th edition. St. Louis: Mosby Year Book Publishers; 1992.
4. Sutton D. A Textbook of Radiology and Imaging, Volume 1 and 2, 5th edition. London: Churchill Livingstone; 1993.
5. Swischuk LE. Imaging of the Newborn, Infant, and Young Child, 3rd edition. Philadelphia: Williams & Wilkins; 1990.

Appendix-1

GROWTH CHARTS [FIG. 11.5 (1 TO 21)]

Chart 1

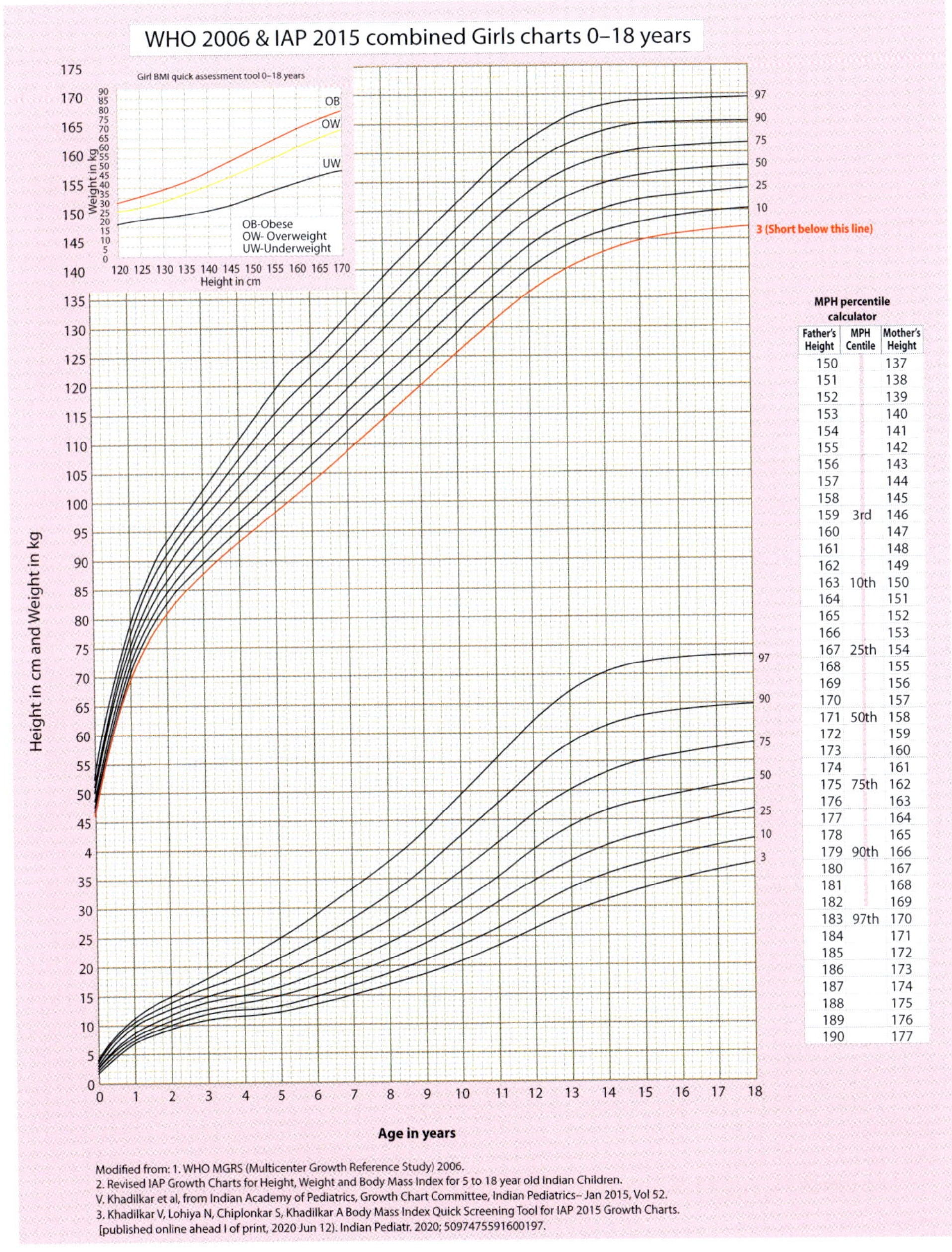

Father's Height	MPH Centile	Mother's Height
150		137
151		138
152		139
153		140
154		141
155		142
156		143
157		144
158		145
159	3rd	146
160		147
161		148
162		149
163	10th	150
164		151
165		152
166		153
167	25th	154
168		155
169		156
170		157
171	50th	158
172		159
173		160
174		161
175	75th	162
176		163
177		164
178		165
179	90th	166
180		167
181		168
182		169
183	97th	170
184		171
185		172
186		173
187		174
188		175
189		176
190		177

Appendix-1, Fig. 11.5: Chart 1—WHO 2006 & IAP 2015 combined girls charts 0–18 yr (height and weight).

Chart 2

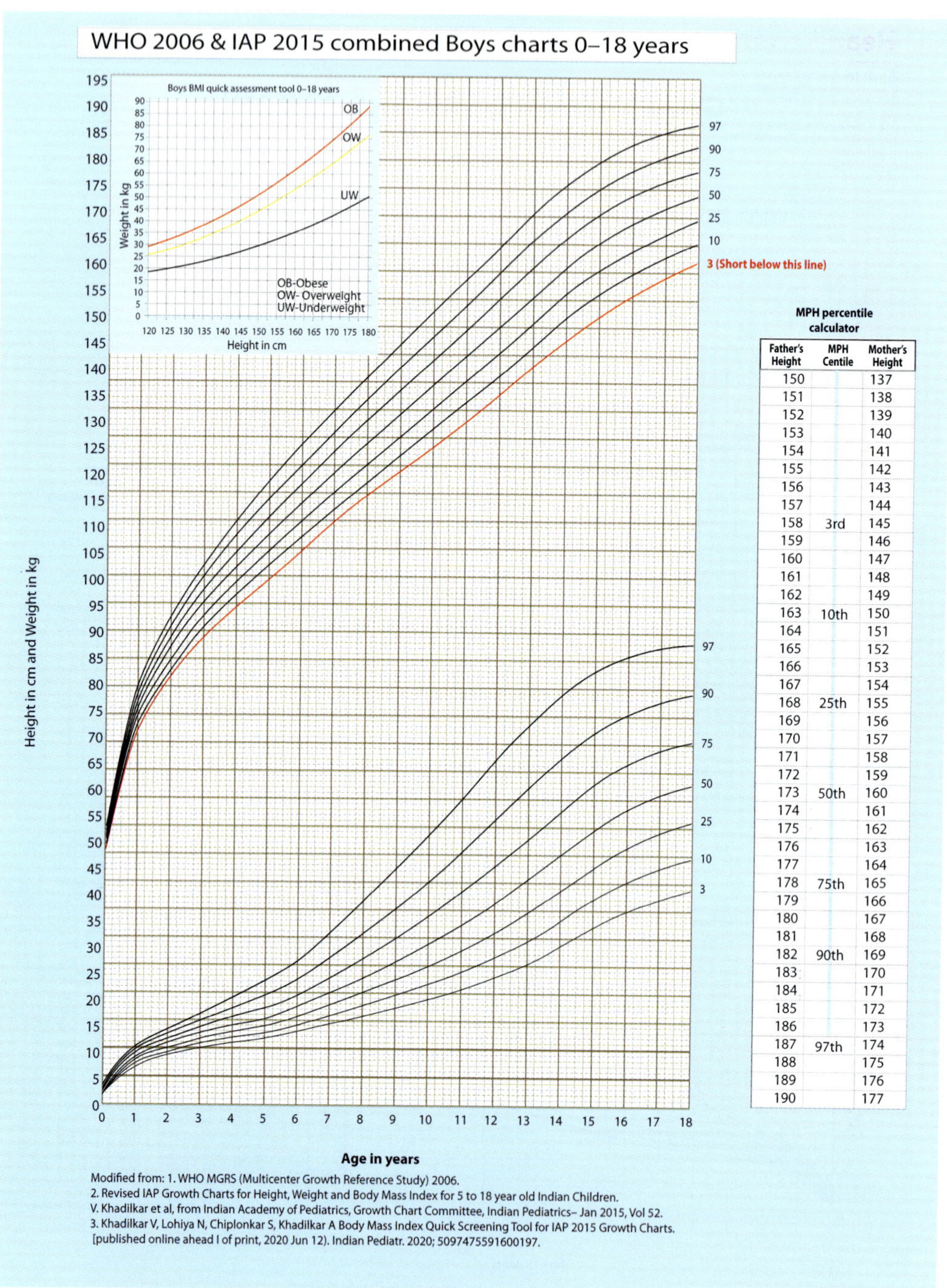

MPH percentile calculator

Father's Height	MPH Centile	Mother's Height
150		137
151		138
152		139
153		140
154		141
155		142
156		143
157		144
158	3rd	145
159		146
160		147
161		148
162		149
163	10th	150
164		151
165		152
166		153
167		154
168	25th	155
169		156
170		157
171		158
172		159
173	50th	160
174		161
175		162
176		163
177		164
178	75th	165
179		166
180		167
181		168
182	90th	169
183		170
184		171
185		172
186		173
187	97th	174
188		175
189		176
190		177

Appendix-1, Fig. 11.5: Chart 2–WHO 2006 & IAP 2015 combined boys charts 0–18 yr (height and weight).

Chart 3

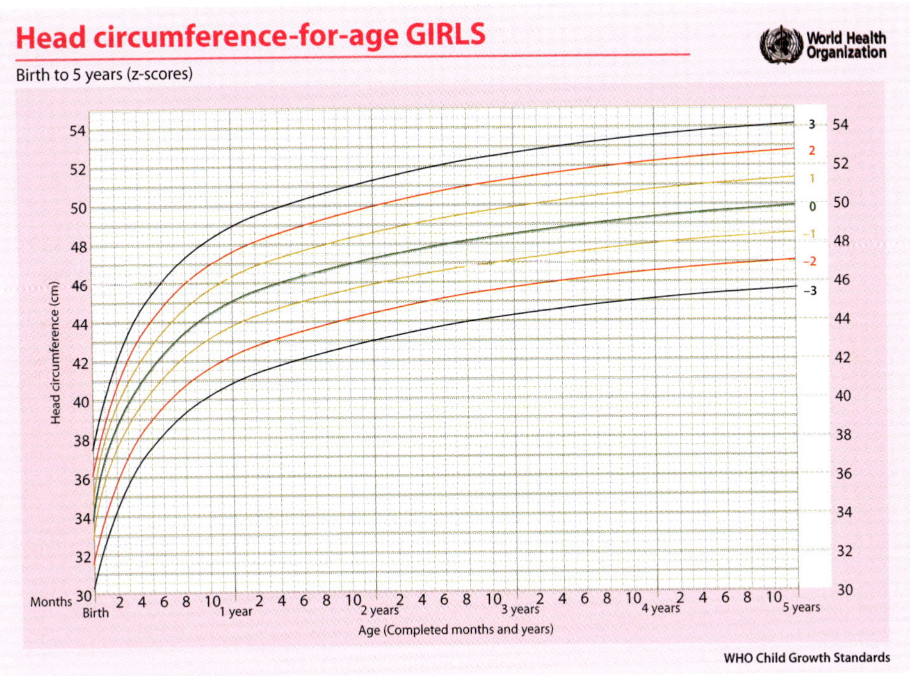

Appendix-1, Fig. 11.5: Chart 3—WHO—Head circumference-for-age Girls 0–5 yr.

Chart 4

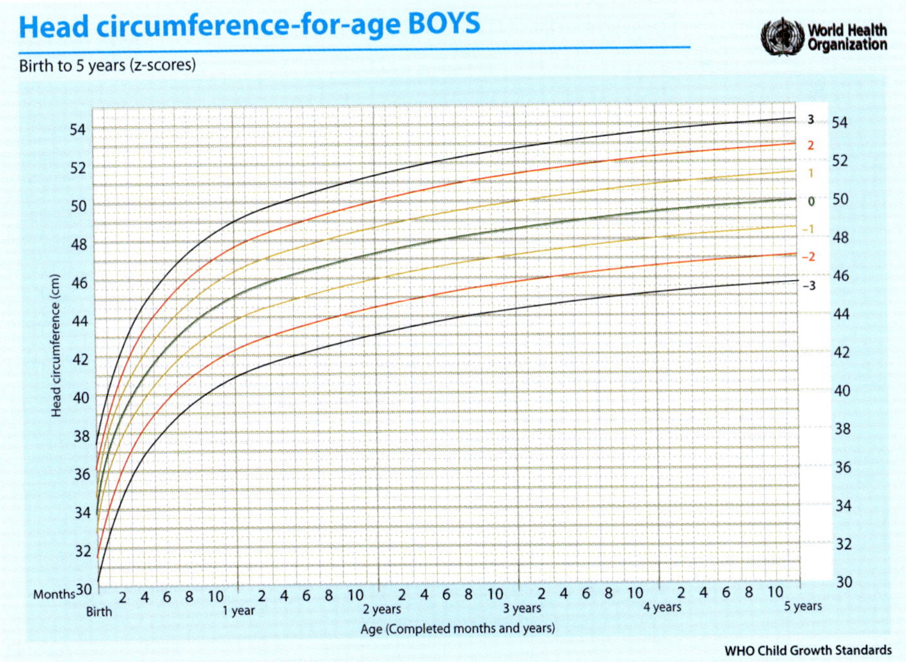

Appendix-1, Fig. 11.5: Chart 4—WHO—Head circumference-for-age Boys 0–5 yr.

Chart 5

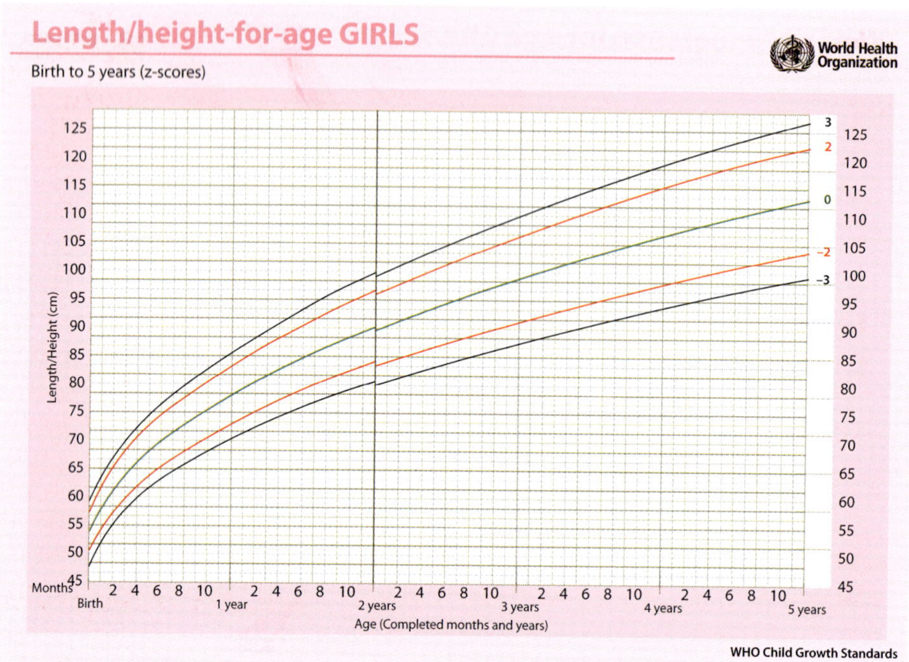

Appendix-1, Fig. 11.5: Chart 5—WHO—Length/height-for-age Girls 0–5 yr.

Chart 6

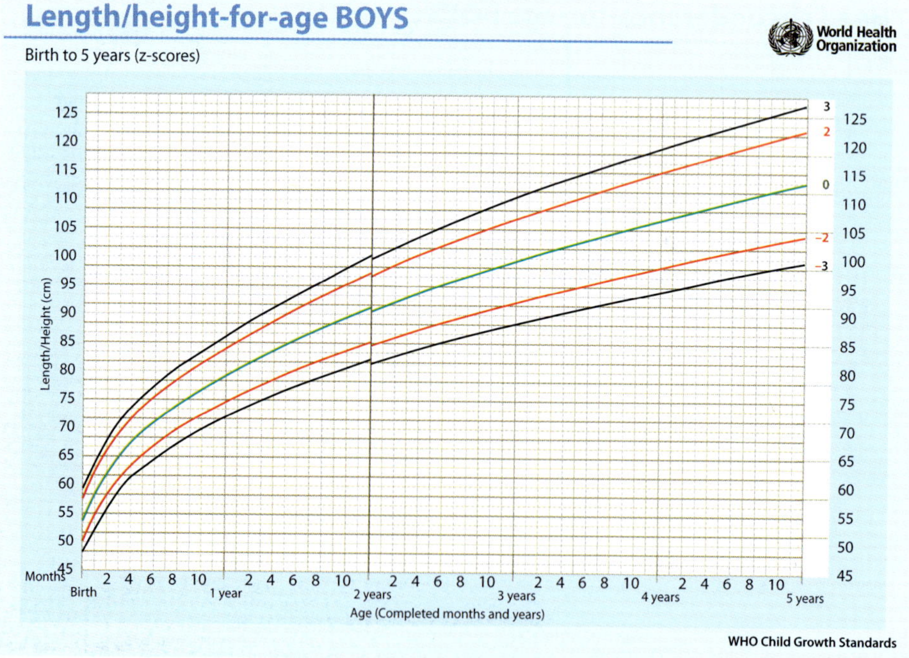

Appendix-1, Fig. 11.5: Chart 6—WHO—Length/height-for-age Boys 0–5 yr.

Chart 7

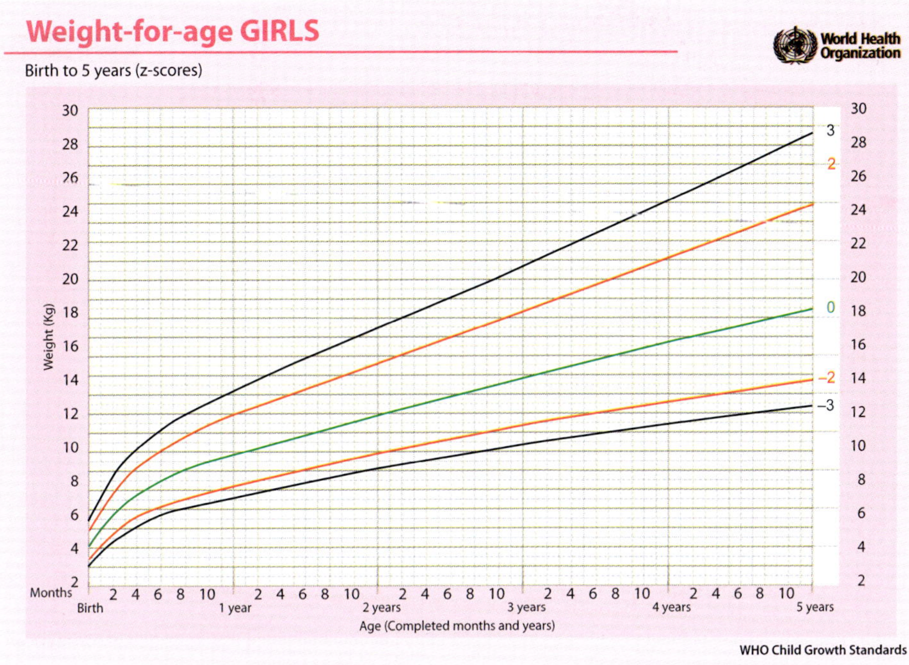

Appendix-1, Fig. 11.5: Chart 7—WHO—Weight-for-age Boys 0–5 yr.

Chart 8

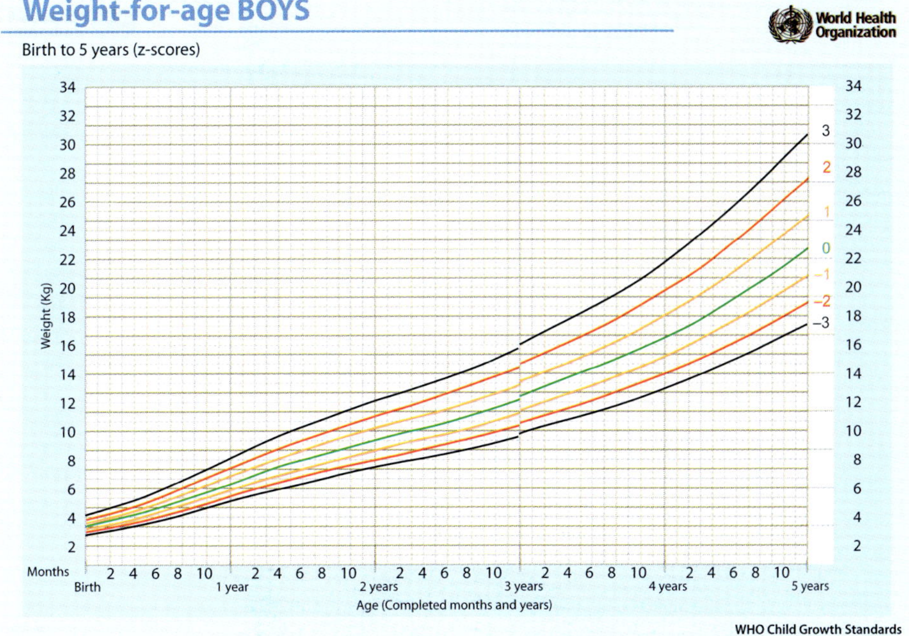

Appendix-1, Fig. 11.5: Chart 8—WHO—Weight-for-age Girls 0–5 yr.

Chart 9

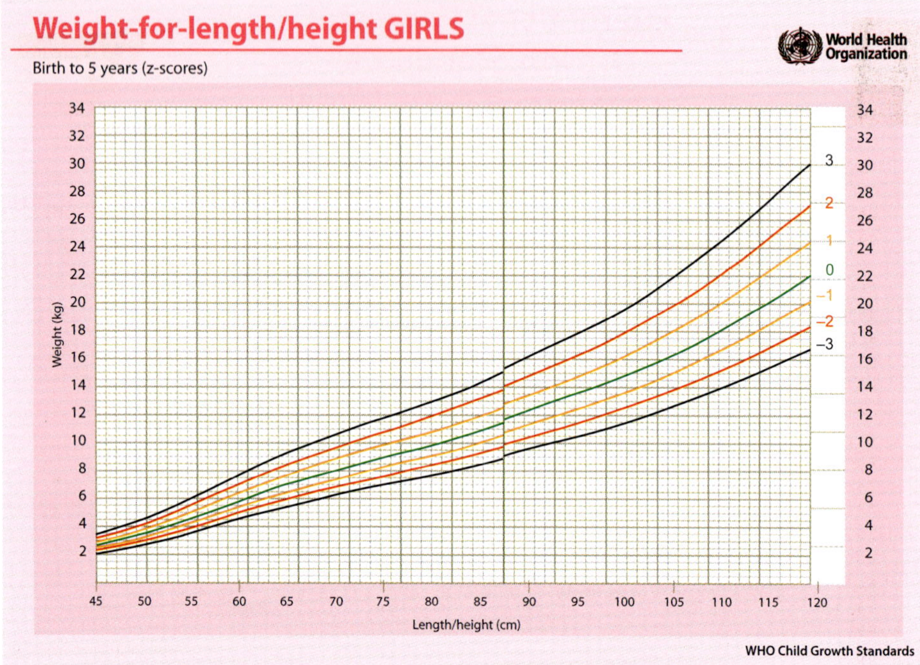

Appendix-1, Fig. 11.5: Chart 9—WHO—Weight-for-length/height Girls 0–5 yr.

Chart 10

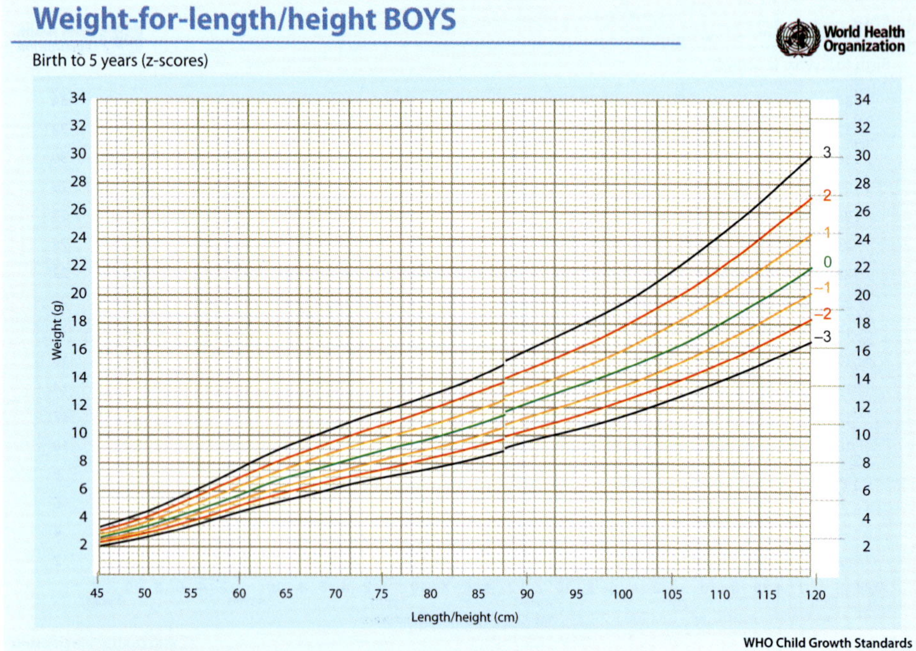

Appendix-1, Fig. 11.5: Chart 10—WHO—Weight-for-length/height Boys 0–5 yr.

Chart 11

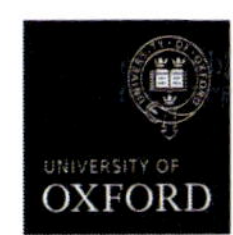

International Postnatal Growth Standards for Preterm Infants (Girls)

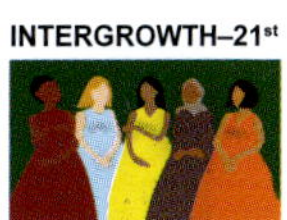

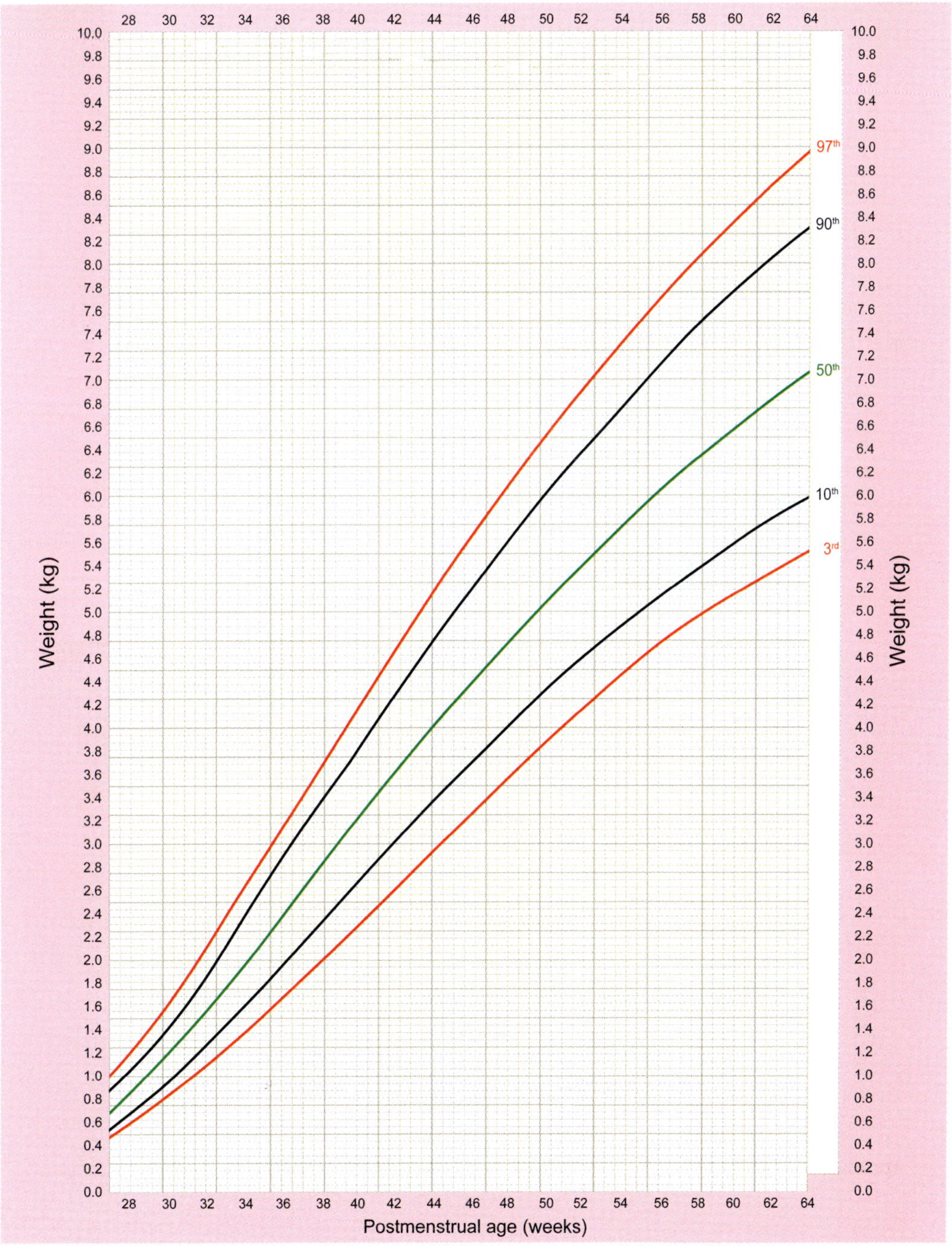

Weight (kg)

10.0 9.8 9.6 9.4 9.2 9.0 8.8 8.6 8.4 8.2 8.0 7.8 7.6 7.4 7.2 7.0 6.8 6.6 6.4 6.2 6.0 5.8 5.6 5.4 5.2 5.0 4.8 4.6 4.4 4.2 4.0 3.8 3.6 3.4 3.2 3.0 2.8 2.6 2.4 2.2 2.0 1.8 1.6 1.4 1.2 1.0 0.8 0.6 0.4 0.2 0.0

97th 90th 50th 10th 3rd

28 30 32 34 36 38 40 42 44 46 48 50 52 54 56 58 60 62 64

Postmenstrual age (weeks)

Appendix-1, Fig. 11.5: Chart 11—International Postnatal Growth Standards for Preterm Infants.

Chart 12

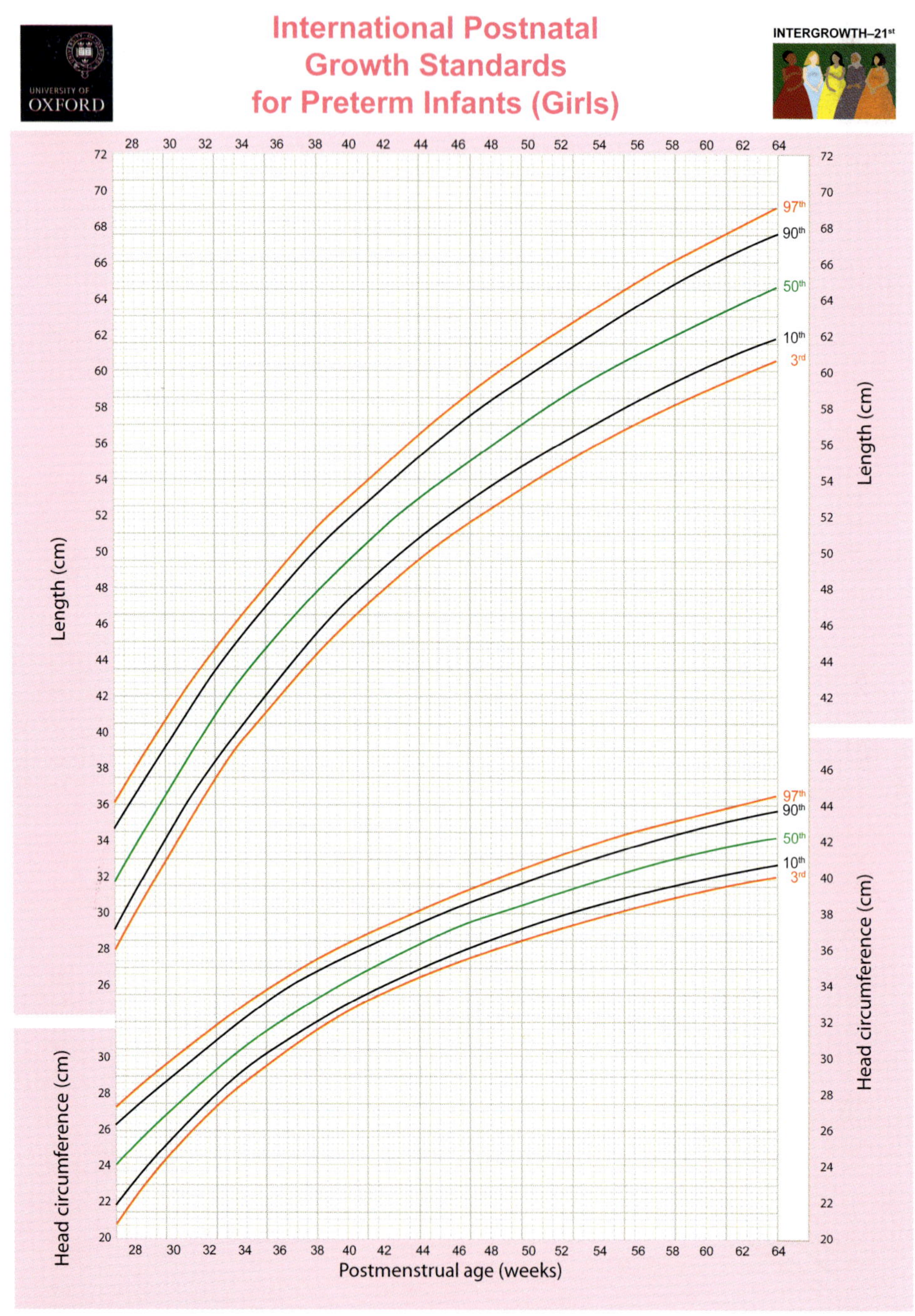

Appendix-1, Fig. 11.5: Chart 12—International Postnatal Growth Standards for Preterm Infants.

Chart 13

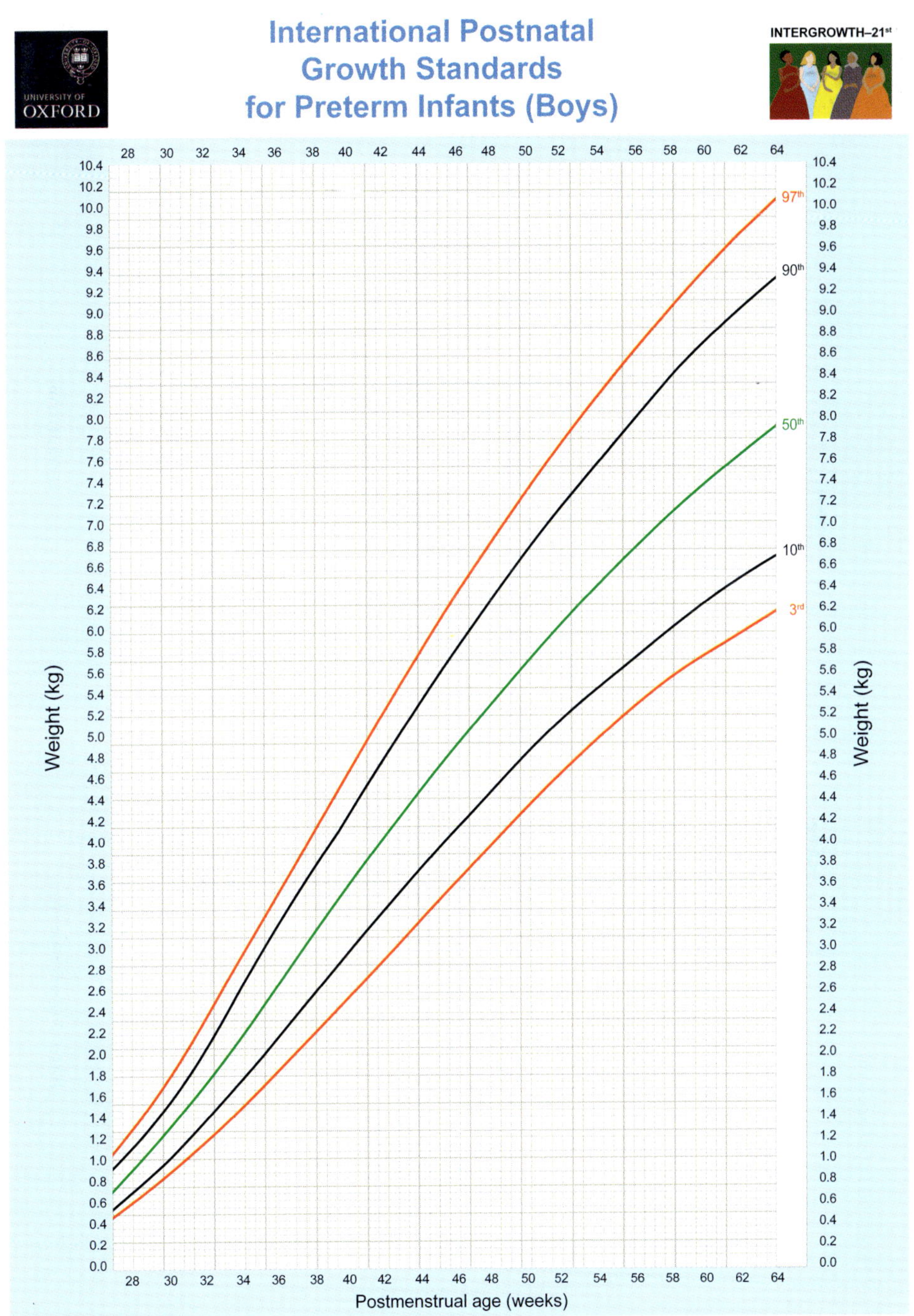

Appendix-1, Fig. 11.5: Chart 13—International Postnatal Growth Standards for Preterm Infants.

Chart 14

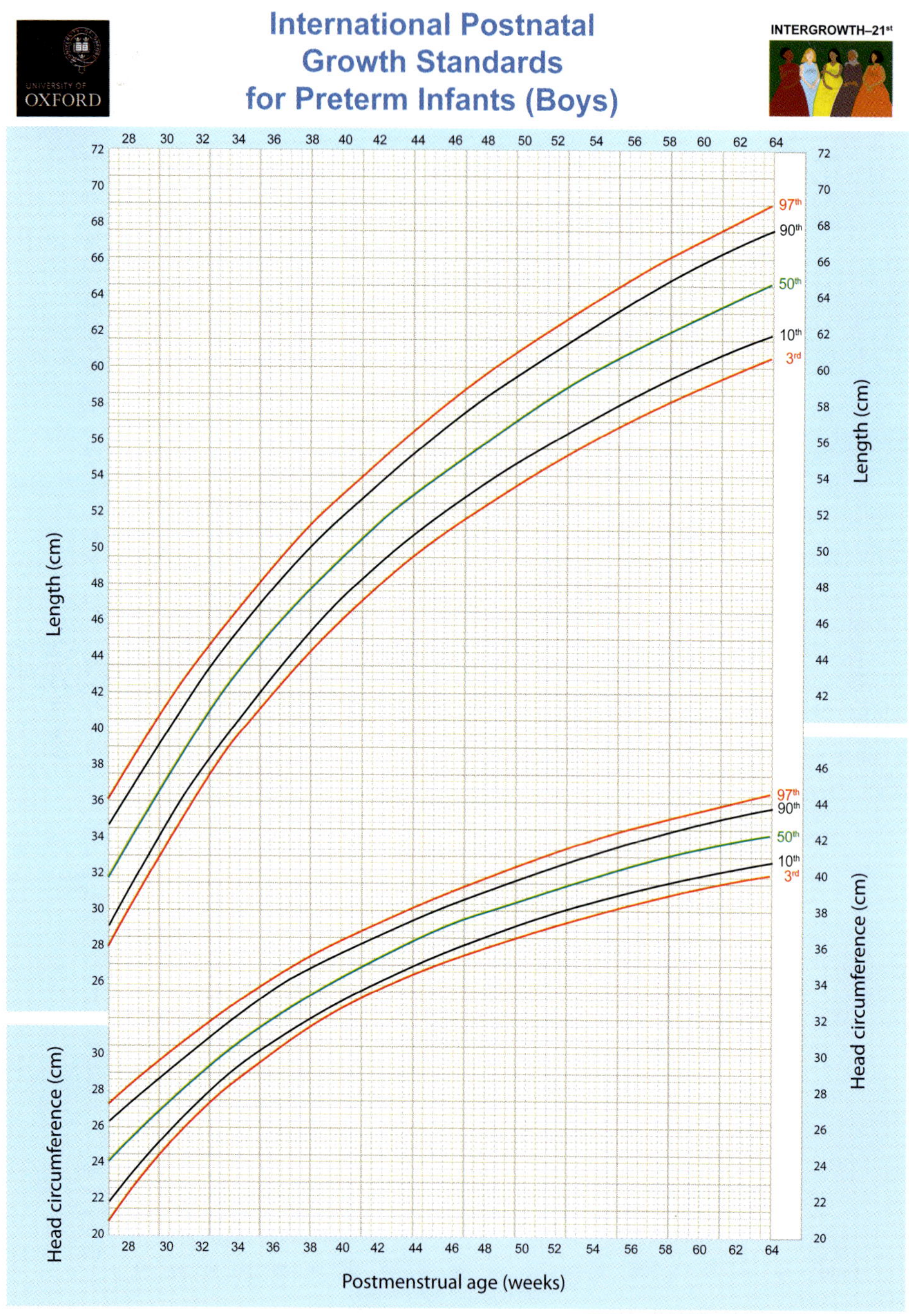

Appendix-1, Fig. 11.5: Chart 14—International Postnatal Growth Standards for Preterm Infants.

Chart 15

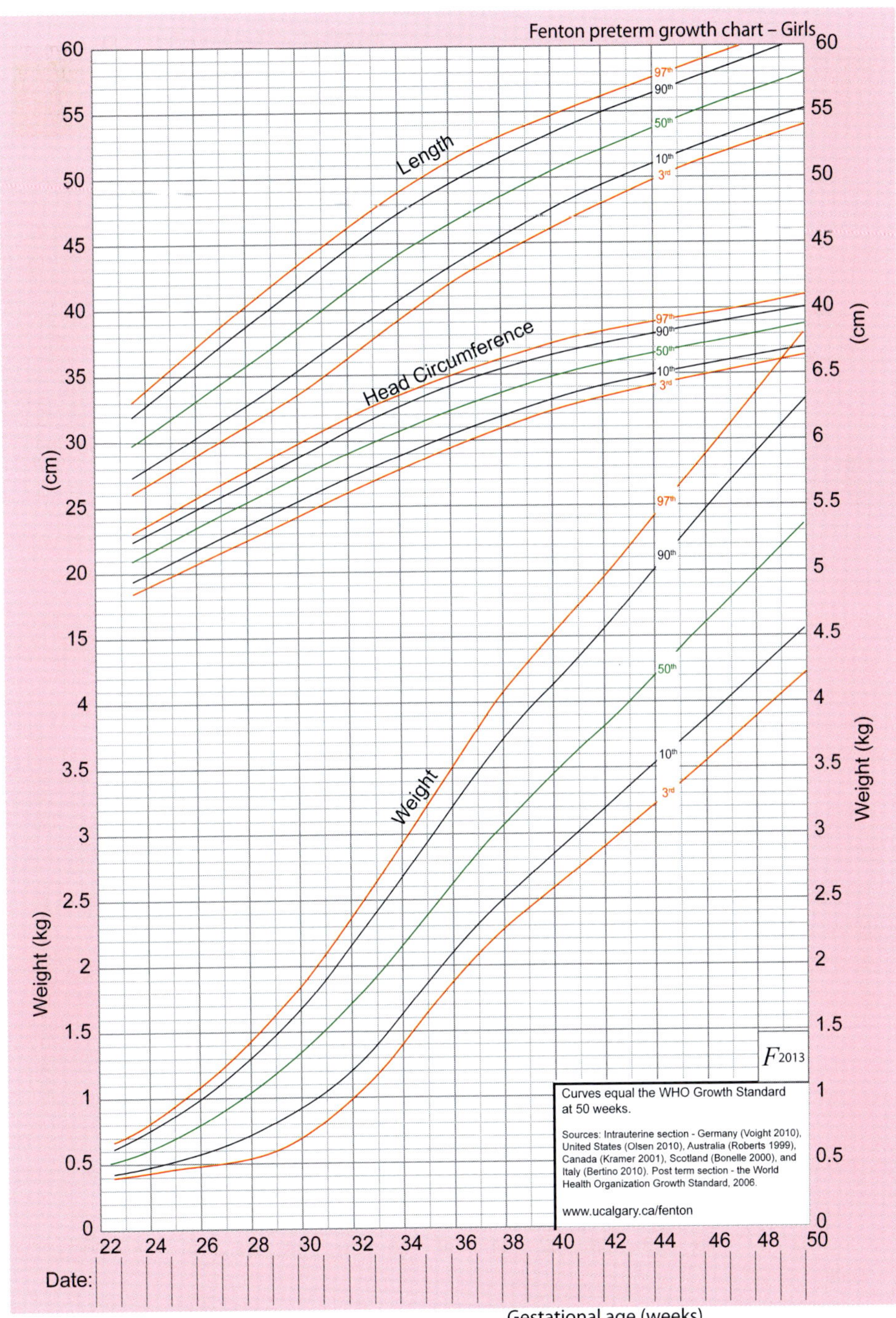

Appendix-1, Fig. 11.5: Chart 15—Fenton Preterm Growth Charts: (Girls)—Fenton Preterm Growth Chart (22 w of gestation to 10 w postnatal)—Girls

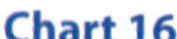

Chart 16

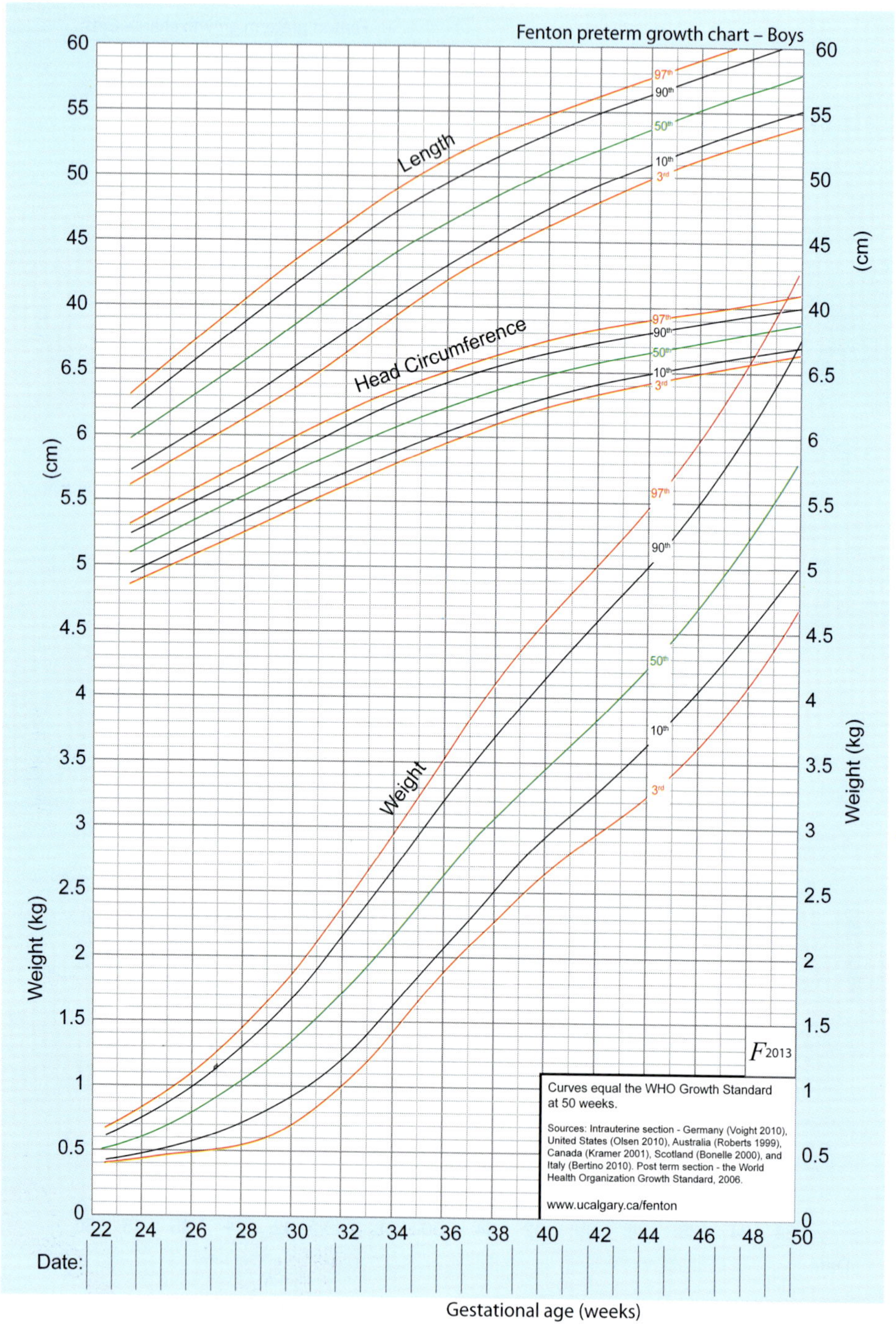

Fenton preterm growth chart – Boys
Length
Head Circumference
Weight
97th
90th
50th
10th
3rd
(cm)
Weight (kg)
60
55
50
45
40
6.5
6
5.5
5
4.5
4
3.5
3
2.5
2
1.5
1
0.5
0
22
24
26
28
30
32
34
36
38
40
42
44
46
48
50
Date:
F2013
Curves equal the WHO Growth Standard at 50 weeks.
Sources: Intrauterine section - Germany (Voight 2010), United States (Olsen 2010), Australia (Roberts 1999), Canada (Kramer 2001), Scotland (Bonelle 2000), and Italy (Bertino 2010). Post term section - the World Health Organization Growth Standard, 2006.
www.ucalgary.ca/fenton
Gestational age (weeks)

Appendix-1, Fig. 11.5: Chart 16—Fenton Preterm Growth Charts: (Boys)—Fenton Preterm Growth Chart (22 w of gestation to 10 w postnatal)—Boys

Chart 17

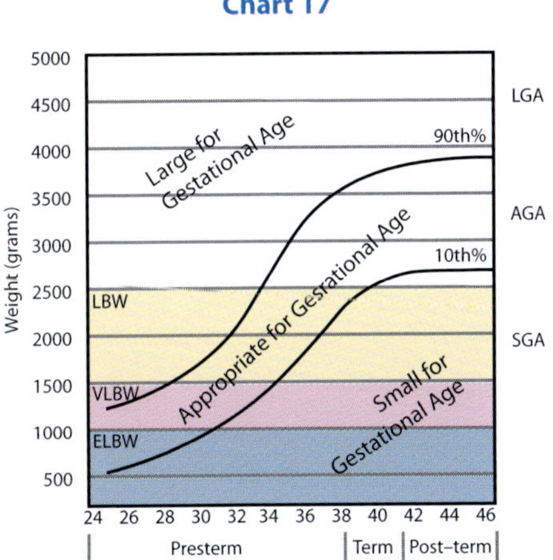

Appendix-1, Fig. 11.5: Chart 17—Intrauterine Growth chart.

Chart 18

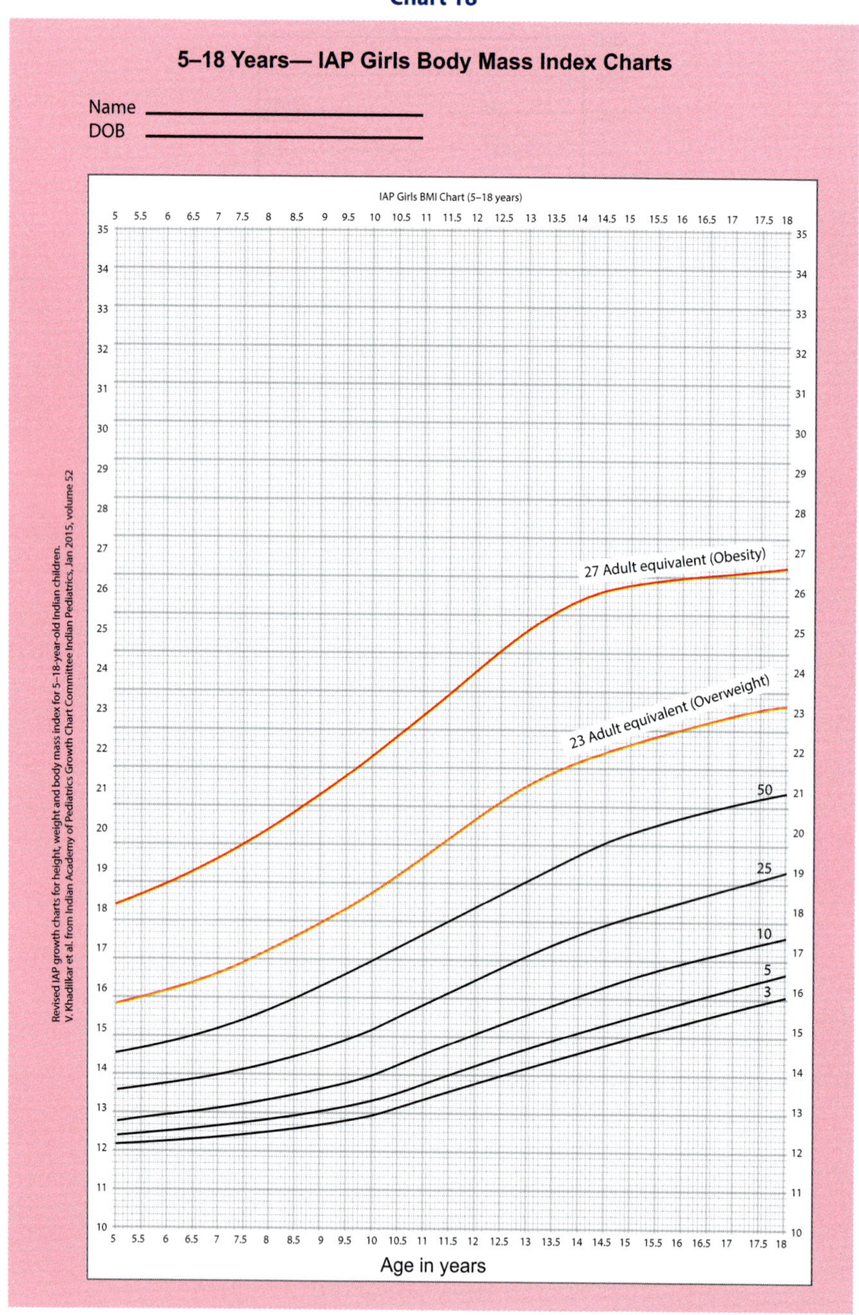

Appendix-1, Fig. 11.5: IAP Growth Charts 18 Body Mass Index—Girls 5–18 yr.

Chart 19

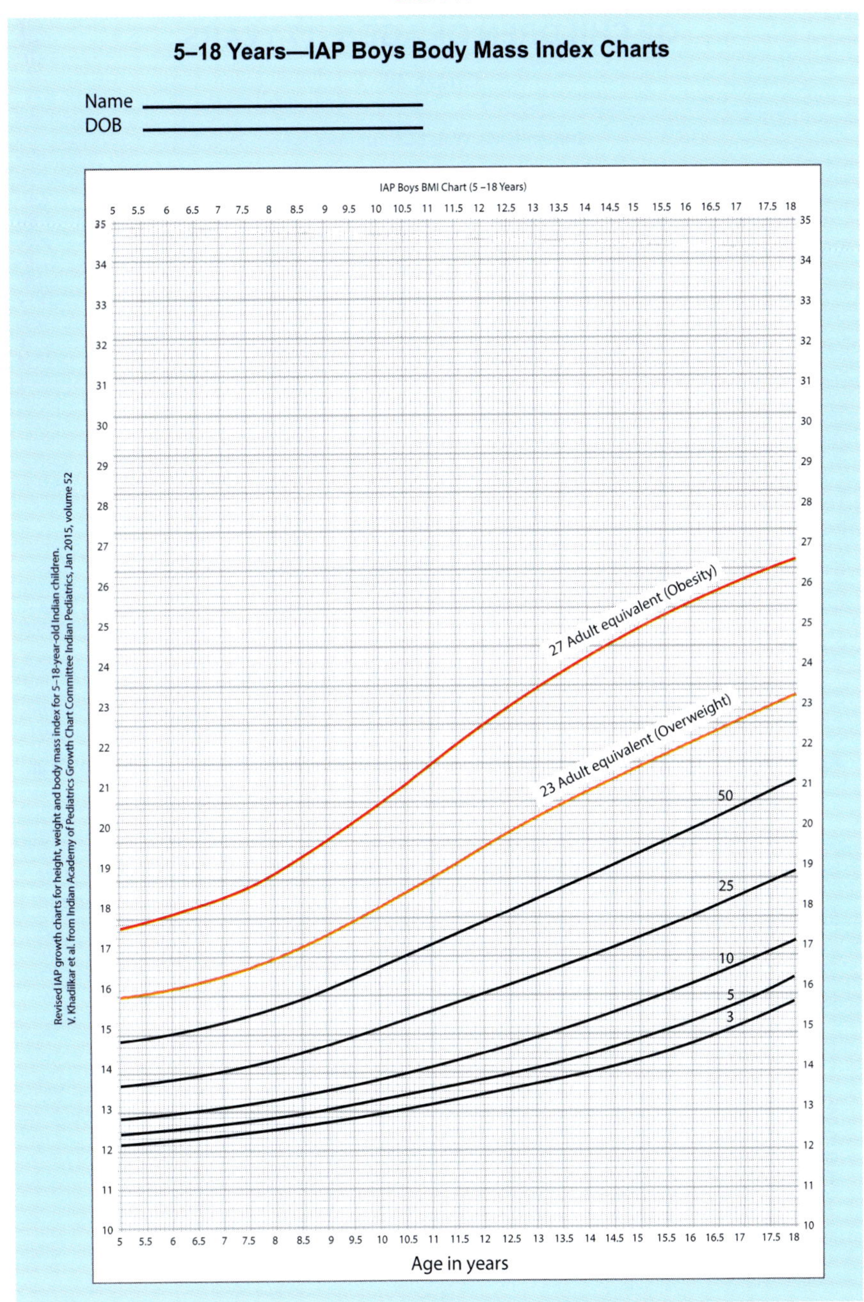

Appendix-1, Fig. 11.5: IAP Growth Charts 19 Body Mass Index—Boys 5–18 yr.

PERCENTILES OF WAIST CIRCUMFERENCE (WC) OF CHILDREN OF AGE 5–17 YEARS

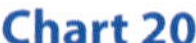

Chart 20

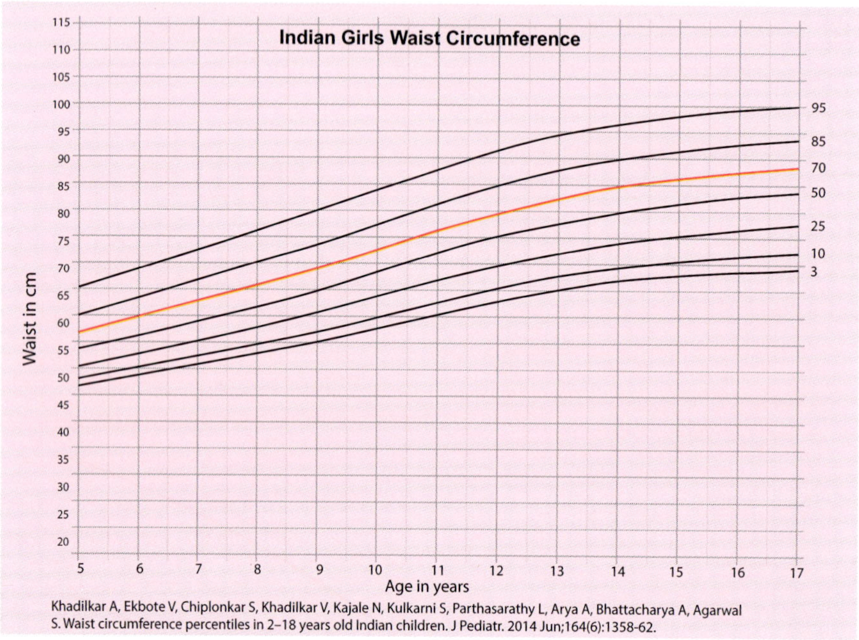

Appendix-1, Fig. 24.5: Growth Chart 20—Waist Circumference—Indian Girls 5–17 yr.

Chart 21

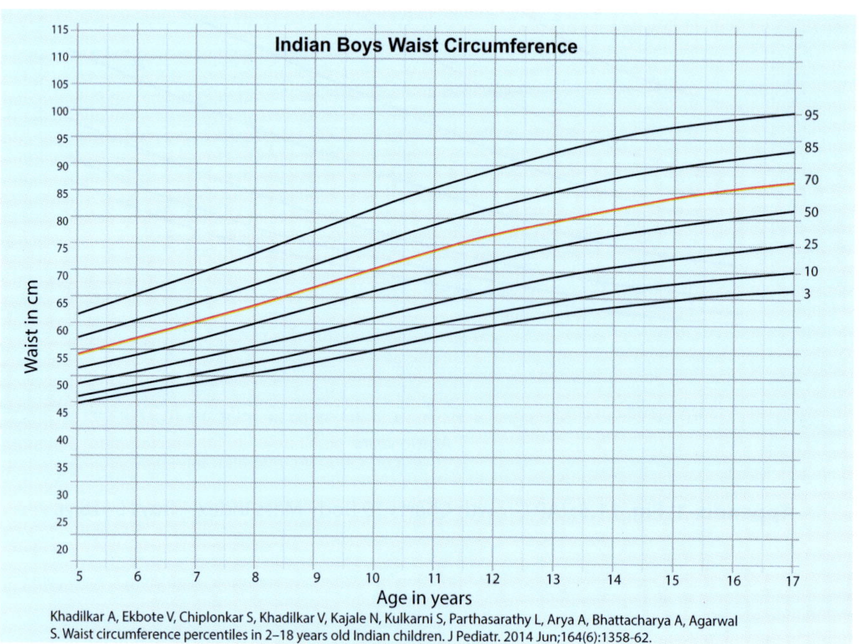

Appendix-1, Fig. 24.5: Growth Chart 21—Waist Circumference—Indian Boys 5–17 yr.

Appendix-2

TABLE 1: Height (cm) Centiles and Standard Deviation for Boys (5–18 yr).								
Age	***3***	***10***	***25***	***50***	***75***	***90***	***97***	***SD***
5.0	99.0	102.3	105.6	108.9	112.4	115.9	119.4	5.7
5.5	101.6	105.0	108.4	111.9	115.4	119.0	122.7	5.3
6.0	104.2	107.7	111.2	114.8	118.5	122.2	126.0	5.6
6.5	106.8	110.4	114.0	117.8	121.6	125.4	129.3	5.5
7.0	109.3	113.0	116.8	120.7	124.6	128.6	132.6	5.9
7.5	111.8	115.7	119.6	123.5	127.6	131.7	135.9	5.7
8.0	114.3	118.2	122.3	126.4	130.5	134.8	139.1	6.3
8.5	116.7	120.8	124.9	129.1	133.4	137.8	142.2	6.1
9.0	119.0	123.2	127.5	131.8	136.3	140.7	145.3	6.4
9.5	121.3	125.6	130.0	134.5	139.1	143.7	148.3	6.4
10.0	123.6	128.1	132.6	137.2	141.9	146.6	151.4	6.8
10.5	125.9	130.5	135.2	139.9	144.7	149.5	154.4	6.5
11.0	128.2	133.0	137.8	142.7	147.6	152.5	157.5	7.6
11.5	130.7	135.6	140.6	145.5	150.5	155.6	160.6	7.3
12.0	133.2	138.3	143.3	148.4	153.5	158.6	163.7	8.1
12.5	135.7	141.0	146.2	151.4	156.5	161.7	166.8	7.9
13.0	138.3	143.7	149.0	154.3	159.5	164.7	169.9	9.0
13.5	140.9	146.4	151.8	157.2	162.4	167.6	172.7	8.4
14.0	143.4	149.0	154.5	159.9	165.1	170.3	175.4	9.0
14.5	145.8	151.5	157.0	162.3	167.6	172.7	177.7	7.8
15.0	148.0	153.7	159.2	164.5	169.7	174.8	179.7	7.9
15.5	150.0	155.7	161.2	166.5	171.6	176.5	181.4	6.6
16.0	151.8	157.4	162.9	168.1	173.1	178.0	182.7	7.2
16.5	153.4	159.1	164.5	169.6	174.5	179.3	183.8	6.7
17.0	155.0	160.6	165.9	171.0	175.8	180.4	184.8	6.9
17.5	156.6	162.1	167.3	172.3	177.0	181.5	185.8	6.1
18.0	158.1	163.6	168.7	173.6	178.2	182.5	186.7	6.9

TABLE 2: Weight (kg) Centiles and Standard Deviation for Boys (5–18 yr).								
Age	***3***	***10***	***25***	***50***	***75***	***90***	***97***	***SD***
5.0	13.2	14.3	15.6	17.1	19.0	21.3	24.2	3.2
5.5	13.8	15.0	16.5	18.2	20.3	22.9	26.1	2.9
6.0	14.5	15.8	17.4	19.3	21.7	24.6	28.3	3.6
6.5	15.3	16.8	18.6	20.7	23.3	26.6	30.8	3.8
7.0	16.0	17.6	19.6	21.9	24.9	28.6	33.4	4.2
7.5	16.7	18.5	20.7	23.3	26.6	30.8	36.2	4.9
8.0	17.5	19.5	21.9	24.8	28.5	33.2	39.4	5.7
8.5	18.3	20.5	23.2	26.4	30.5	35.7	42.6	6.5
9.0	19.1	21.5	24.3	27.9	32.3	38.0	45.5	6.3
9.5	19.9	22.4	25.6	29.4	34.3	40.5	48.6	7.0
10.0	20.7	23.5	26.9	31.1	36.3	43.0	51.8	7.9
10.5	21.6	24.6	28.3	32.8	38.5	45.8	55.2	8.3
11.0	22.6	25.9	29.8	34.7	40.9	48.7	58.7	8.9
11.5	23.8	27.3	31.6	36.9	43.5	51.8	62.5	9.3
12.0	24.9	28.7	33.3	39.0	46.0	54.8	66.1	10.0
12.5	26.1	30.2	35.1	41.2	48.6	57.8	69.5	10.6
13.0	27.5	31.8	37.0	43.3	51.1	60.7	72.6	11.3
13.5	29.0	33.6	39.1	45.7	53.8	63.6	75.6	11.4
14.0	30.7	35.5	41.3	48.2	56.4	66.3	78.3	12.1
14.5	32.6	37.7	43.7	50.8	59.1	69.1	80.9	11.6
15.0	34.5	39.8	45.9	53.1	61.6	71.5	83.1	12.1
15.5	36.1	41.6	47.9	55.2	63.6	73.4	84.7	11.2
16.0	37.5	43.1	49.5	56.8	65.2	74.8	85.8	12.2
16.5	38.7	44.4	50.9	58.2	66.6	76.1	86.8	12.6
17.0	39.8	45.6	52.1	59.5	67.8	77.1	87.5	12.3
17.5	40.8	46.7	53.2	60.6	68.7	77.8	88.0	12.3
18.0	41.8	47.7	54.3	61.6	69.7	78.6	88.4	11.3

TABLE 3: Height (cm) Centiles and Standard Deviations for Girls (5–18 yr).

Age	*3*	*10*	*25*	*50*	*75*	*90*	*97*	*SD*
5.0	97.2	100.5	103.9	107.5	111.3	115.2	119.3	5.4
5.5	99.8	103.2	106.8	110.5	114.4	118.3	122.5	5.7
6.0	102.3	106.0	109.7	113.5	117.4	121.5	125.6	5.8
6.5	104.9	108.7	112.5	116.5	120.5	124.6	128.7	5.5
7.0	107.4	111.4	115.4	119.4	123.5	127.7	131.9	6.1
7.5	110.0	114.1	118.2	122.4	126.6	130.8	135.0	6.0
8.0	112.6	116.8	121.1	125.4	129.6	133.9	138.1	6.2
8.5	115.2	119.6	124.0	128.4	132.7	137.0	141.3	6.8
9.0	117.8	122.4	126.9	131.4	135.8	140.2	144.5	6.9
9.5	120.5	125.2	129.9	134.4	138.9	143.3	147.6	6.6
10.0	123.3	128.1	132.8	137.4	142.0	146.4	150.8	7.8
10.5	126.1	130.9	135.7	140.4	145.0	149.5	153.9	7.3
11.0	128.8	133.7	138.6	143.3	147.9	152.4	156.8	7.9
11.5	131.5	136.4	141.2	145.9	150.6	155.1	159.6	7.1
12.0	134.0	138.9	143.7	148.4	153.0	157.5	162.0	7.0
12.5	136.3	141.1	145.8	150.5	155.1	159.6	164.1	6.7
13.0	138.2	142.9	147.6	152.2	156.8	161.3	165.9	6.9
13.5	139.9	144.5	149.1	153.6	158.2	162.7	167.2	6.0
14.0	141.3	145.8	150.2	154.7	159.2	163.7	168.2	6.6
14.5	142.4	146.8	151.1	155.5	160.0	164.5	169.0	5.9
15.0	143.3	147.5	151.8	156.1	160.5	165.0	169.5	6.6
15.5	144.1	148.1	152.3	156.6	160.9	165.3	169.8	5.9
16.0	144.7	148.6	152.7	156.9	161.2	165.6	170.1	6.1
16.5	145.2	149.1	153.1	157.2	161.4	165.7	170.2	6.4
17.0	145.7	149.5	153.4	157.4	161.6	165.9	170.4	6.5
17.5	146.2	149.8	153.6	157.6	161.7	166.0	170.5	6.7
18.0	146.6	150.2	153.9	157.8	161.9	166.1	170.6	6.6

TABLE 4: Weight (kg) Centiles and Standard Deviations for Girls (5–18 yr).

Age	*3*	*10*	*25*	*50*	*75*	*90*	*97*	*SD*
5.0	12.3	13.4	14.8	16.4	18.5	21.3	25.0	2.5
5.5	13.0	14.3	15.7	17.6	19.9	22.9	27.0	3.5
6.0	13.7	15.1	16.7	18.7	21.3	24.6	29.1	3.4
6.5	14.4	15.9	17.7	19.9	22.7	26.3	31.2	4.1
7.0	15.1	16.8	18.7	21.2	24.2	28.2	33.4	4.4
7.5	15.9	17.7	19.9	22.5	25.9	30.1	35.7	4.8
8.0	16.7	18.7	21.1	24.0	27.6	32.2	38.1	5.2
8.5	17.5	19.7	22.3	25.5	29.5	34.4	40.7	6.4
9.0	18.5	20.9	23.7	27.2	31.5	36.7	43.4	6.4
9.5	19.5	22.1	25.3	29.0	33.6	39.3	46.3	6.9
10.0	20.7	23.5	26.9	31.0	36.0	42.0	49.4	7.7
10.5	22.0	25.1	28.8	33.2	38.4	44.8	52.6	8.3
11.0	23.3	26.7	30.7	35.4	41.0	47.7	55.9	8.5
11.5	24.8	28.4	32.6	37.6	43.6	50.6	59.1	9.1
12.0	26.2	30.0	34.5	39.8	46.0	53.4	62.1	9.0
12.5	27.6	31.6	36.3	41.8	48.2	55.8	64.8	9.7
13.0	28.9	33.1	37.9	43.6	50.2	57.9	67.1	9.4
13.5	30.2	34.4	39.4	45.1	51.8	59.7	69.0	9.8
14.0	31.3	35.6	40.6	46.4	53.2	61.1	70.4	9.6
14.5	32.3	36.6	41.7	47.5	54.3	62.2	71.4	9.4
15.0	33.1	37.5	42.5	48.4	55.1	62.9	72.1	9.6
15.5	34.0	38.3	43.3	49.1	55.8	63.5	72.5	8.7
16.0	34.7	39.1	44.0	49.7	56.3	64.0	72.8	8.7
16.5	35.5	39.8	44.7	50.3	56.9	64.4	73.1	9.2
17.0	36.2	40.5	45.3	50.9	57.3	64.7	73.3	8.8
17.5	36.9	41.1	46.0	51.5	57.8	65.0	73.4	9.5
18.0	37.6	41.8	46.6	52.0	58.2	65.3	73.5	10.2

TABLE 5: Body Mass Index Percentiles and Standard Deviations for Boys.

Age	***3***	***5***	***10***	***25***	***50***	***23***	***27***	***SD***
						Eq(71)	***Eq(90)***	
5.0	12.1	12.4	12.8	13.6	14.7	15.7	17.5	1.6
5.5	12.2	12.4	12.9	13.7	14.8	15.8	17.6	1.5
6.0	12.2	12.5	12.9	13.7	14.9	16.0	17.8	1.8
6.5	12.3	12.5	13.0	13.8	15.0	16.1	18.0	1.8
7.0	12.3	12.6	13.1	13.9	15.1	16.3	18.2	1.9
7.5	12.4	12.7	13.2	14.1	15.3	16.5	18.5	2.2
8.0	12.5	12.8	13.3	14.2	15.5	16.7	18.8	2.5
8.5	12.6	12.9	13.4	14.4	15.7	17.0	19.2	2.8
9.0	12.7	13.0	13.5	14.5	15.9	17.3	19.6	2.6
9.5	12.8	13.1	13.7	14.7	16.2	17.6	20.1	2.8
10.0	12.9	13.2	13.8	14.9	16.4	18.0	20.5	3.1
10.5	13.0	13.3	14.0	15.1	16.7	18.3	21.0	3.2
11.0	13.1	13.5	14.1	15.4	17.0	18.7	21.5	3.2
11.5	13.2	13.6	14.3	15.6	17.3	19.1	22.1	3.3
12.0	13.3	13.8	14.5	15.8	17.7	19.5	22.6	3.4
12.5	13.5	13.9	14.6	16.0	17.9	19.8	23.0	3.6
13.0	13.6	14.0	14.8	16.3	18.2	20.2	23.4	3.5
13.5	13.7	14.2	14.9	16.5	18.5	20.5	23.8	3.7
14.0	13.8	14.3	15.1	16.7	18.7	20.8	24.2	3.7
14.5	14.0	14.5	15.3	16.9	19.0	21.1	24.5	3.5
15.0	14.2	14.7	15.5	17.2	19.3	21.4	24.9	3.7
15.5	14.4	14.9	15.8	17.4	19.6	21.7	25.2	3.4
16.0	14.6	15.1	16.0	17.7	19.9	22.0	25.5	3.7
16.5	14.9	15.4	16.3	18.0	20.2	22.4	25.8	3.8
17.0	15.1	15.6	16.6	18.3	20.5	22.6	26.0	3.8
17.5	15.4	15.9	16.8	18.6	20.8	22.9	26.3	3.6
18.0	15.6	16.2	17.1	18.9	21.1	23.2	26.6	3.2

TABLE 6: Body Mass Index Percentiles and Standard Deviations for Girls.

Age	*3*	*5*	*10*	*25*	*50*	*23*	*27*	*SD*
						Eq(75)	*Eq(95)*	
5.0	11.9	12.1	12.5	13.3	14.3	15.5	18.0	1.4
5.5	11.9	12.2	12.6	13.4	14.4	15.7	18.3	1.7
6.0	12.0	12.2	12.7	13.5	14.5	15.9	18.6	1.7
6.5	12.1	12.3	12.8	13.6	14.7	16.1	18.9	2.0
7.0	12.1	12.4	12.8	13.7	14.9	16.4	19.3	2.1
7.5	12.2	12.5	12.9	13.9	15.1	16.6	19.7	2.2
8.0	12.3	12.6	13.1	14.0	15.3	16.9	20.1	2.3
8.5	12.3	12.7	13.2	14.2	15.6	17.2	20.5	2.7
9.0	12.4	12.8	13.3	14.4	15.8	17.6	21.0	2.7
9.5	12.5	12.9	13.5	14.6	16.1	18.0	21.4	2.8
10.0	12.7	13.1	13.7	14.9	16.5	18.4	21.9	2.9
10.5	12.8	13.2	13.9	15.2	16.8	18.8	22.5	3.1
11.0	13.0	13.4	14.1	15.5	17.2	19.3	23.0	3.1
11.5	13.2	13.7	14.4	15.8	17.6	19.8	23.6	3.3
12.0	13.4	13.9	14.7	16.1	18.0	20.2	24.1	3.2
12.5	13.7	14.2	15.0	16.5	18.4	20.7	24.7	3.3
13.0	13.9	14.4	15.2	16.8	18.8	21.1	25.2	3.2
13.5	14.1	14.6	15.5	17.1	19.1	21.5	25.6	3.5
14.0	14.3	14.9	15.7	17.3	19.4	21.8	25.9	3.4
14.5	14.5	15.1	16.0	17.6	19.7	22.0	26.2	3.3
15.0	14.7	15.2	16.1	17.8	19.9	22.3	26.3	3.4
15.5	14.9	15.4	16.3	18.0	20.1	22.4	26.4	3.1
16.0	15.0	15.6	16.5	18.2	20.3	22.6	26.5	3.1
16.5	15.2	15.8	16.7	18.4	20.4	22.8	26.6	3.2
17.0	15.4	16.0	16.9	18.6	20.6	22.9	26.7	3.0
17.5	15.5	16.1	17.1	18.7	20.8	23.1	26.7	3.1
18.0	15.7	16.3	17.3	18.9	21.0	23.2	26.8	3.6

Source: Indian Academy of Pediatrics Growth Charts Committee; Khadilkar V, Yadav S, Agrawal KK, Tamboli S, Banerjee M, Cherian A, Goyal JP, Khadilkar A, Kumaravel V, Mohan V, Narayanappa D, Ray I, Yewale V. Revised IAP growth charts for height, weight and body mass index for 5- to 18-year-old Indian children. Indian Pediatr. 2015;52(1):47-55. doi: 10.1007/s13312-015-0566-5. PMID: 25638185.

For the Age Group 0- to 5-yr, growth tables (Girls and Boys) can be collected from WHO-MGRS Child Growth Standards table.

Index

Page numbers followed by *b* refer to box, *f* refer to figure, and *t* refer to table.

A

F

G

P

Q

R

S

T

U